1999

The Year Book of VASCULAR SURGERY®

Editor

John M. Porter, M.D.

Professor of Surgery and Head, Division of Vascular Surgery, Oregon Health Sciences University, Portland, Oregon

Mosby

St. Louis Baltimore Boston Carlsbad Naples New York Philadelphia Portland London Madrid Mexico City Singapore Sydney Tokyo Toronto Wiesbaden

Mosby
Dedicated to Publishing Excellence

Associate Publisher: Cynthia Baudendistel
Developmental Editor: Sarah Zagarri
Manager, Periodical Editing: Kirk Swearingen
Production Editor: Pat Costigan
Production Assistant: Karie House
Manager, Literature Services: Idelle L. Winer
Illustrations and Permissions Coordinator: Chidi C. Ukabam

1999 EDITION

Printed in the United States of America
Composition by Reed Technology and Information Services, Inc.
Printing/binding by Maple-Vail

Editorial Office:
Mosby, Inc.
11830 Westline Industrial Drive
St. Louis, MO 63146
Customer Service: customer.support@mosby.com
www.mosby.com/Mosby/CustomerSupport/index.html

International Standard Serial Number: 0749–4041
International Standard Book Number: 0–8151–9801–9

Guest Commentators

Sir Norman L. Browse, M.D., F.R.C.S.

Emeritus Professor of Surgery, United Medical and Dental Schools, University of London; Hon. Consulting Surgeon, St. Thomas' Hospital, London, England

Jack L. Cronenwett, M.D.

Professor of Surgery, Dartmouth Medical School; Chief, Section of Vascular Surgery, Dartmouth-Hitchcock Medical Center, Lebanon, New Hampshire

Anthony E.B. Giddings, M.D., F.R.C.S.

Consultant Surgeon, King's College, Guy's and St. Thomas' Hospitals, London, England

Torben V. Schroeder, M.D., D.M.Sc.

Professor of Surgery, Consultant Vascular Surgeon, Department of Vascular Surgery, University of Copenhagen, Copenhagen, Denmark

Table of Contents

Table of Contents xi

Journals Represented xv

Introduction xvii

1. Basic Considerations 1

- Angiogenesis 1
- Cardiac/Lipids 5
- Claudication 25
- Chlamydia 31
- Coagulation 40
- Diabetes 55
- Estrogen 58
- Homocysteine 61
- Neurologic 69
- Nitric Oxide 75
- Spectroscopy 87
- Vascular Biology 92
- Venous 107

2. Endovascular 119

- Endovascular Grafts 119
- Angioplasty 134

3. Vascular Laboratory and Imaging 151

- Cerebrovascular 151
- Leg Arterial 164
- Venous Imaging 178
- Aortic 188
- Visceral–Renal 191
- Miscellaneous 198

4. Nonatherosclerotic Conditions 207

5. Perioperative Conditions 213

- Coronary Disease 213
- Drug Therapy 216
- Vascular Operations 218

Walking 227
Miscellaneous 229
6. Thoracic Aorta 235
Intimal Disease 235
Innominate Artery 238
Intramural Hematoma 241
Thoracic Aneurysm 245
Thoracoabdominal Aneurysm 247
Miscellaneous 263
7. Aortic Aneurysm 267
Epidemiology 267
Management 271
Miscellaneous 285
8. Aortoiliac Disease 289
9. Visceral Renal Artery Disease 297
Renal Ischemia 297
Visceral Ischemia 304
10. Leg Ischemia 307
Leg Vein Graft 307
Prosthetic Graft 320
Leg Bypass Anesthesia 327
11. Upper Extremity Vascular and Hemoaccess 337
Hemodialysis Access 337
Hand Ischemia 352
12. Carotid and Cerebrovascular Disease 357
Clinical Series 357
Prophylactic Carotid Endarterectomy 369
Epidemiology 376
13. Grafts and Graft Complications 385
Autogenous Vein Grafts 385
Failing Grafts 388
Allografts 394
Prosthetic Grafts 398

14. Vascular Trauma 407
- Arterial 407
- Combined Neural–Vascular 416
- Venous 419

15. Venous Thrombosis and Pulmonary Embolism 421
- Deep Venous Thrombosis 421
- Noninvasive Diagnosis 439

16. Chronic Venous and Lymphatic Disease 451
- Venous Reflux 451
- Subfascial Endoscopic Perforator Vein Surgery 459
- Congenital 461
- Vein Reconstruction 466
- Miscellaneous 470

17. Portal Hypertension 477

SUBJECT INDEX 487

AUTHOR INDEX 527

An intense area of research published in the past year has been the exploration of methods to attempt to reduce neurologic injury in patients with stroke but, by extrapolation, perhaps also in patients undergoing carotid endarterectomy or thoracoabdominal aneurysm repair. The N-methyl-D-aspartate receptor ion channel complex, when stimulated by glutamine, results in a marked worsening of neurologic injury. Intense investigation is ongoing to find drugs to block the receptor, and several candidate drugs have already been identified. In a related area, it appears that ischemic preconditioning of neurologic tissue results in the production of heat shock protein that has significant protective effects against ischemia damage. I suspect we will hear a great deal more about both glutamate receptor and heat shock protein in the immediate future.

Intense interest in the clinical area continues in the placement of endografts for aneurysms. An interesting development in the past year has been the decision of a number of investigators, when dealing with a short infrarenal neck, to deliberately place the proximal anchoring stent directly across the renal artery orifices. They claim this works well with no evidence of renal dysfunction, but I believe extreme caution is indicated in this area. An interesting report during the past year indicated that experimental aneurysms repaired by an endograft that deliberately had a leak left in the endograft, as predicted, resulted in the retention of pulsatility and systemic pressure within the aneurysm sac. In this experiment, the site of leakage was then closed completely by means of coil embolization until there was absolutely no angiographic evidence of continuing leak. Curiously, this did not result in any permanent relief of the elevated pressure within the aneurysm sac. Within a short time, intrasac pressure had returned virtually to systemic levels and pulsatility had returned. This has potentially profound implications for the clinical use of endografts. I have no idea of the explanation for this curious finding, but I suppose a small residual endoleak must have been present that simply could not be visualized with angiography. In an extremely interesting report, Dr. May and associates from Sydney, Australia, who have one of the largest endovascular graft experiences in the world, reported their recent experience on conversion from endoluminal to open repair of aortic aneurysms. Conversion to open repair was required in about 15% of their patients, and the results were not good, with a mortality of almost 25%.

Attempts to improve claudication by superficial femoral artery transluminal angioplasty proved disappointing again this year, as the control group and the angioplasty group 2 years after study entry reported exactly the same symptoms. This is, of course, the identical result that Dr. Creasy and Dr. Collin described from Oxford, most recently in 1994. Carotid angioplasty has been a hot topic in the past year, but little important information has come out. At least one group of investigators used transcranial Doppler US to monitor the middle cerebral microembolic signals during carotid surgery or angioplasty, and they found there were four times as many microembolic signals during angioplasty as during carotid endarterectomy. Other studies have reported that the number of microembolic signals detected per unit of time can be used to accurately predict the likelihood of stroke. Balloon angioplasty for correction of short stenoses in failing lower extremity vein grafts has been revisted. Simply put, the results were dismal, and it appears that enthusiasm for angioplasty of vein graft stenoses is diminishing rapidly.

Power Doppler appears to have come of age. This new technology is capable of producing unbelievably clear images of blood vessels. I, of course, do not know how it is going to sort itself out, but I am certain we shall all hear considerably more about power Doppler in the near future. An area of great interest has been revisiting methods of treating aortic infections or aortic graft infections with in situ replacements. Curiously, the aortic homograft has become a popular method of infected aortic replacement, especially in Europe, as has the impervious Dacron graft bonded to rifampicin. The use of the superficial femoral vein directly in the infected field has given good results. However, none of these results is superior to the old surgical principle of remote grafting through a clean area followed by excision of the infection, if possible. I believe for infrarenal aortic infection that the old way is clearly the best. For suprarenal infection, I suppose we will have to use one of the in situ methods, but presently it is unclear which is superior.

Interesting information this past year indicates that the occurrence of thrombus in a vein graft rapidly results in permanent damage to the underlying graft endothelium. Of special interest is the observation that the removal of thrombus from a lower extremity vein graft by the use of urokinase results in the intermediate term in exactly identical fibrointimal hyperplasia at the site of thrombosis, as if a Fogarty catheter had been used to remove the thrombus. It appears that urokinase is not as benign as many of us thought.

In the field of venous disease, two important topics have recurred. The first is the observation by many that patients who suffer truly idiopathic venous thrombosis have an inordinate likelihood of developing cancer, somewhere in the order of 12% to 25%. This is so worrisome that a number of centers, ours included, have begun to screen patients with idiopathic venous thrombosis for cancer as a matter of routine. The old issue of D-dimer blood level testing has recurred. Two independent groups have concluded that a D-dimer less than 2,000 convincingly excludes the diagnosis of deep vein thrombosis (DVT) and that such patients require no screening or other diagnostic testing. I wonder.

New information indicates that the pneumatic compressive foot pump for prophylaxis of DVT appears as effective as the long leg pneumatic compressive device. This is most interesting information. Another venous area of interest has been the relationship of lower extremity DVT to pulmonary embolism. Many physicians who suspect their patient may have a pulmonary embolism first order a lower extremity noninvasive vascular lab test to detect DVT. A fascinating study this year confirmed that only 9% of such patients actually have DVT, ranging from about 45% in patients with a high-probability V/Q scan, to about 6% to 7% in patients with a low-probability V/Q scan. On balance, it appears that obtaining a duplex study of the lower extremities for DVT provides no assistance in the diagnosis of pulmonary embolism; thus, it should not be obtained.

Again, I express my appreciation to the YEAR BOOK staff at Mosby. I express my special thanks to my loyal assistant, Ms. Heather Morin, who has single-handedly kept up with the enormous amount of data required for the production of this book. Her assistance has been invaluable, and she has my profound thanks.

John M. Porter, M.D.

1 Basic Considerations

Angiogenesis

Therapeutic Angiogenesis: A Comparative Study on the Angiogenic Potential of Acidic Fibroblast Growth Factor and Heparin

Rosengart TK, Budenbender KT, Duenas M, et al (New York Hosp-Cornell Univ)

J Vasc Surg 26:302–312, 1997 1–1

Background.—In vivo studies have shown that acidic basic fibroblast growth factor (aFGF) can include angiogenesis. Heparin appears to be an important cofactor to aFGF and may also stimulate angiogenesis. Angiogenesis plays a key role in the development of collateral vasculature after ischemia. A rat model of hindlimb ischemia was used to evaluate the effects of aFGF or heparin or both on angiogenesis.

Methods.—Rats were subjected to unilateral ligation of the femoral artery. For the next 10 days, they received daily subcutaneous injections with saline solution, 1 mL; heparin, 0.05 mg, or human recombinant aFGF, 1 µg, with or without heparin. Histologic examination was performed to compare the angiogenicity of the various treatments.

Results.—The numbers of vessels per microscopic field in the fibrofatty tissues distal to the point of ligation were 10 with saline solution, 13 with heparin, 26 with aFGF, and 36 with aFGF plus heparin (Fig 5). The distal skeletal muscle tissues showed comparable increases in vascularization. On immunohistochemical study for proliferating cell nuclear antigen, the percentage of total vascular cell nuclei labeled was 7% with saline solution, 21% with heparin, 67% with aFGF, and 83% with aFGF/heparin.

Conclusions.—Heparin appears to accelerate the process of angiogenesis. An even greater acceleration is achieved with aFGF, given with or without heparin. The combination of aFGF and heparin may provide the best clinical approach to enhancing growth of collateral vessels to offset the effects of ischemia.

▶ One of the hottest topics in the entire field of ischemia research is angiogenesis, and the relationship of angiogenic potential in ischemic areas to the administration of various growth factors. The particular factor examined in this study is acidic fibroblast growth factor (aFGF). I really do not know what to make of studies such as this. The tiny vessels that develop in

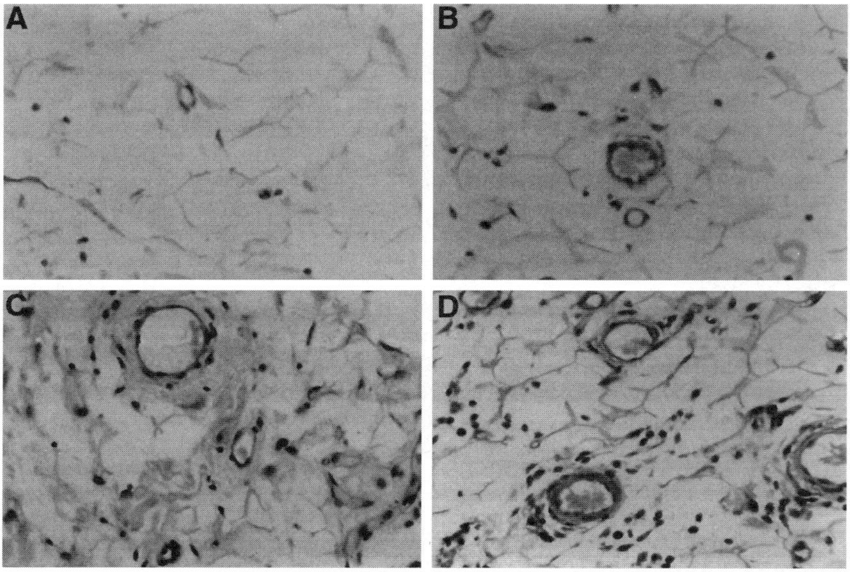

FIGURE 5.—Photomicrographs (original magnification, 400×) of fibrofatty tissue after various treatment regimens. Biopsies of fibrofatty tissues distal to the point of vascular ligation were obtained 10 days after vascular occlusion in animals treated with daily administration of one of the following: 1 mL saline solution (n = 13); 0.05 mg heparin in 1 mL saline solution ((n = 13); 1 µg aFGF (n = 5); of 1 µg recombinant human aFGF and 0.05 mg heparin in 1 mL saline solution (n = 5), and prepared as described in the Methods section. Vascular density compared with saline solution-treated controls (**A**) is increased in heparin-treated rats (**B**), and is increased to a greater extent in aFGF-treated animals (**C**) and aFGF/heparin-treated animals (**D**). *Arrows* depict vasculature. (Courtesy of Rosengart TK, Budenbender KT, Duenas M, et al: Therapeutic angiogenesis: A comparative study on the angiogenic potential of acidic fibroblast growth factor and heparin. *J Vasc Surg* 26:302–312, 1997.)

the ischemic field appear to me capable of carrying about 1 erythrocyte at a time. I am not convinced that these vessels will ever become large enough to make any significant impact on ischemic reperfusion, and I am unaware of any studies showing their growth over time. I do note that in this study the combination of heparin and aFGF produced the most impressive development of new vessels in areas of ischemia, although the new vessels were, as noted above, tiny. I will be most interested to learn in the future if chemical angiogenic stimulation of collateral vessel growth is ever shown to result in any meaningful augmentation of arterial flow.

Reduction of Vein Graft Intimal Hyperplasia and Preservation of Endothelium-dependent Relaxation by Topical Vascular Endothelial Growth Factor

Luo Z, Asahara T, Tsurumi Y, et al (Tufts Univ, Boston)
J Vasc Surg 27:167–173, 1998 1–2

Background.—Intimal hyperplasia may develop in vein grafts after insertion into the arterial circulation. The angiogenic growth factor vascular endothelial growth factor (VEGF) may also have a repair/maintenance or survival function through the modulation of endothelial cell function. The effects of VEGF pretreatment on endothelial function in vein grafts were studied in a rabbit model of vein graft intimal hyperplasia.

Methods.—New Zealand White rabbits with reversed jugular vein-to-common carotid artery interposition grafts were studied. Twenty minute before implantation, the venous conduits were placed in a solution containing 500 μg of $rhVEGF_{165}$ or saline solution. After 28 days, the vein grafts were subjected to histologic examination or isometric tension studies, with the contralateral jugular veins used as a control.

Results.—Intimal area was reduced by 23% in the VEGF-pretreated grafts, and intimal thickness by 30%. In grafts precontracted with norepinephrine, relaxation in response to the endothelium-dependent, receptor-mediated agonist acetylcholine was 0% in control vein grafts vs. 25% in VEGF-pretreated grafts. Response to the calcium ionophore A23187, an endothelium-dependent, receptor-independent agonist, was 123% in control grafts vs. 172% in VEGF-pretreated grafts. The 2 groups had similar responses to the endothelium-independent agonist sodium nitroprusside.

Conclusions.—Preimplantation treatment with VEGF reduces intimal hyperplasia and improves endothelial function in rabbit venous grafts. The mechanism of this effect is unclear, but the effects of VEGF on nitric oxide production may play an important role. Further studies of this simple approach to improving vein graft patency appear warranted.

▶ Dr. Isner's recent work in Boston on human angiogenesis induced by endothelial cell transfection has attracted international interest. He has recently focused on vascular endothelial growth factor (VEGF) as a primary method to stimulate angiogenesis. In this simplistic paper using the rabbit model, vein grafts were immersed in a solution containing VEGF or saline for 20 minutes before implantation. Those immersed in VEGF showed less intimal hyperplasia and preserved endothelium-dependent graft relaxation compared with controls. Dr. Isner uses this information to support his hypothesis that VEGF may be a powerful method of diminishing vein graft intimal hyperplasia. Several problems with this study, of course, include the observation that there was only a single sample time, 28 days, and that the experimental model was the rabbit, hardly a near relative of humans. Perhaps one day we will all spend 20 or 30 minutes soaking our excised vein grafts in a VEGF solution prior to use as a vascular conduit, but not yet.

Treatment of Acute Limb Ischemia by Intramuscular Injection of Vascular Endothelial Growth Factor Gene

Tsurumi Y, Kearney M, Chen D, et al (Tufts Univ, Boston)

Circulation 96:II-382S-II-388S, 1997 1–3

Background.—Ischemic skeletal muscle can take up and express genes transferred as naked plasmid DNA. This suggests that acutely ischemic

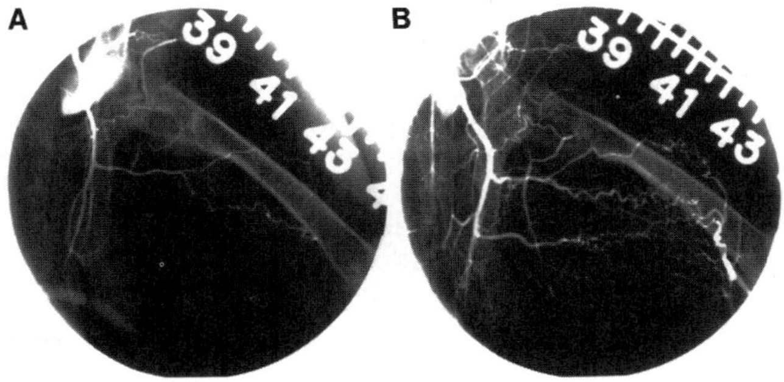

FIGURE 1.—Selective internal iliac angiography at day 30 of control rabbit (**A**) and vascular endothelial growth factor (VEGF)-transfected rabbit (**B**). In contrast to control, angiographic examination of the VEGF-transfected animal discloses extensive collateral artery formation. (Courtesy of Tsurumi Y, Kearney M, Chen D, et al: Treatment of acute limb ischemia by intramuscular injection of vascular endothelial growth factor gene. *Circulation* 96:II-382S–II-388S. Copyright 1997, American Heart Association. Reproduced with permission.)

skeletal muscle could serve as a target for intramuscular gene therapy using naked DNA. A rabbit model of acute hindlimb ischemia was used to assess the effects of IM injection of plasmid DNA encoding the angiogenic vascular endothelial growth factor (VEGF) on development of collateral vessels.

Methods.—Thigh muscle ischemia was produced in New Zealand White rabbits by ligation of the distal external iliac artery. The muscles were then injected with 500 µg of $phVEGF_{165}$. The effects of VEGF injection were assessed by anatomical means, including selective angiography and measurement of capillary density; and by hemodynamic means, including measurements of calf blood pressure and blood flow.

Results.—Thirty days after VEGF injection, the transfected rabbits showed more angiographically apparent collateral vessels and histologically assessed capillaries, compared with controls (Fig 1). The VEGF-transfected animals also showed a less severe hemodynamic deficit, as measured by calf systolic blood pressure ratio and Doppler guidewire measurement of blood flow to the ischemic limb. The ischemic muscles expressed human VEGF mRNA for up to 14 days after gene transfer. Reporter plasmid expression studied suggested that ischemic muscles were transfected up to 6 times more efficiently than nonischemic control muscles.

Conclusions.—Direct IM injection of naked VEGF plasmid DNA may offer a new approach to treatment of acute limb ischemia, these animal findings suggest. The enhanced transfection efficiency of ischemic muscle may be related to the presence of ischemia-induced muscle necrosis/regeneration. Studies of IM gene transfer using $phVEGF_{165}$ in humans are needed.

► I had no idea that injection of naked plasmid DNA fragments into ischemic skeletal muscle would result in expression of the gene product by the muscle. It appears that the ischemic muscle is much more able to express

receptors at least partially mediate the effects of phentolamine on adaptation to ischemia.

▶ The role of ischemic preconditioning in the coronary circulation has attracted the attention of seemingly thousands of investigators in recent years. This sophisticated study of patients undergoing at least 2 episodes of coronary balloon angioplasty randomized to receive intravenous infusion of phentolamine or placebo during the procedure showed a distinct failure of ischemic preconditioning in the group receiving phentolamine, leading the authors to conclude that ischemic preconditioning is at least in significant part mediated by α-adrenergic receptors, a position noted by others.[1] This is potentially important information.

Reference

1. Bankwala Z, Hale SL, Kloner RA: α-Adrenoceptor stimulation with exogenous norepinephrine or release of endogenous catecholamines mimics ischemic preconditioning. *Circulation* 90:1023–1028, 1994.

Myocardial Infarction and Cardiac Mortality in the Bypass Angioplasty Revascularization Investigation (BARI) Randomized Trial

Chaitman BR, on behalf of the BARI Investigators (Saint Louis Univ; Univ of Pittsburgh, Pa; Brown Univ, Providence, RI; et al)

Circulation 96:2162–2170, 1997 1–8

Bacgkround.—Previous comparative studies of coronary artery bypass grafting (CABG) and percutaneous transluminal coronary angioplasty (PTCA) have used the efficacy measures of cardiac mortality and myocardial infarction (MI) rate. Data from a multicenter, randomized trial were used to compare 5-year cardiac mortality and MI rate in patients with multivessel disease undergoing CABG or PTCA.

Methods and Results.—A total of 1,829 patients from the Bypass Angioplasty Revascularization Investigation were studied. Five-year cardiac mortality was approximately 8% in patients randomly assigned to PTCA vs. 5% in those randomly assigned to CABG. Relative risk was 1.55, with a 95% confidence interval of 1.07–2.23. However, on analysis of 1,476 patients without diabetes, cardiac mortality was between 4% and 5% for both groups; relative risk was 1.04, with a 95% confidence interval of 0.65–1.66. Neither was there any significant difference on subgroup analysis by symptoms, left ventricular function, number of diseased vessels, or stenotic proximal left anterior descending artery. The 2 treatments were associated with similar event rates on a combined end point of cardiac death and MI. Patients with MI had a six-fold increase in risk of cardiac mortality, compared with patients without MI. Patients undergoing CABG were more likely to have MI during their hospitalization, whereas those undergoing PTCA had more postdischarge MIs.

Conclusions.—For patients with multivessel disease, 5-year cardiac mortality is significantly higher after initial treatment with PTCA vs. CABG. However, this difference applies mainly to diabetic patients being treated with drugs. There are no significant differences in the composite end point of cardiac mortality MI. For patients without diabetes and other subgroups, there are no significant differences in cardiac mortality. Patients undergoing initial PTCA are more likely to need additional revascularization procedures and hospitalizations. Rigorous studies to determine the long-term impact of new catheter-based approaches to PTCA are recommended.

▶ This is another of the remarkable megatrials funded by the NIH examining patients with coronary disease eligible for either CABG or PTCA with randomization between the 2 therapeutic modalities. A significant 5-year survival benefit was seen in the patients randomly assigned to CABG. Further analysis confirmed that the total difference between the 2 groups was attributable to diabetics who fared much better with CABG. This is further evidence that we should be hesitant to recommend PTCA in diabetic patients. As I have stated in a previous YEAR BOOK, this has been the subject of a Clinic Alert from the NIH.[1] Although diabetics made up only about 10% of this particular cohort, other coronary intervention series have had a much higher percentage of diabetics. This is clearly important information for vascular surgeons.

Reference

1. 1998 YEAR BOOK OF VASCULAR SURGERY, p 12.

Common Carotid Intima-Media Thickness and Risk of Stroke and Myocardial Infarction: The Rotterdam Study

Bots ML, Hoes AW, Koudstaal PJ, et al (Erasmus Univ, Rotterdam, The Netherlands; Utrecht Univ, The Netherlands; Univ Hosp of Rotterdam, The Netherlands)

Circulation 96:1432–1437, 1997 1–9

Background.—Observational studies frequently use noninvasive measurement of intima-media thickness as an intermediate or proxy end point for cardiovascular disease. However, there is limited information on the capability of intima-media thickness to predict cardiovascular disease. The relationship between common carotid intima-media thickness and future strokes and myocardial infarction was examined.

Methods.—In a nested case-control study, ultrasound images of the common carotid artery from 7,983 research subjects aged 55 years or older were analyzed. Research subjects were participants in the Rotterdam Study, and ultrasound images had been stored on videotape. Incident myocardial infarctions and strokes were determined based on hospital discharge records. Logistic regression was based on 98 myocardial infarctions and 95 strokes. The intima-media thickness was measured from the images on videotape in all study participants and in an additional 1,373 research subjects who were free of myocardial infarctions and strokes during follow-up.

Results.—The mean follow-up was 2.7 years, and the results were adjusted for age and sex. The risk of having a stroke increased with increasing intima-media thickness. For strokes, the odds ratio per standard deviation increase was 1.41. For myocardial infarctions, the odds ratio was 1.43. After excluding research subjects with previous myocardial infarctions or strokes, the odds ratio was 1.57 for strokes and 1.51 for myocardial infarctions. After adjusting for several cardiovascular risk factors, the odds ratios decreased to 1.34 for strokes and 1.25 for myocardial infarctions.

Discussion.—These short-term findings demonstrate that an increased common carotid intima-media thickness is associated with future cerebrovascular and cardiovascular events. These results support the use of intima-media thickness measurements as an intermediate or proxy end point in observational studies.

► The carotid intima-media thickness has been used for years as a proxy measurement for generalized atherosclerosis. However, to apply this measurement with confidence, there is a clear need for prospective data showing that increased carotid intima-media thickness is actually associated with an increased level of cerebrovascular and cardiovascular events. In a 4-year follow-up of almost 8,000 subjects, these authors, in fact, did find that there was significantly increased risk of stroke and myocardial infarction in patients who had increased carotid intima-media thickness. This does, in fact, appear to validate the use of this measurement in epidemiologic studies of arteriosclerosis. (See also Abstract 1–10.)

Atherosclerotic Changes in the Carotid Artery Bulb as Measured by B-Mode Ultrasound Are Associated With the Extent of Coronary Atherosclerosis

Hulthe J, Wikstrand J, Emanuelsson H, et al (Göteborg Univ, Gothenburg, Sweden; Erasmus Univ, Rotterdam, The Netherlands)

Stroke 28:1189–1194, 1997 1–10

Background.—Ultrasound has become a useful study for assessing atherosclerotic changes in the carotid and femoral arteries. There is interest in using measurements of intima-media thickness (IMT) as a marker of generalized atherosclerosis, including coronary atherosclerosis. The link between US measurements of peripheral atherosclerosis and angiographic measurements of coronary atherosclerosis was examined.

Methods.—The study included 32 patients with visible atherosclerosis in at least 2 coronary segments on computer-assisted B-mode US. For each

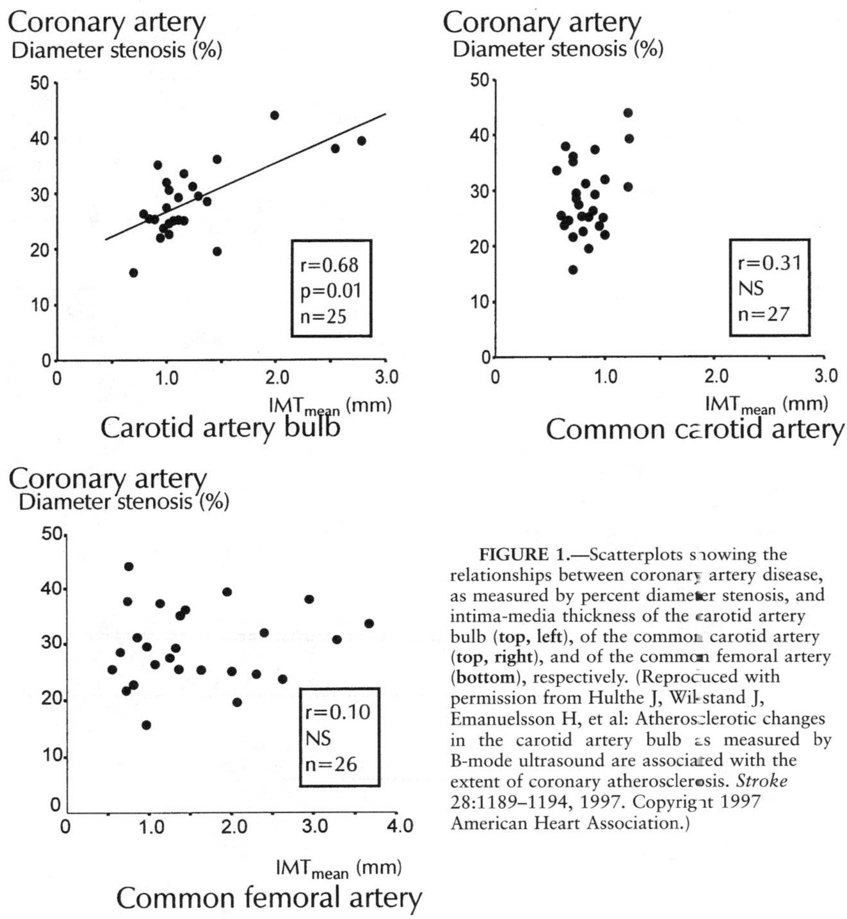

FIGURE 1.—Scatterplots showing the relationships between coronary artery disease, as measured by percent diameter stenosis, and intima-media thickness of the carotid artery bulb (**top, left**), of the common carotid artery (**top, right**), and of the common femoral artery (**bottom**), respectively. (Reproduced with permission from Hulthe J, Wikstand J, Emanuelsson H, et al: Atherosclerotic changes in the carotid artery bulb as measured by B-mode ultrasound are associated with the extent of coronary atherosclerosis. *Stroke* 28:1189–1194, 1997. Copyright 1997 American Heart Association.)

patient, the average diameter stenosis of coronary segments was used to express the extent of coronary atherosclerosis. Measures of peripheral atherosclerosis were IMT and plaque occurrence in the common carotid artery, carotid bulb, and common femoral artery. The relationship between the angiographic and US measurements was analyzed.

Results.—The US-measured IMT of the carotid bulb and the occurrence of carotid plaques were significantly correlated with the diameter stenosis of the coronary segments (Fig 1). However, the diameter stenosis of the coronary segments was unrelated to the IMT of the common carotid artery or common femoral artery or to the presence of femoral artery plaques (Fig 2).

Conclusions.—Ultrasound measurements of atherosclerotic changes in the carotid artery bulb are significantly associated with the extent of coronary atherosclerosis. The same relationship may not exist for US

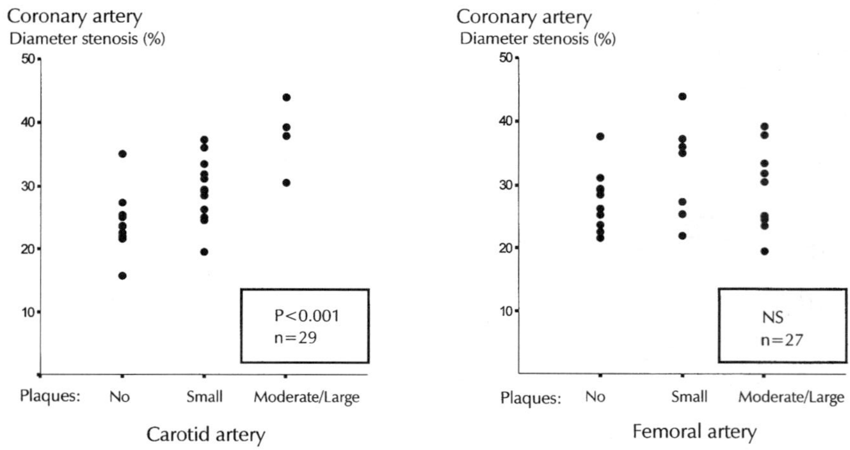

FIGURE 2.—Scatterplots showing the relationships between coronary artery disease, as measured by percent diameter stenosis, and plaque status in the carotid artery (**top**), and in the femoral artery (**bottom**), respectively. (Most of the plaques in the carotid artery were located in the carotid bulb.) (Reproduced with permission from Hulthe J, Wikstand J, Emanuelsson H, et al: Atherosclerotic changes in the carotid artery bulb as measured by B-mode ultrasound are associated with the extent of coronary atherosclerosis. *Stroke* 28:1189–1194, 1997. Copyright 1997 American Heart Association.)

measurements performed in the common carotid artery or femoral artery. Although confirmatory studies in larger numbers of patients are needed, the findings suggest that IMT should be measured and reported separately in the common carotid artery and carotid bulb.

► Periodically, internists rediscover the wheel, invariably taking great pride in this revelation. They herein present convincing evidence that the extent of carotid and femoral artery atherosclerosis correlates with the extent of coronary atherosclerosis. For this belated recognition of what every vascular surgeon already knew, namely that atherosclerosis is a generalized disease, I am pleased to confer upon them the Honorable Mention Camel Dung Award. It is only fair that we should occasionally recognize our dedicated internists.

Blood Viscosity and Elevated Carotid Intima-Media Thickness in Men and Women: The Edinburgh Artery Study

Lee AJ, Mowbray PI, Lowe GDO, et al (Edinburgh Univ, Scotland; Royal Infirmary, Glasgow, Scotland; The Royal Infirmary of Edinburgh, Scotland)
Circulation 97:1467–1473, 1998 1–11

Introduction.—Various hemostatic and rheologic factors have been correlated with incident cardiovascular events. No reports have addressed the association between rheologic factors and early atherosclerosis and carotid intima-media thickness (IMT). The relationship between these factors and carotid IMT were prospectively assessed in a random sample of 1,592 males and females participating in the Edinburgh Artery Study.

Methods.—Fibrinogen, tissue plasminogen activator (tPA), fibrin D-dimer, von Willebrand factor, blood and plasma viscosities, and hematocrit were measured at baseline during 1988–1989. Age range at baseline ranged from 55 to 74 years. At 5-year follow-up, participants underwent B-mode ultrasound scanning to determine IMT, self-administered follow-up questionnaire, and physical examination.

Results.—Valid measurements of IMT were recorded in 1 106 men and women aged 60–80 years at 5-year follow-up. In men, blood viscosity and its primary determinants, plasma viscosity, fibrinogen, and hematocrit were linearly related to IMT. Blood viscosity, fibrinogen, and plasma viscosity continued to be significant on multivariate analysis. Association was not significantly affected when blood viscosity was corrected to a standard hematocrit of 45%. In men, risk was significantly increased for having an IMT above the upper quartile of its distribution for SD increases in blood viscosity, fibrinogen, corrected blood viscosity, and plasma viscosity. Excluding plasma viscosity, these risks were not affected by adjustment for other common cardiovascular risk factors. There was no significant relationship between any of the hemorheologic factors and IMT in women or for tPA, fibrin D-dimer, or vWF in either gender.

Conclusions.—In men, blood viscosity and its major determinants are correlated with incident cardiovascular events and early stages of atherosclerosis. This may help explain the link between rheologic factors and events.

► The link, if any, between rheologic factors and atherosclerosis has remained elusive. This remarkable study examined the carotid IMT in a group of men and women years ago and followed them at least 5 years, and correlated changes observed with plasma viscosity and a number of plasma components of viscosity. While no relationship was seen in women, in men 60–80 years of age blood viscosity and its major components—plasma viscosity fibrinogen and hematocrit—were all clearly related to IMT. Since we know from Abstract 1–9 that IMT does appear to have clinical significance, the demonstration of a rheologic relationship to IMT may prove of real importance.

Cigarette Smoking and Progression of Atherosclerosis: The Atherosclerosis Risk in Communities (ARIC) Study

Howard G, for the ARIC Investigators (Wake Forest Univ, Winston-Salem, NC; Johns Hopkins Univ, Baltimore, Md; Univ of Minnesota, Minneapolis; et al)

JAMA 279:119–124, 1998

1–12

Background.—Cigarette smoking is known to be a strong risk factor for incident heart disease and stroke. However, the association of active and passive smoking with the progression of atherosclerosis has not been determined.

Methods.—A population-based cohort of middle-aged persons from 4 U.S. communities was studied in this longitudinal assessment of the relationship between smoking exposure determined at the initial visit and changes in atherosclerosis 3 years later. A total of 10,914 subjects enrolled in the Atherosclerosis Risk in Communities (ARIC) study between 1987 and 1989 were included.

Findings.—Exposure to cigarette smoke was correlated with progression of atherosclerosis. Compared with persons who never smoked, current smokers had a 50% increase in progression of atherosclerosis after adjustment for demographic factors, cardiovascular risk factors, and lifestyle variables. Past smoking was associated with a 25% increase. Compared with persons not exposed to environmental tobacco smoke (ETS), those exposed to ETS had a 20% increase. The effects of smoking on atherosclerosis progression was greater for persons with diabetes and hypertension. Although a larger number of pack-years of exposure was correlated independently with faster progression, after adjustment for number of pack-years, the progression rates of current and past smokers did not differ.

Conclusions.—Both active smoking and exposure to ETS are correlated with the progression of atherosclerosis. Smoking is especially detrimental to progression of atherosclerosis among patients with diabetes and hypertension. Some adverse effects of smoking may be cumulative and irreversible.

▶ This is a thin slice of salami from the ARIC study. These authorities used carotid intimal-medial thickness as their means of assessment of ASO disease change over a 3-year period. Current cigarette smoking was most strongly associated with an increase in intimal-medial thickness (IMT). Sadly, individuals with exposure to environmental tobacco smoke (passive smoking) also showed a significant increase in carotid IMT compared with those individuals who neither smoked nor had any exposure to ETS. Although hardly surprising, this study does show a clear association between passive smoking and atherosclerotic disease progression. The vigorous effort in America at the present time to completely isolate smokers from individuals who do not smoke appears right on target, despite the unbelievable protests of the tobacco companies.

Randomised Trial of α-Tocopherol and β-Carotene Supplements on Incidence of Major Coronary Events in Men With Previous Myocardial Infarction

Rapola JM, Virtamo J, Ripatti S, et al (Natl Public Health Inst, Helsinki; Natl Cancer Inst, Bethesda, Md; Univ of Helsinki)

Lancet 349:1715–1720, 1997 1–13

Objective.—Whereas data from prospective cohort studies indicate that antioxidants decrease the incidence of coronary heart disease, results of clinical trials do not support these findings. The effects of α-tocopherol and β-carotene supplements on the incidence of major coronary events among men at high risk of a coronary event because of previous myocardial infarction were investigated in the Alpha-tocopherol and Beta-carotene Cancer Prevention (ATBC) Study.

Methods.—Dietary supplements of α-tocopherol (50 mg/day), β-carotene (20 mg/day), both, or placebo were administered to 1,862 male smokers aged 50–69 years, who had a previous myocardial infarction. Individuals completed a questionnaire about their background, smoking, and medical histories, diet, and exercise. Participants were followed up for an average of 5.3 years, 3 times a year. Body mass index was calculated, blood pressure was measured, and blood chemistries were performed. Serum α-tocopherol and β-carotene concentrations were determined. The end point was the first major coronary event.

Results.—Serum levels of α-tocopherol or β-carotene were similar among treatment groups. There were 424 major coronary events, 190 nonfatal and 234 fatal. There was no difference in the total number of coronary events among the 4 groups, although the risk of nonfatal myocardial infarction was lower in the treated groups and significantly lower

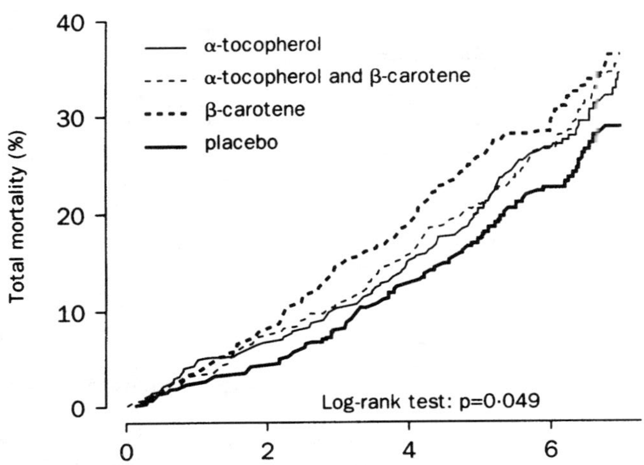

FIGURE 3.—Kaplan-Meier estimates of mortality. (Courtesy of Rapola JM, Virtamo J, Ripatti S, et al: Randomised trial of α-tocopherol and β-carotene supplements on incidence of major coronary events in men with previous myocardial infarction. *Lancet* 349:1715–1720. Copyright 1997, The Lancet Ltd.)

807 men with angiographically documented coronary atherosclerosis. The influence of this DNA variant on cholesterol-lowering therapy was also examined.

Methods.—The presence of the *CETP* gene variant was named B1; its absence was called B2. Patients were randomly assigned to treatment with pravastatin or placebo for 2 years.

Results.—There were no significant between-group differences at baseline with respect to risk factors for coronary artery disease or severity or treatment of coronary atherosclerosis according to TaqIB genotype (Table 1). There was an association between the B1 variant of the *CETP* gene and both higher plasma CETP concentrations and lower HDL cholesterol concentrations. There was a significant dose-dependent correlation between this marker and the progression of coronary atherosclerosis in the placebo group. This correlation was not observed in the pravastatin group. The progression of coronary atherosclerosis was slowed in *B1B1* carriers, but not in *B2B2* carriers (84% and 16% of patients taking pravastatin, respectively).

Conclusions.—There is a significant association between variation at the *CETP* gene locus and the progression of coronary atherosclerosis that is independent of plasma HDL cholesterol levels and the activities of lipolytic plasma enzymes. The *CETP* gene variant seems to predict whether men with coronary artery disease will benefit from treatment with pravastatin to stall the progression of coronary atherosclerosis.

▶ More and more is being learned about the complex interrelationship of lipid metabolism and specific gene products. There is a curious substance known as CETP that appears to have an important role in the metabolism of HDL and individual susceptibility to atherosclerosis. This study suggests that individuals who have a common polymorphism in the CETP protein are relatively resistant to the beneficial effects of pravastatin in delaying the progression of coronary atherosclerosis. This may be the explanation of the observation made repeatedly for years that pravastatin and similar drugs do not prevent myocardial infarctions in a substantial percentage of patients.

Hypercholesterolemia Alters the Gene Expression of Novel Components of the Extracellular Matrix in Experimental Vein Grafts

Dattilo JB, Dattilo MPM, Yager DR, et al (Virginia Commonwealth Univ, Richmond)

Ann Vasc Surg 12:168–173, 1998 1–18

Introduction.—The success rate of vascular bypass surgeries is compromised by development of intimal hyperplasia (IH). It is well known that hypercholesterolemia accelerates IH in arteries and experimental vein grafts; the etiology remains unclear. Hyaluronic acid synthase (HAS-1) is a transmembrane enzyme that causes the formation of hyaluronan, an important component of the extracellular matrix (ECM). Both HAS-1 and

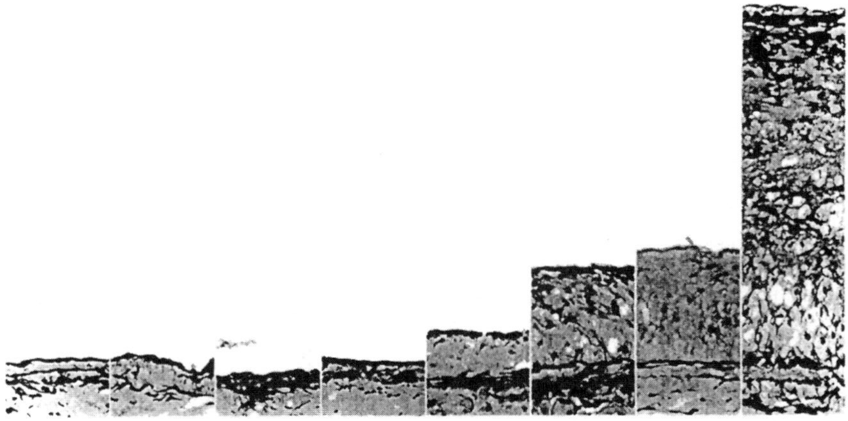

FIGURE 4.—Photomicrograph of histologic sections from normal jugular vein and vein grafts of each group and time points. Sections are stained with Verhoff's elastin stain and viewed using light microscopy at a magnification of 200×. Sections are shown with the internal elastic lamina of each section aligned with one another demonstrating the intimal response (above the lamina) after grafting from each group and time point. (Courtesy of Dattilo JB, Dattilo MPM, Yager DR, et al: Hypercholesterolemia alters the gene expression of novel components of the extracellular matrix in experimental vein grafts. *Ann Vasc Surg* 12(2):168–173, 1998.)

CD-44 (the integrin receptor for hyaluronan) have been examined in the development of ECM of wounds, but have not been analyzed in the ECM of IH within vein grafts. The expression of CD-44 and HAS-1 was assessed to determine whether it increases during the early stages of IH. The effect of cholesterol supplementation on these genes was also evaluated.

Methods.—Forty white male New Zealand rabbits received either cholesterol-supplemented (1% cholesterol chow) or noncholesterol-supplemented chow. Each set of 20 rabbits was further divided into 4 groups of 5 animals: a nonoperative control group and 3 operative groups that underwent a right interposition carotid bypass using jugular vein. Grafts were harvested in groups of 5 each at 3, 7, and 21 days after surgery. Tissues underwent molecular studies, histology examination, and ribonuclease protection assays using ^{32}P-labeled riboprobes for HAS-1, CD-44, and 18s rRNA. The densitometric analysis was expressed as a ratio (riboprobe/rRNA).

Results.—Expression of HAS-1 and CD-44 were significantly higher in the vein grafts, compared with normal jugular vein. Cholesterol supplementation caused a further rise in CD-44 gene expression vs. nonsupplemented vein grafts (Fig 4).

Conclusions.—These findings establish a role for CD-44 and HAS-1 transcription in vein graft IH, which is further changed by cholesterol supplementation. These data may explain differences observed in the development of IH with hypercholesterolemia and ultimately provide improved treatment approaches for alleviating this process.

► Perhaps hyaluronic acid and its integrin receptor CD-44 have an important role in the production of intimal hyperplasia, as suggested by this study. Interestingly, the detrimental effects appear to be enhanced by elevated cholesterol. Not surprisingly, the components of the extracellular matrix within vein grafts appear to have an important role in graft behavior. However, as a nominee for relieving vein graft intimal hyperplasia, I have major reservations.

Claudication

Claudication Distance Is Poorly Estimated and Inappropriately Measured

Watson CJE, Phillips D, Hands L, et al (Univ of Oxford, England)
Br J Surg 84:1107–1109, 1997 1–19

Background.—Reduced waking distance, although clearly a disability, causes a handicap only if it interferes with a patient's usual activities. Intervention is indicated for those whose intermittent claudication represents a handicap. A prospective study was conducted to compare patients' estimate of claudication distance (the distance walked before the onset of pain) with claudication distance as measured objectively on a patient-controlled corridor walk and a fixed-speed level treadmill walk.

Methods.—Study participants were 70 patients referred over a 6-month period for intermittent claudication. None had rest pain or ulceration. The patients were asked to estimate their claudication distance, their maximum walking distance (MWD)—defined as the distance walked before ischemic muscle pain becomes unbearable—and the time taken to walk these distances. Claudication distance and MWD were also measured by observation of patients walking a 30-m–long corridor and on a horizontal treadmill at 3 km/hr or slower. Patients were stopped at 800 mm on the corridor and treadmill tests.

Results.—The median age of the study group was 69 years; 74% were men. Five patients were excluded from walking analysis when their claudication was found to have a neurologic cause. In most cases, the claudication distance reported by patients did not correspond with that reported in their referral letters or subsequent clinic letters. No correlation was observed between the estimated distance and actual distance walked on either the corridor walk or the fixed-speed treadmill walk. Although 14 patients had a median corridor speed of less than 3 km/hr, only 8 of these could not walk at 3 km/hr on the treadmill. Two thirds of the 50 patients who stopped at what they claimed to be their MWD on the corridor were able immediately to walk a further 15 to 45 m back to the rest room.

Conclusion.—Neither clinical signs of occlusive arterial disease nor the findings at angiography are indicative of disability, which requires direct assessment of the distance that a patient can walk. Because patients often substantially underestimate their claudication distance and MWD, objective measurements of the handicap caused by reduced walking distance are needed before intervention is undertaken.

▶ Dr. Jack Collin at Oxford University has a way with words. As he mellifluously notes, "Claudication distance is spuriously estimated, inaccurately reported, falsely recorded, inappropriately measured, and usually misinterpreted." In other words, the patient's statement as to how far he can walk seems to have little or no relationship to how far he can actually walk. This is, of course, of great importance because our assessment of the handicap presented to patients by walking impairment is fundamental in formulating treatment decisions. These authors further note that exclusive reliance on treadmill as a substitute for real terrain walking may result in considerable distortion. On balance, Dr. Collin, as always, has brought up a very important subject. Because we make many therapeutic decisions in our patients with claudication based on the patient's statement of how far he can walk, we would best serve our patients by a critical assessment of the accuracy of their judgment. Dr. Collin's suggestion that real terrain walking is ideal may be true, but it is also difficult to perform in hospital settings. The take-away message from this paper is that we should have a healthy suspicion of whatever distance the patients tell us they can walk. In all likelihood, their real walking distance is considerably greater than they report.

Exercise Training for Intermittent Claudication: Does It Adversely Affect Biochemical Markers of the Exercise-induced Inflammatory Response?

Tisi PV, Hulse M, Chulakadabba A, et al (Royal South Hants Hosp, Southampton, England; Selly Oak Hosp, Birmingham, England)

Eur J Vasc Endovasc Surg 14:344–350, 1997 1–20

Purpose.—Repeated episodes of calf or buttock pain in patients with intermittent claudication may reflect low-grade ischemia-reperfusion injury. The clinical significance of these repeated low-grade inflammatory events remains unknown. Measurement of transient acute inflammatory markers is impractical for use in routine clinical practice. A stable biochemical marker of disease severity in intermittent claudication was identified, and its use in evaluating the effects of therapeutic exercise training was assessed.

Methods.—The first part of the study measured plasma fibrinogen, serum amyloid A protein (SAA), C-reactive protein (CRP), and urinary albumin-creatinine ratio (ACR) in 67 patients with stable intermittent claudication and 15 controls. The results were correlated with walking distances. Thirty-nine patients were then randomly assigned to undergo either supervised exercise training or observation. Follow-up measurements of inflammatory markers were performed at 3, 6, and 12 months.

Results.—At baseline, median fibrinogen level was 3.7 g/L in patients with claudication vs. 3.5 g/L in controls. Values for CRP in patients were 4.7 mg/L vs. 2.1 mg/L in controls, and values for SAA in patients were 72

TABLE 3.—Change in Clinical and Biochemical Parameters in Patients Undergoing Exercise Training (*EX*) and Observation (*OBS*)

Parameter	Rx	Baseline		3 months		6 months		12 months	
Fibrinogen (g/L)	EX	3.7	(3.4–4.0) (*n* = 22)	3.8	(3.6–4.3) (*n* = 21)	3.8	(3.2–4.4) (*n* = 17)	3.9	(3.4–4.6) (*n* = 10)
	OB	4.0	(3.7–4.6) (*n* = 17)	4.2	(3.3–4.6) (*n* = 13)	4.4	(3.8–4.6) (*n* = 12)	4.0	(3.5–4.8) (*n* = 9)
CRP (mg/L)	EX	5.3	(2.8–10.5)	4.4	(1.8–7.2)*	6.6	(3.4–9.0)	4.8	(2.2–9.3)
	OB	5.6	(2.7–8.9)	4.8	(2.1–9.2)	5.4	(1.8–12.6)	2.0	(0.8–15.0)
SAA (mg/L)	EX	70	(54–118)	52	(31–84)	20	(5–64)†	23	(16–102)
	OX	94	(39–167)	106	(32–285)	68	(38–104)	44	(24–206)
ABPI	EX	0.66	(0.02)	0.64	(0.03)	0.65	(0.03)	0.64	(0.05)
	OB	0.70	(0.03)	0.69	(0.03)	0.72	(0.05)	0.74	(0.07)
PFWD (m)	EX	70	(45–87)	106	(72–145)‡	94	(82–273)‡	112	(103–258)†
	OB	80	(44–91)	75	(60–89)§	77	(56–93)	107	(67–137)†
MWD (m)	EX	104	(72–148)	182	(116–238)‡	166	(94–313)†	175	(103–258)†
	OB	110	(81–148)	109	(81–135)§	93	(82–148)§	126	(104–156)†

Note: Results are shown as the median (interquartile range), except for ankle-brachial pressure index (*ABPI*) which is shown as the mean (SEM). Statistics are shown for change with time in comparison to baseline (*$P < 0.05$, †$P < 0.01$, ‡$P < 0.001$) and across time between exercise and observation groups (§$P < 0.05$ for exercise>observation).

Abbreviations: PFWD, pain-free walking distance; *MWD*, maximum walking distance; *CRP*, C-reactive protein; *SAA*, serum amyloid A protein.

(Courtesy of Tisi PV, Hulse M, Chulakadabba A, et al: Exercise training for intermittent claudication: Does it adversely affect biochemical markers of the exercise-induced inflammatory response? *Eur J Vasc Endovasc Surg* 14:344–350. Copyright 1997, W.B. Saunders Company Limited, London.)

mg/L vs. 30 mg/L in controls. Treadmill exercise training produced an increase in urinary ACR for patients, compared with no change for controls. The exercise-training group showed a reduction in SAA at 6 months, a reduction in CRP at 3 months, and a progressive decline in the postexercise increase in ACR (Table 3).

Conclusions.—Serum acute-phase proteins are increased in response to repetitive, low-grade inflammatory events in patients with intermittent claudication. C-reactive protein and SAA protein appear to be useful markers of disease severity, showing correlation with known risk factors for cardiovascular disease and symptoms. As symptoms improve with exercise training, the inflammatory markers decrease. The results do not support the notion that exercise has adverse systemic effects in patients with intermittent claudication.

▶ Some have suggested in recent years that calf or buttock pain with exercise should be regarded as a low-grade ischemia reperfusion injury. They have hypothesized further that repeated episodes of claudication may lead to a complex biochemical sequence of events involving oxygen-derived free-radical formation, neutrophil activation, and endothelial damage, all resulting in a systemic inflammatory response. These investigators sought to identify a stable biochemical marker of disease severity. They found that C-reactive protein was one of the best discriminates, as was serum amyloid A protein. Urinary albumin creatinine ratio increased in claudicants after treadmill exercise. Interestingly, exercise training reduced these markers of inflammation at 3–6 months. Clearly this information is preliminary, but it certainly presents an interesting new area for inquiry. (See also Abstract 1–71.)

Near Infrared Spectroscopy for Noninvasive Assessment of Claudication

Kooijman HM, Hopman MTE, Colier WNJM, et al (Univ of Nijmegen, The Netherlands)
J Surg Res 72:1–7, 1997 1–21

Objective.—Near-infrared spectroscopy (NIRS) has been used to measure blood flow and oxygen consumption in patients with peripheral arterial occlusive disease (PAOD). Muscle oxygen consumption is best measured during and after walking. An investigation was made of the capability of NIRS to assess muscle blood flow oxygen consumption, arterial inflow capacity, oxygen resaturation, and recovery times at rest, under ischemic and hyperemic conditions, and continuously during and after walking exercise in claudicants complaining of intermittent claudication and in matched nonclaudicants.

Methods.—The total hemoglobin signal was measured using NIRS in 11 claudicants (4 women), aged 43 to 74 years, and in 15 nonclaudicants during and after at 4-minute walking test on a treadmill at 3.2 kM/hr and a gradient of 6 degrees (Fig 2). The more affected leg was studied in

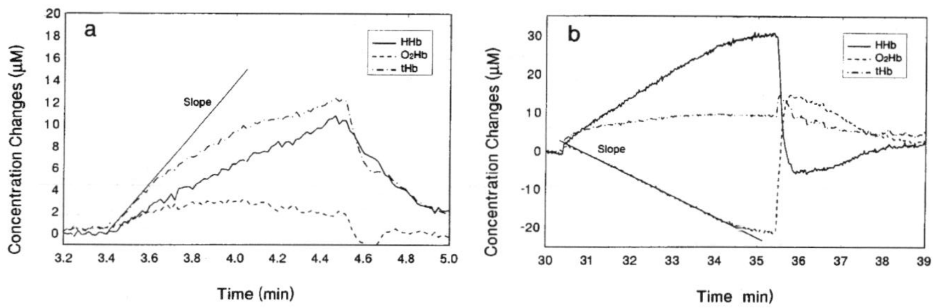

FIGURE 2.—(a) during venous occlusion, blood flow was determined by calculating the initial slope of the total hemoglobin signal (*tHb*). (b) during arterial occlusion, oxygen consumption ($\dot{V}O_2$) was determined by calculating the slope of the linear decrement of the oxyhemoglobin signal (O_2Hb). *Abbreviation: HHb*, deoxyhemoglobin. (Courtesy of Kooijman HM, Hopman MTE, Colier WNJM, et al: Near infrared spectroscopy for noninvasive assessment of claudication. *J Surg Res* 72:1–7, 1997.)

claudicants. The walking test was repeated to measure recovery times of ankle-brachial systolic blood pressure index (ABI) and NIRS signal. Data were compared.

Results.—Blood flow at rest and after walking and oxygen consumption at rest were similar in the 2 groups. One minute after walking, oxygen consumption increased by a factor of 4.1 in claudicants and 1.7 in nonclaudicants. The resaturation rate after arterial occlusion and after walking exercise was significantly lower in claudicants than in nonclaudicants. During walking, claudicants had significantly higher hemoglobin deoxygenation than nonclaudicants. The ABI of claudicants was significantly decreased after occlusion and after exercise, and recovery times were

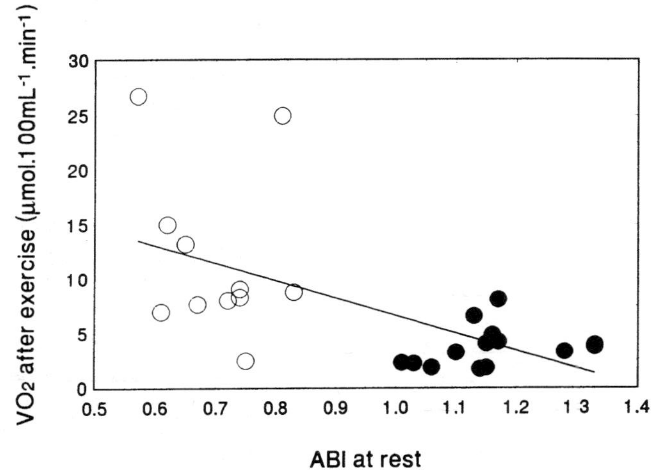

FIGURE 3.—There is a negative relationship between the ankle-brachial systolic blood pressure index (*ABI*) at rest and arterial occlusion oxygen consumption ($\dot{V}O_2$) after walking exercise in all subjects ($r^2 = 0.37$, *P* less than 0.005). *Solid circles* represent controls. *Open circles* represent patients. (There are 2 missing values in the control group). (Courtesy of Kooijman HM, Hopman MTE, Colier WNJM, et al: Near infrared spectroscopy for noninvasive assessment of claudication. *J Surg Res* 72:1–7, 1997.)

significantly longer in claudicants than in nonclaudicants. An increase in oxygen consumption was significantly correlated with a decrease in ABI (Fig 3). The oxygen resaturation rate and deoxygenation after and during walking exercise correlated significantly with ABI. Hemoglobin deoxygenation during exercise and ABI were significantly negatively correlated.

Conclusion.—Near-infrared spectroscopy is an effective and noninvasive method for determining the extent of PAOD at rest and during walking exercise.

▶ Determination of ankle brachial index and ankle pressure decrease with treadmill walking have been the mainstay of the vascular laboratory assessment of claudication. In recent years, we have had the ability to use duplex to determine arterial flow in the lower extremity, although this does not give a particularly accurate hemodynamic indication of muscle ischemia. Other methods, used from time to time, include venous occlusion plethysmography and more recently magnetic resonance spectroscopy which allows determination of the rate of recovery of high-energy phosphates following exercise. Laser Doppler fluxmetry and transcutaneous oxygen tension remain suspect. MRI volume flow determination will probably be no more useful than duplex volume flow determination. Described herein is a new technique attracting increasing attention—namely, near infrared spectroscopy, which depends upon the existence of chromophores in biological tissues whose light-absorbing properties vary with oxygenation. This permits calculation of muscle blood flow, oxygen consumption, and oxygen resaturation after exercise. Striking differences between normals and claudicants are described. Will this technique become an important tool for our future objective assessment of claudication? I have no idea, but it appears to be a technique with which we should all have at least passing familiarity.

Gait Characteristics of Patients With Claudication

Scherer SA, Bainbridge JS, Hiatt WR, et al (Univ of Colorado, Denver)
Arch Phys Med Rehabil 79:529–531, 1998 1–22

Introduction.—Intermittent claudication of the lower extremity vessels causes pain during ambulation. Walking patterns of patients with intermittent claudication were compared with those of healthy controls in a nonrandomized case-control trial.

Methods.—The differences in step length, cadence, and speed during free-speed walking were compared in 19 men with peripheral arterial disease (PAD) and 11 male controls. Eighteen of 19 patients with PAD reported claudication. Research subjects were evaluated as they walked at a self-selected speed for 20 m on a level, indoor surface. During 5 trials each, walking velocity and number of steps were averaged; from these, step length was calculated.

Results.—Compared with controls, patients with claudication had significantly slower gait, shorter step length, and reduced cadence (Table 1). There was no significant correlation between disease severity, peak walking time, step length, cadence, or speed.

considerable attention. This hypothesis has been stimulated by the finding that patients who demonstrate antibodies to *Chlamydia* are at increased risk for cardiovascular disease and that atherosclerotic plaque is frequently immunoreactive to anti-chlamydial antibodies. Although *Chlamydia* is a ubiquitous pathogen, it is extremely difficult to culture because it is an obligate intracellular bacterium. By using new culture techniques, these authors were able to document the presence of live *Chlamydia* in 16% of coronary atherosclerotic lesions from 70 patients, and chlamydial DNA in 30%.

The $64 question is whether this is a cause or effect phenomenon. Because *Chlamydia* is a common respiratory pathogen that infects virtually everyone during their lifetime, it is possible that live *Chlamydia* gain access to atherosclerotic lesions by infected monocytes, which could be vectors for their dissemination. As the authors point out, to establish an etiologic role, it will be important to establish an animal model in which to test the effect of *Chlamydia* on atherosclerotic lesion development.

This is a significant report using new culture techniques to demonstrate live *Chlamydia* organisms in coronary atherosclerotic plaque. The authors' conclusion, however, that *Chlamydia* "commonly" thrive in these lesions, when *Chlamydia* were found in only 16% of samples seems somewhat excessive. Their additional conclusion that this finding justifies a controlled investigation of antimicrobial treatment benefit for coronary artery disease appears premature in contrast to the otherwise excellent science in this report.

J.L. Cronenwett, M.D.

► See also Abstracts 1–27 and 1–28. The antimicrobials have already reared their ugly head!

J.M. Porter, M.D.

Infection With *Chlamydia pneumoniae* Accelerates the Development of Atherosclerosis and Treatment With Azithromycin Prevents It in a Rabbit Model

Muhlestein JB, Anderson JL, Hammond EH, et al (Univ of Utah, Salt Lake City)

Circulation 97:633–636, 1998 1–27

Background.—Infectious agents may serve as an additional risk factor for coronary disease. Serologic studies have suggested that *Chlamydia pneumoniae* infection may be associated with atherosclerosis, and *C. pneumoniae* antigen has been detected in plaque. The effects of *C. pneumoniae* infection and treatment with azithromycin on the rate of development of atherosclerotic lesions were studied in rabbits.

Methods.—Three groups of New Zealand White rabbits were fed a diet enriched with 0.25% cholesterol. At 3-week intervals, the rabbits received separate intranasal inoculations of *C. pneumoniae* or saline. After their final inoculation, all animals were randomized to receive 7 weeks of

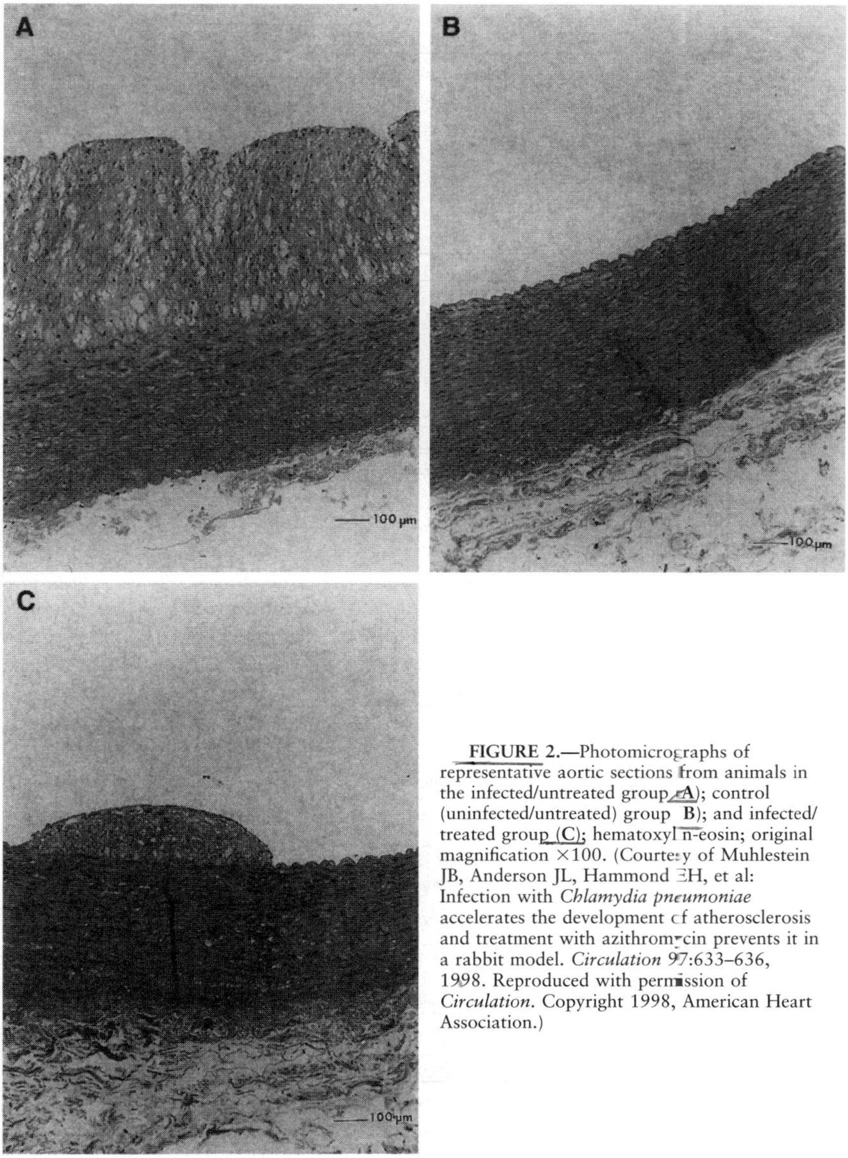

FIGURE 2.—Photomicrographs of representative aortic sections from animals in the infected/untreated group (A); control (uninfected/untreated) group (B); and infected/treated group (C); hematoxylin-eosin; original magnification ×100. (Courtesy of Muhlestein JB, Anderson JL, Hammond EH, et al: Infection with *Chlamydia pneumoniae* accelerates the development of atherosclerosis and treatment with azithromycin prevents it in a rabbit model. *Circulation* 97:633–636, 1998. Reproduced with permission of *Circulation*. Copyright 1998, American Heart Association.)

azithromycin therapy or no treatment. The animals were killed for examination 3 months after their final inoculation. Thoracic aortic sections were investigated for maximal intimal thickness, percentage of luminal circumference involved, and plaque area index. Direct immunofluorescence studies for the presence of vascular chlamydial antigen were performed as well.

Results.—The rabbits inoculated with *C. pneumoniae* had a greater increase in maximal intimal thickness (0.55 mm) than the uninfected controls or the infected but antibiotic-treated rabbits (about 0.2 mm in each). The infected rabbits also had a greater plaque area index and a tendency toward a greater percentage of luminal circumference involved (Fig 2). Two of the untreated and 3 of the treated rabbits had chlamydial antigen. None was found in the control animals.

Conclusion.—In rabbits fed a moderately cholesterol-enhanced diet, infection with *C. pneumoniae* leads to accelerated intimal thickening. This effect is prevented by treatment with azithromycin. The results add to the evidence suggesting that *C. pneumoniae* is an etiologic factor in atherosclerosis. The authors call for further studies, including trials of antibiotic therapy in humans.

▶ The repeated message is that *C. pneumoniae* is frequently found in atherosclerotic plaques, where it may have a causative role rather than acting as a passive fellow traveler. In the interesting experiment described herein, rabbits were actually infected with inoculations of *C. pneumoniae* followed by a high cholesterol diet. Certain animals were begun on a 7 week course of the antibiotic azithromycin, which is lethal for *C. pneumoniae.* Interestingly, aortic thickness was the same in the infected rabbits receiving antibiotics as in the control rabbits who were never infected. The infected rabbits without antibiotics had much more wall thickening. The authors conclude, and I suspect correctly, that this study strengthens the etiologic link between *C. pneumoniae* and atherosclerosis. I suspect that we are very close to a large clinical antibiotic trial with azithromycin, despite Dr. Cronenwett's curmudgeonly complaint in Abstract 1–26. See also Abstract 1–28 for the report of the first clinical azithromycin trial.

Elevated *Chlamydia pneumoniae* Antibodies, Cardiovascular Events, and Azithromycin in Male Survivors of Myocardial Infarction

Gupta S, Leatham EW, Carrington D, et al (St George's Hosp Med School, London)

Circulation 96:404–407, 1997 1–28

Background.—The clinical significance of associations between elevated anti–*Chlamydia pneumoniae* antibody titers and coronary heart disease has not been established. The relationship between antibodies against *C. pneumoniae* and future cardiovascular events in male survivors of myocardial infarction was analyzed. The effect of antibiotic therapy with azithromycin was also evaluated in a subgroup of patients.

Methods.—Of 220 consecutive male survivors of myocardial infarction screened for anti–*C. pneumoniae*, 213 were divided into 3 groups: group Cp–ve consisted of 59 patients with no detectable *C. pneumoniae* antibodies, group Cp-I consisted of 74 patients with intermediate titers ranging from 1/8 to 1/32 dilution, and group Cp+ve consisted of 80 patients

TABLE 2.—Odds Ratios for CV Events in Groups of Patients With Seronegativity and Seropositivity

Group	Total CV Events, n (%)	Unadjusted OR (95% CI)	Adjusted OR (95% CI)
Cp-ve (n=59)	4 (7)		
Cp-I (n=74)	11 (15)	2.4 (0.7–8.0)	2.0 (0.6–6.8)
Cp+ve-NR/P (n=40)	11 (28)	5.2 (1.5–17.8)*	4.2 (1.2–15.5)†
Cp+ve-A (n=40)	3 (8)	1.1 (0.2–5.3)	0.9 (0.2–4.6)

Note: Comparisons of CV events are for all groups relative to group Cp-ve (expressed as OR [95% CI]). Adjusted ORs calculated after controlling for the following variables: age, diabetes mellitus, smoking status, hypertension, hyperlipidemia, and previous coronary revascularization.

$^*P = 0.008$.

$^\dagger P = 0.03$ vs. group Cp-ve.

Abbreviations: CV, cardiovascular; *OR*, odds ratios; *CI*, confidence interval; *Cp, Chlamydia pneumoniae*; *Cp-ve*, seronegative group of patients; *Cp-I*, group with intermediate antibody titres; *Cp+ve-NR/P*, group with elevated antibody titres either randomized to receive placebo or not randomized; *Cp+re-A*, group with elevated antibody titres randomized to receive azithromycin.

(Courtesy of Gupta S, Leatham EW, Carrington D, et al: Elevated *Chlamydia pneumoniae* antibodies, cardiovascular events, and azithromycin in male survivors of myocardial infarction. *Circulation* 96:404–407, 1997. Reproduced with permission *Circulation*. Copyright 1997 American Heart Association.)

who were seropositive at 1/64 dilution or greater. Patients with persistent seropositivity of 1/64 dilution or greater were randomized to receive oral azithromycin or placebo (group Cp+ve-P, 20 patients). There were 2 azithromycin regimens: 500 mg/day for 3 days or 500 mg/day for 6 days. An additional group designated Cp+ve-NR consisted of 20 patients not treated with the antibiotic. The mean follow-up was 18 months.

Results.—The incidence of adverse cardiovascular events increased with increasing anti–*C. pneumoniae* titers: 7% of patients in group Cp–ve, 15% of patients in group Cp-I, 30% of patients in group Cp+ve-NR, and 25% of patients given placebo (Table 2). A fourfold higher risk of adverse cardiovascular events was seen in patients in the Cp+ve-NR and placebo groups compared with patients in the Cp–ve group. The odds ratio for cardiovascular events in patients given azithromycin was the same as in patients in the Cp–ve group. Patients given azithromycin had a higher incidence of decreased IgG anti–*C. pneumoniae* titers than did patients given placebo.

Discussion.—These results indicate that increased anti–*C. pneumoniae* titers may predict future adverse cardiovascular events in male survivors of myocardial infarction. Short-term treatment with azithromycin may lower this risk, perhaps by acting against *C. pneumoniae*.

► Looking at the opposite side of the coin, these investigators screened 220 male survivors of myocardial infarction for anti-*Chlamydia pneumoniae* antibodies. Overall, they detected such antibodies in about three fourths of patients. Patients with high serum antibody titers were randomized to receive azithromycin in 2 dose ranges vs. placebo. The incidence of adverse cardiovascular events over a mean follow-up of 18 months in patients with *Chlamydia* titer receiving azithromycin was lower than observed in patients with *Chlamydia* titers who received either placebo or no treatment. Thus, at least preliminary information suggests that the use of a new macrolide antibiotic, which appears to be well tolerated and achieves high concentration in tissues, may have a beneficial effect in patients whose atherosclerotic plaques contain *C. pneumoniae*. Stay tuned. There surely will be a great deal more on this subject.

Coagulation

Profound and Sustained Inhibition of Platelet Aggregation by Fradafiban, a Nonpeptide Platelet Glycoprotein IIb/IIIa Antagonist, and Its Orally Active Prodrug, Lefradafiban, in Men

Müller TH, Weisenberger H, Brickl R, et al (Ctr of Clinical Pharmacology, Biberach, Germany)
Circulation 96:1130–1138, 1997 1–29

Background.—One of the requirements for platelet thrombus formation is platelet aggregation, and the platelet glycoprotein (GP) IIb/IIIa complex helps cross-link platelets into aggregates. To determine whether GP IIb/IIIa complex antagonists would be useful in inhibiting platelet aggregation in men, orally active drugs are needed. These authors examined fradafiban, an intravenously administered drug that is known to bind selectively to the human platelet GP IIb/IIIa complex, and its orally active prodrug, lefradafiban, to determine their effects on platelet inhibition in men.

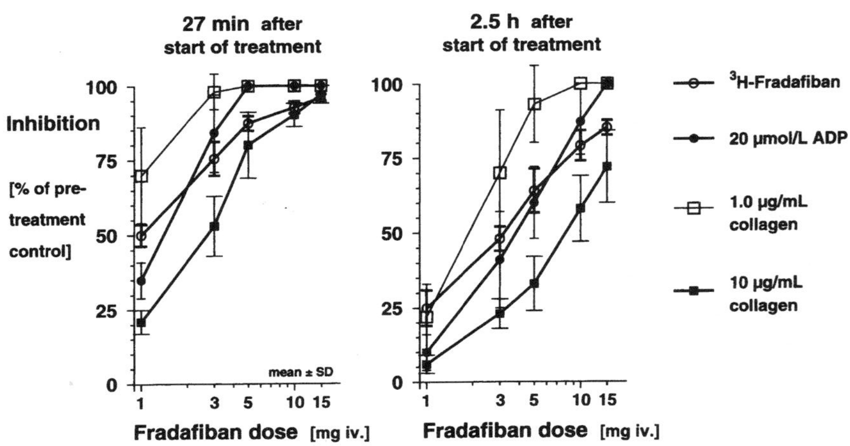

FIGURE 1.—Dose-response relations for the GP IIb/IIIa-antagonistic and the anti-aggregatory activity ex vivo after continuous infusion of 1 to 15 mg fradafiban over 30 minutes. Measurements were performed in platelet-rich plasma prepared from the blood of 8 subjects per dose group at 27 minutes and 2.5 hours after the start of the fradafiban infusion. Mean plus or minus SD values are presented for each dose. (Courtesy of Müller TH, Weisenberger H, Brickl R, et al.: Profound and sustained inhibition of platelet aggregation by fradafiban, a nonpeptide platelet glycoprotein IIB/IIIa antagonist, and its orally active prodrug, lefradafiban, in men. *Circulation* 96:1130–1138, 1997. Reproduced with permission, American Heart Association.)

Methods.—Three double-blind, placebo-controlled, dose-escalation studies were performed. The subjects were 130 healthy men with normal platelet aggregation. Blood samples to determine the inhibition of platelet aggregation ex vivo in platelet-rich plasma in response to collagen, adenosine diphosphate, or a thrombin receptor agonist peptide were drawn at regular intervals in all 3 studies. In study 1, intravenous doses of fradafiban from 1–15 mg were infused for 30 minutes. In study 2, a single oral dose of lefradafiban from 10–150 mg was administered. In study 3, multiple oral doses of lefradafiban from 25–100 mg were given every 8 hours for 7 days.

Findings.—In study 1, intravenous fradafiban significantly inhibited platelet aggregation in a dose-related manner (Fig 1). In study 2, single oral lefradafiban doses of 50 mg or higher significantly inhibited platelet aggregation as early as 4 hours after administration. The effects by 32 hours after dosing were no longer significant. The concentration-response curves for platelet inhibition after single oral doses of Lefradafiban were identical to those after intravenous fradafiban. In study 3, multiple oral lefradafiban doses of 50 mg or higher significantly inhibited platelet aggregation by 2 hours after dosing. Continued anti-aggregatory activity even after 19 dosings (day 7) indicates that the platelets did not desensitize after prolonged treatment.

Conclusions.—Fradafiban and its oral prodrug, lefradafiban, reproducibly and reversibly inhibit platelet aggregation ex vivo in a similar manner. Furthermore, continuous oral doses of lefradafiban maintained anti-aggregatory activity for 1 week. Further studies of lefradafiban are needed to determine its role in the treatment of thromboembolic disease.

► The final pathway in platelet activation consists of binding of fibrinogen and other multi-valent ligands, such as von Willebrand factor, to the platelet GP IIb/IIIa complex on the surface of activated platelets. To date, the only available IIb/IIIa complex inhibitor has been the intravenous C7E3FAB, a humanized monoclonal antibody directed against the human platelet glycoprotein. Currently, there are no approved oral preparations available. Reported herein is the use of one of the very early oral preparations, lefradafiban. The fascinating phase I pharmacology study reported here shows that the administration of the prodrug lefradafiban maintains potent GP IIb/IIIa antagonism during treatment of healthy subjects without signs of loss of antiplatelet activity. On balance, it appears that the GP Ib/IIIa receptor blockers will be superior to all other antiplatelet drugs currently available. I suspect these drugs will have an important role in clinical practice in the near future.

CAST: Randomised Placebo-controlled Trial of Early Aspirin Use in 20 000 Patients With Acute Ischaemic Stroke

Chen Z-M, for the CAST Collaborative Group (Radcliffe Infirmary, Oxford, England)

Lancet 349:1641–1649, 1997 1–30

Background.—In China, about 15 million people are expected to die of stroke during the current decade, and many others are expected to have stroke-related disabilities. Aspirin is effective in treating acute myocardial infarction, and long-term, low-dose aspirin therapy is effective in preventing serious vascular events among survivors of stroke and myocardial infarction. There is little evidence for the benefits and risks of early aspirin therapy during the acute phase of ischemic stroke.

Methods.—The Chinese Acute Stroke Trial, a randomized, placebo-controlled trial, enrolled 21,106 patients with acute ischemic stroke a mean of 25 hours after onset of symptoms. The mean age of patients was about 63. Before random assignment, 87% of patients underwent a CT scan. Treatment was continued in the hospital for as long as 4 weeks. Main

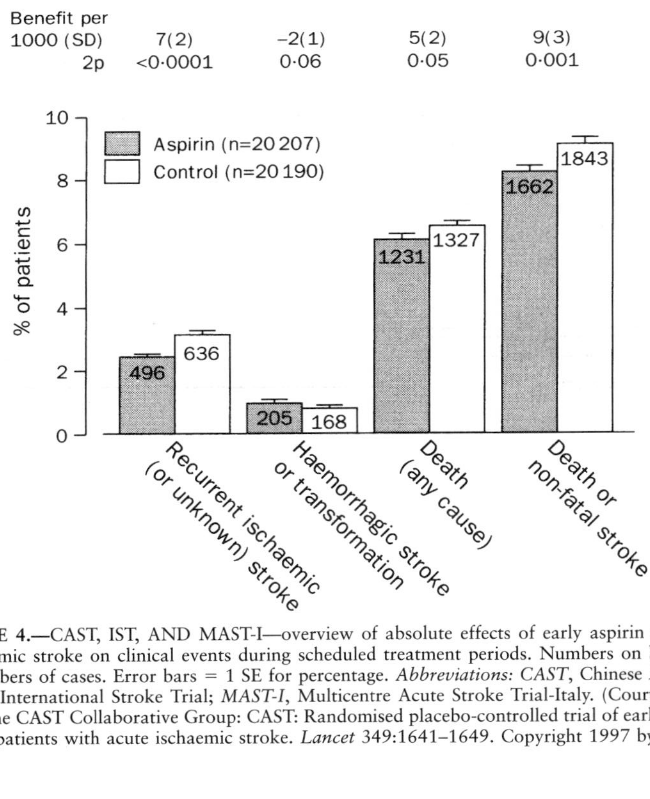

FIGURE 4.—CAST, IST, AND MAST-I—overview of absolute effects of early aspirin treatment in acute ischemic stroke on clinical events during scheduled treatment periods. Numbers on bars indicate actual numbers of cases. Error bars = 1 SE for percentage. *Abbreviations: CAST,* Chinese Acute Stroke Trial; *IST,* International Stroke Trial; *MAST-I,* Multicentre Acute Stroke Trial-Italy. (Courtesy of Chen Z-M, for the CAST Collaborative Group: CAST: Randomised placebo-controlled trial of early aspirin use in 20 000 patients with acute ischaemic stroke. *Lancet* 349:1641–1649. Copyright 1997 by The Lancet Ltd.)

outcome measures were death from any cause and death or dependence at discharge; analyses were according to intention to treat.

Results.—During the treatment period, a significant 14% decrease in mortality rate was observed. In the group treated with aspirin, there were significantly fewer cases of recurrent ischemic stroke but somewhat more cases of hemorrhagic stroke. In the group treated with aspirin, there was a 12% reduction in risk of death or nonfatal stroke at 4 weeks; this resulted in an absolute difference of 6.8 fewer cases per 1,000 patients. At discharge, 3,153 patients given aspirin and 3,266 patients given placebo were dead or dependent.

Discussion.—The results of this trial were to be reported with results of the concurrent International Stroke Trial of 20,000 patients with acute stroke from other countries (Fig 4). The results of the Chinese Acute Stroke Trial and the International Stroke Trial show small but definite benefits of early in-hospital aspirin treatment for patients with acute ischemic stroke. About 9 fewer deaths or nonfatal strokes occurred per 1,000 patients, and 13 fewer patients per 1,000 were dead or dependent after several weeks or months of follow-up.

► This is a monumental study from China reporting the randomization of 20,000 patients with acute ischemic strokes to either aspirin or no aspirin during initial hospitalization. Without question, aspirin started early in the hospital course produced a small but definite net benefit, with a 14% reduction in mortality during the study, and a 12% reduction in the combined end points of death or nonfatal recurrent stroke. These data, combined with those of the International Stroke Trial[1] conducted in other countries, reliably demonstrate that aspirin started early in the hospital course of acute stroke produces a small but definite patient benefit.

Reference

1. International Stroke Trial Collaborative Group: The International Stroke Trial (IST): A randomized trial of aspirin, subcutaneous heparin, both or neither among 19,435 patients with acute ischemic stroke. *Lancet* 349:1569–1581, 1997.

Coronary Stent Placement in Patients With Acute Myocardial Infarction: Comparison of Clinical and Angiographic Outcome After Randomization to Antiplatelet or Anticoagulant Therapy

Schömig A, Neumann FJ, Walter H, et al (Technische Universität München, Munich)

J Am Coll Cardiol 29:28–34, 1997 1–31

Introduction.—The Intracoronary Stenting and Antithrombotic Regimen trial is a randomized analysis of antiplatelet with anticoagulant therapy after coronary Palmaz-Schatz stent placement. Stenting is a common treatment option for acute myocardial infarction. The optimal antithrombotic regimen after stent implantation has not been determined. Early and

Long-term Oral Anticoagulation Reduces Bone Mass in Patients With Previous Hemispheric Infarction and Nonrheumatic Atrial Fibrillation

Sato Y, Honda Y, Kunoh H, et al (Futase Social Insurance Hosp, Iizuka, Japan; Kurume Univ, Japan)

Stroke 28:2390–2394, 1997 1–35

Background.—Vitamin K is essential to the synthesis of plasma clotting proteins and the carboxylation of bone matrix proteins. Warfarin reduces the risk of stroke by inhibiting vitamin K–dependent blood clotting. Whether the reduction in vitamin K with long-term warfarin therapy also affects bone mineral density in stroke patients with nonrheumatic atrial fibrillation was determined.

Methods.—The participants were hemiplegic stroke patients who had been taking warfarin for at least 1 year (n = 64, mean age 70.6 years), hemiplegic stroke patients who had not received warfarin (n = 63, mean age 71.1 years), and healthy controls (n = 39, mean age 71.6 years). None of the participants had rheumatic atrial fibrillation. On the day that bone mineral density was measured, serum samples were collected and assayed for vitamins K_1 and K_2, bone G1a protein, 25-hydroxyvitamin D, and 1,25-dihydroxyvitamin D. A densitometer was used to measure the bone mineral density of the second metacarpal in both hands.

Findings.—Bone mineral density was significantly lower in both patient groups compared with the controls (control: hemiplegic side, 2.806 mm Al; intact side, 2.817 mm Al). Furthermore, bone mineral density was significantly lower in the patients treated with warfarin compared with the patients who did not receive warfarin (hemiplegic side, 1.264 vs. 2.035 mm Al; intact side, 1.348 vs. 2.303 mm Al). Similarly, vitamin K_1 concentrations were significantly lower in both patient groups compared with controls (warfarin group, 0.237 ng/mL; nonwarfarin group, 0.329 ng/mL; controls, 0.553 ng/mL), but K_2 levels did not differ between groups. Bone G1a protein levels were significantly lower in patients treated with warfarin compared with the patients who did not receive warfarin (1.241 vs. 4.476 ng/mL). Furthermore, levels of 25-hydroxyvitamin D and 1,25-dihydroxyvitamin D were significantly lower in patients treated with warfarin (11.1 ng/mL and 28.0 pg/mL, respectively) compared with the patients who did not receive warfarin (11.8 ng/mL and 25.8 pg/mL). Statistical analysis revealed significant correlations between bone mineral density on both the affected and unaffected sides in patients taking warfarin, and the concentrations of vitamin K_1 and bone G1a protein.

Conclusions.—Compared with patients who did not receive warfarin, patients who had been taking long-term oral warfarin had significantly lower bone mineral density in both hands and significantly reduced levels of vitamin K_1, bone G1a protein, and vitamin D. Note that the patients taking warfarin had avoided eating green leafy vegetables containing vitamin K as part of their treatment. Thus, supplementation with vitamins K and D may be advisable to prevent fractures in poststroke hemiplegic patients with nonrheumatic atrial fibrillation.

► In this well-designed study, the authors demonstrated a 40% reduction in the bone mineral density of stroke patients who had been receiving warfarin for treatment of atrial fibrillation for an average of 5 years. This was true not only on the hemiplegic side (where reduced bone density results from disuse even without warfarin), but also on the normal side. Because hemiplegic patients with lower bone density are known to be at higher risk for hip fracture, this study suggests that warfarin therapy may also increase fracture risk. Unfortunately, such patients are caught between the proverbial rock and hard-place, because warfarin has been shown to dramatically reduce stroke risk and other embolism risks in patients with nonrheumatic atrial fibrillation. Comparing possible hip fracture vs. stroke, most patients would prefer to take warfarin to prevent stroke and take their chances with fractures. The authors point out, however, that vitamin D and bisphosphonate supplementation may reduce bone density loss in such patients, and thus is probably advisable in elderly patients receiving warfarin.

J.L. Cronenwett, M.D.

Heparin Inhibits Thrombin-induced Mitogen-activated Protein Kinase Signaling in Arterial Smooth Muscle Cells

Hedin U, Daum G, Clowes AW (Univ of Washington, Seattle; Karolinska Hosp, Stockholm)

J Vasc Surg 27:512–520, 1998 1–36

Objective.—Whereas it is known that heparin interferes with smooth muscle cell (SMC) proliferation that contributes to atherosclerosis, the mechanism of this interference is poorly understood. The effect of heparin on the activity of the mitogen-activated protein kinase (MAPK) pathway and DNA synthesis was investigated in baboon SMCs stimulated with thrombin and other G-protein agonists.

Methods.—The SMCs isolated from baboon aortic media were cultured and serum-starved for 72 hours. Then they were stimulated with thrombin, angiotensin II, endothelin-1, or lysophosphatidic acid with or without heparin. The MAPK activity was measured using duplicate in-gel assays, MAPK kinase-1 (MAPKK-1) activity was measured using immunoprecipitation methods, and DNA synthesis was analyzed using ^{3}H-thymidine labeling.

Results.—Heparin completely inhibited DNA synthesis by thrombin and inhibited thrombin-induced MAPK activity by a protein kinase C–independent pathway (Fig 4). Heparin inhibited G-protein–dependent mitogenic pathways. Heparin completely blocked DNA synthesis by thrombin, angiotensin II, endothelin-1, and lysophosphatidic acid.

Conclusions.—Heparin inhibits DNA synthesis by thrombin, angiotensin II, endothelin-1, and lysophosphatidic acid by preventing induction of

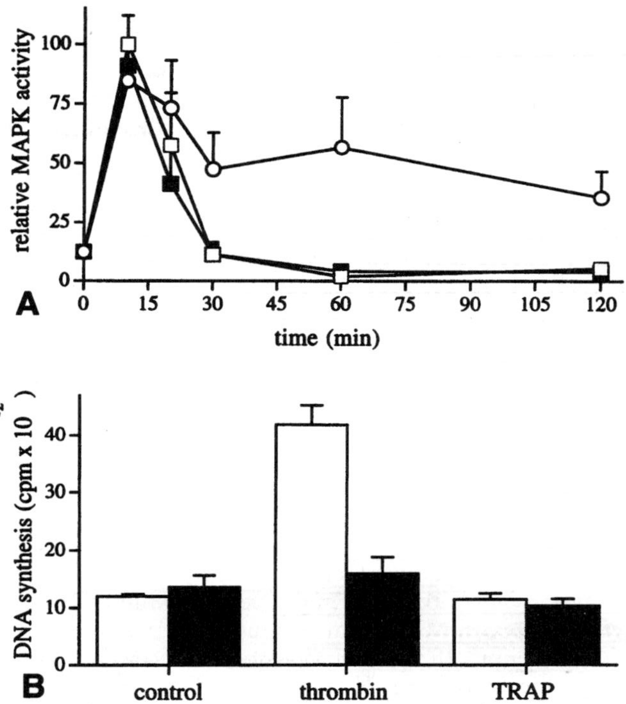

FIGURE 4.—Insufficient growth signaling by thrombin receptor agonist peptide in baboon smooth muscle cells. A, serum-starved cells were stimulated with 10 nmol/L thrombin (*open circles*) or 10 μmol/L thrombin receptor agonist peptide SFLLRNPNDKYEPF (TRAP) in presence (*solid squares*) or absence (*open squares*) of 0.1 mg/mL heparin and mitogen-activated protein kinase (*MAPK*) activity analyzed as described in Methods. Data obtained by phosphoimager analysis are related to maximum activity and presented as mean ± SD of 3 experiments. **B**, DNA synthesis induced by thrombin and TRAP in presence or absence of 0.1 mg/mL heparin was analyzed by ^{3}H-incorporation during 48 hours, and results are presented as mean ± SD of quadruplicate samples. (Courtesy of Hedin U, Daum G, Clowes AW: Heparin inhibits thrombin-induced mitogen-activated protein kinase signaling in arterial smooth muscle cells. *J Vasc Surg* 27:512–520, 1998.)

MAPK activity. This information could prove useful in the prevention of lesion development after vascular surgery.

► In an attempt to understand the mechanism by which heparin inhibits the growth of smooth muscle cells, the University of Washington group reported that heparin inhibits the activation of MAPK by serum, but not by platelet-derived growth factor or fibroblast growth factor.[1] This led the authors to conclude that the effect of heparin on smooth muscle cell growth depended on the specific mitogen, but that when heparin inhibited smooth muscle proliferation, it did so by preventing activation of MAPK kinase-1. It is known that activation of G-proteins stimulates the MAPK pathway Thus, the authors' finding in this follow-up study that heparin inhibited growth of baboon smooth muscle cells stimulated by thrombin or other G-protein activators is not surprising, but rather predictable in light of their previous observations.

Nonetheless, this study adds a little additional information about the precise mechanism of heparin inhibition of smooth muscle cell growth that might facilitate future development of specific agents to reduce intimal hyperplasia through this mechanism. The search for the magic bullet continues!

J.L. Cronenwett, M.D.

Reference

1. Daum G, Hedin U, Wang T, et al: Diverse effects of heparin on mitogen-activated protein kinase dependent signal transduction in vascular smooth muscle cells. *Circ Res* 81:17–23, 1997.

Activated Protein C Resistance, Factor V Leiden and Peripheral Vascular Disease

Foley PWX, Irvine CD, Standen GR, et al (Bristol Royal Infirmary, England)
Cardiovasc Surg 5:157–160, 1997 1–37

Background.—Activated protein C resistance is a thrombophilia disorder caused by a specific amino acid substitution at the protein C cleavage site of factor V. The resultant mutant factor (factor V Leiden) is 10 times more resistant to deactivation than normal. Previous studies have indicated that the activated protein C resistance caused by this mutation can predispose patients to venous thromboembolism. The prevalence of activated protein C resistance and factor V Leiden in patients with peripheral vascular disease was studied.

Methods.—The participants were 45 patients (26 men and 19 women, mean age 66.8 years) with peripheral vascular disease and 45 age- and sex-matched controls with no known peripheral vascular disease or venous thromboembolism. Warfarin was being used by 12 of the patients. All participants underwent venesection, and levels of factor VIIIc, protein C, protein S, plasminogen, and antithrombin III were measured in controls and in the 33 patients not taking warfarin. Activated protein C resistance was expressed as a ratio of clotting time with activated protein C/calcium chloride solution divided by the clotting time with calcium chloride. A ratio of less than 2.2 defined such resistance. Polymerase chain reaction was used to genotype the patients' factor V Leiden status, and to determine the activated protein C resistance ratio in patients taking warfarin.

Findings.—The patients not taking warfarin had normal plasma levels of antithrombin III, proteins C and S, and plasminogen. Their levels of factor VIIIc were elevated, but they did not correlate with the activated protein C ratio. The patients not taking warfarin had significantly lower activated protein C resistance ratios than controls (median 2.82 [range 1.36–3.83] vs. 2.97 [range 2.24–4.11]), and 8 of these patients (24%) had activated protein C resistance, with a ratio of less than 2.2. Five of these 8 patients were heterozygous for the factor V Leiden mutation, 1 was homozygous for this mutation, and 1 patient taking warfarin had the mutation, for an overall frequency of mutation of 17.8% (8 of 45 patients). (Previous reports show a prevalence of this genotype in Britain of 3.5%.) In the detection of factor V Leiden, an activated protein C resistance ratio of 2.2 had a specificity of 93% and a sensitivity of 97%. Graft patency did not differ significantly between patients who had and did not have the factor V Leiden mutation.

Conclusions.—Almost one fifth of patients with peripheral vascular disease had activated protein C resistance. Furthermore, the patients were about 5 times more likely to have factor V Leiden than were controls. These findings suggest that activated protein C resistance is a cofactor for the development of peripheral vascular disease.

► A surprising number of patients with both venous thrombosis and arterial occlusive disease possess inherited factor V resistance to activated protein C (factor V Leiden). While many have suggested such abnormalities are causative in venous thrombosis, the evidence linking these abnormalities to arterial disease is far weaker. In this study, while a significant number of patients with arterial disease possess the abnormality, it did not appear to adversely affect their outcome. Not so in other studies. I believe a fair conclusion at present is that a significant number of patients with arterial disease possess the factor V Leiden abnormality, but it is as yet unproven whether this has an adverse impact upon the patient's clinical course.

A Comparison of Low-Molecular-Weight Heparin With Unfractionated Heparin for Unstable Coronary Artery Disease

Cohen M, for the Efficacy and Safety of Subcutaneous Enoxaparin in Non–Q-Wave Coronary Events Study Group (Allegheny Univ, Philadelphia; Hôpital St Sacrement, Quebec; Instituto de Cardiologia y Cirugia, Buenos Aires, Argentina; et al)

N Engl J Med 337:447–452, 1997 1–38

Introduction.—Standard therapy for patients hospitalized with unstable angina or non–Q-wave myocardial infarction consists of IV unfractionated heparin plus oral aspirin. Because of the substantial failure rate of this treatment, a randomized trial was conducted to assess the efficacy of low–molecular weight heparins in this setting. Previous trials have documented the advantages of the low–molecular weight heparins, including their more predictable anticoagulant effect.

Methods.—Patients were enrolled from October 1994 to May 1996 at 176 centers in the United States, Canada, South America, and Europe. The double-blind study assigned 3,171 patients to receive either enoxaparin (1 mg/kg of body weight administered subcutaneously twice daily) or continuous IV unfractionated heparin. Patients were treated for at least 48 hours to a maximum of 8 days. The primary outcome was the composite triple end point of death, myocardial infarction (or reinfarction), or recurrent angina at 14 days of follow-up. Data on coronary end points were

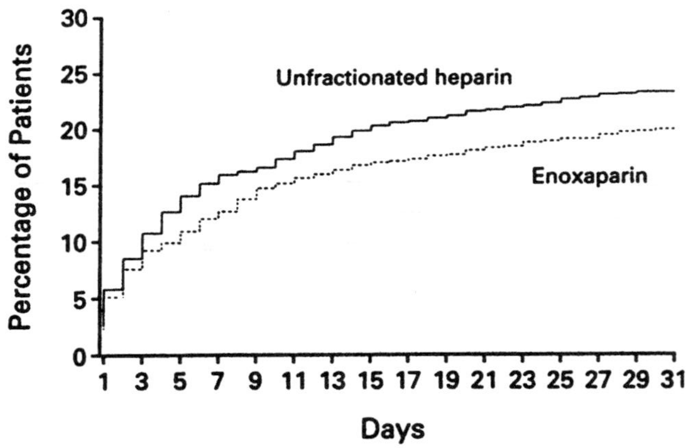

FIGURE 1.—Kaplan-Meier plots of the time to a first event over a period of 30 days for the composite end point of death, myocardial infarction, or recurrent angina. (Reprinted by permission of *The New England Journal of Medicine* from Cohen M, for the Efficacy and Safety of Subcutaneous Enoxaparin in Non–Q-Wave Coronary Events Study Group. A comparison of low-molecular-weight heparin with unfractionated heparin for unstable coronary artery disease. *N Engl J Med* 337:447–452, 1997.)

collected during a period of 30 days. The targeted activated partial-thromboplastin time was 55 to 85 seconds.

Results.—The 2 treatment groups were similar in baseline variables. Assigned therapies were initiated within 12 hours of randomization in 96% of patients, and both trial therapies were continued for a median of 2.6 days. At 14 days, patients randomized to enoxaparin had a significantly lower risk of death, myocardial infarction, or recurrent angina (16.6%) than those randomized to unfractionated heparin (19.8%). The risk of this composite end point continued to be significantly lower (Fig 1) in the enoxaparin group at 30 days (19.8% vs. 23.3%). Enoxaparin treatment was also associated with a significantly less frequent need for revascularization procedures but a significantly higher incidence of bleeding overall.

Conclusion.—Enoxaparin plus aspirin was a more effective antithrombotic therapy than unfractionated heparin plus aspirin for patients hospitalized with unstable angina or non–Q-wave myocardial infarction. The risk of death, myocardial infarction, or recurrent angina was significantly reduced at both 14 and 30 days in patients randomized to enoxaparin. Minor bleeding was the only adverse effect reported for enoxaparin.

► I continue to regard low–molecular weight heparin (LMWH) as an important new therapeutic principle. Numerous articles previously included in the *Year Book* series have convincingly demonstrated that LMWH appears at least as effective as unfractionated heparin (UFH), both in the prophylaxis and treatment of venous thrombosis. Some of the studies have suggested superiority for LMWH. In this remarkable study of over 3,000 patients with unstable angina who were randomized to LMWH or UFH, benefits at 14 days, as measured by the incidence of death, myocardial infarction, or recurrent angina, were significantly greater in the patients assigned to the LMWH group. Benefits remained significant at 30 days, and the need for revascularization procedures was significantly less in the patients randomized to LMWH. In this very large, important randomized study, antithrombotic therapy with LMWH was clearly more effective than therapy with UFH. All patients in the study received aspirin. More and more randomized studies suggest a therapeutic superiority in favor of LMWH. I would not be at all surprised if in the next 3 or 4 years UFH becomes an infrequently used clinical drug.

Diabetes

Metabolic Control and Prevalent Cardiovascular Disease in Non–Insulin-Dependent Diabetes Mellitus (NIDDM): The NIDDM Patient Outcomes Research Team

Meigs JB, Singer DE, Sullivan LM, et al (Harvard Med School, Boston; New England Med Ctr, Boston; Boston Univ; et al)

Am J Med 102:38–47, 1997 1–39

Background.—Although it is known that non–insulin-dependent diabetes mellitus (NIDDM) is associated with an increased risk of cardiovascular disease, the mechanism involved in its contribution to large-vessel atherosclerosis is not well understood. This report describes a cross-sectional analysis of the association between glycemic control and cardiovascular disease in NIDDM patients.

Methods.—The participants of this study were enrolled in the NIDDM Patient Outcome Research Team (PORT) study at the Puget Sound site. Patients with NIDDM who were at least 30 years of age were eligible to participate. Patient information was collected from a self-administered questionnaire completed by the 1,539 patients who made up the study group. Glycohemoglobin, glucose, and lipid values were determined as part of routine care. The independent association of risk factors and cardiovascular disease were evaluated by multiple logistic regression.

Results.—The average duration of NIDDM in the study population was 9 years. Average glycohemoglobin level was 10.6%. In this population, 60% reported hypertension, 16% reported smoking, and the average total high-density lipoprotein (HDL) cholesterol ratio was 5.7. Although 51% of the participants reported cardiovascular disease, the prevalence remained constant across increasing quartiles of glycohemoglobin for both men and women. Prevalent cardiovascular disease was associated with established cardiovascular risk factors, including age, hypertension, cigarette smoking, and total HDL cholesterol ratio. Cardiovascular disease was also associated with NIDDM duration.

Conclusions.—This large cross-sectional study of cardiovascular disease in patients with NIDDM found no association between glycemic control and cardiovascular disease. In contrast, established cardiovascular risk factors had significant, independent, positive associations with cardiovascular disease in this population. Duration of NIDDM was also independently associated with cardiovascular disease. Intensive management of cardiovascular risk factors may be the best way to reduce the cardiovascular complications associated with NIDDM.

▶ I find the basic message of this article quite interesting, namely, that glycemic control in type II diabetes mellitus appears unrelated to prevalent cardiovascular disease in a large patient cohort. I note with concern, however, that the entire database was obtained from patient surveys, which, in my opinion, are inherently suspect and have the potential for significant study bias. Nonetheless, it is more than fascinating to observe that these patients with NIDDM had precisely the anticipated relationship between established risk factors and cardiovascular disease and showed no relationship between glucose control and macrovascular cardiovascular disease. If true, massive efforts to micromanage glucose control in patients with diabetes may have always been futile.

Relationship Between Insulin and Carotid Atherosclerosis in the General Population: The Bruneck Study

Bonora E, Willeit J, Kiechl S, et al (Univ of Verona, Italy; Hosp of Bruneck, Italy; Univ of Innsbruck, Austria)

Stroke 28:1147–1152, 1997 1–40

Objective.—Hyperinsulinemia increases the risk of cardiovascular problems. The relationship between serum insulin and carotid atherosclerosis (CA) has not been prospectively investigated. The relationships between serum insulin and CA were investigated cross-sectionally and prospectively in a large population-based sample of men and women aged 40–79 years.

Methods.—Serum insulin was measured at fasting in 888 individuals (450 men); 811 of these individuals also had serum insulin measured at 2 hours after oral glucose loading (known diabetics were excluded). After 5 years, 804 individuals were available for analysis. Carotid arteries were examined by duplex sonography at baseline and at 5-year follow-up.

Results.—At baseline, 159 women and 218 men had CA (prevalence of 36.2% and 48.4%, respectively). Prevalence rates increased by decade from 5.6% at ages 40–49, to 31.7% at ages 50–59, to 57.3% at ages 60–69, and to 79.5% at ages 70–79. Logistic regression analysis revealed a significant relationship between insulin levels and CA with age and sex even after correcting for glucose tolerance, body mass index, physical activity level, smoking habits, alcohol intake, socioeconomic status, and lipid profile. Fasting insulin levels showed a U-shaped relationship to atherosclerosis risk that was increased in quintiles I–II and IV–V. Results for fasting glucose or 2-hour glucose or HbA_{1c} were similar.

Conclusions.—Both hyperinsulinemia and hypoinsulinemia appear to increase the risk for CA.

mortality was prospectively examined in patients with coronary artery disease.

Methods.—A total of 587 patients with coronary artery disease, all confirmed by angiography, were studied. Coronary risk factors, including homocysteine levels, were assessed during 1991–1992. Subsequent treatment consisted of coronary artery bypass grafting in 318 patients, percutaneous transluminal coronary angioplasty in 120, and medical treatment in 149. Median follow-up was 5 years.

Results.—Eleven percent of patients died during follow-up. Four-year mortality was 3.8% for patients with homocysteine levels of less than 9 µmol/L, compared with 24.7% for those with homocysteine levels of 15 µmol/L. There was no strong relationship between homocysteine level and extent of coronary artery disease. However, homocysteine levels were strongly related to history of myocardial infarction, left ventricular ejection fraction, and serum creatinine levels. Homocysteine levels were strongly related to mortality even after adjustment for confounders. Compared with patients having homocysteine levels of less than 9 µmol/L, mortality ratio was 1.9 for those with homocysteine levels of 9.0–14.9 µmol/L, 2.8 for those with levels of 15.0–19.9 µmol/L, and 4.5 for those with levels of 20.0 µmol/L or greater (Fig 1).

Conclusions.—A strong relationship exists between plasma total homocysteine levels and mortality among patients with angiographically confirmed coronary artery disease. In this group, homocysteine levels are the most powerful modifiable predictor of overall and cardiovascular mortality. No causal association can be assumed, but further trials of homocysteine-reducing therapy are called for.

▶ This study provides information beyond the simple relationship that patients with high homocysteine levels have more symptomatic coronary disease and a higher mortality than patients with low homocysteine levels. While these investigators did confirm that basic, but well-known relationship, they further confirmed that homocysteine levels were only weakly related to the extent of coronary artery disease on coronary arteriography, but were strongly related to a history of myocardial infarction. The observation that the mortality for patients with homocysteine levels below 9 µmol/L after 4 years was only 3.8%, compared with 24.7% for those with homocysteine levels greater than 15 µmol/L. Homocysteine levels only weakly related to the extent of disease on coronary arteriography must lead one to consider possibilities other than a simple relationship between homocystinuria and arteriosclerosis obliterans. We are now beginning to wonder whether the mortality of chronic hyperhomocysteinemia may be more related to the induction of thrombosis rather than the anatomical progression of atherosclerosis. More studies are beginning to point in this direction. Nonetheless, the adverse relationship between hyperhomocysteinemia and cardiovascular health appears established beyond reasonable doubt. We desperately need a large-volume therapeutic trial of folate vs. placebo with detailed follow-up of a large patient cohort to confirm the anticipated benefits.

Myocardial Infarction in Young Women in Relation to Plasma Total Homocysteine, Folate, and a Common Variant in the Methylenetetrahydrofolate Reductase Gene

Schwartz SM, Siscovick DS, Malinow MR, et al (Univ of Washington, Seattle; Oregon Regional Primate Research Ctr, Beaverton; Univ Hosp, Leiden, The Netherlands; et al)

Circulation 96:412–417, 1997 1–45

Background.—Homocysteine is a methionine metabolite with atherogenic and thrombotic properties. Elevated levels of plasma total homocysteine (tHCY) are a risk factor for cardiovascular disease. Low levels of folate in the blood appear to be a determinant of tHCY levels in some populations. Genetic factors also contribute to tHCY levels. A common C to T change at nucleotide 677 of the 5,10-methylenetetrahydrofolate reductase (MTHFR) enzyme gene is associated with elevated tHCY level and may be a risk factor for cardiovascular disease. The relationship of plasma tHCY level, plasma folate concentration, and this MTHFR polymorphism to the risk of acute myocardial infarction (MI) among young women was examined in a population-based case-control study.

Methods.—The participants for this study came from a study of incident cardiovascular disease among women aged 18 to 44 residing in 3 counties in Washington state. Women in whom a first MI was diagnosed between July 1991 and February 1995, with no prior history of cardiovascular disease, were eligible to participate. After 79 patients had been recruited, random-digit telephone dialing was used to obtain 386 age-matched women from the same counties to serve as controls. Participants were interviewed about cardiovascular risk factors, smoking, height and weight, menstrual history, contraceptive use, alcohol consumption, physical activity, history of MI in first-degree relatives, and demographic characteristics. A venous blood specimen was also obtained. Plasma tHCY concentrations were obtained by high-pressure liquid chromatography and electrochemical detection. Plasma folate and vitamin B_{12} concentrations were obtained with the Quantaphase II Assay system. Genomic DNA was extracted for MTHFR genotyping. Cholesterol and triglyceride levels were also assessed.

Results.—Case patients had higher average tHCY levels and lower average folate concentrations than controls. There was no difference in vitamin B levels between these 2 groups. After adjustment for known cardiovascular risk factors, women with a tHCY level of at least 15.6 mmol/L had about twice the risk of MI as women with a tHCY level of less than 10.0 mmol/L. Women with a folate level of at least 8.39 nmol/L had half as much risk of MI as women with less than 5.27 nmol/L of plasma folate. Approximately 10% of both case patients and controls were homozygous for the MTHFR-677 polymorphism, and these women had higher plasma tHCY levels and lower plasma folate concentrations than women with other genotypes. There was no association of homozygosity with risk of MI.

Conclusions.—These data support other studies indicating an association of elevated plasma tHCY levels and reduced plasma folate concentrations with increased risk of myocardial infarction among young women. Homozygosity for MTHFR T^{677} was associated with elevated plasma tHCY levels and reduced plasma folate levels, but was not associated with an increased risk of acute MI in this population. The relationship between plasma tHCY level, plasma folate concentration, the MTHFR T^{677} allele, and cardiovascular disease requires further clarification.

▶ Both low serum folate and a high total homocysteine concentration were related to a significantly increased risk of myocardial infarction in young women in this study. The high homocysteine and low folate levels were, of course, inversely related. The MTHFR T^{677} allele appeared significantly associated with increased plasma homocysteine, but there was not an observed increase of MI among women who had this particular genotype. Thus, we have another well-characterized association between elevated homocysteine and cardiovascular disease and further evidence that MTHFR T^{677} is not a risk factor for MI in this population.

Folate and Vitamin B$_6$ From Diet and Supplements in Relation to Risk of Coronary Heart Disease Among Women

Rimm EB, Willett WC, Hu FB, et al (Harvard School of Public Health, Boston; Brigham and Women's Hosp, Boston; Harvard Med School, Boston)

JAMA 279:359–364, 1998 1–46

Objective.—Moderately elevated blood homocysteine levels have been linked to coronary heart disease (CHD). Whereas it is known that folate with or without vitamins B_6 and B_{12} reduces homocysteine levels, there are no prospective data on the relationship of intake of these vitamins and risk of CHD. The relation of intake of folate and vitamin B_6 to risk of CHD was examined in 80,082 women enrolled in the Nurses' Health Study and followed prospectively for 14 years (1980–1994).

Methods.—Women from the study completed a food frequency questionnaire designed to measure intake of folate and vitamin B_6. End points were nonfatal myocardial infarction (MI) and fatal CHD confirmed by World Health Organization (WHO) criteria.

Results.—During 14 years of follow-up, there were 658 cases of nonfatal MIs and 281 cases of fatal CHD. Compared with women in the lowest quintile of folate intake, women in the highest quintile had an age-adjusted relative risk (RR) of CHD of 0.53. When smoking was controlled for, the RR was 0.61; when vitamin E consumption was controlled for, the RR was 0.65; and when cardiovascular risk factors were accounted for, the RR was 0.69 for folate and 0.67 for vitamin B_6. There was an RR of 0.89 for each additional 200-µg increase in dietary intake of folate. Women in the highest folate and vitamin B_6 quintile had an RR of

0.55 compared with women in the lowest quintile. Women taking multiple vitamins had an RR of 0.76 for CHD. Women with high folate intakes who had up to 1 alcoholic drink per day had an RR of 0.69, whereas woman who had more than 1 alcoholic drink per day had an RR of 0.27.

Conclusions.—Folate and vitamin B_6 intake above the recommended dietary allowance (RDA) appears to confer additional protection against CHD in women.

► This study has all the flaws of a mail questionnaire. The conclusion that the intake of folate and vitamin B_6 above currently recommended dietary allowances may be important in the primary prevention of coronary heart disease among women may be correct, but it is awfully hard to prove from weak data such as these. We may properly regard this as another thin slice of salami from the Nurses' Health Study.

Prospective Study of Hyperhomocysteinemia as an Adverse Cardiovascular Risk Factor in End-stage Renal Disease

Moustapha A, Naso A, Nahlawi M, et al (Cleveland Clinic Found, Ohio)

Circulation 97:138–141, 1998 1–47

Objective.—Elevated total plasma homocysteine (tHcy) levels increased the risk for vascular events in patients receiving dialysis. The association between tHcy and cardiovascular events were examined prospectively in patients with end-stage renal disease.

Methods.—Baseline predialysis tHcy levels and total fasting cholesterol concentrations were measured in 130 patients receiving hemodialysis and in 46 patients receiving peritoneal dialysis. Cardiovascular events and causes of mortality were recorded, and predictors of those events were

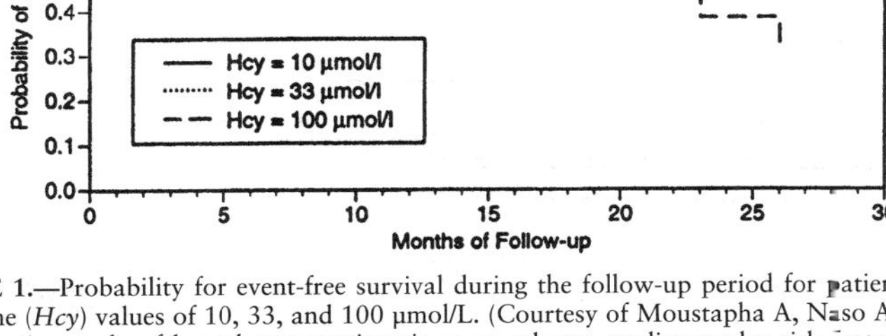

FIGURE 1.—Probability for event-free survival during the follow-up period for patients with mean homocysteine (*Hcy*) values of 10, 33, and 100 µmol/L. (Courtesy of Moustapha A, Naso A, Nahlawi M, et al: Prospective study of hyperhomocysteinemia as an adverse cardiovascular risk factor in end-stage renal disease. *Circulation* 97:138–141. Copyright 1998, American Heart Association. Reproduced with permission.)

identified using Cox regression analysis. Patients were followed up for an average of 17.4 months.

Results.—There were 167 patients (93% male) available for follow-up. During follow-up, 55 patients (33%) had 1 or more cardiovascular events. There were 31 deaths (19%), 12 (8%) from cardiovascular causes. Levels of tHcy were higher in patients who had adverse cardiovascular events than in patients who did not (43.0 vs. 26.9 µmol/L, respectively). Both cardiovascular events and deaths were more common in patients in the highest tHcy quartile than in the other 3 quartiles (45% vs. 29%, respectively). Both diabetes mellitus and tHcy were independent predictors of cardiovascular complications, according to Cox regression analysis. This corresponds to an increase of relative risk for cardiovascular events by 1% per µmol/L increase in tHcy level. When arteriovenous fistula thrombotic events were excluded from cardiovascular events, tHcy (RR 1.01) and diabetes (RR 2.27) remained independent predictors of cardiovascular events (Fig 1).

Conclusions.—Increased levels of tHcy in dialysis patients increases their risk of cardiovascular events.

► In 1996, these authors reported a case-controlled study of 176 dialysis patients and concluded that total plasma homocysteine concentration is an independent risk factor of atherosclerotic complications of end-stage renal disease.[1] It is reassuring that the same authors have confirmed these observations in the same group in this study, in which they analyzed cardiovascular events that occurred in the 17 months since their original report. Interestingly, the most frequent "cardiovascular complication" in these dialysis patients was thrombosis of the hemoaccess fistula. Excluding this end point, hyperhomocysteinemia was still an independent predictor of worse outcome, although the relative risk was only 1.01. Diabetes was a much stronger predictor of worse outcome with a relative risk of 2.27. The question remains as to whether reduction of homocysteine levels by treatment with folic acid, vitamin B_6, or vitamin B_{12} will reduce cardiovascular complications. It's time to perform such a trial and stop reporting additional studies that only confirm the well-established fact that hyperhomocysteinemia is an independent risk factor for cardiovascular end points.

J.L. Cronenwett, M.D.

Reference

1. Robinson K, Gupta A, Dennis V, et al: Hyperhomocysteinemia confers an independent increased risk of atherosclerosis in end-stage renal disease and is closely linked to plasma folate and pyridoxine concentrations. *Circulation* 94:2743–2748, 1996.

► Right on, you silver-tongued devil.

J.M. Porter, M.D.

Levels of Prothombin Fragment F1+2 in Patients With Hyperhomocysteinemia and a History of Venous Thromboembolism

Kyrle PA, Stümpflen A, Hirschl M, et al (Univ of Vienna; Hanuschkrankenaus, Vienna; Wilhelminenspital, Vienna; et al)

Thromb Haemost 78:1327–1331, 1997 1–48

Background.—Patients with clotting abnormalities, such as inherited defects in the antithrombin or protein C anticoagulant pathways, may show increased thrombin generation. The same finding may occur in patients with thrombosis who lack a specific clotting abnormality. Patients with hyperhomocysteinemia (H-HC) are at elevated risk of venous thromboembolism (VTE). Thrombin generation was investigated in patients with a history of VTE and H-HC.

Methods.—Forty-eight patients with H-HC and 183 patients without H-HC were prospectively studied. Median ages were 62 and 50 years, respectively. Plasma samples were obtained for measurement of prothrombin fragment F1+2, an indicator of thrombin generation. Plasma F1+2 was measured during and after treatment with oral anticoagulants.

Results.—Median F1+2 levels while the patients were receiving anticoagulants were 0.4 nmol/L in the H-HC group vs. 0.3 nmol/L in the non–H-HC group. After oral anticoagulant treatment was stopped, F1+2 levels rose to above-normal levels in 20% of H-HC patients and 5% to 6% of non–H-HC patients, compared with age- and sex-matched controls (Fig 1). Sixteen percent of patients in the H-HC group either had at least 2 H-HC measurements above the upper limit of normal or an elevated F1+2 measurement followed by recurrent VTE, compared with 4% of the non–H-HC group.

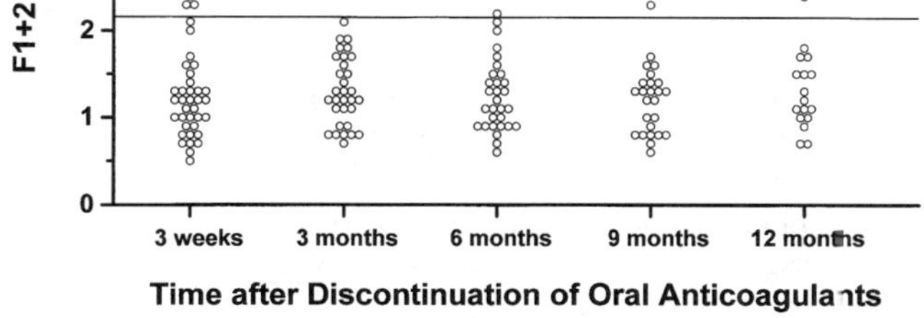

FIGURE 1.—Levels of prothrombin fragment 1+2 (F1+2) at several time points after discontinuation of oral anticoagulants in patients with hyperhomocysteinemia. The *dashed line* indicates the upper normal limit (mean + 2 standard deviations) obtained from 34 age- and sex-matched healthy control subjects. (Courtesy of Kyrle PA, Stümpflen A, Hirschl M, et al: Levels of prothrombin fragment F1+2 in patients with hyperhomocysteinemia and a history of venous thromboembolism. *Thromb Haemost* 78:1327–1331, 1997.)

Conclusions.—In some patients with H-HC and a history of VTE, permanent activation of the hemostatic system is detected after discontinuation of oral anticoagulant therapy. Patients with H-HC may need higher than conventional doses of oral anticoagulants for effective secondary thromboprophylaxis.

▶ We have increasingly come to suspect in recent years that one of the primary adverse effects of H-HC may be alteration of the coagulation status. This interesting prospective study found that 20% of patients with H-HC and 5% of patients without H-HC had elevated levels of prothrombin fragments 1 + 2 well above the upper limits of normal controls on at least 2 occasions. The authors' conclusion that a permanent activation of the hemostatic system is detectable in a number of patients with H-HC may be correct. We desperately need more accurate information in this titillating area. We also need to know whether oral anticoagulation will suppress the apparent hypercoagulable activities of H-HC. Stay tuned. There will surely be much more to follow.

Hyperhomocyst(e)inemia Is a Risk Factor for Arterial Endothelial Dysfunction in Humans

Woo KS, Chook P, Lolin YI, et al (Chinese Univ of Hong Kong; Royal Prince Alfred Hosp, Sydney, Australia)

Circulation 96:2542–2544, 1997 1–49

Background.—Epidemiologic evidence of an association between hyperhomocysteinemia and premature vascular disease has accumulated. In experimental systems, high homocysteine levels have been shown to cause endothelial cell injury, which may be involved in atherogenesis or thrombosis. The association between hyperhomocysteinemia and arterial endothelial dysfunction was investigated in symptom-free adults.

Methods.—The study participants were part of an ongoing community atherosclerosis study performed at the Prince of Wales Hospital in Hong Kong. From November 1995 to August 1996, 81 Chinese volunteers, aged 40 to 70, without any history of cardiovascular disease were recruited into the study group. After a 14-hour fast, each participant visited the hospital for a detailed history, physical examination, and blood sampling for measurement of fasting plasma cholesterol, creatinine, homocysteine, vitamin B_{12}, and folate levels. From this group, 14 nonsmoking hyperhomocysteinemic adults and 14 age- and sex-matched controls were selected for endothelium-dependent flow-mediated dilation (EDD) and endothelium-independent nitroglycerin-induced dilation (GTN) high-resolution ultrasound assays.

Results.—Endothelium-dependent dilation was significantly lower in hyperhomocysteinemic symptom-free volunteers than in those with low homocysteine levels; GTN responses were similar for these 2 groups.

Multivariate analysis confirmed homocysteine level as the strongest independent predictor of decreased EDD in this group of volunteers.

Conclusions.—Impairment of EDD was detected in symptom-free adult volunteers with no known vascular risk factors other than hyperhomocysteinemia. The mechanism of EDD impairment by hyperhomocysteinemia is not known. Inasmuch as endothelial dysfunction is an important early event in atherogenesis, these findings may have important clinical implications. High homocysteine levels may be treated with oral folate, betaine, or pyridoxine therapy, and such treatments may have a role in the treatment of atherogenesis. Prospective studies to examine this possibility are currently under way.

► The relationship, if any, between elevated homocysteine and arterial wall vasoreactivity is substantially unknown, as is the importance of any observed changes. These authors suggest that endothelium-dependent dilatation in upper extremity arteries is diminished in patients with hyperhomocysteinemia. Prior studies in our laboratory had suggested an alteration in α-adrenoceptor function. It appears appropriate at the present time to conclude that hyperhomocysteinemia constitutes an independent risk factor for arterial endothelial dysfunction in otherwise healthy adults. The significance of this dysfunction, however, is unclear at present.

Neurologic

Effect of CP101,606, a Novel NR2B Subunit Antagonist of the *N*-Methyl-*D*-Aspartate Receptor, on the Volume of Ischemic Brain Damage and Cytotoxic Brain Edema After Middle Cerebral Artery Occlusion in the Feline Brain

Di X, Bullock R, Watson J, et al (Virginia Commonwealth Univ, Richmond; Pfizer Central Research, Groton, Conn)

Stroke 28:2244–2251, 1997 1–50

Background.—CP101,606 is a newly discovered and potent *N*-methyl-D-aspartate receptor antagonist. Its neuroprotective effects in neurotrauma and hemorrhagic stroke are well recognized. This study evaluated the effects of CP101,106 in ischemic stroke.

Methods.—Ischemic stroke was induced in cats by transorbital middle cerebral artery occlusion. One group of animals was treated with CP101,106. The ability of CP101,106 to ameliorate the increase in lactate, delay the development of cytotoxic edema, and decrease the volume of infarct after ischemic stroke was investigated.

Results.—In the control group, dialysate lactate was increased by 15.5% at 30 minutes and 332% at 1 hour after middle cerebral artery occlusion, compared with the CP101,606-treated animals. The rate of decline in the apparent diffusion coefficient at 1 and 5 hours was significantly different between the 2 groups. The findings of infarct volume measurement on triphenyltetrazolium chloride–stained sections showed a

number of deaths at follow-up varied significantly among trials. Reasons for this may have included differences in the use of antithrombotic therapy in the first 24 hours after thrombolysis, differences in the severity of stroke, time to thrombolysis, and thrombolytic dose. None of the studies directly compared tissue plasminogen activator (t-PA) with streptokinase or urokinase. Poor outcomes in patients treated with streptokinase may have involved the presence of more severe strokes, the greater use of antithrombotic drugs, the use of higher dosages, and the longer time to treatment than with t-PA.

Conclusions.—The best available evidence suggests that thrombolytic therapy for patients with acute ischemic stroke is of uncertain benefit and associated with considerable risk. There are still questions about the timing of effective thrombolytic therapy in this situation. Additional randomized trials are needed, including studies to establish the safety of t-PA vs. streptokinase.

▶ I have previously expressed reservations about the quality of current data on the role of t-PA in the early treatment of thromboembolic ischemic stroke. These authors have performed a preliminary meta-analysis reviewing all available completed randomized trials of thrombolytic therapy in this setting. Surprisingly, they were able to find 12 trials that included more than 3,000 patients. Thrombolytic therapy was associated with a significant excess of early death and intracranial hemorrhage, but nevertheless there was a significant reduction in the number of patients in the combined outcome of dead or dependent in this group. These authors display the classic use of language that we have come to expect from those from the United Kingdom, concluding that thrombolysis for acute ischemic stroke requires further testing and large randomized trials "because the risk seems substantial, the benefits uncertain, and the time window for effective treatment remains unclear." God bless the British.

Nitric Oxide

Inducible Nitric Oxide Synthase Expression in Human Vein Grafts

Dattilo JB, Dattilo MPM, Spratt JA, et al (Virginia Commonwealth Univ, Richmond)

Am J Surg 174:177–180, 1997 1–55

Introduction.—The high incidence of restenosis severely limits the long-term results of coronary and lower extremity revascularization procedures. Intimal hyperplasia is a major event in the restenosis of vein grafts. In vascular physiology and pathophysiology, nitric oxide is known to play a critical role, but little is known regarding the role of nitric oxide in vein bypass grafts. The enzyme responsible for nitric oxide synthesis is inducible nitric oxide synthase. Whether human saphenous vein and vein bypass grafts express the gene for inducible nitric oxide synthase, and whether this expression is different in aortocoronary and infrainguinal bypass grafts was investigated.

Methods.—Harvesting and processing for RNA isolation was conducted with nonthrombosed sections from 5 aortocoronary vein grafts, 5 infrainguinal vein bypass grafts, and 4 control saphenous veins. With the use of ^{32}P radioactively end labeled primers, quantitative reverse transcription-polymerase chain reaction was performed on these samples. The internal control was glyceraldehyde-3-phosphate-dehydrogenase, and results were expressed as inducible nitric oxide synthase pmol/ glyceraldehyde-3-phosphate-dehydrogenase pmol.

Results.—In the aortocoronary vein grafts, there was a significant increase in the inducible nitric oxide synthase gene (0.049±0.01) when compared with normal saphenous veins (0.011±0.002) and infrainguinal vein bypass grafts (0.019±0.001). Between normal vein and the infrainguinal grafts, there was no significant difference. There was 84% homology with the available gene bank human sequence, which was confirmed by sequencing of a fragment of the amplified 428 bp gene product.

Conclusion.—In human vein bypass grafts, inducible nitric oxide synthase is expressed. In human aortocoronary vein grafts, there is significant elevation of inducible nitric oxide synthase message when compared with normal saphenous veins or infrainguinal vein bypass grafts. The unique vascular beds supplied by these grafts may account for this difference. In these grafts, manipulation of inducible nitric oxide synthase expression may lead to therapies to alleviate intimal hyperplasia.

▶ As the importance of nitric oxide in human vascular biology has become clearer, 2 primary questions have been posed in reference to vein grafts. In the first place, are vein grafts capable of making nitric oxide, and in the second place, what is the significance of any locally manufactured nitric oxide? This study seems to conclusively answer the first question, namely, that vein grafts placed in either the coronary circulation or in the infrainguinal arterial circulation in humans most assuredly are capable of making nitric oxide. Interestingly, the grafts in the coronary system seem to make about 4 times as much as the grafts in the infrainguinal system, the reasons for which are totally unclear. The normal saphenous vein contains inducible nitric oxide synthase, the enzyme responsible for synthesizing nitric oxide. Although the authors gratuitously suggest that manipulation of inducible nitric oxide synthase expression in vein grafts may one day lead to therapies to alleviate graft intimal hyperplasia, I suspect that day is miles and miles away, if that close. (See also Abstract 1–56.)

Dilatation of Saphenous Vein Grafts by Nitric Oxide

Golledge J, Hicks RCJ, Ellis M, et al (Charing Cross & Westminster Med School, London)

Eur J Vasc Endovasc Surg 14:41–47, 1997 1–56

Introduction.—The success of use of saphenous vein as an arterial bypass conduit may partially depend on the ability of the graft to simulate the responses of healthy arteries to variations in blood flow. The response of infrainguinal vein grafts to flow-dependent vasodilation was assessed. The ability of nitric oxide donors to dilate vein grafts to improve the flow through graft stenoses was assessed.

Methods.—Change in the external diameter of mature patent vein grafts was measured by duplex US to assess vasodilation in response to reactive hyperemia and glyceryl trinitrate (GTN). Severity ratio (ratio of proximal systolic velocity, V1, to peak systolic velocity at the stenosis, V2, of vein graft stenoses) was assessed by duplex US before and 24 hours after placement of a GTN patch on the skin at the site overlying the graft stenosis.

Results.—In postocclusion hyperemia, the diameter of 7 patent distal vein grafts increased to a maximum of 112% of resting diameter 2 minutes after release of thigh cuffs and to 117% of resting value after oral GTN. The velocity ratio, V2/V1, through graft stenoses decreased by 20% after application of GTN patches in 6 patients. This happened mainly as a result of decrease in V2. Changes in response to GTN were more obvious for proximal than for distal vein graft stenoses.

Conclusion.—Flow-induced vasodilation responses, which may be attributed to the endothelial release of nitric oxide, are sustained in patent vein grafts. The grafts dilate even more in response to GTN. The placement of GTN patches close to a vein graft stenosis seems to decrease the velocity ratio through vein graft stenosis. Placement of GTN patches might be helpful in decreasing the risk of graft occlusion when there is a delay between the detection and treatment of hemodynamically significant graft stenoses.

► While these authors purport to show that vein grafts in humans respond to nitric oxide stimuli by dilation, I am not totally convinced. The amount of dilatation was only 12% in 1 group of experiments, and 17% in the other. This conclusion was based upon calculation using duplex US, a measuring device in which I have never had total confidence. On balance, however, I think it interesting to observe that human saphenous veins after a mean implant time of 6 to 9 months show evidence of endothelial release of nitric oxide. I wish I knew whether or not this was important.

Local Effects of Nitric Oxide Supplementation and Suppression in the Development of Intimal Hyperplasia in Experimental Vein Grafts

Fulton GJ, Davies MG, Barber L, et al (Duke Univ, Durham, NC; Univ of Bergen, Norway)

Eur J Vasc Endovasc Surg 15:279–289, 1998 1–57

Objective.—Intimal hyperplasia, a common occurrence in arterial vein bypass grafts, is characterized by the loss of endothelium-dependent nitric oxide–mediated relaxation. The effects of a single dose, local application by pluronic gel of a nitric oxide donor, S-nitroso-N-acetylpenicillamine

TABLE 1.—Dimensional Analysis

	Control (n=6)	Gel control (n=6)	SNAP (n=6)	L-NAME (n=6)	p-value
Lumen (mm²)	13.9±2	26.9±2.8*	28.2±3.4*	24.6±2.9	0.005
Intima (mm²)	0.98±0.11	1.38±0.11	0.83±0.08†‡	1.42±0.23	0.02
Media (mm²)	0.97±0.07	1.14±0.09	1.36±0.09	1.49±0.37	0.28
Intimal ratio	0.49±0.03	0.54±0.03	0.41±0.03*†‡	0.53±0.05	0.01
Luminal index	29.6±3.1	44.1±3.1	59.4±7.7**‡	38.9±4.4	0.003

The area of the lumen, the intimal and medial layers from the control, gel encased and S-nitroso-N-acetylpenicillamine (*SNAP*) and nitro-L-arginine methyl ester (*L-NAME*) treated grafts. The intima ratio (intimal area/intimal + medial areas) and luminal index (luminal diameter/cross-sectional wall thickness) are also shown. Values are the mean ± SEM. Statistical differences between groups were tested by Kruskal-Wallis nonparametric analysis of variance (ANOVA) with *post hoc* Dunn's multiple comparison test (*P < 0.5 and **P < 0.01 vs. control, †P < 0.05 vs. gel control, ‡P < 0.05 vs. L-NAME).

(Courtesy of Fulton GJ, Davies MG, Barber L, et al: Local effects of nitric oxide supplementation and suppression in the development of intimal hyperplasia in experimental vein grafts. *Eur J Vasc Endovasc Surg* 15:279–289. Copyright 1998, W.B. Saunders Company Limited, London.)

(SNAP), and a nitric oxide synthase inhibitor, nitro-L-arginine methyl ester (L-NAME), on the formation of intimal hyperplasia were examined.

Methods.—Right common carotid artery bypass grafting was performed on 40 New Zealand white rabbits. Ten animals were controls, 10 had the outer surface of the graft coated with 30% pluronic gel, and the remainder were immersed for 15 minutes in Ringer lactate with 10^{-3} mol/L SNAP or L-NAME and coated with 2.5 mL of gel containing either SNAP (10^{-3} mol/L) (n = 10) or L-NAME (10^{-3} mol/L) (n = 10), which allows for sustained delivery for up to 6 hours. On postoperative day 28, vein grafts were harvested for morphology by electron microscopy, dimensional analysis by videomorphometry, and isometric tension studies.

Results.—Intimal hyperplasia was apparent in all vein grafts under light microscopy. Whereas application of pluronic gel or L-NAME did not affect either intimal or medial thickness, local treatment with SNAP significantly decreased intimal thickness by 36% (72 μm vs. 45 μm) but did not affect medial thickness (Table 1).

Conclusions.—Nitric oxide appears to exert a protective effect against vascular injury. Treatment with a nitric oxide synthase has no effect.

▶ These investigators have long been interested in studying the factors affecting vein graft adaptation in experimental animals. The rather complex experiment described herein indicates that nitric oxide has a protective effect against the development of intimal hyperplasia in New Zealand white rabbits. Perhaps. I certainly hope that one day we can bring one of the hundreds of compounds that seem to be effective in diminishing intimal hyperplasia in animals successfully to humans. (See also Abstract 1–55.)

Flow-induced Arterial Enlargement is Inhibited by Suppression of Nitric Oxide Synthase Activity In Vivo

Guzman RJ, Abe K, Zarins CK (Stanford Univ, Calif)

Surgery 122:273–280, 1997 1–58

Background.—Endothelial nitric oxide (NO) mediates acute changes in arterial diameter in response to flow. However, its action in adaptive enlargement induced by chronic flow is unknown. A study was performed in rats to examine the contribution of NO in arterial adaptation to increased blood flow.

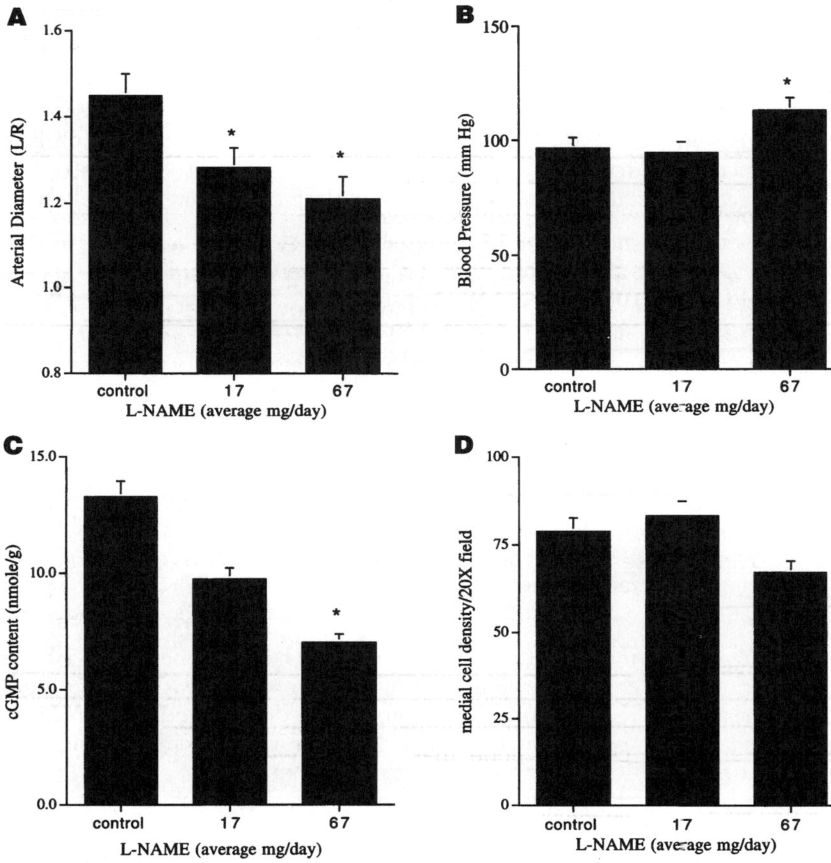

FIGURE 3.—A, L/R iliac diameter in rats receiving L-NAME. Both low and high doses of L-NAME cause significant decrease in flow-induced arterial dilation. (ANOVA, $P < 0.05$). B, Blood pressure in rats receiving L-NAME. Blood pressure is significantly higher only in animals treated with high dose, with no difference seen at lower dose. C, cGMP content in left iliac arteries of rats exposed to L-NAME. D, cell density in iliac segments of rats exposed to L-NAME. (*$P < 0.05$ vs. control). (Courtesy of Guzman RJ, Abe K, Zarins CK: Flow-induced arterial enlargement is inhibited by suppression of nitric oxide synthase activity in vivo. *Surgery* 122:273–280, 1997.)

Methods.—A left femoral arteriovenous fistula was created in adult male rats to increase blood flow in the iliac artery. Measurements of left iliac artery blood flow and diameter were made, and wall shear stress was calculated. The rats received either vehicle or the NO synthase inhibitor N^{ω}-nitro-L-arginine-methyl ester (L-NAME) (0.5 or 2.0 mg/mL) in drinking water. Twenty-one days later, arterial diameter, blood pressure, and medial cell density were determined again. In another group of rats, cyclic guanosine monophosphate (cGMP) content was measured in the left iliac artery.

Results.—Arteriovenous fistula formation caused an immediate 4-fold increase in left iliac artery blood flow and wall shear stress. Within 7 days, the artery had become enlarged. Measurements at 42 days indicated normalization of wall shear stress. In both doses, L-NAME treatment inhibited flow-induced arterial enlargement. Only the high-dose group had blood pressure elevation, however. Rats treated with L-NAME had lower cGMP content in the left iliac artery (Fig 3).

Conclusions.—This study in rats shows that suppression of NO inhibits flow-induced iliac artery enlargement. Thus, NO appears to be involved in flow-induced arterial remodeling; other signaling mediators probably play a role as well.

▶ This report is especially important because it appears to be the first description of direct in vivo measurements of flow-dependent NO using a novel NO-specific electrode. The results are exactly as predicted in other abstracts in this section, namely that an increase in flow increases NO concentration. The real importance of information, to me, is not in the conclusions, but in the methods.

Role of Nitric Oxide and Tumor Necrosis Factor on Lung Injury Caused by Ischemia/Reperfusion of the Lower Extremities

Tassiopoulos AK, Carlin RE, Gao Y, et al (State Univ of New York, Syracuse)
J Vasc Surg 26:647–656, 1997 1–59

Background.—Acute aortic occlusion with ischemia–reperfusion of the lower extremities can cause lung injuries, although the pathophysiologic characteristics of these injuries have not been determined. The role of tumor necrosis factor and nitric oxide in lung injuries caused by ischemia–reperfusion of the lower extremities was investigated.

Methods.—In a rat model, the infrarenal aorta was cross-clamped for 3 hours, and reperfusion was performed for 1 hour. Rats were randomly assigned to 1 of 5 groups: group 1 had the aorta exposed but not clamped; group 2 had the aorta clamped for 3 hours and then had 1 hour of reperfusion; group 3 received 1 mg/kg dexamethasone before the aorta was clamped; group 4 received 25 mg aminoguanidine before the aorta was clamped (aminoguanidine is a specific inducible nitric oxide synthase inhibitor); and group 5 received 2 mg/kg tumor necrosis $factor_{bp}$ before the aorta was clamped (tumor necrosis $factor_{bp}$ is a PEG-ylated dimeric form of the high-affinity p55 tumor necrosis factor receptor I). Nitric oxide concentrations in exhaled gas were measured at 30-minute intervals during ischemia–reperfusion as an index of nitric oxide production by the lung. Serial arterial blood samples were collected for tumor necrosis factor assays. The lungs were removed at the end of the experiment and examined for histologic evidence of injury.

Results.—In group 2, nitric oxide concentrations in exhaled gas increased from 0.7 parts per billion (ppb) at baseline to 54.3 ppb at the end of ischemia and remained stable during reperfusion. Production of nitric oxide concentrations in exhaled gas was blocked by aminoguanidine, dexamethasone, and tumor necrosis $factor_{bp}$ administered before aortic occlusion. In groups 2, 3, and 4, serum tumor necrosis factor rapidly increased during early ischemia, reached its peak 60 minutes after occlusion of the aorta, slowly decreased to baseline values at the end of ischemia, and remained low during reperfusion. When tumor necrosis $factor_{bp}$ was administered before aortic occlusion, it decreased serum tumor necrosis factor concentrations significantly. Histologic examination of the lungs showed that aminoguanidine, dexamethasone, and tumor necrosis $factor_{bp}$ had a protective effect.

Discussion.—Serum tumor necrosis factor rapidly increases during ischemia of the lower extremities and increases the production of nitric oxide by the lungs by upregulating aminoguanidine. Increased nitric oxide production was associated with a more severe lung injury. The blocking of aminoguanidine had a protective effect on the lungs. The blocking of tumor necrosis factor before the occurrence of ischemia decreases the production of nitric oxide by the lungs and lessens lung injury. These findings show that the nitric oxide concentration in exhaled gas is an early indicator of lung injury caused by ischemia–reperfusion of the lower extremities.

► It has been recognized for years that revascularization of severely ischemic lower extremities predisposes to lung injury. Although pathophysiologic mechanisms have not been well-described, noxious cytokines have been suspected. These investigators, using an animal model, incriminate tumor necrosis factor as the noxious agent involved in this type of lung injury. Interestingly, tumor necrosis factor appears to increase the production of nitric oxide from the lung by upregulating an inducible NO synthase. I certainly did not know previously that increased NO production by the lungs caused lung damage, but that is the conclusion reached by these authors.

Acute Lung Injury After Aortic Surgery: The Relation Between Lung and Leg Microvascular Permeability to ^{111}Indium-labelled Transferrin and Circulating Mediators

Raijmakers PGHM, Groeneveld ABJ, Rauwerda JA, et al (Free Univ, Amsterdam Red Cross Blood Transfusion Service, Amsterdam)

Thorax 52:866–871, 1997 1–60

Background.—Aortic surgery is a risk factor for acute lung injury, which may be related to ischemia–reperfusion of the lower extremities and release of inflammatory mediators. Changes in microvascular protein permeability and circulating inflammatory mediators after aortic surgery were defined.

Methods.—There were 11 consecutive patients who had elective aortic surgery. Microvascular permeability in the lung and leg was determined before and a median of 2.8 hours after surgery using ^{111}indium-labeled transferrin and ^{99m}technetium-labeled red blood cells. This resulted in a protein leak index specific for protein permeability. Circulating leukocyte counts and inflammatory mediator levels were also calculated.

Results.—In the lung, the protein leak index increased from a median of 0.6×10^{-3}/min before surgery to 5.4×10^{-3}/min after surgery. In the leg, the protein leak index increased from a median of 0.3×10^{-3}/min before surgery to 5.0×10^{-3}/min after surgery (Fig 1). The increases in the protein leak index in the lung and leg were related. No change was seen in levels

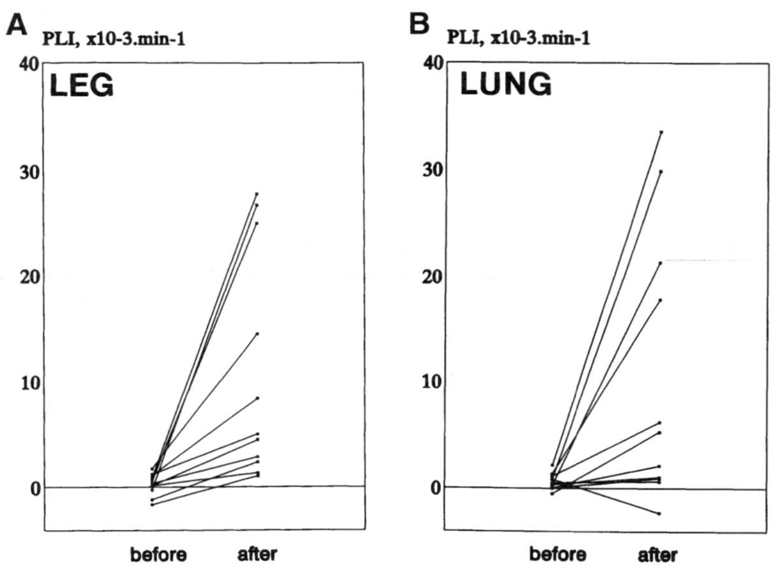

FIGURE 1.—Protein leak index (PLI) in the leg (**A**) and lung (**B**) before and after aortic surgery. Postoperative vs. preoperative values: in the leg, $P < 0.005$; and in the lung, $P < 0.02$. (Courtesy of Raijmakers PGHM, Groeneveld ABJ, Rauwerda JA, et al: Acute lung injury after aortic surgery: The relation between lung and leg microvascular permeability to ^{111}indium-labeled transferrin and circulating mediators. *Thorax* 52:866–871, 1997 BMJ Publishing Group.)

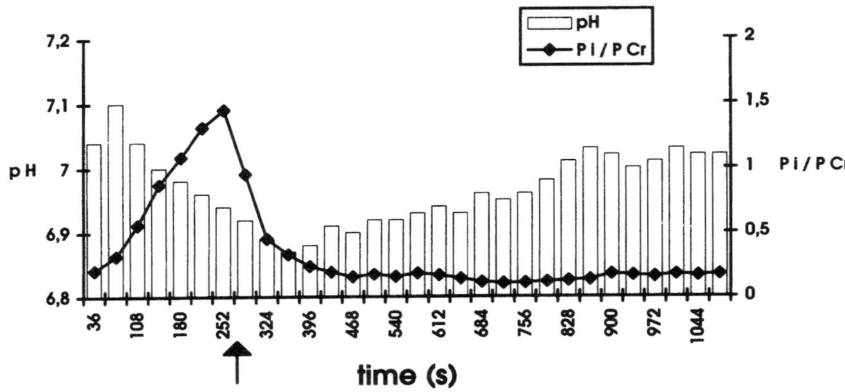

FIGURE 3.—Course of inorganic phosphate/phosphocreatine and pH during and after isotonic exercise of the right quadriceps muscle in a patient with arterial occlusive disease (stage IIb; the *arrow* indicates the end of the exercise). (Courtesy of Schunk K, Romaneehsen B, Mildenberger P, et al: Dynamic phosphorus-31 magnetic resonance spectroscopy in arterial occlusive disease: Correlation with clinical and angiographic findings and comparison with healthy volunteers. *Invest Radiol* 32:651–659, 1997.)

tients had a higher phosphomonoester (PME)/β-ATP ratio than nondiabetic patients (0.86 vs. 0.63), and AOD patients had a significantly higher ratio than controls (0.66 vs. 0.48). Although controls exercised significantly longer than patients, dynamic ^{31}PMRS exercise results were similar for both groups. Relative to P_i/PCr values, AOD patients had significantly higher acidosis than controls, resulting in a steeper linear regression line (m = −0.33 vs. −0.14). Recovery of P_i/PCr was significantly faster in controls than in AOD patients (80 vs. 25 seconds for isometric exercises and 70 vs. 37 seconds for isotonic exercises). Recovery of pH was only slightly faster in controls than in patients. Recovery rate of P_i/PCr was correlated with stage of AOD (r = 0.17), severity of vascular disease (r = 0.20), and extent of atherosclerosis (r = 0.30).

Conclusions.—Recovery rate of P_i/PCr, as assessed by dynamic ^{31}PMRS, is an excellent measure of muscle metabolism, which is significantly lengthened in AOD patients. There were no significant differences between patients and controls in other exercise-induced changes except for an elevated PME/β-ATP in AOD patients.

▶ Magnetic resonance spectroscopy focused on phosphorus-31 is a well-established technique to investigate muscle metabolism. Because of the unique spectroscopic characteristics of the different phosphate-containing muscle metabolites (e.g., phosphocreatine, inorganic phosphate, ATP), their relative distribution and even intramuscular pH can be determined.

This technique has been well established and applied to experimental studies of muscle metabolism for more than 10 years. In fact, in 1986, Hands et al.[1] noted a significantly greater depletion of phosphocreatine and a fall in pH during exercise in the calf muscle of patients with severe claudication compared with normal volunteers. They also demonstrated a much slower recovery of pH after exercise in these patients. Also in 1986, Zatina et al.[2]

studied 214 limbs in patients with peripheral vascular disease and demonstrated impairment of oxidative metabolism at rest in patients with severe ischemia (ankle/brachial index < 0.4) and with exercise in patients with less severe ischemia. These authors also demonstrated the worsening consequences of multilevel occlusive disease and demonstrated that return of normal muscle metabolism after revascularization is quite prolonged.

In comparison with these early pioneering studies, the current study by Schunk et al. adds little if any new information. Unfortunately, the current authors attempted to correlate muscle metabolism with arteriographic findings in their patients, rather than quantitating the ischemia with pressure measurements. Not surprisingly, they found relatively low correlations between metabolic patterns and Fontaine level of disease or arteriographic patterns. They conclude that muscle metabolism is influenced by "microangiopathia," by which they mean diabetes, despite the fact that they could not control for this variable in their study.

One interesting finding in this study was that the maximum duration of quadriceps exercise in normal subjects was 6 times longer than in patients with occlusive disease, but that both groups had similar muscle metabolic changes upon completing exercise. This suggests that maximal exercise tolerance is strongly influenced by the same end points of muscle metabolism, whether in ischemic or normal extremities. With the exception of this finding, interested readers are referred to the earlier articles cited above, which provided a comprehensive and insightful analysis of this subject more than 10 years ago.

J.L. Cronenwett, M.D.

References

1. Hands L, Bore P, Galloway G, et al: Muscle metabolism in patients with peripheral vascular disease investigated by ^{31}P nuclear magnetic resonance spectroscopy. *Clin Sci* 71:283–290, 1986.
2. Zatina M, Berkowitz H, Gross G, et al: ^{31}P NMR spectroscopy: Noninvasive biochemical analysis of the ischemic extremity. *J Vasc Surg* 3:411–420, 1986.

Biochemical Composition of Human Peripheral Arteries Examined With Near-Infrared Raman Spectroscopy

Salenius JP, Brennan JF III, Miller A, et al (MetroWest Med Ctr, Framington, Mass; Massachusetts Inst of Technology, Cambridge; Harvard Med School, Boston)

J Vasc Surg 27:710–719, 1998 1–65

Objective.—Whereas plaques rich in extracellular lipids covered by a thin fibrous cap are known to be vulnerable to rupture, there are no methods for identifying and examining such lesions. The lipid and calcium salt contents of human peripheral arteries were evaluated by Raman spectroscopy.

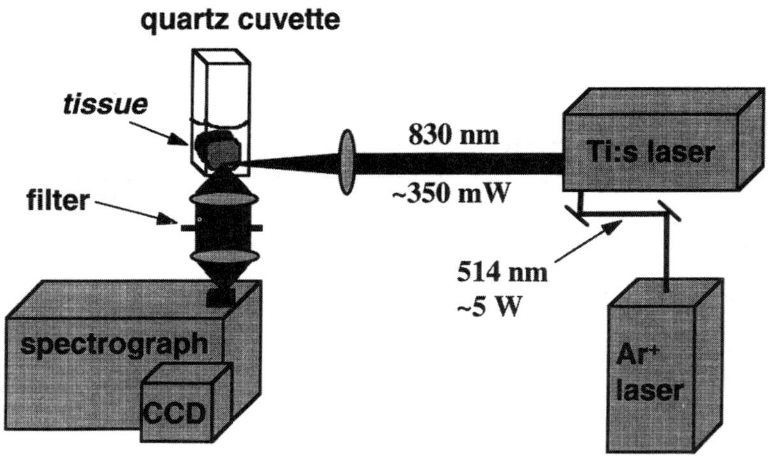

FIGURE 1.—Block diagram of Raman spectroscopy system. *Abbreviation: CCD*, change-coupled device. (Courtesy of Salenius JP, Brennan JF III, Miller A, et al: Biochemical composition of human peripheral arteries examined with near-infrared Raman spectroscopy. *J Vasc Surg* 27:710–719, 1998.)

Methods.—Raman spectra were taken of 167 specimens of carotid and femoral artery wall in various pathologic states (Fig 1). Cholesterol and calcium content determined from Raman spectra were compared with values obtained histologically.

Results.—Spectroscopic and histologic findings were significantly correlated (Fig 2). The spectra revealed the presence of disease as well as the degree of transformation of the arterial wall involved with atherosclerotic disease.

Conclusions.—Raman spectroscopy provides accurate, reliable information about the location, extent, and composition of peripheral and coronary artery plaques.

▶ This is a technique that generates frequency-shifted light. Incident light causes the molecule to change from one vibrational energy to another, and the re-emitted light is shifted in frequency by the molecular vibrational frequency. The studies reported herein examined ex vivo specimens, and generally the spectroscopic spikes appeared to correlate with the quantitative analysis of the lipid within the specimen. With in vivo use, Raman spectroscopy appears to have the ability to detect material only to a depth of about 1.5 mm and laterally about 1 mm displaced from the 100-μm irradiated spot. I have no idea whether this will ever prove clinically useful.

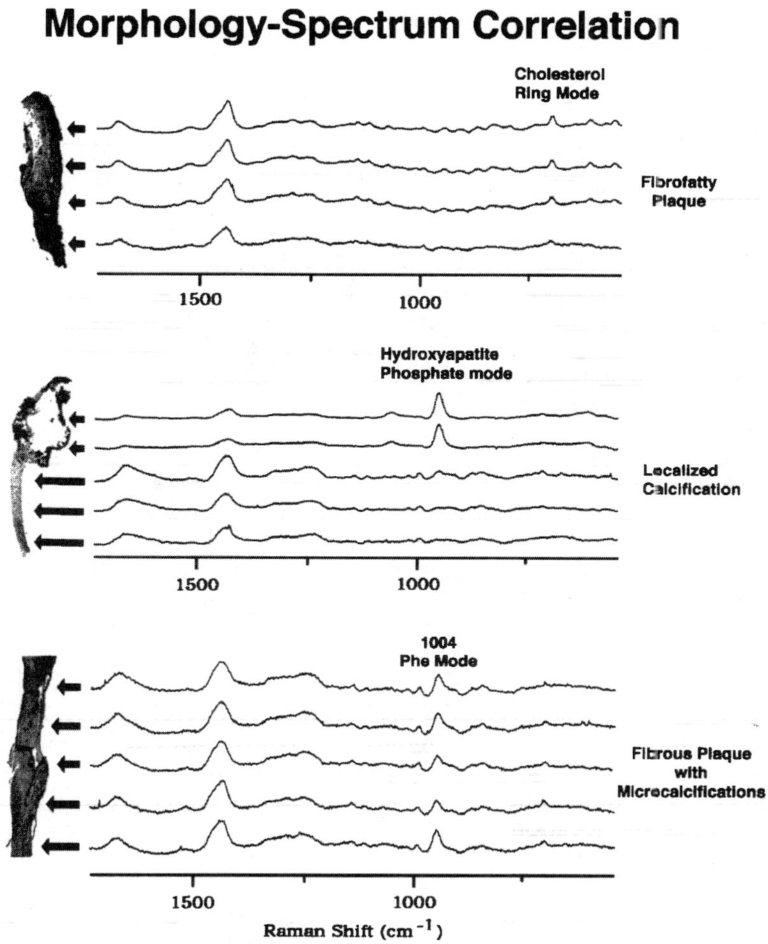

FIGURE 2.—Low-power photomicrograph (original magnification, ×20) of cross sections from 3 typical arterial lesions and their corresponding spectra. **Top,** fibrofatty plaque with lipid core in the upper part of the lesion. Corresponding cholesterol ring-related spectra diminish from **top** to **bottom. Center,** plaque with heavy calcification in the upper portion of the lesion and corresponding strong phosphate peak. **Bottom,** fibrous plaque with scattered microcalcifications. (Courtesy of Salenius JP, Brennan JF III, Miller A, et al: Biochemical composition of human peripheral arteries examined with near-infrared Raman spectroscopy. *J Vasc Surg* 27:710–719, 1998.)

Vascular Biology

Platelet-derived Growth Factor and Extracellular Matrix Proteins Provide a Synergistic Stimulus for Human Vascular Smooth Muscle Cell Migration

Nelson PR, Yamamura S, Kent KC (Harvard Med School, Boston)
J Vasc Surg 26:104–112, 1997 1–66

Background.—After arterial injury, smooth muscle cells (SMCs) are stimulated by factors within the arterial wall to migrate. The influence of various growth factors and extracellular matrix (ECM) proteins on SMCs has been studied, but the effect of combinations of these factors, more similar to in vivo conditions, has not been evaluated. In this study, the effect on SMC migration of growth factors combined with ECM proteins was evaluated in vitro.

Methods.—Human SMCs were harvested from saphenous veins and cultured. Modified Boyden-chamber migration assays were used to assess the effect on SBC migration of platelet-derived growth factor (PDGF)-AB, basic fibroblast growth factor (bFGF), or epidermal growth factor (EGF) in combination with 1 of the ECM proteins: fibronectin, laminin, collagen type I, or collagen type IV. Intracellular calcium changes were measured by spectrofluorometer. The expected additive effect of combinations of growth factors and ECM proteins was calculated and compared with the actual effect on SMC migration to look for synergy.

Results.—There was a simple additive effect of ECM proteins and either bFGF or EGF. In the case of PDGF and ECM proteins, there was a synergistic effect on SMC chemotaxis. This synergy could be detected for all collagen concentrations but was detected only at higher concentrations of fibronectin and laminin. Although exposure of SMC to ECM proteins did not increase their intracellular calcium levels, the presence of ECM proteins augmented the early intracellular calcium peak induced by PDGF.

Conclusions.—After vascular reconstruction injury, smooth muscle cells are exposed to many growth factors, extracellular matrix proteins, cytokines, and mediators. To better understand the influence of these factors on SMCs, SMCs were exposed in vitro to combinations of growth factors and ECM proteins. Both PDGF and ECM proteins stimulated SMC migration, but exposure to both resulted in a synergistic stimulation of SMC migration. The mechanism of this synergistic effect is not known. Alterations in intracellular calcium may be involved, inasmuch as ECM proteins increase the early intracellular calcium increase provoked by exposure to PDGF, which is necessary for its stimulation of SMC migration. An understanding of this synergy and its underlying mechanism may permit the design of more effective inhibitors of intimal hyperplasia to prevent restenosis after vascular reconstruction.

▶ Our understanding of the sophistication of vascular wall biology appropriately increases with time. These investigators accurately note that arterial smooth muscle cells exist in a complex environment, with simultaneous exposure to many different growth factors and extracellular matrix proteins. Clearly, the way smooth muscle cells migrate in vitro in response to any one of these agents may be quite different from its in vivo behavior in response to a simultaneous mixture of agents. In fact, in this study the authors present evidence that platelet-derived growth factor acts synergistically with extracellular matrix proteins to promote smooth muscle cell migration. As we move from the infancy of vascular wall biologic research to a slightly more developed phase, we are going to require more complex studies such as this.

Smooth Muscle Cell Migration and Proliferation Are Mediated by Distinct Phases of Activation of the Intracellular Messenger Mitogen-activated Protein Kinase

Nelson PR, Yamamura S, Mureebe L, et al (Beth Israel/Deaconess Med Ctr, Boston; Harvard Med School, Boston)
J Vasc Surg 27:117–125, 1998 1–67

Objective.—Vascular smooth muscle cell (SMC) proliferation and migration are necessary for intimal plaque formation. Both proliferation and migration are stimulated by platelet-derived growth factor (PDGF). Whether mitogen-activated protein kinase (MAPK) activation is necessary for this process is not well understood. The role of MAPK in PDGF-induced migration and proliferation of human vascular SMCs was investigated.

Methods.—Human saphenous vein SMCs were harvested and grown in serum-free medium for 72 hours. Migration was assayed by microchemotaxis for 4 hours. Proliferation was assayed using ^{3}H-thymidine uptake. Cell counts were determined after stimulation with PDGF, in the presence and absence of the inhibitor PD098059, and temporal phases of MAPK activation were determined.

Results.—PD098059 significantly inhibited MAPK activation by PDGF-BB in SMCs. PDGF-BB increased SMC chemotaxis by 3.5–4.5 times. The concentrations of PD098059 necessary to inhibit chemotaxis and MAPK were similar, indicating that MAPK activation is necessary for SMC chemotaxis (IC_{50} for both processes was 10 μmol/L, with complete inhibition at 50 μmol/L). Growth factor stimulation of SMCs results in early and prolonged MAPK activation for up to 24 hours. Smooth muscle cells treated simultaneously with PD098059 and PDGF did not undergo chemotaxis. Addition of PD098059 5 minutes after PDGF stimulation partially inhibited chemotaxis, and addition of the inhibitor 15 minutes or later after PDGF stimulation resulted in no inhibition of chemotaxis. Mitogen-activated protein kinase activity in the first 15 minutes is associated with SMC migration, whereas MAPK activity between 1 and 4 hours is identified with SMC proliferation.

Conclusions.—Mitogen-activated protein kinase activity is involved in both the migration and proliferation of SMCs. Because distinct phases of enzyme activation are necessary to stimulate these 2 separate cellular events, it may be possible to prevent intimal hyperplasia by inhibiting this enzyme.

▶ Here we have another candidate compound for inhibition of intimal hyperplasia, namely MAPK. I hereby conclude that there is no limit to the number of compounds that can be shown in the laboratory to be promising agents for use in the suppression of human intimal hyperplasia. Now if only one of these could be proved successful in humans.

Activation of pp60$^{c\text{-}src}$ Is Necessary for Human Vascular Smooth Muscle Cell Migration

Mureebe L, Nelson PR, Yamamura S, et al (Harvard Med School, Boston)

Surgery 122:138–145, 1997 1–68

Purpose.—Migration of vascular smooth muscle cells (SMCs) into the intima is a necessary step in the development of intimal plaque. Though agonists of SMC migration are recognized, the intracellular pathways they activate remain unclear. The protein pp60$^{c\text{-}src}$ (src) is the most widely distributed nonreceptor tyrosine kinase, but its role as an intracellular signaling protein in cell migration is unknown. This study evaluated the role of src in migration of human vascular SMCs.

Methods.—The study used a microchemotaxis chamber assay with videomicroscopy to assess SMC migration. Phosphorylation of p34^{cdc2}, a specific substrate for src, was used as a measure of src kinase activity. Cytoplasmic microinjection was performed to introduce blocking antibodies to src.

Results.—When SMCs were stimulated with platelet-derived growth factor (PDGF)-BB and PDGF-AB, src activation increased significantly. However, PDGF-AA stimulation had no consistent effect on src activity. Smooth muscle cell chemotaxis increased by more than 7-fold in response to PDGF-BB and 5-fold in response to PDGF-AB. However, injection of a blocking antibody significantly inhibited SMC migration in response to PDGF-BB and serum.

Conclusions.—Agonist-induced activation of the protein tyrosine kinase src is associated with SMC chemotaxis, these findings demonstrate. Migration of SMCs is greatly inhibited by an antibody that blocks src activation. The results suggest that src activation plays an essential role in SMC migration. Molecular or pharmacologic src blockers could become an important part of strategies to control intimal hyperplasia.

▶ Dr. Kent and his associates continue to focus on the development of intimal hyperplasia as a cause of the failure of peripheral vascular reconstructions. They have developed a clever microchemotaxis chamber assay which purports to study directly the migration of vascular smooth muscle cells, believed essential for the development of intimal hyperplasia. They present herein rather convincing evidence that a non-receptor tyrosine kinase, pp60$^{c\text{-}src}$, is essential for SMC migration. They go on to hypothesize that inhibitors of this specific tyrosine kinase may be useful in the control of intimal hyperplasia. Perhaps. Here we have another candidate compound for prevention of intimal hyperplasia. The list is massive and growing.

Proliferation and Extracellular Matrix Production by Human Infragenicular Smooth Muscle Cells in Response to Interleukin-1β

Forsyth EA, Aly HM, Neville RF, et al (George Washington Univ, Washington DC; Georgetown Univ, Washington DC)

J Vasc Surg 26:1002–1008, 1997 1–69

Objective.—Interleukin (IL)-1β is thought to play a role in induction of cellular proliferation. Because the proliferation of vascular smooth muscle cells (VSMCs) is one of the first steps in the formation of atherosclerotic plaques, the effects of IL-1β on the proliferation of human infragenicular VSMCs and on the production of extracellular matrix proteins, fibronectin, collagen type IV, and laminin in culture were investigated.

Methods.—Vascular smooth muscle cells obtained from atherosclerotic infragenicular arteries of 5 individuals with diabetes during below-the-knee amputations were incubated for 48 hours with concentrations of IL-1β ranging from 0.5 to 10 ng/mL and then counted. Cells from subconfluent cultures were seeded into 6-well plates at 10,000 cells per well, incubated for 48 hours, serum-starved for 24 hours, and then incubated with 1 ng/mL of IL-1β daily for 96 hours. Samples were counted and results compared with those of matched control samples incubated in serum-free media. Extracellular matrix protein production was studied with and without IL-1β, stained with fluorescein-labeled antibody specific for an extracellular protein, and analyzed using immunofluorescent microscopy.

Results.—Compared with control samples, IL-1β significantly increased VSMC cellular proliferation in a dose-dependent fashion at all time points. Interleukin-1β significantly increased cell numbers within 96 hours by a factor of 2 compared with control samples, increased production of fibronectin and of extracellular matrix proteins, and decreased production of laminin. Interleukin-1β did not affect production of collagen type IV.

Conclusions.—Interleukin-1β stimulates VSMC production by increasing fibronectin deposition while not affecting collagen type IV production. Interleukin-1β enhances the phenotypic transformation of VSMCs from the contractile to the synthetic state that hastens the formation of atherosclerotic plaques.

► The obvious problem with this study is the absence of an active control, namely VSMCs derived from other sites in the body. The authors have

timal and medial wall thickness were performed, and mean intimal/medial thickness ratios were calculated. Four days and 2 weeks after balloon injury, 5-Bromo-2'-deoxyuridine labeling was performed to assess medial cell proliferation in arteries treated with adenoviral gene transfer of antisense bFGF (Ad.ASbFGF) and Ad.lacZ.

Results.—After 14 days, the Ad.ASbFGF-treated arteries showed significant inhibition of intimal thickening, compared with Ad.lacZ- and PBS-treated controls. The intimal-medial thickness ratio was 0.22 with Ad.ASbFGF vs. 1.03 with Ad.lacZ and 0.86 with phosphate-buffered saline solution (Fig 3). Four days after injury, the proliferation indices of vessels in the Ad.ASbFGF and Ad.lacZ groups were not significantly different. However, the Ad.ASbFGF-treated vessels showed a significant increase in apoptosis.

Conclusion.—In rabbits with femoral artery balloon injury, inhibition of new bFGF synthesis via ASbFGF RNA gene transfer causes significant inhibition of the neointimal response. Thus, continued bFGF synthesis after injury plays an important role in the arterial response to injury. The results suggest that gene transfer therapy with ASbFGF could help to reduce the intimal hyperplastic response to vascular reconstructive surgery.

► In the rabbit model, the intramural Ad.AsbFGF resulted in a significant decrease in subsequent intimal hyperplasia at sites of arterial injury. Thus, bFGF must be put on our list of things to consider as we ponder methods to clinically modulate intimal hyperplasia after vascular grafting. I wonder how a combination of vascular endothelial growth factor and bFGF would do?

Fatty Acids Augment Endothelium-dependent Dilation in Hand Veins by a Cyclooxygenase-dependent Mechanism

Stepniakowski KT, Lu G, Davda RK, et al (Med Univ of South Carolina, Charleston)

Hypertension 30:1634–1639, 1997 1–74

Background.—Obesity is associated with insulin resistance, increased vascular α-adrenergic reactivity, and hypertension. Obese patients have elevated plasma levels of nonesterified fatty acids (NEFAs). These observations suggest a link between insulin resistance, defects in NEFA metabolism, and increased neurovascular tone in these obese hypertensive patients. It has been proposed that elevated plasma NEFA levels inhibit endothelial NO and prostacyclin synthesis, which contributes to increased neurovascular reactivity and blood pressure. To determine whether NEFA elevation has this effect, the effect of local increases in plasma levels of NEFA on the dorsal hand venodilator response to endothelium-dependent and -independent dilators was evaluated.

Methods.—The study group consisted of 8 healthy normotensive volunteers, age 23 to 45 years. This group consisted of 6 women and 2 men of whom 5 were white and 3 were black. After an overnight fast, dorsal hand vein distensibility was measured with the linear variable differential transducer technique. After reproducibility was established, responses to dilators were assessed under control (saline) conditions in 1 hand and with elevated NEFAs (10% intralipid) in the contralateral hand, after the vein diameter was first reduced 60% with phenylephrine. These studies were repeated with indomethacin to block the production of cyclooxygenase products.

Results.—Local elevation of plasma NEFAs in vivo increased venodilator responses to the endothelium-dependent dilators, acetylcholine, and methacholine. The response to the endothelium-independent dilator nitroglycerin was not affected by the elevated NEFA levels. Indomethacin attenuated the NEFA-induced increase in endothelium-dependent venodilator response.

Conclusions.—Local increases in plasma levels of NEFAs increased the response to endothelium-dependent venodilators by a cyclooxygenase-dependent mechanism. This study does not support the idea that increased plasma levels of NEFAs in obese hypertensive patients increase α-adrenoceptor–mediated constriction by inhibiting NO synthesis.

► NEFAs have been hypothesized to have a major role in altering α-adrenergic reactivity in blood vessels. The in vitro human experiments described here indicate that raising NEFAs locally augments endothelium-dependent vasodilation by a cyclooxygenase-dependent mechanism. There is no evidence that NEFAs augment α1–adrenoceptor-mediated reactivity by reducing nitric oxide synthesis. It does appear that NEFAs may have an important modulating function on α-adrenoceptor activity.

Photodynamic Therapy Inactivates Extracellular Matrix–Basic Fibroblast Growth Factor: Insights to Its Effect on the Vascular Wall

LaMuraglia GM, Adili F, Karp SJ, et al (Harvard Med School, Boston; Boston Univ)

J Vasc Surg 26:294–301, 1997 1–75

Background.—Experimental studies suggest that photodynamic therapy (PDT) may inhibit the development of intimal hyperplasia. The host response to PDT promotes favorable vascular wall healing without inflammation and proliferation. The findings suggest that PDT may cause changes in the extracellular matrix. The effects of PDT on basic fibroblast growth factor (bFGF), a potent, matrix-resident mitogen, were studied.

Methods.—Photodynamic therapy was performed to inactivate bFGF in vitro and in vivo using the photosensitizing agent chloroaluminum sulfonated phthalocyanine. The effects on bFGF in solution and on endothelial cell-derived ECM were assessed. After treatment with PDT or extraction from the ECM, bFGF was quantitated with an enzyme-linked immunosorbent assay. Smooth muscle cell mitogenesis by ^{3}H-thymidine incorporation was used to assess functional activity of matrix-associated bFGF. In addition, immunohistochemical studies were performed in rat carotid arteries treated with PDT.

Results.—In solution, bFGF was undetectable after PDT. In ECM, PDT significantly reduced matrix-bound bFGF from 27.5 to 1.0 pg/mL, while reducing vascular smooth muscle cell mitogenesis by 52%. When PDT-treated matrix was replenished with exogenous bFGF, proliferation returned to baseline levels. In PDT-treated carotid arteries, bFGF staining was reduced compared with untreated arteries.

Conclusions.—These experiments demonstrate the inactivation of matrix-resident bFGF, and possibly other bioactive molecules, by PDT. The findings may provide a mechanism of PDT's ability to suppress smooth muscle cell proliferation in the blood vessel wall. Matrix alteration, mediated by free radicals, could play a role in the favorable vascular healing observed when PDT is used to inhibit injury-induced intimal hyperplasia.

► PDT, the light activation of photosynthesizer dyes for the production of oxygen and other free-radical moieties without the generation of heat, continues to hover around the edges of medical practice. Among its many attributes has been suggested the possibility (surprise, surprise) that it may inhibit the development of intimal hyperplasia. These authors suggest that photodynamic therapy may function in part by inactivating a matrix resident fibroblast growth factor. Of course, the use of photodynamic therapy does require the use of a photosynthesizer dye, in this case chloroaluminum sulfonated phthalocyanine. While I am impressed with the persuasiveness of the authors' work, I do note that PDT has been around for years and to date has failed to make any material impression on the clinical problem of intimal hyperplasia. I am doubtful that it ever will.

Apolipoprotein(a) Induces Monocyte Chemotactic Activity in Human Vascular Endothelial Cells

Poon M, Zhang X, Dunsky KG, et al (Mount Sinai School of Medicine, New York)

Circulation 96:2514–2519, 1997 1–76

Background.—Previous studies have shown an association between elevated levels of lipoprotein(a) [Lp(a)] and premature atherosclerosis, but not the mechanism of this relationship. In the atherogenic process, monocyte recruitment to the blood vessel wall is an early event. The effects of Lp(a) on induction of monocyte chemotactic activity (MCA) were studied in human umbilical vein endothelial cells (HUVECs) and in coronary artery endothelial cells.

Methods and Results.—In HUVECs, unoxidized Lp(a) induced MCA, whereas low-density lipoprotein (LDL) did not have the same effect under the same condition. Lipoprotein (a) had no direct MCA, in the absence of HUVECs. Induction of MCA did not result from endotoxin. The HUVEC response to Lp(a) was inhibited by actinomycin D and cycloheximide, suggesting the need for protein and RNA synthesis. The response appeared to depend on the apolipoprotein(a) [apo(a)] portion of Lp(a). Monocyte chemotactic activity in human coronary artery endothelial cells was also induced by Lp(a) and apo(a). The Lp(a)-conditioned medium showed no detectable granulocyte-monocyte colony-stimulating factor. Neither was monocyte chemoattractant protein-1 mRNA found in Lp(a)-induced HUVECs.

Conclusions.—Monocyte recruitment to the blood vessel wall appears to involve Lp(a). This may help to explain the involvement of Lp(a) in the atherogenic process. High levels of Lp(a) may recruit circulating monocytes to the vascular endothelium, thus promoting atherosclerosis.

▶ The evil activities ascribed to LP(a) elevation are legendary. An elevated blood concentration of this substance has been associated with an increased risk of myocardial infarction, stroke, restenosis of saphenous coronary grafts, and restenosis after balloon angioplasty. To date, however, the actual mechanism of harm has never been fully elucidated. This fascinating study indicates that LP(a) induced endothelial cells to secrete monocyte chemotactic activity, leading these authors to conclude that LP(a) appears to be involved in the recruitment of monocytes to the vessel wall, and that this may be its primary mechanism of interaction in the atherosclerotic process. I note that a number of lipid experts, including those at our institution, do not believe that elevated LP(a) is significant in the absence of hyperlipidemia.

Integrin Signaling Transduces Shear Stress–Dependent Vasodilation of Coronary Arterioles

Muller JM, Chilian WM, Davis MJ (Univ of Missouri, Columbia; Med College of Wisconsin, Milwaukee; Texas A&M Univ, College Station)

Circ Res 80:320–326, 1997 1–77

Background.—Shear stress in blood vessels is directly related to endothelium-dependent nitric oxide (NO)-mediated vasodilation. It is unknown how shear stress is transduced to the biochemical signals leading to NO production. The possible involvement of interaction between integrins and extracellular matrix proteins in this process was investigated.

Methods.—The investigators hypothesized that binding of integrin to Arg-Gly-Asp (RGD) peptide sequences in extracellular matrix proteins plays a key role in the sequence by which shear stress activates endothelial tyrosine kinase and causes isolated arterioles to dilate. Coronary arterioles were isolated and exposed to increasing shear strength. This was done in the presence of GRGDNP, a synthetic peptide that competitively inhibits integrin binding to extracellular matrix proteins containing RGD peptide sequences.

Results.—In intraluminal concentrations of 0.1, 0.5, and 1.0 mmol/L, GRGDNP inhibited shear stress–induced vasodilation in concentration-dependent fashion (Fig 1). Endothelium-dependent relaxation to substance

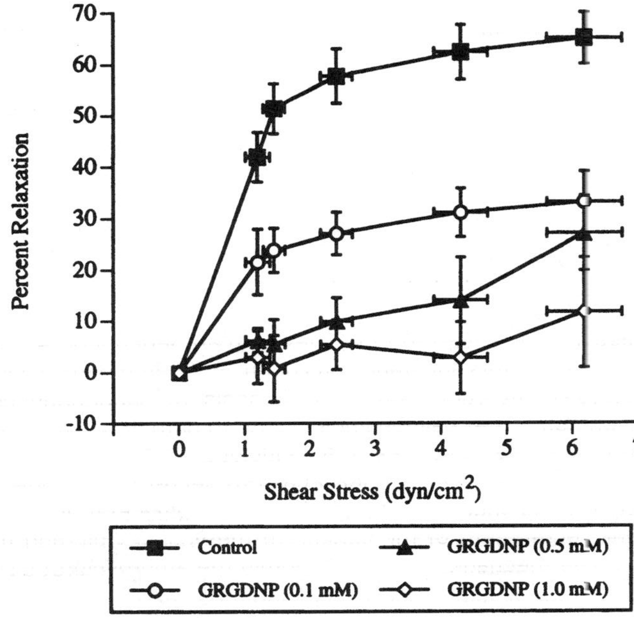

FIGURE 1.—Shear stress-induced vasodilation of coronary arterioles under control conditions and in the presence of 0.1 mmol/L (n = 5), 0.5 mmol/L (n = 8), and 1.0 mmol/L (n = 6) GRGDNP. Diameter changes were expressed as a percentage of the maximal dilation determined in the presence of 100 μmol/L sodium nitroprusside. At 0.5 and 1.0 mmol/L, GRGDNP significantly reduced the shear stress-induced vasodilation ($P < 0.05$). (Courtesy of Muller JM, Chilian WM, Davis MJ: Integrin signaling transduces shear stress–dependent vasodilation of coronary arterioles. *Circ Res* 80:320–326. Copyright 1997, American Heart Association. Reproduced with permission.)

P was unaffected by GRGDNP. Induction of vasodilation by shear stress was unaffected by the inactive structural analogue GRGESP. When a blocking antibody was administered to the integrin β_3 chain, the vasodilatory response was significantly inhibited. Antiphosphotyrosine binding studies showed a significant increase in tyrosine kinase activity in association with shear stress. Under shear stress, GRGDNP reduced antiphosphotyrosine kinase activation during integrin signaling.

Conclusions.—Interactions between integrin and the extracellular matrix appear to play a key role in shear stress–induced vasodilation. These interactions may take place at focal adhesions. The findings suggest a possible association between integrin binding and tyrosine kinase activation and the intracellular signaling cascade, leading to endothelium-dependent NO release and thus to vasodilation.

► It is virtually an item of faith today that increased shear stress induces endothelium-dependent NO-mediated vasodilation of blood vessels. However, to date the mechanism of shear stress transduction remains largely unknown. This sophisticated study concludes that the primary transduction mechanism for shear stress in vasodilation is binding of integrins to RGD peptide sequences in the extracellular matrix. The authors suggest that the β-$_3$ integrins are specifically involved. Perhaps β-$_3$ integrin binding to RGD extracellular matrix proteins is in fact an intermediate step in the transduction of shear stress to vascular dilation.

Serum-Elastin-Peptides as a Predictor of Expansion of Small Abdominal Aortic Aneurysms

Lindholt JS, Heickendorff L, Henneberg EW, et al (Aarhus Univ, Denmark)
Eur J Vasc Endovasc Surg 14:12–16, 1997 1–78

Introduction.—The size of abdominal aortic aneurysms (AAAs) determines when surgery should be performed. However, especially as more small AAAs are diagnosed, it would be useful to have more accurate surgical indications. Serum elastin peptide (SEP) levels were analyzed as a possible predictor of expansion of small AAAs.

Methods.—The study included 3,334 elderly men, aged 65–73, who were screened for AAA. An AAA was detected in 141 subjects. Of these, 19 had AAAs >5 cm in diameter; all were referred for immediate surgery. The remaining 122 subjects were given an opportunity for annual follow-up. Eighty-three patients provided a blood sample for measurement of SEP using an enzyme-linked immunosorbent assay. All follow-up scans were read without knowledge of the SEP results.

Results.—The AAAs expanded at an average rate of 2.6 mm/yr. About 8% of AAAs grew to >5 cm during follow-up, and the patients were referred for surgery. Significant predictors of AAA expansion on multiple regression analyses were AAA size, SEP, β-agonist treatment, and forced expiratory volume in 1 second. β-Blocker treatment was not a significant predictor (Table 3).

TABLE 3.—Multiple Linear Regression Analysis: Annual Expansion of Small Abdominal Aortic Aneurym as a Dependent Variable

Independent variable	Beta-coefficient	95% CI	Partial F-test
Initial AAA-size	0.21	0.12–0.29	23.10*
S-elastin peptides	0.09	0.04–0.14	13.22*
FEV1	0.01	0.00–0.02	5.89*
Beta-agonist treatment	2.19	0.23–4.15	4.76*
Steroid-treatment	1.74	−0.01–3.49	3.80
Diastolic blood pressure	0.03	−0.01–0.06	2.43
Smoking	0.11	−0.85–1.06	0.04
ABI	−0.01	−0.02–0.02	0.14
Beta-blockers	−0.55	−1.87–0.78	0.66
BMI	−0.01	−0.13–0.11	0.03

*$P < 0.05$.

Abbreviation: ABI, ankle blood pressure/systolic blood pressure.

(Courtesy of Lindholt JS, Heickendorff L, Henneberg EW, et al: Serum-elastin-peptides as a predictor of expansion of small abdominal aortic aneurysms. *Eur J Vasc Endovasc Surg* 14:12–16. Copyright 1997, by permission of WB Saunders Company Limited, London.)

Conclusions.—In patients with smaller AAAs, SEP appears to be a fairly strong predictor of aneurysmal growth. However, larger studies with longer follow-up are needed before any recommendations are made.

► This study was performed to determine if SEP levels may be a predictor for the expansion of small AAAs. In fact, it appears that indeed it was a predictor of aneurysm expansion. Over the years, many investigators have looked at many variables as possible predictors of aneurysm expansion. Some of these include systolic blood pressure, diastolic blood pressure, β-agonist treatment, β-blocker treatment, and original aneurysm size. Interestingly, randomized trials with propranolol are now under way in Canada and Denmark. On balance, the observation herein that SEP levels were significantly higher among expanding aneurysms compared with nonexpanding aneurysms is interesting and suggests a possible future clinical use for this determination.

Venous

Reduced Growth of Dermal Fibroblasts From Chronic Venous Ulcers Can Be Stimulated With Growth Factors

Stanley AC, Park H-Y, Phillips TJ, et al (Boston Med Ctr)
J Vasc Surg 26:994–1001, 1997 1–79

Background.—Venous ulcers are known to heal slowly, but the nature of the underlying healing defect is unknown. Fibroblasts play an important role in all stages of wound repair. Differences in fibroblasts from venous ulcers vs. normal tissue were assessed.

Methods.—The analysis included biopsy specimens from 6 patients with chronic venous ulcers, with samples taken from the wound margins and from normal upper thigh tissue. Dermal fibroblasts were isolated and plated; total cells per plate were counted over time to construct growth curves. The effects of supplementing the growth medium with additional calf serum and with various growth factors were assessed.

Results.—Cell replication was more rapid in normal fibroblasts than in wound fibroblasts. The wound fibroblasts also had different morphological characteristics, including a larger size, polygonal shape, and less uniform nuclei. Adding calf serum increased the growth of normal fibroblasts but did not affect wound fibroblast growth. The growth of wound fibroblasts was enhanced by the addition of basic fibroblast growth factor and epidermal growth factor; interleukin-1β stimulated growth in most specimens, but the difference was not significant.

Conclusions.—Fibroblasts from chronic venous ulcers proliferate more slowly than normal fibroblasts and have different morphological characteristics. These characteristics are similar to those observed in aged or senescent cells. Slow growth may help to explain the slow healing rate of these ulcers. Growth factors appear to enhance the growth of wound fibroblasts; exogenous growth factor administration may aid ulcer healing in some patients.

▶ The cause of delayed healing of chronic venous ulcers is unknown. Using biopsy samples, these authors concluded that fibroblasts taken from the edge of venous ulcers behaved in a distinctly abnormal fashion, compatible with aging fibroblasts. Their performance in tissue cultures was markedly enhanced by the use of fibroblast or epidermal growth factors, leading these authors to conclude that the exogenous administration of specific growth factors to indolent venous ulcers may promote healing. Perhaps, but hasn't this been tried multiple times in the past with inconclusive results?

Endothelial Activation in Patients With Chronic Venous Disease

Saharay M, Shields DA, Georgiannos SN, et al (Univ College London)

Eur J Vasc Endovasc Surg 15:342–349, 1998 1–80

Objective.—White cell trapping resulting from endothelial activation has been proposed as the cause of skin damage in patients with chronic venous disease. Endothelial activation was assessed by measuring the plasma levels of endothelial leukocyte adhesion molecule-1 (ELAM-1), intracellular adhesion molecule-1 (ICAM-1), vascular cell adhesion molecule-1 (VCAM-1), and von Willebrand factor (vWf) before and after short-term venous hypertension in controls and in patients with chronic venous disease.

Methods.—Blood samples were taken from the foot veins of 25 normal controls (12 female), aged 20–59 years, and 30 patients (15 female), aged 29–73 years, with chronic venous disease before and after venous hypertension was induced. Fifteen patients had varicose veins with skin changes and 15 had varicose veins only. Plasma levels of ELAM-1, ICAM-1, and VCAM-1 were measured using enzyme-linked immunosorbent assay (ELISA). Von Willebrand factor was assayed using a noncommercial ELISA method.

Results.—Baseline levels of all 3 adhesion molecules were significantly higher in patients than in controls. Plasma concentrations of ELAM-1, ICAM-1, and VCAM-1 rose significantly in both groups after induction of venous hypertension (Table 2). Baseline VCAM-1 levels, the amount of VCAM-1 increase, and vWf were higher in patients with skin changes than in patients without skin changes. Levels of ICAM-1 and ELAM-1 were similar in both patient groups.

Conclusions.—Venous hypertension may promote endothelial activation leading to increased levels of adhesion molecules. Patients with skin changes show higher baseline levels of VCAM-1 and vWf, which may be markers for increased microcirculatory damage.

▶ Here we have the 93rd entry into the Pantheon of Dr. Coleridge Smith's monument to activated cells in chronic venous disease. He concludes here

compression devices—applied for 120 minutes in random order. Venous blood was obtained for various assays before, during, and after IPC.

Results.—All 5 devices caused a sharp rise in fibrinolytic activity at 180 minutes in both groups. The postthrombotic group had significantly lower baseline and stimulated fibrinolytic activity, however. Plasma tissue plasminogen activator (tPA) antigen decreased by 12% in normal individuals and by 17% in postthrombotic individuals, although only the normal individuals had a 4% increase in tPA activity (Fig 2). Both groups had a reduction in plasminogen activator inhibitor-1 (PAI-1) antigen—13% in the normal group and 12% in the postthrombosis group—and a dramatic reduction in PAI-1 activity (Fig 5). Von Willebrand factor was unaffected by IPC. Only the postthrombotic group showed an increase in α-2–antiplasmin complexes.

Conclusions.—In individuals with and without a history of thrombosis, IPC is associated with stimulation of endogenous fibrinolytic activity. However, postthrombotic patients have a reduced baseline and overall fibrinolytic response. Reduced PAI-1—causing an increase in tPA activity—is the most likely explanation of the increased fibrinolytic activity with IPC.

▶ I do not know how to interpret this paper. Before we all rush to the conclusion that intermittent pneumatic leg compression causes enhanced fibrinolysis, we must consider that the measured changes were extremely small and that a number of equally apparently valid studies have found no difference in fibrinolysis after pneumatic compression. I remain unconvinced that fibrinolytic alterations underlie the thromboprophylactic effects of IPC of the legs.

Effect of Intraluminal Thrombus on Abdominal Aortic Aneurysm Wall Stress

Mower WR, Quiñones WJ, Gambhir SS (Univ of California, Los Angeles)
J Vasc Surg 26:602–608, 1997 1–83

Background.—When the wall stresses of an abdominal aortic aneurysm (AAA) are greater than the strength of the wall tissue, aneurysm rupture occurs. Intraluminal thrombi may absorb some of these stresses, but the extent of protection possible has not been evaluated. Finite element analysis is capable of modeling stresses in complex physical structures. Finite element analysis was used to assess the effect of intraluminal thrombus on AAA wall stress.

Methods.—Computer simulations were used to model aneurysms as axially symmetric structures of revolution with walls constructed of homogeneous and isotropic materials with linear elastic deformation properties. Analyses were performed to examine the importance of thrombus size, thrombus strength, aneurysm strength, aneurysm size, and thrombus inhomogeneity. Peak Von Mises stresses were compared between modified

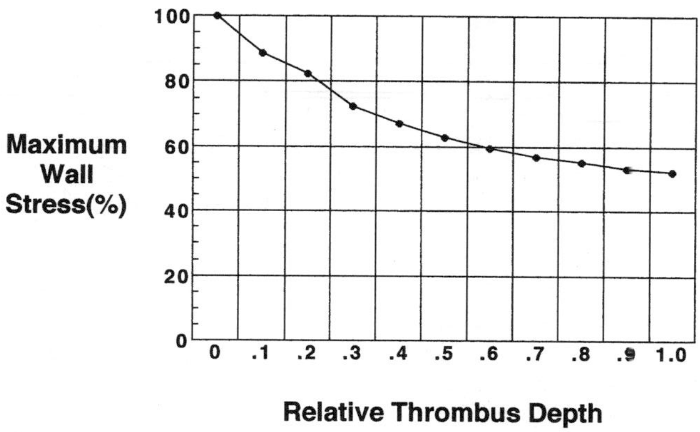

FIGURE 2.—Maximum wall stress decreases as the size of the intraluminal thrombus increases (maximum stress values are expressed as a percentage of the stresses found in an aneurysm with no intraluminal thrombus). (Courtesy of Mower WR, Quiñones WJ, Gambhir SS: Effect of intraluminal thombus on abdominal aortic aneurysm wall stress. *J Vasc Surg* 26:602–608, 1997.)

and unmodified aneurysms. Stress reduction greater than 25% was considered significant.

Results.—Intraluminal thrombi reduced AAA wall stress in all models. The amount of stress reduction was related to thrombus size (Fig 2), thrombus strength (Fig 3), aneurysm strength, and aneurysm size. Inhomogeneity had little affect on aneurysm wall stress.

Conclusions.—Intraluminal thrombus can significantly reduce wall stresses in abdominal aortic aneurysms. This effect is strongest for large, well-organized thrombi in pliant aneurysms.

► Using complex modeling and computer simulations, these investigators performed detailed analyses of a variety of factors related to AAAs. They

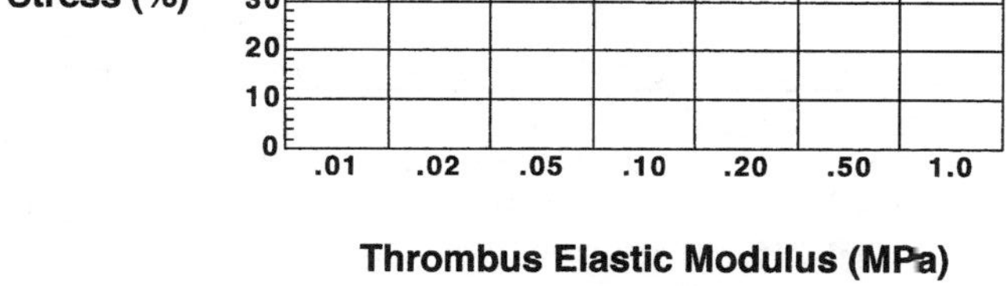

FIGURE 3.—Maximum wall stress decreases as the strength of the intraluminal thrombus increases (maximum stress values are expressed as a percentage of the stresses found in an aneurysm with no intraluminal thrombus). (Courtesy of Mower WR, Quiñones WJ, Gambhir SS: Effect of intraluminal thombus on abdominal aortic aneurysm wall stress. *J Vasc Surg* 26:602–608, 1997.

were specifically interested in stress on the aneurysm wall. Their conclusion that intraluminal thrombus can significantly reduce AAA wall stress, while interesting, does not appear to be of any particular use to vascular surgeons at the present time. While a majority of aneurysms contain abundant thrombus, we all encounter occasional large aneurysms with no thrombus at all. Are these more prone to rupture? Perhaps, but it would appear premature to use this information to influence treatment decisions.

Mast Cell Distribution, Activation, and Phenotype in Atherosclerotic Lesions of Human Carotid Arteries

Jeziorska M, McCollum C, Woolley DE (Manchester Royal Infirmary, England; Withington Hosp, Manchester, England)

J Pathol 182:115–122, 1997 1–84

Background.—Recent evidence has accumulated for mast cell (MC) involvement in the development of atherosclerotic lesions. This study is the first report of MC distribution, activation, and tryptase/chymase phenotype in 250 samples of type I to VI atherosclerotic human carotid artery lesions.

Methods.—Carotid artery samples were collected from 51 male and 30 female patients undergoing therapeutic interventions for atherosclerotic changes. Age-matched carotid arteries were obtained from routine postmortems as controls. Monoclonal antibodies to MC tryptase and MC chymase were used to identify MCs.

Results.—Healthy, control carotid arteries contained few intimal MCs, while atherosclerotic lesions had increased numbers of MCs with focal accumulations. MCs could be detected at the earliest atherosclerotic stages and were especially common in the shoulder regions of fully formed atheroma. They were detected in association with HAM56+ macrophages, extracellular lipid, and at sites of foam cell formation. MCs were also detected within new calcification sites and near small calcified deposits. Diffuse extracellular tryptase staining, indicative of extensive MC activation/degranulation, was common in advanced atherosclerotic plaques complicated by fissure, hemorrhage, and thrombus, often associated with local edema and stromal matrix disruption. MCs containing both tryptase and chymase (MC_{TC} phenotype) accounted for 80–95% of the observed MCs.

Conclusions.—This study is the first to reveal significant numbers and focal accumulations of mast cells in all developmental stages of atherosclerotic carotid arteries. As MCs contain and express many potent mediators, they may have a multifunctional role in the development and pathogenesis of atherosclerosis. Further studies are required to examine the contribution of MCs to specific stages of plaque development.

▶ Increasing evidence suggests that mast cells have an important role in atherosclerosis.[1] This remarkable paper documents the intimate association of mast cells, macrophages, extracellular lipids, and foam cells at all stages of atherosclerotic lesion development. Mast cells are especially prominent at the shoulder regions of fully formed atheroma, an observation confirmed by many investigators. Mast cells contain potent proteolytic enzymes and are quite capable of degranulation with extrusion of these enzymes into the local environment. The conclusion that mast cells appear to have an important role in both atherosclerotic plaque development and fibrous cap rupture appears inescapable.

Reference

1. 1997 Year Book of Vascular Surgery, p 32.

Dissolution of Thrombotic Arterial Occlusion by High Intensity, Low Frequency Ultrasound and Dodecafluoropentane Emulsion: An In Vitro and In Vivo Study

Nishioka T, Luo H, Fishbein MC, et al (Ground Self Defense Force Med School, Tokyo; Cedars-Sinai Med Ctr, Los Angeles, Calif)

J Am Coll Cardiol 30:561–568, 1997 1–85

Background.—Although thrombolytic therapy is commonly used to recanalize occluded coronary arteries in patients with myocardial infarction, there is a risk of hemorrhagic complications. A noninvasive technique that rapidly dissolved blood clots without a risk of hemorrhagic complications would be useful. The use of ultrasound to dissolve clots has been investigated for many years. The most likely mechanism of clot dissolution is acoustic cavitation or microbubbles. The addition of transpulmonary echo contrast agents that form microbubbles at physiologic conditions might enhance this effect. Use of ultrasound and contrast agent microbubbles to dissolve clots was investigated both in vitro and in vivo.

Methods.—For the in vitro study, whole blood was obtained from volunteers and allowed to clot. Serum was aspirated and the clots were cut into pieces, weighed, and placed into a plastic cassette. Clots were exposed to either saline solution or the contrast agent, EchoGen, composed of 2% dodecafluoropentane (DDFP) emulsion, with or without ultrasound. The reduction of clot weight was used to calculate clot disruption. The clot-containing solution was collected after each procedure and analyzed by flow cytometer to measure particulate debris. The in vivo study employed 22 thrombotically occluded arteries in 11 adult rabbits. One artery was exposed to ultrasound, and the contralateral artery was exposed to ultrasound plus EchoGen. Angiography was performed to assess patency.

Results.—The clot-disruption rate of ultrasound was significantly increased by the addition of EchoGen both in vitro and in vivo. No vessel was recanalized by EchoGen alone, and only 1 artery was patent after treatment with ultrasound alone. After treatment with both ultrasound and EchoGen, 82% of rabbit ileofemoral arteries were recanalized. Recanalized arteries had only minimal focal mural thrombus, and no vessel wall damage was observed histologically. Rabbit dermis and subcutaneous tissue was injured.

Conclusions.—The clot-dissolving effect of low-frequency ultrasound was significantly increased with the addition of the microbubble contrast agent, EchoGen, both in vitro and in vivo. This suggests that the combination of transcutaneous ultrasound and microbubble contrast agent has clinical potential as a clot-disrupting therapy for patients with thrombotic arterial occlusions.

► Catheter-delivered low-frequency ultrasound has been reported successful in dissolving clots, both in vitro and in vivo in animal models and in patients sporadically over the past 20 years. Transcutaneous exposure to US energy has been reported to enhance the effect of thrombolytic agents in vitro and in vivo in animal models. The actual mechanism of US-induced clot disruption is not known but appears related to acoustic cavitation. This study used transcutaneously administered ultrasound with or without the echo contrast agent dodecafluoropentane. Remarkable success in clot disruption was reported with the use of ultrasound in combination with dodecafluoropentane. The potential clinical application of this method is apparent. Time will tell.

2 Endovascular

Endovascular Grafts

Abdominal Aortic Aneurysms: Treatment With Juxtarenal Placement of Covered Stent-Grafts

Duda SH, Raygrotzki S, Wiskirchen J, et al (Eberhard-Karls-Universität Tübingen, Germany)

Radiology 206:195–198, 1998 2–1

Introduction.—The need for a sufficiently sized proximal aortic neck has always been emphasized for placement of stent-grafts in patients with abdominal aortic aneurysms (AAAs). The technical feasibility and clinical outcome of juxtarenal placement of covered stent-grafts for endovascular treatment of AAAs with a proximal neck less than 15 mm long were evaluated.

Methods.—Fourteen patients with AAAs were treated with polyester-covered nitinol stent-grafts. In 7 patients with proximal necks of the AAA

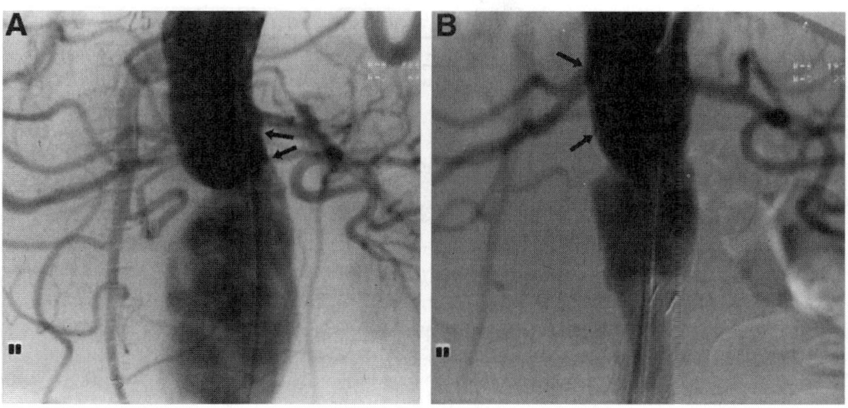

FIGURE 2.—Patient 7. **A**, intra-arterial digital subtraction angiogram shows a type E abdominal aortic aneurysm with a proximal neck of 9 mm (*arrows*). **B**, control angiogram obtained after juxtarenal implantation of a bifurcated aortic prosthesis demonstrates successful exclusion of the abdominal aortic aneurysm. Both renal arteries are perfused through the interstices of the nitinol wire mesh in the uncovered portion of the stent-graft. The *V-shaped metal markers* denote the beginning and end of the uncovered portion of the stent-graft (*arrows*). (Courtesy of Duda SH, Raygrotzki S, Wiskirchen J, et al: Abdominal aortic aneurysms: Treatment with juxtarenal placement of covered stent-grafts. *Radiology* 206:195–198. Copyright 1998, Radiological Society of North America.)

of less than 15 mm, the stent-graft was placed across the renal arteries (juxtarenal). The other 7 patients underwent standard infrarenal stent-graft placement. Computed tomography and laboratory values were used to assess clinical outcome in all 14 patients. The 7 patients who underwent juxtarenal placement were also evaluated by captopril renography (Fig 2).

Results.—Transfemoral placement of polyester-nitinol stent-grafts was technically effective in all 14 patients, and conversion to open procedure was not needed. Two of 7 patients who underwent juxtarenal stent-graft placement had minor perfusion of the aneurysm by collateral vessels immediately after the procedure. Another patient in the juxtarenal group had a persistent major endoleak along the distal part of the stent-graft and required revision with a bifurcated prosthesis 6 months after the original procedure. One patient in the infrarenal stent-graft group had minor retrograde perfusion of 10% of the AAA volume after the procedure. At a mean follow-up of 10.1 months, all patients were symptom-free with no incidence of major bleeding or distal embolization.

Conclusions.—It is possible to successfully exclude AAAs located closer than 15 mm to the orifices of the renal arteries using juxtarenal placement of the uncovered portion of the stent in the abdominal portion of the aorta.

▶ There currently appears to be 2 approaches to a short infrarenal aortic aneurysm neck in patients considered for an endovascular graft. Some investigators deem these patients ineligible for the procedure, as described in Abstract 2–5. Other investigators, as represented by this group, simply place the uncovered portion of the stent directly across the renal orifices. While this may provide secure purchase for the proximal stent, it does, of course, force renal blood flow to be sieved across a chicken wire mesh. Although these investigators have gotten away with this in the short-term, I have no enthusiasm for this technique. There is something distinctly nonphysiologic about sieving renal artery flow through chicken wire. Any build-up of cellular debris on the wire would have the potential to impair renal artery flow, and also a real potential for renal artery embolization. I doubt this will be a satisfactory long-term solution.

Endovascular Treatment of Infrarenal Abdominal Aneurysms by the Stentor System: Preliminary Results of 79 Cases

Mialhe C, for the Stentor Restrospective Study Group (Polyclinique Notre-Dame, Draguignan, France; Polyclinique d'Essey les Nancy, France; Université Paris Val de Marne, Créteil, France)

J Vasc Surg 26:199–209, 1997 2–2

Introduction.—The Stentor system offers a variety of endovascular grafts, including a bifurcated graft. The initial French multicenter experience with the Stentor system in patients undergoing endovascular treatment of abdominal aortic aneurysm (AAA) was reported.

Methods.—The Stentor system was used to treat 79 consecutive patients with AAAs. Seventy-one bifurcated grafts and 8 straight grafts were placed. Mean follow-up was 5.7 months (range, 1–18 months).

Results.—No patients required surgical conversion. Four patients (4.8%) died after surgery. Of these, 2 were considered inoperable by the standard technique. Postoperative complications included pulmonary complications in 4 patients, colonic ischemia in 3 patients, postoperative fever in 45 patients, and transitory thrombocytopenia in 8 patients. The aneurysm was immediately excluded in 66 patients (83%); exclusion was definitive in 62 patients (78%). There were 13 initial and 6 delayed endoleaks in 17 patients. The initial endoleak sealed temporarily in 2 patients and resumed after 1 year of follow-up. These endoleaks required an additional straight, covered stent. Seven leaks were successfully treated by an additional endovascular graft, 1 needed a lumbar artery embolization, 8 sealed spontaneously, and 1 was untreated. There was no incidence of aneurysm rupture. Two patients died of causes unrelated to AAA or its treatment.

Conclusions.—Short-term follow-up indicates that the Stentor system can safely and effectively treat AAAs. Patients will need to be followed up closely in the long-term to detect delayed endoleak and efficacy of this method in preventing AAA rupture.

▶ Here is another testimonial for yet another commercial endovascular graft. The authors modestly report a surgical mortality of 4.8%, pulmonary complications in 4.8% of patients and colon ischemia in 3.7%. Twenty-four percent of recipients developed an endograft leak, one-third of which occurred in a delayed fashion. On balance, this does not appear to be the stuff dreams are made of, although perhaps it is an accurate description of the current state of the art of endovascular grafting. As you may have guessed, I am not impressed. I note that endovascular aortic grafts have been with us now for at least 7 years, and the long promised giant leap forward in technical innovation has yet to appear. We still seem to be having about the same number of complications that we were having years ago. I sometimes wonder if the king is wearing any clothes at all.

Endoleak After Endovascular Graft Repair of Experimental Aortic Aneurysms: Does Coil Embolization With Angiographic "Seal" Lower Intraaneurysmal Pressure?

Marty B, Sanchez LA, Ohki T, et al (Albert Einstein College of Medicine, New York)

J Vasc Surg 27:454–462, 1998 2–3

Background.—The presence of flow outside the graft (endoleaks) is one of the main concerns with the use of endovascular grafts in the treatment of aneurysmal aortic disease. The effect on intra-aneurysmal pressure

sitating dialysis occurred in 3 patients, and there were 3 perioperative deaths and 1 late death. These authors presciently observe that conversion of an endoluminal to an open aneurysm repair may require technical modifications of the standard operative technique and results in a much higher than generally accepted morbidity and mortality rates. Overall, 15% to 17% of patients required conversion to open repair. In patients in a high-risk group, rejected initially for conventional aneurysm repair, the mortality rate associated with conversion to open repair was a remarkable 43%. It remains my opinion that endoluminal aneurysm repair is going to have to improve considerably before it is ready for prime time.

Modular Bifurcation Endoprosthesis for Treatment of Abdominal Aortic Aneurysms

White RA, Donayre CE, Walot I, et al (Univ of California, Los Angeles; Stanford Univ, Palo Alto, Calif)
Ann Surg 226:381–391, 1997 2–7

Background.—Recent years have seen several reports of successful exclusion of abdominal aortic aneurysms (AAAs) with endovascular prostheses. A phase I trial of a new self-expanding, modular, bifurcated device for the treatment of AAAs is reported.

Methods.—The study device was the Medtronic AneuRx, an endoluminal prosthesis consisting of self-expanding nitinol stents lined by a polyethylene terephthalate fiber prosthesis (Fig 1). This device was used to treat 16 patients with AAAs, 15 men and 1 woman, average age 72. The patients' conditions were American Society of Anesthesiologists grades 2 through 4. The average diameter of their AAAs was 57 mm.

Results.—Endoprosthetic treatment was successful in all patients; none required conversion to open surgery. Predischarge contrast CT scans showed no endovascular leaks or aneurysmal enlargement, nor did 1-month follow-up duplex US scans. Of 13 patients examined at 6 months, 12 were still free of such leaks. The remaining did have a small leak related to an area traumatized when the device was deployed. One patient died of septic complications related to a gangrenous gallbladder, which was recognized 1 day after device placement; the procedure-related mortality rate was thus 6%. There were no deaths related to the device itself, however.

There were 2 cases of iliac artery dissection, 2 of groin wound infection, and 2 of transient elevation of serum creatinine. The procedure took a median of 5 hours; the patients stayed in the ICU for a median of 1 day and in the hospital for 4.5 days, and median blood loss was 1,100 mL. All of these values decreased with experience. Most patients' blood replacement needs were managed with autotransfusion or banked autologous blood replacement. The 6-month follow-up data showed an average 5.6 mm reduction in the maximum diameter of the aneurysm. The average decrease in maximal cross-sectional area was 20.3% (Fig 3).

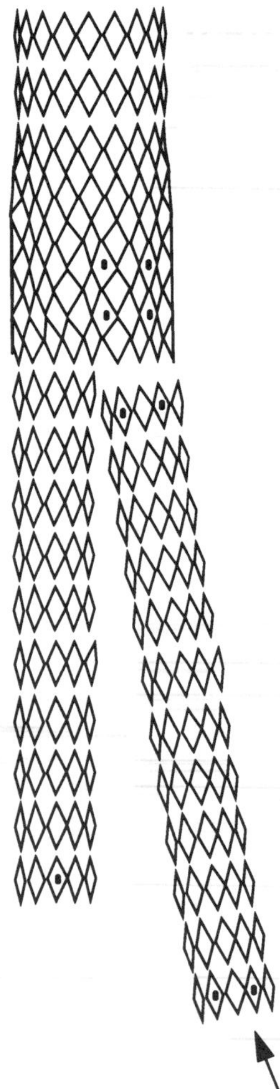

FIGURE 1.—Diagram of the segmented (nickel-titanium alloy) stent superstructure of the endograft showing the bifurcated body and integral leg and the contralateral iliac limb component. The polyethylene terephthalate fiber inner lining of the prosthesis is not shown. (Courtesy of White RA, Donayre CE, Walot I, et al: Modular bifurcation endoprosthesis for treatment of abdominal aortic aneurysms. *Ann Surg* 226:381–391, 1997.)

Conclusions.—A trial of endovascular prosthetic exclusion of AAAs with the AneuRx self-expanding modular device was successful. Though confirmatory studies are needed, this device may offer an effective alternative for patients who would otherwise need surgical management.

▶ The number of commercial endovascular grafts continually popping up appears limited only by the number of surgeon-entrepreneurs in our ranks. This particular AneuRx graft is a modular graft in which the second limb is

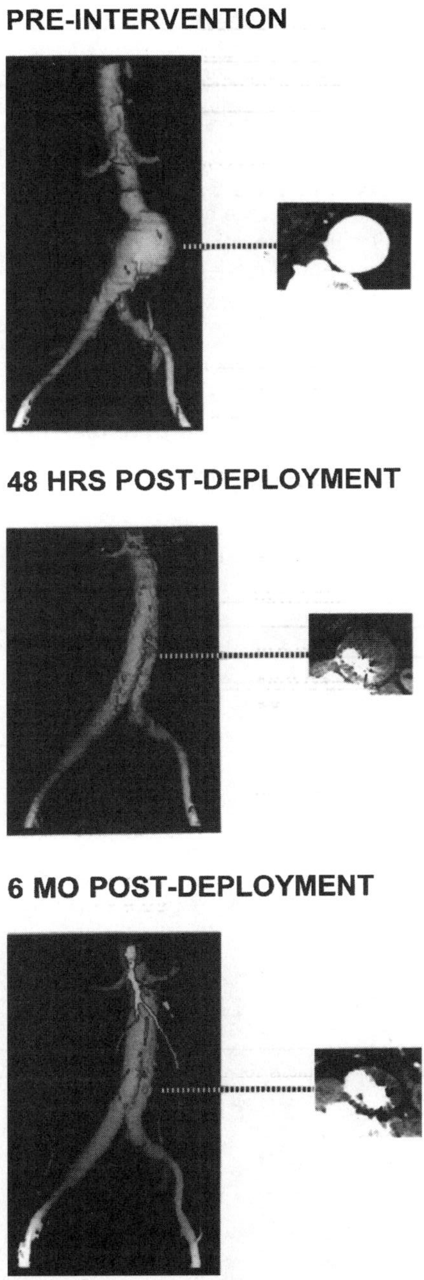

FIGURE 3.—Computed tomography angiograms and cross-sectional axial views of an AAA preintervention at 48 hours after deployment of a bifurcated Medtronic AneuRx device (Medtronic AneuRx, Inc, Cupertino, Calif.), and at 6 months after deployment showing nearly complete regression of the aneurysm. (Courtesy of White RA, Donayre CE, Walot I, et al: Modular bifurcation endoprosthesis for treatment of abdominal aortic aneurysms. *Ann Surg* 226:381–391, 1997.)

inserted separately. Although the results reported here for 16 patients are generally satisfactory, they are not all that good. One patient died, complications included 2 iliac artery dissections, 2 groin wound infections, and 2 transient elevations of creatinine level. The procedure took a median time of 5 hours and required an ICU stay of 1 day, a postprocedure hospitalization of 4.5 days, and carried a blood loss of 1,100 mL. At present, I simply have no idea where the endograft is going to fit in the future treatment of our patients with vascular problems. One must remember when considering the use of these inherently complex and unproven devices that we do have a very satisfactory operative procedure for the treatment of aortic aneurysms, producing a mortality rate of 2% to 4% and a low rate of serious complications. I have no idea whether the AneuRx modular graft will be superior to the multiple other designs or not.

Endovascular Treatment of Abdominal Aneurysmal Aortitis in Behçet's Disease

Vasseur M-A, Haulon S, Beregi JP, et al (Cardiologic Hosp, Lille, France)
J Vasc Surg 27:974–976, 1998 2–8

Background.—Arterial complications of Behçet's disease (BD), affecting mainly the aorta and iliac arteries, are rare. The most common complication is perforation of the arterial wall, which predisposes to false aneurysm or rupture. Open surgical repair is difficult. In addition, anastomotic false aneurysms occur frequently because of aortic wall fragility. The use of a bifurcated stent in the treatment of aortoiliac false aneurysms in 1 patient was reported.

Case Report.—Man, 37, given a diagnosis of BD in 1984, experienced sudden back and abdominal pain associated with ileus

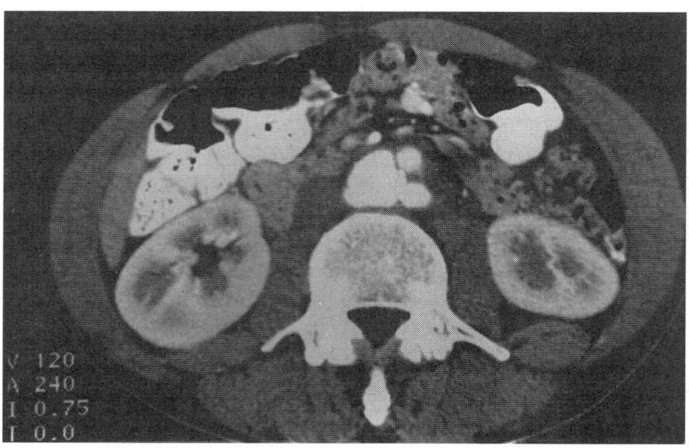

FIGURE 1.—Preoperative CT. (Courtesy of Vasseur M-A, Haulon S, Beregi JP, et al: Endovascular treatment of abdominal aneurysmal aortitis in Behçet's disease. *J Vasc Surg* 27:974–976, 1998.)

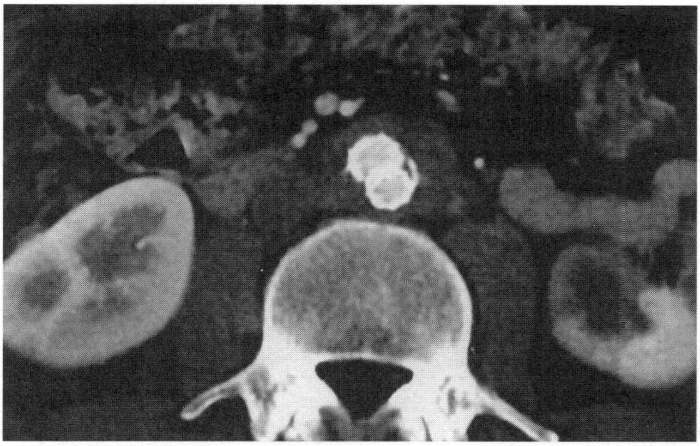

FIGURE 3.—Postoperative CT: thrombosis of the aortic aneurysm and limbs of the endoprosthesis. (Courtesy of Vasseur M-A, Haulon S, Beregi JP, et al: Endovascular treatment of abdominal aneurysmal aortitis in Behçet's disease. *J Vasc Surg* 27:974–976, 1998.)

during a strenuous effort in 1997. Abdominal contrast-enhanced CT revealed aortic and iliac false aneurysms (Fig 1). Treatment consisted of a bifurcated stent placed below the renal arteries through a right groin incision and left percutaneous femoral approach. A thermic memory form self-expandable device was used. The device had 2 components: an aortic section, with a single limb inserted in an 18-F introducer. At the trailing of the aortic section, the second contralateral limb was inserted in a short branch through a 10-F introducer. Once in place, the nitinol stent was expanded by gentle manual inflation with a 10-mm balloon filled with diluted contrast medium. Thrombosis of the aneurysms was demonstrated on a final angiography. The patient recovered uneventfully, with an excellent outcome (Fig 3). He was discharged from the hospital 4 days after the procedure, with prescriptions for 300 mg aspirin, 60 mg prednisone, and 1 mg colchicine per day. At his 6-month follow-up, complete regression of the aorta iliac false aneurysms and good graft patency were demonstrated.

Conclusion.—The endovascular approach may be a new form of treatment for aneurysmal manifestations of BD. This apporach has yielded excellent short-term results in the patient described above. Long-term outcomes have yet to be determined.

► Some heritable and inflammatory aortopathies present almost insurmountable surgical challenges. Ones ability to suture a graft replacement of an aneurysm in BD or Ehlers-Danlos disease is extremely limited. I congratulate these authors on their successful deployment of an endograft in a patient with BD. We had a somewhat similar patient with Ehlers-Danlos disease type IV with recurrent aneurysms, in which a large infrarenal abdominal aortic aneurysm finally developed. This was successfully excluded by a carefully placed endograft, which functioned well for several years until the patient's death. I believe that the heritable and inflammatory arteriopathies are a valid indication for use of an endograft.

Fatal Colonic Ischaemia After Stent Graft for Aortic Aneurysm

Sandison AJP, Edmondson RA, Panayiotopoulos YP, et al (Guy's Hosp, London)

Eur J Vasc Endovasc Surg 13:219–220, 1997 2–9

Background.—New technological advances have led to renewed interest in the treatment of infrarenal aortic aneurysms by endovascular techniques. However, any new technique has a learning curve. Fatal colonic ischemia associated with a stent graft used to treat a symptomatic abdominal aortic aneurysm was reported.

Case Report.—Man, 73, sought medical attention for a 4-day history of central abdominal pain radiating to the back. A tender, 4-cm abdominal aortic aneurysm was noted on examination. Seven years earlier, the patient had had a myocardial infarction, and 2 weeks before his current admission, he had had severe chest pain at rest. An urgent CT scan confirmed an infrarenal aortic aneurysm and revealed a large mass, which appeared to be malignant, posterior to the heart. Treatment with an endoluminal graft stent was selected. Bilateral iliac angioplasties were done to gain access to the aorta, and the next day a straight Palmaz aortic stent was successfully deployed through a right common femoral arteriotomy under general anesthesia. The stent graft partially covered the origin of the left common iliac artery. A kissing balloon technique was used, with catheters placed in the origins of both common iliac arteries for correct stent graft positioning.

Immediately after surgery, the patient's left foot was noted to be ischemic. Despite continuous IV infusion of iloprost, the circulation in his foot deteriorated over time. With the patient under general anesthesia, both the dorsalis and posterior tibial arteries were explored and found to be occluded with fresh thrombus. Through embolectomy, good inflow was established. On the following day, a chemical lumbar sympathectomy was performed, improving circulation to the proximal part of the foot. However, the toes became nonviable, and the pain in the foot prevented the patient from mobilizing. A pyrexia developed on the fourth day after surgery. A chest radiograph showed pneumonia. Bronchoscopy failed to show the nature of the patient's chest mass. Although IV antibiotics initially resulted in improvement, the patient's condition again deteriorated when lower abdominal pain and diarrhea developed. A repeat CT scan showed that the stent graft was in a good position, with no leaks.

During the next 4 days, the patient became increasingly septic. Renal function began to deteriorate. Severe abdominal pain with peritonitis developed on day 11, and a laparotomy was performed. The left part of the colon was necrotic, and a Hartmann's procedure was done. Multiple sequential organ failure developed, and the patient died on day 15. Postmortem examination showed that the stent graft was correctly placed. The first 1 cm of inferior mesenteric artery was occluded with thrombus. The chest mass was a mesothelioma.

Conclusion.—As new technology is developed, enabling endovascular treatment of abdominal aortic aneurysms, clinicians must continue to adhere to the basic principles of open repair. An awareness of the risks of embolization, resulting in colonic ischemia—especially in the presence of a previously patent inferior mesenteric artery, may permit early recognition and intervention, thus avoiding the potentially fatal consequences that occurred in the patient described.

▶ This case of fatal colonic ischemia occurring after deployment of an infrarenal aortic stent graft reminds us, once again, that embolization of debris from within the aneurysm during stent graft deployment is a very real and ever present danger. This particular patient also had infarction of the distal portion of his left foot. Although such misadventures can occur after traditional surgical aneurysmectomy, they seem much more frequent with endografts. Clearly, this is another problem to be overcome. (See also Abstract, 2–10.)

Postoperative Fever, Bowel Ischaemia and Cytokine Response to Abdominal Aortic Aneurysm Repair: A Comparison Between Endovascular and Open Surgery

Syk I, Brunkwall J, Ivancev K, et al (Malmö Univ, Sweden; Lund Univ, Sweden; Sahlgrenska Univ, Sweden; et al)

Eur J Vasc Endovasc Surg 15:398–405, 1998 2–10

Background.—Because transfemorally placed endoluminal grafting (TPEG) for aortic aneurysms requires no clamping of the aorta, this procedure may result in less intraoperative splanchnic ischemia than open surgery. Regardless of the method used, occlusion of a patent inferior mesenteric artery increases the risk of a postoperative ischemia in the sigmoid colon, particularly when flow through the internal iliac vessels is compromised. This study assessed the occurrence of bowel ischemia in TPEG for abdominal aortic aneurysms, as well as its relationship to cytokine response or postoperative fever.

Methods.—Fourteen patients undergoing conventional surgery and 23 undergoing endovascular procedures for infrarenal abdominal aortic aneurysm repair were studied prospectively. Tonometry was used to determine sigmoid colon pH and enzyme-linked immunosorbent assays were used for serum interleukin (IL)-6.

Findings.—In both groups, mucosal pH in the sigmoid colon declined significantly during clamping and reperfusion. The lowest-measured sigmoid colon pH values in the open and TPEG groups were 7.1 and 7.2, respectively. Serum IL-6 concentrations peaked after 4 hours of reperfusion, at 249 pg/mL in the open group and 89 pg/mL in the TPEG group. High IL-6 levels in the postoperative period and persisting low sigmoidal pH were associated with serious complications. Postoperative temperature did not differ significantly between groups, and there were no correlations with sigmoid colon pH or IL-6 levels.

Conclusion.—In patients undergoing TPEG, perioperative bowel ischemia was less pronounced, indicating an advantage of this procedure over conventional surgery. Splanchnic ischemia was uncorrelated with postoperative fever, IL-6, or tumor necrosis factor response.

▶ The authors purport to show differences in colonic pH and the serum level of IL-6 in a group of patients with aneurysm treated by either endograft placement or conventional surgery. I quickly lost interest in this article when I learned that 3 of the 23 patients undergoing endovascular grafting died, and that 2 of the 14 patients undergoing conventional surgery required resection of bowel infarction which occurred as a complication of the aneurysmectomy. With surgical results this poor, I am not interested in any detailed metabolic comparisons between the 2 groups.

Angioplasty

Is Intermittent Claudication Improved by Percutaneous Transluminal Angioplasty? A Randomized Controlled Trial

Whyman MR, Fowkes FGR, Kerracher EMG, et al (Univ of Edinburgh, Scotland; Royal Infirmary of Edinburgh, Scotland)

J Vasc Surg 26:551–557, 1997 2–11

Introduction.—The use of and indications for percutaneous transluminal angioplasty (PTA) for the treatment of peripheral arterial disease are expanding. However, there have been few controlled studies to support its benefits. A randomized, controlled trial of PTA versus conventional medical therapy for patients with mild to moderate intermittent claudication is reported.

Methods.—Of 600 patients screened, 62 were randomly assigned to study groups. Forty-seven had short-segment femoral artery stenoses or occlusions and 15 had iliac stenoses. One group received PTA plus medical therapy; the other received only medical therapy, consisting of low-dose aspirin and advice regarding smoking and exercise. After 2 years, the groups were compared for differences in outcome, including patient-reported maximum walking distance, treadmill walking distance to onset of claudication, treadmill maximum walking distance, ankle-brachial pressure index, quality of life, and duplex US assessment of occlusive disease.

Conclusion.—Carotid endarterectomy is established as a successful procedure with a durable result. In this study, costs were considerably higher for PTAS than for CEA (25% in the lowest cost comparison). The greater cost of PTAS appears to be related to the difference between a procedure in a cardiac catheterization laboratory and one in an operating room.

▶ The University of Alabama cardiologists, under the leadership of Dr. Roubin, have been leading proponents of internal carotid balloon stent angioplasty in this country. The vascular surgeons at the same institution present here an analysis of total hospital charges for patients undergoing carotid angioplasty vs. those undergoing CEA. Interestingly, the authors found that charges for the CEA group were about 30% less than charges for the carotid angioplasty group. While these results are interesting, I am not sure just how important they really are, as the charges for angioplasty will doubtless go down in the future of HMO contracts. I note with concern that no representative of cardiology was included on the list of authors. I am always concerned about reporting other people's patients when the other people are not included in the authorship.

Comparison of Hemodynamic Cerebral Ischemia and Microembolic Signals Detected During Carotid Endarterectomy and Carotid Angioplasty

Crawley F, Clifton A, Buckenham T, et al (St George's Hosp, London; Atkinson Morley's Hosp, London)

Stroke 28:2460–2464, 1997 2–15

Introduction.—Carotid percutaneous transluminal angioplasty (PTA) is regarded as a promising treatment for carotid stenosis. However, it has been suggested that carotid PTA may be associated with a higher risk of cerebral ischemia than carotid endarterectomy (CEA). Transcranial Doppler was used to study cerebral hemodynamics and microembolization during the 2 procedures.

Methods.—Twenty-eight patients undergoing carotid PTA and 14 undergoing CEA with a shunt were studied. During the procedure, the middle cerebral artery of each group was monitored with transcranial Doppler. Total occlusion time was determined by adding the periods in which the internal carotid artery was occluded by the PTA balloon or by a clamp without the shunt in place. The time in which middle cerebral artery velocity decreased to one third of baseline or less was defined as the ischemic time. Microembolic signal counts were made during each procedure.

Results.—Mean individual occlusion time was 168 minutes with CEA vs. 20 minutes with PTA. Mean total occlusion time was 337 vs. 26 minutes, respectively, while ischemic time was 165 vs. 17 minutes. The mean number of microembolic signals was 52 with CEA vs. 202 with PTA.

Conclusions.—In patients with carotid stenosis, PTA produces less hemodynamic ischemia but more microembolization. The study permits no conclusions about how ischemic time and microembolism are related to stroke. Clinical trials to determine neurologic and neuropsychological outcomes after PTA and CEA are needed.

► With the use of transcranial Doppler to monitor the middle cerebral artery, these investigators determined that there were 4 times as many microembolic signals during carotid angioplasty as during CEA. I continue to have considerable concern about the emboli generated by carotid angioplasty. It is now widely reported that "minor" stroke occurs in 6% to 10% of patients undergoing carotid angioplasty, but most patients rapidly recover in several days. I wonder. Dead neurons are dead neurons, and even though motor and sensory function may recover, you have got to be concerned about intellectual function. Because most carotid endarterectomies are now done as morning-admit surgery with no ICU stay and patients are discharged 1 or 2 days later with a combined mortality-stroke rate of 2% to 5%, I am simply unable to clearly perceive the putative benefit of carotid stent angioplasty. Perhaps my failure to appreciate the importance of this dramatic new work is a sign of increasing age.

Carotid Endarterectomy Performed After Progressive Carotid Stenosis Following Angioplasty and Stent Placement

Vale FL, Fisher WS III, Jordan WD Jr, et al (Univ of Alabama, Birmingham)
J Neurosurg 87:940–943, 1997 2–16

Background.—Carotid endarterectomy (CEA) is the treatment of choice for internal carotid artery (ICA) stenosis of greater than 60%. Recently, percutaneous transluminal angioplasty (PTA) with stent placement has been proposed as 1 treatment option. The outcome of CEA performed after PTA with stent placement in 1 patient was reported, together with pathologic findings.

Case Report.—Woman, 55, with insulin-dependent diabetes mellitus reported symptoms of a left hemispheric transient ischemic attack. A high-grade stenosis in the left ICA and a probable right ICA occlusion was diagnosed, and a left CEA was performed with no complications. The patient was then referred for further assessment. High-resolution angiography showed that the right ICA was not occluded completely but was severely stenosed, allowing only a trickle flow distally (Fig 1). The right external carotid artery showed 50% to 60% stenosis. After a standard CEA, surgical intervention was difficult because of the length of the exposure needed to dissect the metallic stent, the difficulty with opening and cutting the artery, and the care needed to remove the stent to avoid vessel wall perforation (Fig 2). Pathologic assessment of the specimen showed classic atherosclerotic changes that indicated persis-

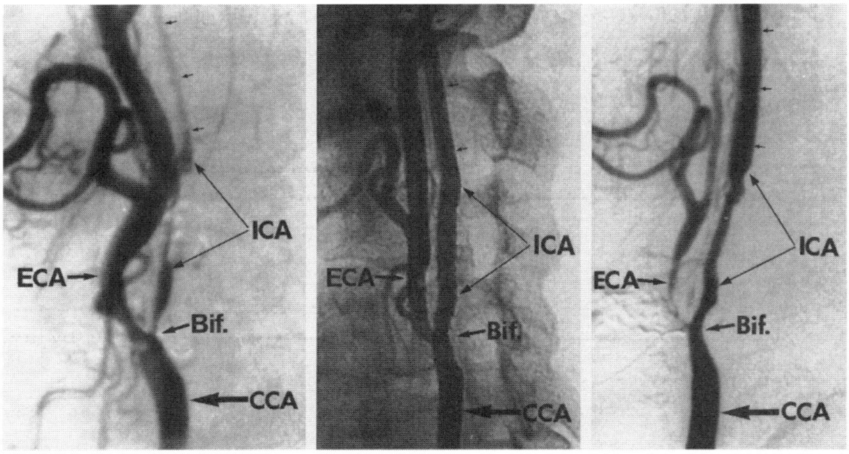

FIGURE 1.—**Left**: angiogram obtained at presentation after left carotid endarterectomy, shows the almost completely occluded right internal carotid artery (*ICA*) and faintly visualized distal ICA (*small black arrows*). Bifurcation (*Bif.*) refers to bifurcation of the common carotid artery (*CCA*). **Center**, angiogram shows appearance of the right (Bif., ICA, and external carotid artery (*ECA*) immediately after angioplasty with stent placement. Normal flow through the distal ICA (*small black arrows*) is restored. **Right**, follow-up angiogram obtained 6 months later reveals restenosis within the Bif., ICA, and ECA. Blood flow through the distal ICA (*small black arrows*) is maintained. (Courtesy of Vale FL, Fisher WS III, Jordan WD Jr, et al: Carotid endarterectomy performed after progressive carotid stenosis following angioplasty and stent placement. *J Neurosurg* 87:940–943, 1997.)

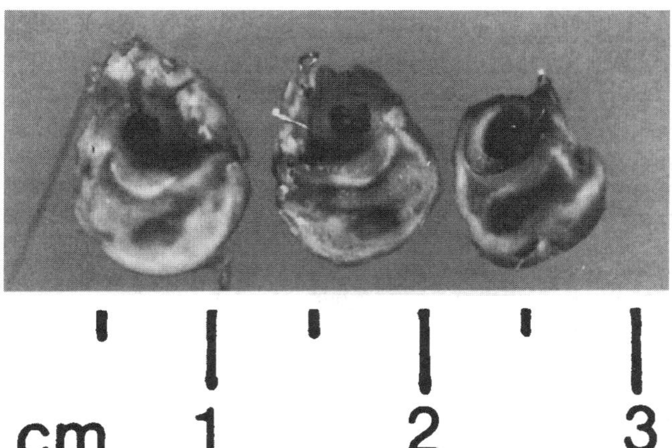

FIGURE 2.—Photograph shows cross-sectional views of en bloc plaque in and around the stent removed from the right internal carotid artery. Note the size of the retained plaque, which can cause external compression of the external carotid artery during internal carotid artery balloon expansion. (Courtesy of Vale FL, Fisher WS III, Jordan WD Jr, et al: Carotid endarterectomy performed after progressive carotid stenosis following angioplasty and stent placement. *J Neurosurg* 87:940–943, 1997.)

tence of native disease. The metallic stent was embedded in the plaque.

Conclusion.—Carotid endarterectomy of a stent-containing carotid artery is a feasible alternative that should be considered when stenosis recurs after PTA. Many questions regarding the physiologic and biological changes that occur in the carotid vessel wall after PTA with stent placement remain unanswered.

▶ Sufficiently few CEAs have been performed after carotid stent angioplasty that I include this single case report as a novelty. The surgeons concluded that the operation was made technically more difficult by the presence of the stent, including the requirement for additional dissection. Interestingly, the surgeons described the stent as being deeply imbedded within the plaque. I suppose we had all best get prepared, because we are all going to be called upon to perform surgery in more and more stented carotid arteries in the future.

Management of Upper Extremity Central Venous Obstruction Using Interventional Radiology

Kalman PG, Lindsay TF, Clarke K, et al (Univ of Toronto)
Ann Vasc Surg 12:202–206, 1998 2–17

Background.—Significant morbidity is associated with upper extremity central vein stenosis/occlusion. The use of interventional radiologic techniques in the management of upper extremity central venous obstruction was reported.

Methods.—All 59 radiologic interventions for central vein stenosis/occlusion performed between 1991 and 1996 were reviewed. Ten patients had thrombolytic therapy only; 40 had percutaneous transluminal angioplasty, and 9 had deployment of a venous stent. The involved vein was the subclavian, axillary, or innominate in 45 patients and the superior vena cava in 14. The cause was an indwelling foreign body in 90%. The mean follow-up after treatment was 17.2 months. The cumulative success rate at follow-up was analyzed by the Kaplan-Meier method.

Findings.—The cumulative success rate at 2 years was 70%. Thereafter, this rate declined rapidly. Twenty-five percent of interventions failed by 17 months, 50% by 26.6 months, and 75% by 33.8 months. No significant differences among subgroups were noted (Fig 1).

Conclusion.—Clinicians should consider interventional radiologic techniques when symptoms from upper extremity central vein stenosis/occlusion are severe and disabling or when veno-access or maintenance of patency of an ipsilateral arteriovenous access is needed. These data suggest that the short- to medium-term outcomes are acceptable.

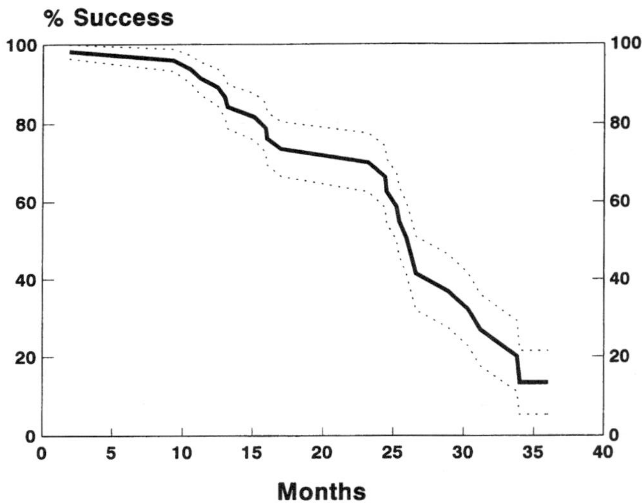

FIGURE 1.—Cumulative percentage success for 59 radiologic interventions (Kaplan-Meier). (Courtesy of Kalman PG, Lindsay TF, Clarke K, et al: Management of upper extremity central venous obstruction using interventional radiology. *Ann Vasc Surg* 12(3):202–206, 1998.)

► This is a generally favorable report of a large number of cases of central venous obstruction of the upper extremities treated by interventional radiology. Most cases, as predicted, were caused by indwelling catheters. I find it noteworthy that after variable treatment with thrombolytic therapy or angioplasty, the cumulative success rate was 70% at 2 years, with a rapid decline thereafter. A 70% success rate at 2 years actually seems quite good to me. I commend the authors on their results.

Balloon Angioplasty Combined With Primary Stenting Versus Balloon Angioplasty Alone in Femoropopliteal Obstructions: A Comparative Randomized Study

Vroegindeweij D, Vos LD, Tielbeek AV, et al (Catharina Hosp, Eindhoven, The Netherlands)

Cardiovasc Intervent Radiol 20:420–425, 1997 2–18

Introduction.—Results of balloon angioplasty (BA) in the treatment of occluded femoropopliteal arteries have been disappointing, for patency is often short lived. The introduction of vascular stents to prevent recoil after dilation has been considered a promising method for improving patency and reducing restenosis. A prospective randomized study compared outcome after BA alone with BA combined with stenting (ST).

Methods.—Fifty-one patients with femoropopliteal obstructive disease and claudication ranging from mild to severe were recruited for the study. Twenty-seven were randomized to BA alone and 24 to BA with ST. Excluded were patients with multisegmental disease and with no runoff

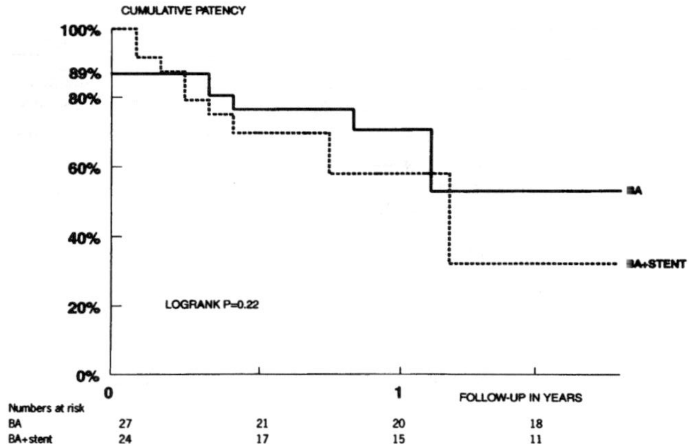

FIGURE 2.—Cumulative patency rates indicated by a peak systolic velocity ratio of 2.5 or less in patients treated by balloon angioplasty alone (*BA*) and those treated by balloon angioplasty combined with stenting (*BA + STENT*). Numbers represent patients at risk at different intervals. (Courtesy of Vroegindeweij D, Vos LD, Tielbeek AV, et al: Balloon angioplasty combined with primary stenting versus balloon angioplasty alone in femoropopliteal obstructions: A comparative randomized study. *Cardiovasc Intervent Radiol* 20:420–425, copyright 1997, Springer-Verlag.)

and those with lesions larger than 5 cm. In the ST group, Palmaz stents were placed at angiographically identified lesions and expanded by BA. At follow-up evaluation, patients were assessed by ankle blood pressure measurements at rest and after graded treadmill exercise and by color-flow duplex US. Primary patency rates were determined by the life-table method.

Results.—The 2 patient groups were similar in most risk factors for peripheral arterial disease and characteristics of the lesions. Four severely obese patients had to be crossed over from ST to BA. The BA and ST groups did not differ in early clinical/hemodynamic improvement. Eight patients (30%) treated by BA and 9 (43%) treated by ST experienced a clinical deterioration after 1 year. In both groups the ankle-brachial blood pressure index showed only a modest deterioration during follow-up. Residual stenosis (30% diameter reduction or greater) occurred in 3 BA patients. The cumulative rate of clinical and hemodynamic success after 1 year was 74% with ST and 85% with BA. Primary patency at 1 year (Fig 2), as assessed by color-flow duplex US, was 62% in the ST group and 74% in the BA group. Occlusion rates were 21% with ST vs. 7% with BA alone.

Conclusion.—The addition of ST to balloon angioplasty did not improve clinical and hemodynamic outcome in patients with femoropopliteal obstruction. Those treated with ST had a higher occlusion rate.

▶ By the authors' own admission, a significant majority of patients in this study had "mild to moderate intermittent claudication." There were no patients with rest pain. Maximal lesion length for study inclusion was 5 cm, and very few complete occlusions were included. The overall patency rate at one year was in the 60% to 70% range, but one must keep in mind that these were the most favorable patients one could possibly have selected. The message of the paper is that stenting was no better than angioplasty alone. There continues to be a dramatic dearth of information concerning the superiority of stenting over angioplasty without stenting. The long-promised publication from Germany describing the superiority of stenting continues to be long-promised, and, as of this writing, it has not yet been published anywhere. For the time being, it appears that stents do not convey any benefit over angioplasty and that both give distinctly inferior results compared with well-performed surgery. As exemplified by this series, the best results are achieved predictably in patients who need intervention least—in this case, a large preponderance of "mild to moderate claudicators." I consider endovascular surgical intervention in patients with "mild to moderate" claudication unconscionable. Is that clear enough? (See also Abstract 2–11.)

Is Balloon Angioplasty Indicated for "Short" Stenoses of Failing Vein Grafts?

Rua I, Calligaro KD, Dougherty MJ, et al (Univ of Pennsylvania Hosp, Philadelphia)

Ann Vasc Surg 12:134–137, 1998 2–19

Introduction.—Balloon angioplasty is reported to yield a good outcome in the treatment of short (less than 2 cm) stenoses in a failing peripheral vein graft. To determine whether balloon dilatation is preferable to surgery in such cases, researchers reviewed their experience of 19 failing peripheral vein grafts in 16 patients.

Methods.—Procedures were performed at the study institution between August 1, 1993 and December 31, 1996. All bypasses had been performed for limb salvage, and balloon angioplasty was the first intervention in each patient. Six grafts had 2 lesions and 13 had a single lesion; 20 lesions were 1 cm or less and 5 were between 1 and 2 cms. There were 18 severe (greater than 75% luminal diameter narrowing) and 7 moderate (50% to 75% narrowing) stenoses. Ten lesions were located at an anastomosis and 10 in the body of the graft; 5 were peri-anastomotic. Fifteen procedures were performed percutaneously, and 4 required angioplasties.

Results.—All 19 grafts showed less than 20% residual stenosis at the completion arteriogram. The cumulative 1-year primary patency rate was 39%; the 1-year assisted primary patency rate was 73%. During follow-up ranging from 7–20 months, only 5 grafts remained patent. Two hematomas requiring surgical repair occurred after the percutaneous approach. The use of anticoagulation in the postintervention period did not appear to affect outcome.

Conclusion.—Compared with patency rates reported for short (less than 2 cm) stenoses of failing peripheral vein grafts treated surgically, the long-term patency rate of these lesions treated with balloon angioplasty was disappointing. In most cases, these short lesions are better treated surgically.

► Treatment of short segment stenosis in vein grafts with balloon angioplasty has attracted the attention of interventionalists for years. This has never made any particular sense to me, as we have been informed repeatedly that the mechanism of benefit of balloon angioplasty is the fracture of intimal plaque with "controlled" wall dissection. Without question, stenoses in vein grafts are collagenous. Collagen, of course, does not stretch. Once bursting strength is exceeded, collagen simply tears. I have never been able to understand how tearing collagen can produce a durable dilatation. These authors apparently found the same thing, with a primary patency at 1 year after segmental graft dilatation of only 39% and an assisted primary patency of 73%. This is contrasted with our experience at surgical revision of threatened reversed infrainguinal vein grafts.[1] We found a 1-year patency of 99% with surgical revision, indeed a remarkable improvement over that reported here. I continue to regard balloon angioplasty as inappropriate therapy for segmental vein graft stenosis.

Reference

1. 1996 Year Book of Vascular Surgery, p 266.

Laparoscopic Aortobifemoral Bypass

Ahn SS, Hiyama DT, Rudkin GH, et al (Univ of California, Los Angeles)

J Vasc Surg 26:128–132, 1997 2–20

Background.—Laparoscopic techniques have been widely accepted in many fields of surgery, though there have been significant obstacles to the use of laparoscopy for intra-abdominal vascular procedures. In a pig model, the feasibility of totally laparoscopic aortofemoral bypass with carbon dioxide peritoneal insufflation has previously been demonstrated. Initial experience with the laparoscopic intra-abdominal insertion of an aortofemoral grafts is reported.

Case.—Man, 49, with left thigh and calf claudication underwent laparoscopic aortobifemoral bypass. The patient was reluctant to undergo open surgery. The procedure was performed with carbon dioxide pneumoperitoneum induced with a Veress needle (United States Surgical Corp., Norwalk, Conn.) and maintained at 9 to 16 mm Hg. The procedure used a 30-degree–angled endoscope introduced through a central epigastric subxiphoid port, along with 6 additional Versaports (United States Surgical; Fig 1). After a 3 cm arteriotomy was made in the infrarenal aorta, a bifurcated polyethylene terephthalate fiber graft was sutured to the aorta end-to-side in continuous running fashion. The procedure took a total of

Middle Cerebral Artery Blood Velocity, Embolisation, and Neurological Outcome During Carotid Endarterectomy: A Prospective Comparison of the Javid and the Pruitt-Inahara Shunts

Wilkinson JM, Rochester JR, Sivaguru A, et al (Northern Gen Hosp, Sheffield, England; Royal Hallamshire Hosp, Sheffield, England)

Eur J Vasc Endovasc Surg 14:399–402, 1997 3–2

Background.—Shunt design has a critical effect on internal carotid artery blood flow. The Javid and Pruitt-Inahara devices are commonly used carotid shunts that yield good results but that have very different design characteristics. The in vivo hemodynamic performance and neurologic outcomes of these 2 shunts were documented.

Methods.—One hundred sixty-three consecutive patients undergoing carotid endarterectomy for symptomatic carotid disease were randomly assigned to receive the Javid or Pruitt-Inahara shunt. The main outcome measures were middle cerebral artery velocity (MCAV) before and during clamping, during shunting, and after flow restoration; embolic episodes; and neurologic outcomes.

Findings.—The 2 groups had similar MCAVs preoperatively, at carotid clamping, and postoperatively. During shunting, the patients with the Pruitt-Inahara shunt had a significantly lower MCAV. Fifty-nine percent of the Javid shunts and 34% of the Pruitt-Inahara shunts maintained MCAV at preoperative levels. Seventy-three percent of those receiving Javid shunts had emboli at declamping, compared with 41% of the patients receiving the Pruitt-Inahara shunt, a significant difference. Four patients with a Javid shunt and 1 with a Pruitt-Inahara shunt had disabling thromboembolic strokes. Overall, the thromboembolic stroke rate was 3.7%. The between-group difference in stroke rates was nonsignificant (Table 2).

Conclusion.—The Pruitt-Inahara shunt was unable to maintain preoperative MCAV in 66% of the patients. The Javid shunt was associated with a greater incidence of emboli on declamping. Although these factors may

TABLE 2.—Middle Cerebral Artery Blood Velocities

	Javid (n=73) Median (range)	Pruitt (n=73) Median (range)	Mann-Whitney (2-tailed p-test)
Pre	38 (3–85)	39 (19–87)	0.43
Clamp	25 (0–67)	26 (0–73)	0.76
Shunt	40 (16–109)	33 (12–90)	<0.005
Post	48 (13–120)	52 (15–93)	0.47

Note: Blood velocities are given in centimeters per second.

result in an increased risk of stroke, the numbers needed for statistical confirmation would be large.

▶ This study is impossible to interpret accurately. The Pruitt shunt seems to carry less blood, but its removal is associated with far fewer emboli. We made the decision years ago to primarily use the Pruitt shunt and have found no reason to change our opinion. I find the Javid arterial clamp to be quite damaging to the artery, and I have no desire to use this clamp on a regular basis. I regard this paper as interesting, albeit inconclusive. (See also Abstract 3–1.)

Predictive Ability of Duplex Ultrasonography for Internal Carotid Artery Stenosis of 70%–99%: A Comparative Study

Chen JC, Salvian AJ, Taylor DC, et al (Univ of British Columbia, Vancouver, Canada)

Ann Vasc Surg 12:244–247, 1998 3–3

Background.—The use of carotid endarterectomy (CEA) without angiography necessitates duplex US criteria that accurately predict stenosis of 70% or greater to minimize the performance of unnecessary surgery. An investigation was made of the accuracy of published duplex US criteria in identifying 70% to 99% internal carotid artery (ICA) stenosis using the North American Symptomatic Carotid Endarterectomy Trial (NASCET) method of measurement.

Methods.—Between March and December 1995, all patients considered for CEA were assessed with carotid duplex US and carotid angiography

TABLE 1.—Duplex US Criteria and Their Reported Sensitivity and Specificity for Inferring Internal Carotid Artery Stenosis of 70% or Greater According to NASCET

Author	Velocity criteria (cm/sec)	Sensitivity (%)	Specificity (%)
Browman et al.*	PSV > 175 or PSV < 40	91	60
Hunink et al.*	PSV > 230	80	90
Moneta et al.*	Ratio of ICA to CCA PSVs > 4	91	87
Faught et al.*	PSV > 130 plus EDV > 100	81	98
Neale et al.*	PSV > 270 plus EDV > 110	96	91
Strandness et al.*	PSV > 125 plus EDV > 135	99*	84*

Note: Information is according to North American Symptomatic Carotid Endarterectomy Trial Criteria.

*Result of comparison to angiography in which the degree of stenosis was determined using the normal carotid bulb diameter as the denominator.

Abbreviations: PSV, peak systolic velocity; *EDV*, end diastolic velocity; *ICA*, internal carotid artery; *CCA*, common carotid artery.

(Courtesy of Chen JC, Salvian AJ, Taylor DC, et al: Predictive ability of duplex ultrasonography for internal carotid artery stenosis of 70%–99%: A comparative study. *Ann Vasc Surg* 12:244–247, 1998.)

within 1 month of the US study. Duplex measurement of ICA peak systolic velocity (PSV), end diastolic velocity (EDV), and the ratio of the ICA to common carotid artery (CCA) PSVs were noted. The degree of stenosis was determined angiographically using NASCET criteria.

Findings.—Ninety-nine patients with a total of 185 carotid bifurcations were included in the final analysis. The duplex criteria for determining NASCET-defined 70% to 99% ICA stenosis were ICA PSV exceeding 175 cm/sec or PSV of less than 40 cm/sec, PSV of greater than 230 cm/sec, ratio of ICA to CCA PSV exceeding 4, PSV of greater than 130 cm/sec plus EDV of greater than 100 cm/sec, and PSV exceeding 270 cm/sec plus EDV of greater than 110 cm/sec. Compared with angiography, the calculated PPVs for these criteria were 71%, 81%, 86%, 88%, and 90%, respectively. The University of Washington criteria for critical stenosis—PSV of greater than 125 cm/sec plus EDV of greater than 135 cm/sec—have the highest PPV (91.6%) (Table 1).

Conclusion.—Carotid duplex US without angiography can be used to identify patients with 70% to 99% angiographic stenosis with an acceptable margin of error. This margin of error can be minimized by using the University of Washington criteria for critical stenosis.

► There is more to testing than positive predictive value. Although the University of Washington criteria (using the bulb, not the distal ICA) produced a high positive predictive value, it had the lowest sensitivity, namely 76%. I believe I would prefer a high sensitivity, even if it had a somewhat lower positive predictive value. Dr. Moneta of our group defined the criteria for NASCET as an ICA-CCA PSV ratio of greater than 4.0, with a sensitivity of 92%, a specificity of 80%, and a positive predictive value of 86%. This has been good enough for us, and I believe I will stick with it.

Duplex Imaging Findings Predict Stenosis After Carotid Endarterectomy

Golledge J, Cuming R, Ellis M, et al (Charing Cross and Westminster Med School, London)

J Vasc Surg 26:43–48, 1997 3–4

Background.—Duplex surveillance identifies restenosis in up to 20% of patients after carotid endarterectomy. Early duplex scanning has proven useful in evaluating the need for repeat surgery in patients with acute symptoms after carotid endarterectomy. The ability of this technique to predict the occurrence of restenosis was evaluated.

Methods.—Participants were 92 symptomatic patients, with a median age of 67 years, undergoing carotid endarterectomy. All were studied with color duplex scanning at 1 day and 1 week after surgery. These imaging studies were done to identify minor residual disease, arterial kinking, and suture kinking. The external and luminal diameters of the carotid bulb and distal internal carotid artery were measured at the same time. Prospective

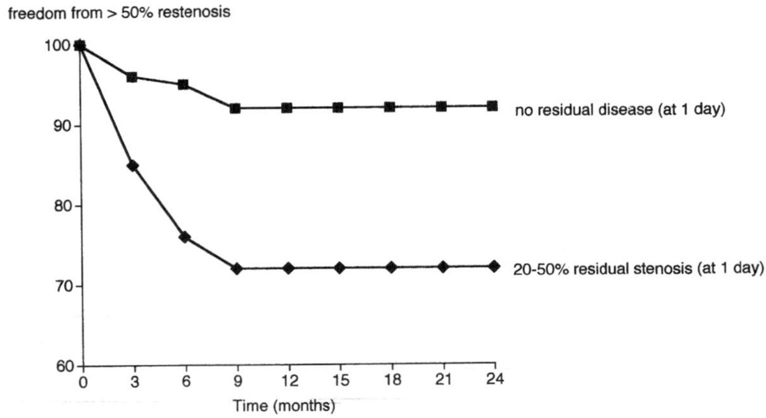

Numbers at risk

Time (months)	0	3	6	9	12	18	24
no residual disease	163	155	140	109	104	83	67
20-50% residual stenosis	25	19	16	13	13	13	12

FIGURE 1.—Development of restenosis in relation to residual disease identified 1 day after carotid endarterectomy. (Courtesy of Golledge J, Cuming R, Ellis M, et al: Duplex imaging findings predict stenosis after carotid endarterectomy. *J Vasc Surg* 26:43–48, 1997.)

duplex surveillance was then carried out for a median of 24 months for the occurrence of greater than 50% restenosis.

Results.—Duplex imaging identified stenoses in 13% of patients: residual stenoses in 4 patients at 1 day and restenosis in 21 patients at a median of 6 months. Multiple logistic regression analysis suggested that restenosis of greater than 50% was related to minor residual stenosis on the day after surgery and to small luminal diameter of the distal internal carotid artery at 1 week after surgery (Fig 1). On life-table analysis, the rate of restenosis at 24 months was 18% for patients with a carotid bulb external diameter of below the median vs. 5% for those with a diameter above the median.

Conclusions.—In patients undergoing carotid endarterectomy, duplex scanning performed within 1 week postoperatively can identify residual stenosis of greater than 50%. This imaging technique can also identify minor residual stenosis of 25% to 50%, as well as small carotid dimensions. All of these are good predictors of greater than 50% restenosis at 6 months.

▶ This interesting article concluded that greater than 50% recurrent carotid stenosis within 6 months of carotid endarterectomy was accurately predicted by finding a minor residual stenosis or a small luminal diameter of the distal internal carotid artery on duplex exam 7 days after surgery. While interesting, and probably accurate, I am not sure just how important this information really is. We follow-up our postoperative carotids routinely by duplex, and do not operate unless we find recurrent symptoms or extremely high-grade asymptomatic stenosis, certainly far in excess of the 50% described by these authors. This article can be added to a growing pile suggesting that less-than-perfect perioperative duplex results are associated with an increased risk of recurrent stenosis with time. Someday I may become sufficiently motivated to begin routine postoperative duplex surveillance or angiography in the operating room. But not yet.

Power Doppler Imaging of Carotid Artery Stenosis: Comparison With Color Doppler Flow Imaging and Angiography

Steinke W, Ries S, Artemis N, et al (Univ of Heidelberg, Germany)

Stroke 28:1981–1987, 1997 3–5

Background.—Power Doppler imaging (PDI) is a new technique in vascular imaging. The intravascular color signals generated by PDI depend on the number of red blood cells present. This means that the PDI color display is independent of the angle of insonation and of the direction of blood cell movement. As such, PDI may visualize the continuity of blood flow in arterial stenoses with improved sensitivity. The value of PDI for diagnosis of internal carotid artery (ICA) stenosis was assessed, including comparisons with color Doppler flow imaging (CDFI) and angiography.

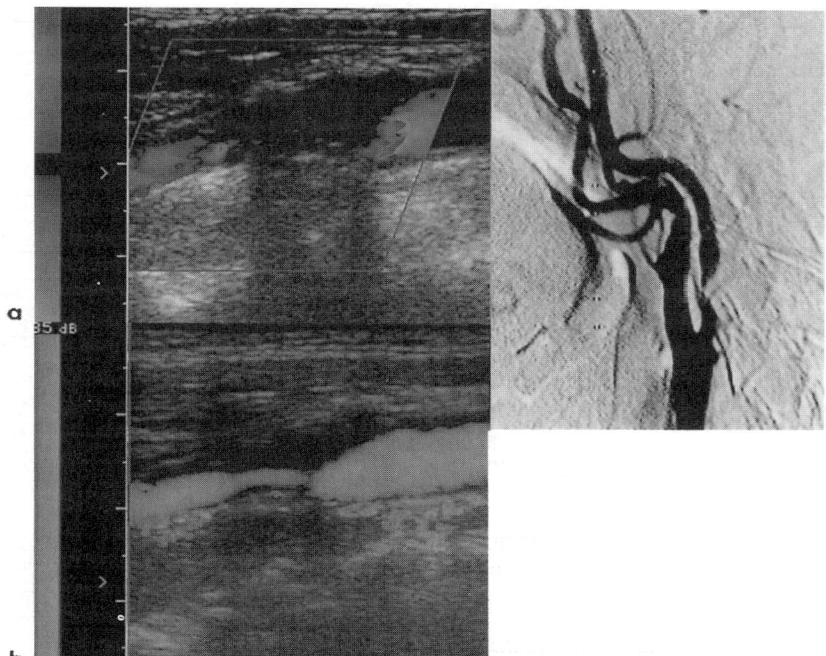

FIGURE 3.—High-grade ICA stenosis. A, poor display on CDFI without visualization of the residual stenotic lumen as a result of a calcified plaque at the anterior vessel wall with a dense echo shadow. B, color signals of PDI contrast the stenotic vascular lumen and the plaque surface. C, angiogram corresponds to PDI. (Steinke W, Ries S, Artemis N, et al: Power Doppler imaging of carotid artery stenosis: Comparison with color Doppler flow imaging and angiography. *Stroke* 1997, 28:1981–1987. Reproduced with permission *Stroke* Copyright 1997 American Heart Association.)

Methods.—The study sample comprised 128 ICA stenoses (at least 50%) and 12 complete occlusions in 100 patients. All patients underwent both PDI and CDFI. Forty-eight also underwent intra-arterial angiography. On PDI and CDFI, the diameter of stenosis was calculated by measuring the intrastenotic lumen on longitudinal views, whereas the area of stenosis was calculated from measurements made on transverse views. Standard methods were used to angiographically determine the degree of stenosis.

Results.—The view of the intrastenotic lumen was rated as good to excellent in 92% of cases with PDI, compared to 79% with CDFI. The advantage of PDI was particularly apparent in complicated, high-grade stenoses (Fig 3). The 2 sonographic techniques showed high overall correlation in terms of diameter and area of stenosis. Agreement was best for vessels with 80% to 99% area of stenosis. Angiography tended to underclassify stenoses when the North American Symptomatic Carotid Endarterectomy Trial method was used and to overclassify them when the European Carotid Surgery Trial and common carotid methods were used. Thus, there was only moderate correlation between the sonographic techniques and angiography.

Conclusions.—In the evaluation of ICA stenosis, PDI offers better visualization of the stenotic vascular lumen than does CDFI. Both sonographic techniques permit direct measurement of local stenosis, whereas angiography is more dependent on the method used for evaluation. The roles of PDI and CDFI in making decisions about carotid endarterectomy need further study.

▶ PDI is arguably one of the most important developments in vascular laboratory technology in recent years. It generates intravascular color signals according to reflected echo amplitude, which in turn depends almost exclusively on the number of red blood cells within the sample volume. The reflected echo amplitude is significantly independent of the angle of insonation and, more important, the velocity and direction of moving blood cells. The benefit of PDI, of course, is to produce a superior image, allowing detection of stenosis. In the comparative study described here, PDI provided significantly more good or excellent displays of the stenotic carotid lumen than did CDFI. Considerable additional information suggests they are correct.

Color Duplex Ultrasonography in the Diagnosis of Temporal Arteritis

Schmidt WA, Kraft HE, Vorpahl K, et al (Clinic of Rheumatology, Berlin-Buch; Klinikum Buch, Berlin)

N Engl J Med 337:1336–1342, 1997 3–6

Introduction.—A temporal artery biopsy is usually recommended to confirm the clinical diagnosis of temporal arteritis, but the procedure may lead to complications, and false-negative findings can occur if the biopsy is taken from an area without lesions. The value of color duplex ultrasonography (US) in diagnosing temporal arteritis in patients with clinically suspected active temporal arteritis or polymyalgia rheumatica was prospectively studied.

Methods.—Thirty patients met at least 3 of the 5 criteria for temporal arteritis. Biopsy was performed in 27 patients and yielded positive findings in 21, negative findings in 4, and insufficient material for analysis in 2. Symptoms of both temporal arteritis and polymyalgia rheumatica were present in 16; 2 had symptoms of temporal arteritis alone and 2 of polymyalgia rheumatica alone. Thirty-seven patients met 3 or more criteria for polymyalgia rheumatica, and 15 patients with negative histologic findings received a diagnosis other than temporal arteritis or polymyalgia rheumatica. Controls were 30 patients with rheumatoid arthritis but no signs of temporal arteritis. Two color duplex US studies performed in each case were read before the biopsy specimens.

Results.—In patients with temporal arteritis, the diameter of the artery wall was significantly larger than in the other groups. The US studies of 22 (73%) patients with temporal arteritis showed a dark halo around the lumen of the temporal arteries, and the halos disappeared after corticosteroid treatment (mean 16 days). Stenoses or occlusions of temporal artery segments were present in 80% of patients; 93% had stenoses, occlusions, or a halo. None of the US studies of patients without temporal arteritis showed a halo, but stenoses or occlusions were observed in 7%. The interrater agreement was 95% for each of the 3 types of abnormalities identified at US.

Conclusions.—Color duplex US visualizes characteristic signs of temporal arteritis with a sensitivity and specificity that may provide a diagnosis without the need for temporal artery biopsy. A dark halo is the most specific sign; patients with strong clinical evidence of temporal arteritis but no clear halo should still undergo biopsy.

▶ Most of us are asked on occasion to biopsy temporal arteries to establish the diagnosis of temporal arteritis. This interesting study suggests that between 70% and 75% of patients with positive biopsies will show a specific temporal artery ultrasonographic pattern consisting of a dark halo around the lumen. This halo may be caused by edema of the arterial wall, although no one knows for sure. The authors suggest that this sign may be sufficiently specific to allow the initiation of steroid treatment without the necessity for temporal artery biopsy. This may represent a real step forward in the diagnosis of temporal arteritis.

Echo-Lucency of Computerized Ultrasound Images of Carotid Atherosclerotic Plaques Are Associated With Increased Levels of Trigylceride-rich Lipoproteins as Well as Increased Plaque Lipid Content

Grønholdt MM, Nordestgaard BG, Wiebe BM, et al (Rigshospitalet, Copenhagen; Herlev Hosp, Denmark; Gentofte Hosp, Denmark; et al)

Circulation 97:34–40, 1998 3–7

Background.—Carotid artery plaques that are echolucent (i.e., that weakly reflect B-mode ultrasound) are associated with higher plasma levels of triglyceride-rich lipoproteins. Furthermore, echolucent plaques have a higher lipid content, which increases their likelihood of rupture. The authors examined whether measurements of plasma triglyceride-rich lipo-

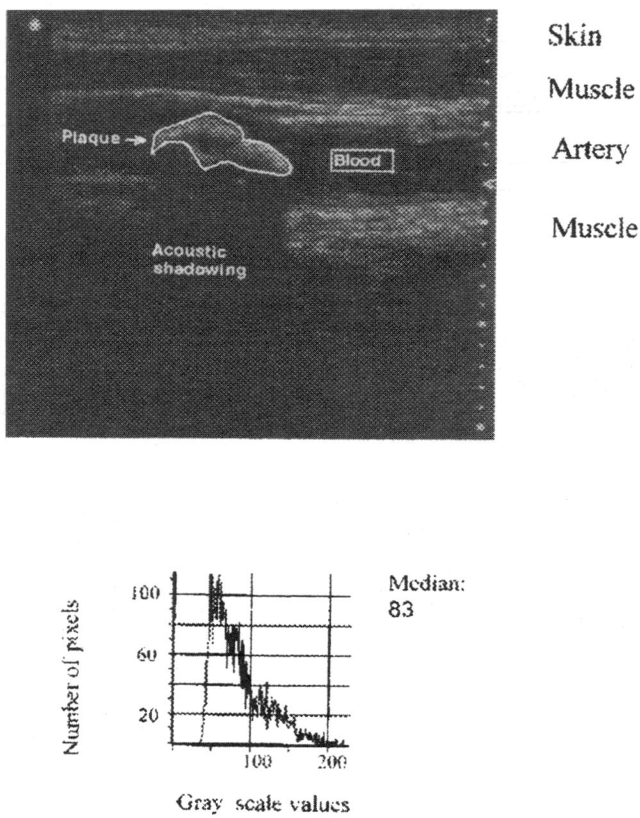

FIGURE.—Ultrasound B-mode image of a carotid artery plaque. *Outline* (excluding the *acoustic shadowing*) shows the plaque area where gray-scale levels of all pixels are used to construct the histogram showing distribution of gray-scale level among pixels. Median of the gray-scale level is used for further analysis. (Courtesy of Grønholdt MM, Nordestgaard BG, Wiebe BM, et al: Echo-lucency of computerized ultrasound images of carotid atherosclerotic plaques are associated with increased levels of triglyceride-rich lipoproteins as well as increased plaque lipid content. *Circulation* 97:34–40, 1998.)

TABLE 1.—Results of the Kappa Analysis and the Level of Accuracy Achieved in Detecting Normal (0% to 49%), Stenosed (50% to 99%), and Occluded (100%) Infrapopliteal Arteries

	Distinguishing normal from occluded arteries			Distinguishing normal, stenosed, and occluded arteries		
	Kappa value	95% Confidence Interval	Accuracy (%)	Kappa value	95% Confidence Interval	Accuracy (%)
Angio 1 vs. Angio 2	0.80	0.70–0.89	91	0.70	0.61–0.79	82
Angio 1 vs. Duplex	0.61	0.49–0.74	84	0.50	0.39–0.62	72
Angio 2 vs. Duplex	0.63	0.50–0.74	84	0.50	0.39–0.61	72

(Reprinted from Sensier Y, Fishwick G, Owen R, et al: A comparison between color Duplex ultrasonography and arteriography for imaging infrapopliteal arterial lesions. *Eur J Vasc Endovasc Surg* 15:44–50. Copyright 1998, by permission of the publisher, WB Saunders Company Limited, London.)

infrapopliteal arteries or the full length of each tibial and peroneal artery. The ability of color duplex US to identify patent, stenotic, and occluded infrapopliteal arteries was examined.

Methods.—The infrapopliteal vasculature in 51 limbs was assessed by color duplex US and digital subtraction angiography. All arteries from the distal popliteal to the pedal were examined, for a total of 204 individual arterial segments. Each segment was classified as 0% to 49% diameter reduced, 50% to 99% diameter reduced, or occluded. Stenosis classification on US was achieved by observing peak systolic velocity ratios. A doubling of peak systolic velocity indicated a 50% or greater diameter-reducing stenosis. When no Doppler signal was evident, the vessel was assumed to be occluded. Two radiologists independently evaluated disease extent on angiographic studies for each infrapopliteal artery, noting areas of 50% or greater diameter reduction and occlusion.

Findings.—The overall Kappa level of agreement between US and angiographic assessment for distinguishing patent from occluded segments was 0.61. The agreement between the radiologists' interpretations was 0.8. The lowest agreement was for US assessments of the peroneal and tibioperoneal trunk arterial segments (Table 1).

Conclusion.—Moderate levels of agreement were observed between US and arteriography in distinguishing patent, stenosed, and occluded run-off arteries. These levels of agreement did not differ significantly from those of the 2 radiologists interpreting the same arteriograms. Thus, color duplex US can be used to assess infrapopliteal artery patency.

▶ The authors emphasize that few previous reports have assessed the infrapopliteal vessels systematically or differentiated between patent, stenotic, and, occluded vessels to evaluate whether reconstructive surgery can be based alone on duplex US. Consequently, it would have been of considerable interest had the study addressed whether a surgical plan based on duplex US differed from that based on angiography. Moreover, to be accepted as a reasonable alternative to an established procedure—i.e., arteriography—it is important to consider essential methodologic problems.

The fact that 5 arterial segments were not examined because of time constraints indicates that time consumption related to the procedure might be a problem. I assume that the authors have left the 5 not-examined segments out of the analysis, which can be criticized according to the principle of intention to treat. Duplex US is an investigator-dependent technique. Consequently, it would have been of interest to also assess the variability among the 4 ultrasonographers who performed the examinations. On balance, this study is unconvincing.

T.V. Schroeder, M.D., D.M.Sc.

Duplex Assessment of Run-off Before Femorocrural Reconstruction

Wilson YG, George JK, Wilkins DC, et al (Derriford Hosp, Plymouth, England)
Br J Surg 84:1360–1363, 1997 3–12

Background.—The quality of distal vascular runoff has a major impact on the results of femorotibial reconstruction for occlusive vascular disease. Contrast arteriography is the "gold standard" for preoperative assessment, but supplemental techniques are sought to help in identifying the optimal run-off vessel before surgery. Color duplex imaging was evaluated for use in assessing distal runoff before femorocrural reconstruction.

Methods.—A total of 43 consecutive patients with critical ischemia who were to undergo infrapopliteal bypass for limb salvage were studied. There were 33 men and 10 women, whose mean age was 78 years. Twelve patients had diabetes; 1 was undergoing bilateral reconstruction. Preoperatively, the patients underwent 3 separate runoff assessments: Doppler examination performed by a vascular surgeon, arteriography performed by a radiologist, and color duplex imaging performed by a vascular technologist. Each study was performed without knowledge of the other results. The results of duplex imaging were compared with the intraoperative findings and graft results, and with the arteriographic findings.

TABLE 2.—Comparative Performance of Dependent Doppler, Contrast Arteriography, and Duplex Scanning in the Preoperative Detection and Selection of a Suitable Run-off Vessel as Verified by Intraoperative Findings and Follow-up

	Dependent Doppler	Arteriography	Duplex
Suitable vessel selected	21 (48)	32 (72)	44 (100)
Equivocal	4 (9)	6 (14)	0
Failed	19 (43)	3 (7)	0
Suboptimal vessel selected	0	3 (7)	0

Values in parenthesis are percentages.

(Courtesy of Wilson YG, George JK, Wilkins DC, et al: Duplex assessment of run-off before femorocrural reconstruction. *Br J Surg* 84:1360–1363.)

Results.—Thirty-day primary cumulative graft patency was 86%. A suitable runoff vessel was correctly identified by dependent Doppler in 47% of cases. However, the Doppler results were indeterminate in 10% of limbs and unrecordable in 43%. With arteriography, a suitable runoff vessel was correctly identified in 73% of cases; the results were indeterminate in 14%, and no runoff was demonstrated in 7%. In 7% of cases, the vessel identified by arteriography was suboptimal for bypass. Duplex imaging correctly identified a suitable runoff vessel in 100% of cases (Table 2).

Conclusions.—In patients with critical leg ischemia, preoperative color duplex imaging is superior to arteriography in defining the distal tibial and pedal runoff. Duplex imaging for noninvasive preoperative assessment of runoff may avoid the need for blind surgical exploration or on-table arteriography.

▶ The answer, dear reader, is simple to me. Duplex takes too long and simply cannot reliably detect patent vessels in the lower limb. Dedicated arteriography performed by professionals using a variety of techniques including, but not limited to, downstream injection, pharmacologic dilatation, limb hyperemia, etc., in my experience can visualize 99.9% of all vessels available for arterial bypass. I am convinced a high-quality preoperative arteriogram is the best way to ensure optimal surgical results. Thirty-day cumulative graft patency reported in this paper of only 86% is worrisome.

Distal Lower Extremity Arteries: Evaluation With Two-dimensional MR Digital Subtraction Angiography

Lee HM, Wang Y, Sostman HD, et al (Cornell Univ, New York)

Radiology 207:505–512, 1998 3–13

Background.—Two-dimensional time-of-flight (TOF) MR angiography is of value for imaging the tibial runoff vessels of the calf and foot. However, various artifacts lead to reduced image quality and diagnostic accuracy. Two-dimensional MR digital subtraction angiography avoids these limitations. Magnetic resonance digital subtraction angiography was compared with TOF MR angiography for imaging of distal lower extremity arteries.

Methods.—A total of 23 consecutive patients undergoing MRI of the foot and ankle for clinical indications were studied prospectively. Thirty-seven extremities were imaged with both 2-dimensional TOF MR angiography and MR digital subtraction angiography. The scans were read in randomized, blinded fashion, with attention to 7 potential arterial segments and the number of digital arteries visualized. The 2 studies were compared for overall image quality and for ability to demonstrate patent arterial segments.

Results.—Both patent arterial segments and digital arteries were better imaged by MR digital subtraction angiography than by TOF MR angiog-

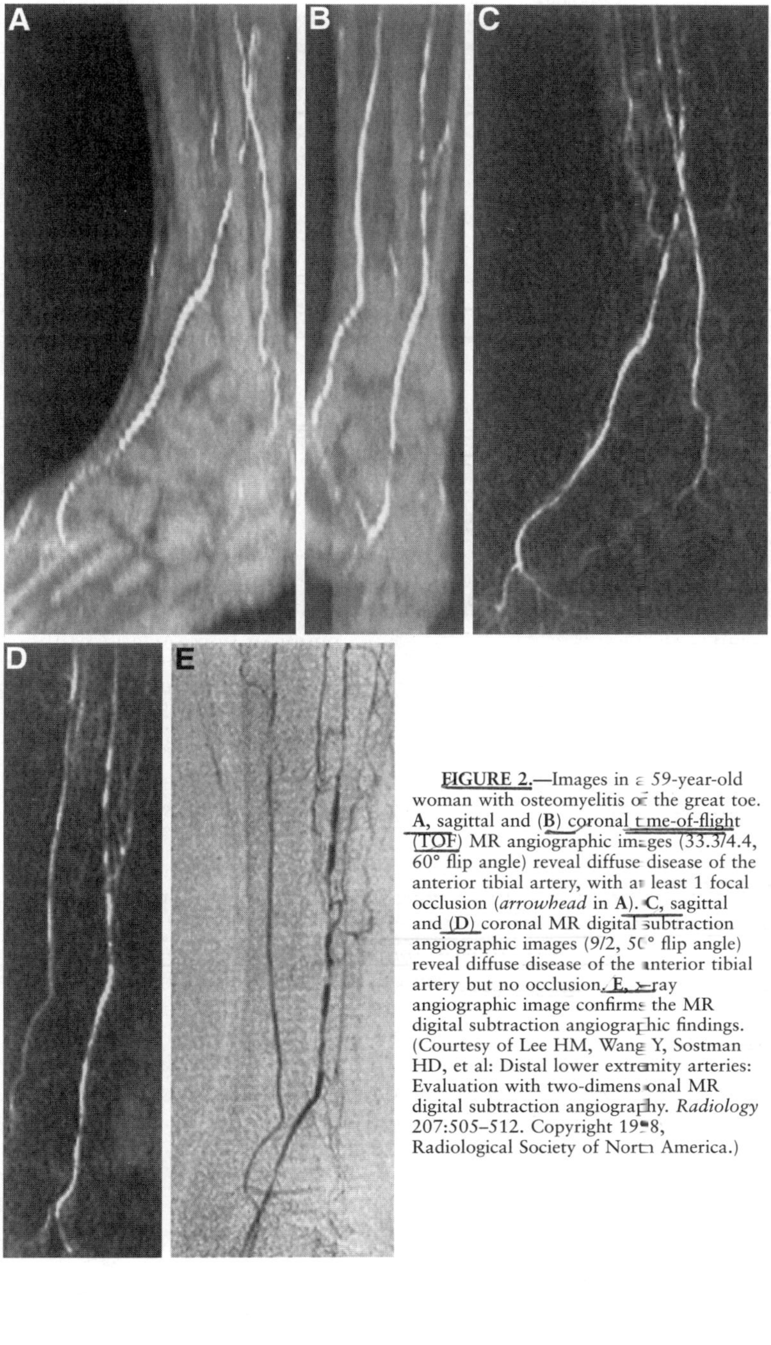

FIGURE 2.—Images in a 59-year-old woman with osteomyelitis of the great toe. A, sagittal and (B) coronal time-of-flight (TOF) MR angiographic images (33.3/4.4, 60° flip angle) reveal diffuse disease of the anterior tibial artery, with at least 1 focal occlusion (*arrowhead* in A). C, sagittal and (D) coronal MR digital subtraction angiographic images (9/2, 50° flip angle) reveal diffuse disease of the anterior tibial artery but no occlusion. E, x-ray angiographic image confirms the MR digital subtraction angiographic findings. (Courtesy of Lee HM, Wang Y, Sostman HD, et al: Distal lower extremity arteries: Evaluation with two-dimensional MR digital subtraction angiography. *Radiology* 207:505–512. Copyright 1998, Radiological Society of North America.)

raphy. Image quality was higher with MR digital subtraction angiography as well (Fig 2).

Conclusions.—In MR examination of the distal lower extremity, 2-dimensional MR digital subtraction angiography is more effective than TOF MR angiography in demonstrating patent arterial segments in the tibial runoff vessels. The authors call for larger studies using conventional angiography to establish the diagnostic accuracy of MR digital subtraction angiography.

▶ While 2-dimensional TOF MR angiography has enjoyed considerable clinical utility, it is limited by a number of artifacts, including spin saturation from in-plane flow, artifacts from turbulent flow, and stepladder motion artifacts of reformatted intensity images. Even venous saturation pulses may eliminate arterial signals when the arterial flow is retrograde. Two-dimensional MR digital subtraction angiography using gadolinium has none of these limitations and appears to be superior. I do hope we will soon come to the day when we can reliably obtain high-quality MR angiography. I continue to believe we would be best served if all arterial imaging modalities, including MR, contrast CT, and arteriography were under the control of the same radiologic physicians. They could then pick the modality best suited for the study and the patient without turf considerations. Perhaps one day we shall arrive at this version of nirvana.

Lower Extremity Arterial Evaluation: Are Segmental Arterial Blood Pressures Worthwhile?

Gale SS, Scissons RP, Salles-Cunha SX, et al (Jobst Vascular Ctr, Toledo, Ohio)

J Vasc Surg 27:831–839, 1998 3–14

Background.—The severity of lower extremity arterial disease can be assessed using blood flow waveform analysis and blood pressure measurements. Segmental blood pressures (SEGPs) are commonly measured at the thigh, calf, and ankle; however, little is known about their diagnostic value. The effects of SEGP data on diagnostic accuracy in the noninvasive lower extremity arterial evaluation were assessed.

Methods.—Participants included 81 patients in whom continuous-wave Doppler velocity waveforms were recorded at the levels of the common femoral artery (CFA), the popliteal artery (POP), and the dorsal pedal and posterior tibial (TIB) arteries (Fig 1). Systolic SEGP measurements were performed at the upper thigh, upper calf, and ankle. Fourteen technologists or physicians interpreted the waveforms alone and with the addition of ankle-brachial indices (ABIs) and SEGP data, without knowledge of the clinical and arteriographic findings. The presence of severe (75% or greater) stenosis was assessed for the iliofemoral artery (CFA), the superficial-femoral artery (SFA), the popliteal artery (POP), and the infrapopliteal artery (TIB). The analysis included a total of 9,072 segments.

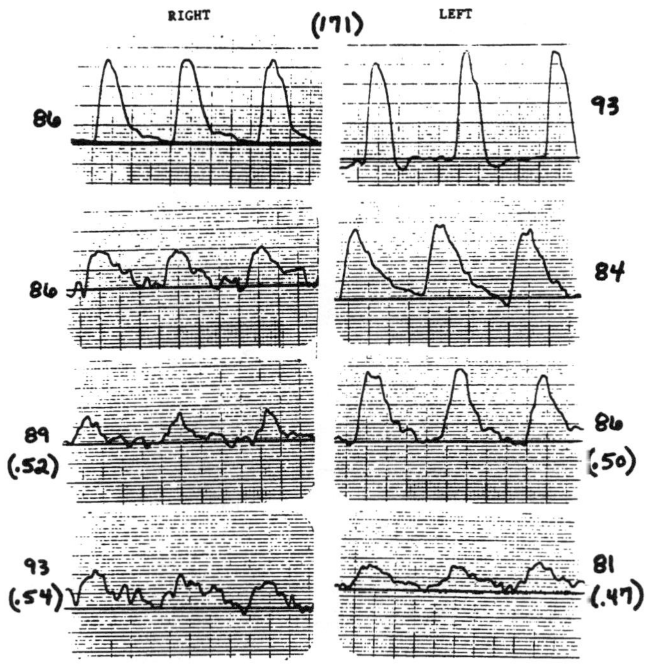

FIGURE 1.—Lower extremity arterial physiologic testing. Blood flow velocity waveforms at the right and left common femoral, popliteal, posterior tibial, and dorsal pedal arteries are shown from **top** to **bottom**. The highest right or left arm pressure and right and left thigh, upper calf, and ankle pressures are also presented from **top** to **bottom** with ankle-brachial indices within parentheses. (Courtesy of Gale SS, Scissons RP, Salles-Cunha SX, et al: Lower extremity arterial evaluation: Are segmental arterial blood pressures worthwhile? *J Vasc Surg* 27:831–839, 1998.)

Results.—Waveform analysis was 83% accurate in demonstrating severe stenosis at or proximal to the CFA, 79% for the SFA, 64% for the POP, and 73% for the TIB. The addition of ABI to waveform analysis significantly improved accuracy at all sites: 88% at the CFA, 86% at the SFA, 70% at the POP, and 85% at the TIB. The results were not as good with the combination of waveform analysis and SEGP: 86% at the CFA, 85% at the SFA, 70% at the POP, and 80% at the TIB (Table 3).

Conclusions.—The addition of ABI data to Doppler waveform analysis significantly improves the accuracy of noninvasive lower extremity arterial evaluation. No such improvement is noted when SEFP measurements are added to waveform analysis. The findings suggest that SEGP measurements performed above the level of the ankle are neither clinically useful nor cost-effective.

► We have always used 4 cuff leg pressures as part of the vascular lab peripheral arterial examinations and find them helpful, although we recognize they are not the final word. I do not waste time with arterial waveform analysis, because I consider this little more than subjective. I suppose, however, if you are using arterial waveform analysis as the gold standard,

TABLE 3.—Comparison of Physiologic Assessment and Arteriography for Lower Extremity Arterial Occlusive Disease

*Assessment**	*CFA*	*SFA*	*POP*	*TIB*
Accuracy				
Waveforms	83%	79%	64%	73%
plus ABI	88%	86%	70%	85%
plus SEGP	86%	85%	70%	80%
Sensitivity				
Waveforms	86%	77%	51%	75%
plus ABI	87%	86%	69%	90%
plus SEGP	89%	87%	57%	85%
Specificity				
Waveforms	82%	81%	67%	67%
plus ABI	88%	85%	70%	69%
plus SEGP	85%	82%	73%	65%
Positive predictive value				
Waveforms	49%	80%	30%	89%
plus ABI	59%	85%	39%	91%
plus SEGP	55%	83%	37%	89%
Negative predictive value				
Waveforms	97%	79%	83%	44%
plus ABI	97%	86%	89%	67%
plus SEGP	97%	97%	86%	56%

*Location code: significant arterial stenosis (≥75% diameter reduction) at and proximal to the CFA, SFA, POP, and TIB arteries. Assessment code: waveforms obtained at the CFA, POP, distal posterior tibial, and dorsal pedal arteries.

Abbreviations: CFA, common femoral artery; *SFA*, superficial femoral artery; *POP*, popliteal artery; *TIB*, infrapopliteal arteries; *ABI*, ankle systolic pressure ratio (index) obtained at the posterior tibial and dorsal pedal (anterior tibial) arteries; *SEGP*, segmental pressures obtained at the thigh, upper calf, and ankle.

(Courtesy of Gale SS, Scissons RP, Salles-Cunha SX, et al: Lower extremity arterial evaluation: Are segmental arterial blood pressures worthwhile? *J Vasc Surg* 27:831–839, 1998.)

perhaps the addition of ABI will allow you to improve your waveform analysis more easily than the addition of segmental leg pressures. I find this entire study curious and just a wee bit flawed. Our position on segmental waveforms has been published.[1]

Reference

1. Moneta GL, Yeager RA, Lee RW, et al: Noninvasive localization of arterial occlusive disease. *J Vasc Surg* 17:578–582, 1993.

In Vitro Evaluation of Multiple Arterial Stenoses Using Three-dimensional Power Doppler Angiography

Guo Z, Durand L-G, Allard L, et al (George Washington Univ, Washington, DC; Clinical Research Inst of Montreal; John P Robarts Research Inst, London, Ont, Canada)

J Vasc Surg 27:681–688, 1998 3–15

Background.—Doppler spectral analysis is widely used for quantification of lower limb arterial stenoses. There is evidence to suggest that the sensitivity and accuracy of waveform analysis are reduced in limbs with

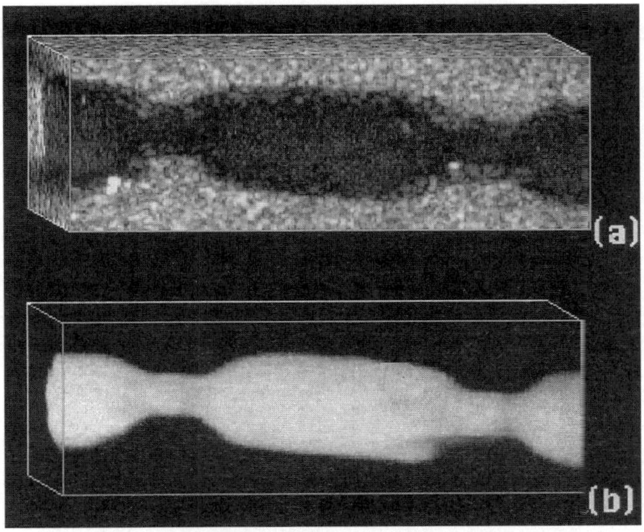

FIGURE 2.—Three-dimensional (3D) B-mode image (A) and 3D power Doppler angiogram (B) of the porcine artery with long stenoses. A steady flow of 25 mL/sec was used to generate the 3D power Doppler angiogram. (Courtesy of Guo Z, Durand L-G, Allard L, et al: In vitro evaluation of multiple arterial stenoses using three-dimensional power Doppler angiography. J Vasc Surg 27:681–688, 1998.)

multisegmental arterial stenoses. Three-dimensional power Doppler angiography was evaluated as a new technique for imaging and measurement of multiple arterial stenoses.

Methods.—The in vitro study used artery phantoms containing multiple stenoses, one made of stenotic porcine arteries and the other designed to evaluate central stenosis of a wall-less agar lumen, controlling for proximal and distal stenoses. Using an experimental 3-dimensional ultrasound imaging system, power Doppler angiograms of the lumens were created at varying rates of steady and pulsatile flow. The computerized system permitted offline 3-dimensional acquisition, reconstruction, and display of ultrasound images. The power Doppler luminal images were compared with measurements made on B-mode ultrasound or with the true geometry of the stenoses.

Results.—Three-dimensional power Doppler angiography created high-quality 3-dimensional images of the flow lumens (Fig 2). Diagnosis of arterial stenoses was possible in the presence of multiple stenoses. The technique was associated with an average error of −10% in estimating 80% area reduction stenoses and −4% in estimating 50% area reduction stenoses (Fig 4).

Conclusions.—Three-dimensional power Doppler angiography is a promising new technique for quantitative grading of multiple lower limb stenoses. It can also produce a map of the vasculature for surgical planning. Clinical studies are needed to compare 3-dimensional power Doppler angiography with 2-dimensional power Doppler imaging and contrast angiography for quantification of multisegmental stenoses.

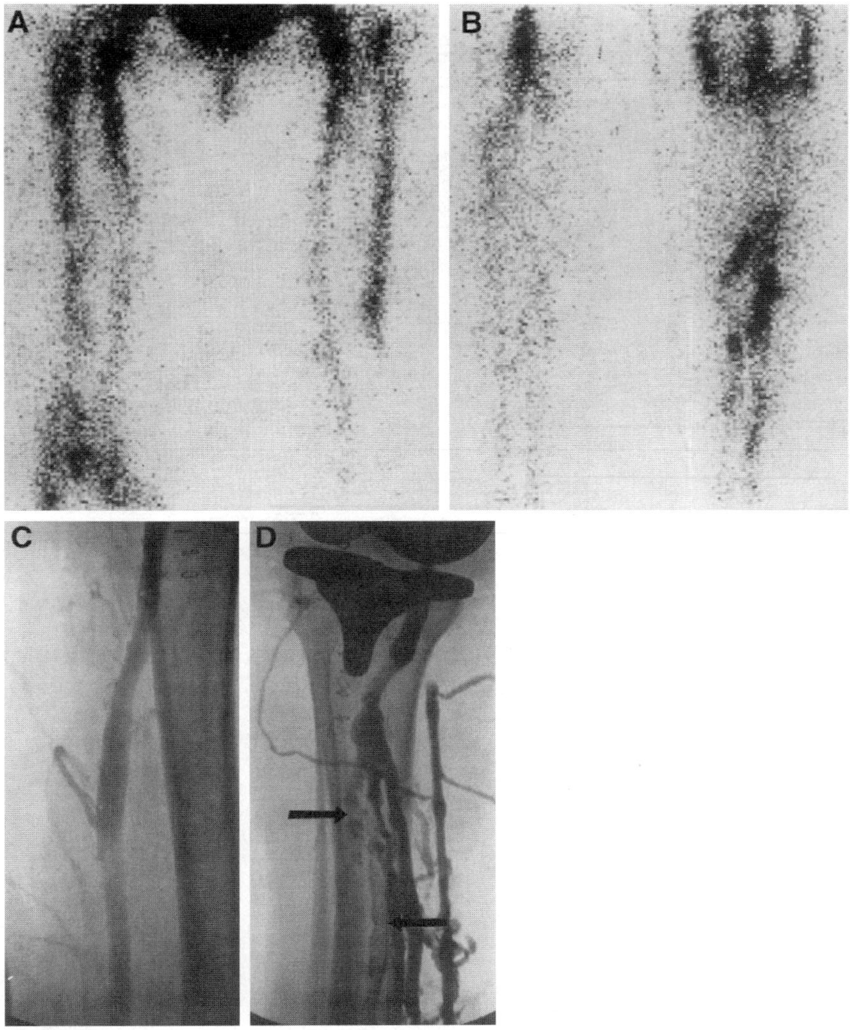

FIGURE 2.—A, anterior thigh image demonstrating symmetrical tracer accumulation in femoral veins. Uptake of tracer surrounding the right total knee replacement and in the bone marrow of the femoral shafts is prominent. **B**, posterior calf scan demonstrating marked accumulation of tracer in the right midcalf region. Minimal tracer uptake is seen in the contralateral calf. **C**, normal contrast venogram of right femoral vein in same patient. **D**, contrast venogram of right calf veins demonstrating thrombosis involving the deep veins of the calf (*arrows*). (Courtesy of Butler SP, Rahman T, Boyd SJ, et al: Detection of postoperative deep-venous thrombosis using technetium-99m-labeled tissue plasminogen activator. *J Nucl Med* 38:219–223, 1997. Reprinted by permission of the Society of Nuclear Medicine.)

plasty patients was evaluated for the presence of DVT by means of scintigraphic scanning with technetium-99m–labeled modified recombinant tissue plasminogen activator (^{99m}Tc-rt-PA).

Methods.—The study group included 53 consecutive patients with a mean age of 71 years; 23 had total knee replacements and 30 had total hip replacements. Scintigraphic scanning with ^{99m}Tc-rt-PA followed by contrast venography was performed before discharge at an average of 7 days after surgery. All were receiving subcutaneous prophylactic heparin at the time of the studies. Scintigraphic scans were viewed by 2 nuclear medicine physicians "blinded" to the results of contrast venography. Positive scintigraphic criteria for femoral, calf, and popliteal veins consisted of increased tracer accumulation in comparison with the contralateral side; for popliteal veins, patients were also to have coexisting calf or femoral thrombosis.

Results.—Contrast venography, the gold standard for detection of DVT, yielded 84 segments of diagnostic quality and 22 that were excluded from analysis as uninterpretable. Thromboses were seen in 15 segments, 1 proximal and 14 distal, and were detected in 65% of total knee replacement patients vs. 13% of total hip replacement patients. All scintigraphic scans were judged to be of diagnostic quality. Fourteen of 15 thrombosed segments had positive scans (Fig 2); 63 of 69 nonthrombosed segments had negative scans. Scintigraphic scanning with ^{99m}Tc-rt-PA had a sensitivity of 93% and a specificity of 91% for the detection of DVT.

Conclusions.—Scintigraphic scanning with ^{99m}Tc-rt-PA provides a noninvasive method of detecting DVT in patients undergoing total hip or knee arthroplasty. Although the technique shows a high level of sensitivity and specificity, bilateral DVT may be difficult to detect because asymmetry is the criterion for a positive scan.

▶ These investigators compared technetium-labeled tissue plasminogen activator as a scanning agent with contrast phlebography in the detection of postoperative venous thrombosis. Without question, the scintigraphic technique worked well, with an overall sensitivity of 93% and specificity of 91%, compared with phlebography. As I review the scintigraphic scans, they appear a bit vague and subjective to me. The authors dismiss the use of duplex scanning for the detection of asymptomatic venous thromboses, basing these conclusions on historic articles published more than 5 years ago. I am convinced from our recent experience that venous duplex has become sufficiently accurate that it most assuredly can be used in the detection of asymptomatic venous thrombosis in all parts of the leg, including the calf. I am sorry the authors did not include venous duplex as one limb of this study. I hope this obscure scintigraphic technique does not catch on as an imaging technique of choice. I think it would be a step backward.

The Role of Air Plethysmography in the Diagnosis of Chronic Venous Insufficiency

Criado E, Farber MA, Marston WA, et al (Univ of North Carolina, Chapel Hill)
J Vasc Surg 27:660–670, 1998 3–20

Background.—Diagnostic investigation of chronic venous insufficiency (CVI) focuses on the demonstration of venous valvular reflux in the various venous systems. The role of air plethysmography (APG) in this process remains unclear. The clinical utility of APG in diagnosing CVI was investigated, including correlations between APG and the clinical severity of disease and the anatomical distribution of reflux.

Methods.—Duplex scanning and venography were performed in 186 limbs of 108 patients. In addition, APG was performed for measurement of venous volume, venous filling index (VFI), ejection fraction, and residual volume fraction. Clinical severity ratings were based on the Society for Vascular Surgery and International Society for Cardiovascular Surgery classifications, and on the anatomical distribution of valvular incompetence on duplex scanning and venography.

Results.—There was no evidence of disease in 61 limbs, mild disease in 60 limbs, and severe disease in 65 limbs. Duplex scanning and venography suggested that reflux was absent in 56 limbs. Fifty-two limbs showed isolated superficial venous reflux; 30 had perforator reflux, with or without superficial reflux; and 19 had deep and perforator reflux, with or without superficial reflux.

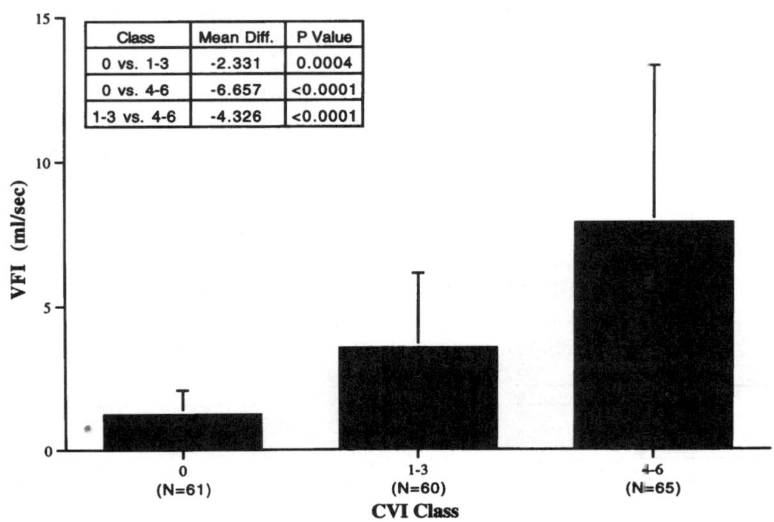

Class	Mean Diff.	P Value
0 vs. 1-3	-2.331	0.0004
0 vs. 4-6	-6.657	<0.0001
1-3 vs. 4-6	-4.326	<0.0001

FIGURE 1.—Comparison of venous filling index (*VFI*) values by severity of disease for 186 limbs studied with air plethysmography. The table depicts mean differences and *P* values for group comparisons. Statistical significance among all 3 groups exists. *Abbreviation: CVI*, chronic venous insufficiency. (Courtesy of Criado E, Farber MA, Marston WA, et al: The role of air plethysmography in the diagnosis of chronic venous insufficiency. *J Vasc Surg* 660–670, 1998.)

For the identification of reflux of any type, VFI offered a sensitivity of 80% and positive predictive value of 99%. This index was capable of distinguishing between limbs of varying clinical severity or different types of reflux (Fig 1). When VFI was normal, deep or perforator reflux was present in only 7% of limbs. In contrast, when VFI was greater than 5, the incidence of deep or perforator reflux was 82%. The incidence of deep or perforator reflux was 72% in 86 limbs with VFI values that were not corrected with the use of a thigh tourniquet, compared with 33% in 15 limbs with tourniquet-corrected VFI values. Air plethysmography did not effectively predict severe disease or ulceration. Disease severity did not vary with ejection fraction or residual volume fraction. These parameters could not differentiate between different types of reflux and did not add to the predictive value of APG.

Conclusions.—Air plethysmographic measurement of VFI is highly effective in predicting the presence of venous reflux and in estimating the clinical severity of disease. It is of some help in predicting the presence of perforator and deep vein reflux but does not correlate with disease severity or the presence of ulceration. The diagnostic value of the ejection fraction and residual volume fraction does not justify their routine clinical performance.

▶ We have been unable to get much mileage out of the air plethysmograph in our unit. I believe this device has basic design flaws, primarily the unrealistic expectation that one size fits all and fits all precisely. These authors found that the VFI measured by the APG was a satisfactory test providing an estimate of the clinical severity of disease, although even they noted that the thigh tourniquet added little, and the predictive value of APG for severe disease or ulceration was poor. The ejection fraction and residual volume fraction individually or in combination with VFI added virtually no important information. We have substantially abandoned the use of the APG in our lab. We depend on duplex insonation of valve sites for reflux, combined with venous recovery time. We simply have no confidence in the air plethysmograph. (See also Abstract 16–2.)

A New Method for the Assessment of Venous Insufficiency in Primary Varicose Veins Using Near-infrared Spectroscopy

Hosoi Y, Yasuhara H, Shigematsu H, et al (Univ of Tokyo)

J Vasc Surg 26:53–60, 1997 3–21

Background.—Venous function in patients with chronic venous insufficiency (CVI) has been evaluated with duplex scanning and plethysmography, but these techniques cannot be used to assess the patient during exercise. It is now possible to measure changes in tissue deoxygenated hemoglobin (DeoHb) and oxygenated hemoglobin during movement noninvasively with the use of near-infrared spectroscopy (NIRS). This tech-

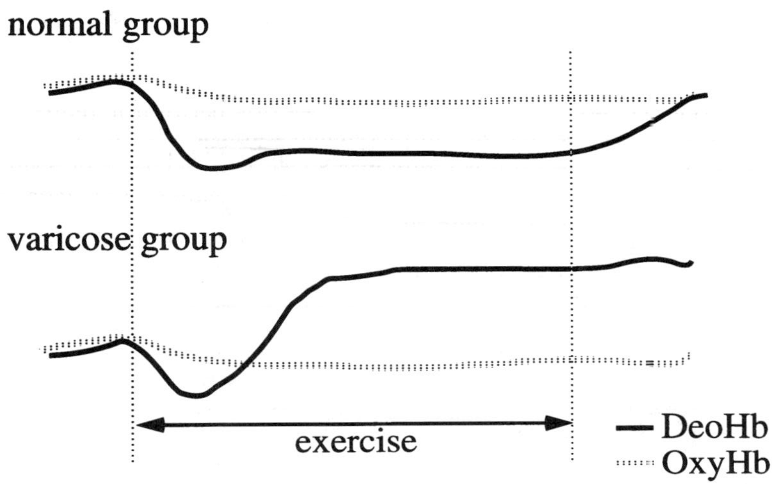

FIGURE 1.—Patterns of serial changes in OxyHb and DeoHb. A difference in waveform was apparent between the normal and varicose groups. *Abbreviations: OxyHb*, oxygenated hemoglobin; *DeoHb*, deoxygenated hemoglobin. (Courtesy of Hosoi Y, Yasuhara H, Shigematsu H, et al: A new method for the assessment of venous insufficiency in primary varicose veins using near-infrared spectroscopy. *J Vasc Surg* 26:53–60, 1997.)

nique was used to examine ambulatory venous function in patients with CVI.

Methods.—Two groups of subjects were studied: 59 patients with a total of 72 primary varicose veins, and 13 volunteers, in whom a total of 20 normal limbs were studied. According to the International Consensus Committee classification, the limbs of the patients with varicose veins were graded as having mild CVI, class 2 or 3, 50 limbs; moderate CVI, class 4, 11 limbs; and severe CVI, class 5 or 6, 11 limbs. During a treadmill walking test, all participants underwent NIRS for continuous measurement of oxygenated hemoglobin and DeoHb. Changes in DeoHb over time were used to compare the ambulatory venous retention index in normal limbs vs. limbs with mild, moderate, or severe CVI. Air plethysmographic data were available for comparison in 19 limbs of 13 patients.

Results.—In normal subjects, calf muscle contraction caused a decrease in the DeoHb level. In contrast, the patients showed increasing DeoHb during exercise, apparently because of venous reflux into the calf muscles (Fig 1). The ambulatory venous retention index did not appear to be related to the ejection fraction. However, it was significantly correlated with the venous filling index and weakly correlated with the residual volume fraction.

Conclusions.—In patients with primary varicose veins, the new technique of NIRS provides an accurate assessment of venous dysfunction during walking. In addition to evaluating the severity of CVI, NIRS may prove useful in assessing the hemodynamic effects of surgery and the natural history of CVI.

▶ This clever article informs us that the pattern of deoxyhemoglobin in the skin of the leg, measured by near-infrared spectroscopy, differs considerably in patients with normal limbs compared with that in patients with venous insufficiency. NIRS would appear to offer yet another method of determining the presence of venous insufficiency, in addition to the duplex determination of venous valvular insufficiency and the venous recovery time. Presently, I have no idea of the accuracy or the cost of the NIRS hardware. (See also Abstract 1–21.)

Acute Pulmonary Embolism: Role of Helical CT in 164 Patients With Intermediate Probability at Ventilation-Perfusion Scintigraphy and Normal Results at Duplex US of the Legs

Ferretti GR, Bosson J-L, Buffaz P-D, et al (Centre Hospitalier Universitaire Grenoble, France)

Radiology 205:453–458, 1997 3–22

Objective.—Helical CT is a minimally invasive technique that has shown good sensitivity and specificity for diagnosing pulmonary embolism (PE). The clinical usefulness of helical CT was prospectively evaluated, and the outcome during 3-month follow-up in patients who did not receive anticoagulant treatment because of normal findings at helical CT was assessed.

Methods.—Helical CT was performed on 164 consecutive patients (55 men), aged 21–90 years, with suspected PE. Exclusion criteria were severe PE, mean time of more than 72 hours between clinical suspicion for PE and performance of helical CT, contraindications to the use of intravenous contrast material, pregnancy, and age younger than 18 years. Patients were required to have an intermediate probability at ventilation-perfusion (V-P) scintigraphy and negative findings at duplex US of the legs. All patients had helical CT, V-P scintigraphy, and duplex US performed within 72 hours after suspected PE.

Results.—Helical CT demonstrated PE in 39 patients (23.8%). Of the 123 patients with high clinical probability, PE was diagnosed in 33 (27%) by helical CT. Of the 41 patients with low probability, PE was diagnosed in 6 (15%) by helical CT. There were no immediate complications. Pulmonary angiography was performed in 15 patients with normal helical CT findings but high clinical probability. Findings at pulmonary angiography demonstrated PE in 1 patient and an isolated subsegmental thrombus. Acute PE was diagnosed in a total of 40 (24.4%) patients. At 3 months, 99 patients were still alive, and PE was diagnosed in 2 patients.

Conclusions.—Helical CT did not detect a subsegmental thrombus but was able to visualize some pulmonary arteries at the segmental level. At 3 months, 3 patients had a recurrence of PE, resulting in 1 death. Initial helical CT scans gave false-negative results in 6 (5.4%) of 112 patients.

▶ Helical CT has been successful in the past for the visualization of central pulmonary emboli but has been rather poor for visualization of peripherally located emboli. Despite that, these authors concluded that helical CT was of considerable value in the diagnosis of PE, and may have an important role in the decision for anticoagulant therapy. Unfortunately, concomitant pulmonary angiography was performed in only 15 patients, so we really don't have any gold standard control for the helical CT. The take-away message, as far as I can tell, is that while helical CT may be of value in the detection of pulmonary emboli, I do not believe it is as good as pulmonary angiography, and I certainly do not intend to use it to replace pulmonary angiography.

"Bull's-eye" Sign on Gadolinium-enhanced Magnetic Resonance Venography Determines Thrombus Presence and Age: A Preliminary Study

Froehlich JB, Prince MR, Greenfield LJ, et al (Univ of Michigan, Ann Arbor)
J Vasc Surg 26:809–816, 1997 3–23

Background.—Gadolinium-enhanced MR venography (MRV) can detect the inflammatory response associated with venous thrombosis. Enhancement appears around the thrombus, the result of gadolinium extravasation into tissues. Patients with deep vein thrombosis (DVT) were studied by MRV to determine whether gadolinium enhancement occurs, and whether it can determine the age of thrombus.

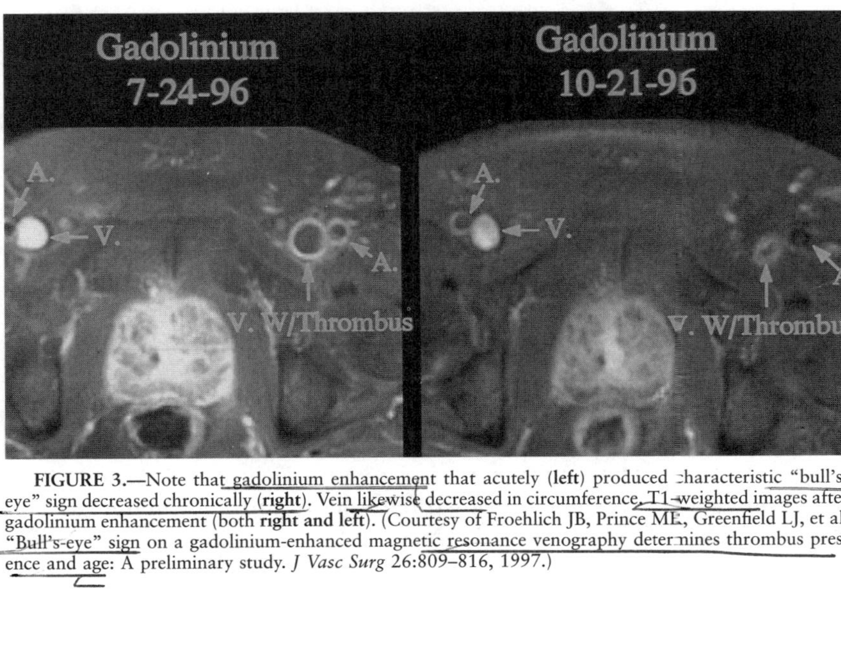

FIGURE 3.—Note that gadolinium enhancement that acutely (**left**) produced characteristic "bull's-eye" sign decreased chronically (**right**). Vein likewise decreased in circumference. T1-weighted images after gadolinium enhancement (both **right and left**). (Courtesy of Froehlich JB, Prince MR, Greenfield LJ, et al: "Bull's-eye" sign on a gadolinium-enhanced magnetic resonance venography determines thrombus presence and age: A preliminary study. *J Vasc Surg* 26:809–816, 1997.)

Methods.—Participants included 14 patients with duplex ultrasound-diagnosed iliofemoral DVT who were undergoing MRV to determine the central extent of the thrombus. Before and after gadolinium injection, T1-weighted images were obtained. After gadolinium enhancement, signal intensity was measured at the periphery of the thrombus, at the center of the thrombosed vein, and in the contralateral normal vein. The data were used to calculate rim-center vein signal intensity ratios in a total of 39 scans.

Results.—The MRV scans showed enlargement of the thrombosed veins, with a "bull's-eye" of enhancement around the peripheral rim. Thrombosed veins had a rim-center ratio of 2.16, compared with 0.66 for normal veins. The rim-center ratio was 2.38 for studies obtained within 14 days, compared with 1.29 for studies obtained after 14 days. Eight patients underwent both early and late MRV. In this group, the rim-center ratio declined from 2.33 to 1.29 (Fig 3). The rim-center ratio increased in a patient with active cancer and recurrent symptoms, suggesting that active thrombosis was occurring.

Conclusions.—In patients with DVT, a "bull's-eye" of gadolinium enhancement can be seen around acutely enhanced veins. The rim-center ratio appears to be a useful indicator of whether the DVT is acute or chronic, which may have therapeutic implications.

▶ We have been searching for years for a technique that will accurately determine the age of a venous thrombus. These investigators found that gadolinium-enhanced MRV showed a characteristic enhanced peripheral rim around the thrombus in the early stages, with the rim diminishing markedly after several weeks. This is an interesting study that may be of real clinical importance in permitting us to date thrombi as less than or greater than 2 weeks old. Even that would help. I look forward to learning more about this technique.

Venous Duplex Scanning for Unilateral Symptoms: When Do We Need a Contralateral Evaluation?

Miller N, Obrand D, Tousignant L, et al (McGill Univ, Montreal)

Eur J Vasc Endovasc Surg 15:18–23, 1998 3–24

Background.—Duplex ultrasound is widely used for the diagnosis or exclusion of deep vein thrombosis (DVT). Duplex scanning is commonly performed in both legs, whereas contrast venography is usually done in the symptomatic limb only. The value of bilateral duplex scanning was assessed prospectively in patients with unilateral symptoms of DVT.

Methods.—Participants were 1,161 consecutive patients with unilateral symptoms of acute DVT, i.e., pain and swelling. All patients underwent bilateral duplex scanning. The proportion of patients with bilateral DVT was assessed, as well as the therapeutic implications of the contralateral cases detected.

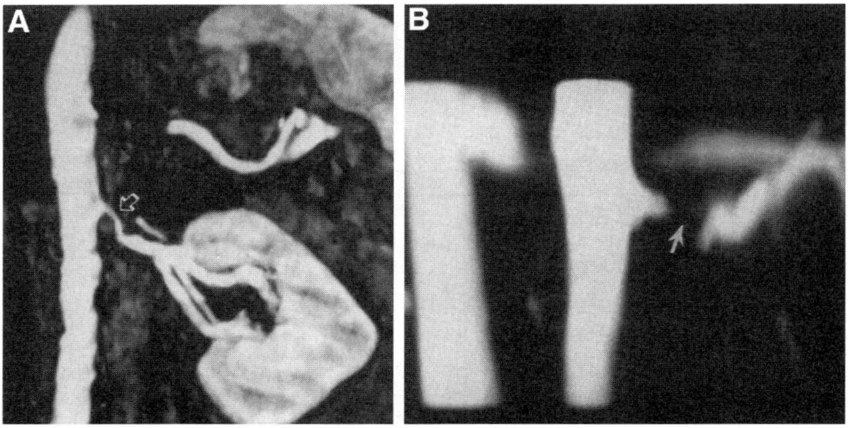

FIGURE 1.—A, coronal oblique maximum intensity projection image from a 3-dimensional dynamic gadolinium-enhanced spoiled gradient-echo angiogram (13.8/2.5, 45-degree flip angle) in a 48-year-old man after a right nephrectomy shows a stenotic left renal artery (*arrow*). B, three-dimensional phase-contrast angiogram (23/7.9, 35-degree flip angle) after injection of contrast material overestimates the severity of the stenosis (*arrow*) because high-velocity, separated flow with swirling eddy currents just distal to the stenosis causes signal loss from intravoxel dephasing. Dephasing was graded as severe in this patient because the signal dropout simulates occlusion. Left renal artery stenosis was confirmed at surgery (without angiography), and the patient's blood pressure control and serum creatinine level improved after revascularization. (Courtesy of Prince MR, Schoenberg SO, Ward JS, et al: Hemodynamically significant atherosclerotic renal artery stenosis: MR angiographic features. *Radiology* 205:128–136, 1997. Radiological Society of North America.)

fibromuscular dysplasia. Forty-seven of the remaining 90 patients underwent renal vascularization. Surgery was performed in 30 of these and balloon angioplasty in 16; 1 patient had surgery after balloon failure. Magnetic resonance angiography included T1-weighted spin-echo, 3-dimensional gadolinium-enhanced spoiled gradient-echo, and 3-dimensional phase-contrast pulse sequences. Kidney length, cortical thickness, parenchymal enhancement, and poststenotic dilatation were measured in 35 patients (52 arteries) who benefited from renal vascularization. Arteries were also examined for dephasing (signal drop-out) on phase-contrast angiograms (Fig 1).

Results.—Thirty-six (59%) of the 52 hemodynamically significant renal artery stenoses had poststenotic dilatation greater than 20%, and 45 (87%) showed severe dephasing. The mean ischemic kidney length was reduced to 9.3 cm (vs. a mean of 10.7 cm for the contralateral normal kidney) in patients with unilateral hemodynamically significant stenosis or occlusion. Also reduced were mean parenchymal thickness (from 1.7 to 1.2 cm) and mean parenchymal enhancement (15% less on the ischemic side). Severe dephasing on phase-contrast angiograms was common in unilateral hemodynamically significant stenoses (9 of 12) but occurred in only 1 contralateral normal renal artery.

Conclusion.—Data from the 35 patients with hemodynamically significant renal artery lesions demonstrate the value of MRI and MR angiography for identifying physiologic changes that indicate the hemodynamic and functional significance of these stenoses.

► These investigators from the University of Michigan analyzed detailed MR angiography findings in patients with proven renal artery stenosis. They restricted their study to 47 patients who underwent renal artery repair with beneficial results, thus appearing to precisely identify patients who really had significant renal stenosis to start with. Among the findings reported are post-stenotic dilatation of greater than 20% in 59% of patients, severe dephasing in 87% of patients, mean ischemic kidney length of 9.3 cm, and reductions in both parenchymal thickness and mean parenchymal enhancement. This article presents a current state-of-the-art analysis of the use of MR angiography in detecting renal artery stenosis. As vascular surgeons become radiologists, we are going to have to know this material.

Renal Hilar Doppler Analysis Is of Value in the Management of Patients With Renovascular Disease

Nazzal MMS, Hoballah JJ, Miller EV, et al (Univ of Iowa, Iowa City)
Am J Surg 174:164–168, 1997 3–28

Background.—There is growing interest in the use of Doppler US and duplex scanning as screening tests for renovascular hypertension. Renal hilar Doppler US (RHDU) was evaluated for use in the assessment of renal artery stenosis and for postoperative follow-up in patients undergoing renal revascularization.

Methods.—The study included 114 patients with suspected renovascular disease, mean age 64. Renal revascularization, most often renal artery bypass, was performed in 72 of these. All patients were studied by RHDU, the results of which were compared with 130 angiograms performed within 1 month. Waveform analysis was performed on Doppler velocity signals recorded in a segmental artery in the renal parenchyma. Indicators of significant renal artery stenosis were an acceleration index (AI) of less than 3.78 KHz/sec/MHz and an acceleration time (AT) of greater than 0.1 second (Figure).

Results.—The RHDU studies were successfully carried out in 94% of patients. Mean AI values were 4.7 KHz/sec/MHz in patients with normal renal arteries versus 1.2 KHz/sec/MHz in those with stenotic renal arteries. Mean values for AT were 0.05 versus 0.12, respectively. The AI had a sensitivity of 89%; specificity of 92%; positive and negative predictive values of 85% and 94%, respectively; and accuracy of 92%. For AT, sensitivity was 63%; specificity was 98%; positive and negative predictive values were 91% and 87%, respectively; and accuracy was 87%. The results of AI and AT agreed extremely well with those of arteriography. Arteriography showed multiple renal arteries in 11% of kidneys; in this group, the accuracies of AI and AT dropped, and their agreement with

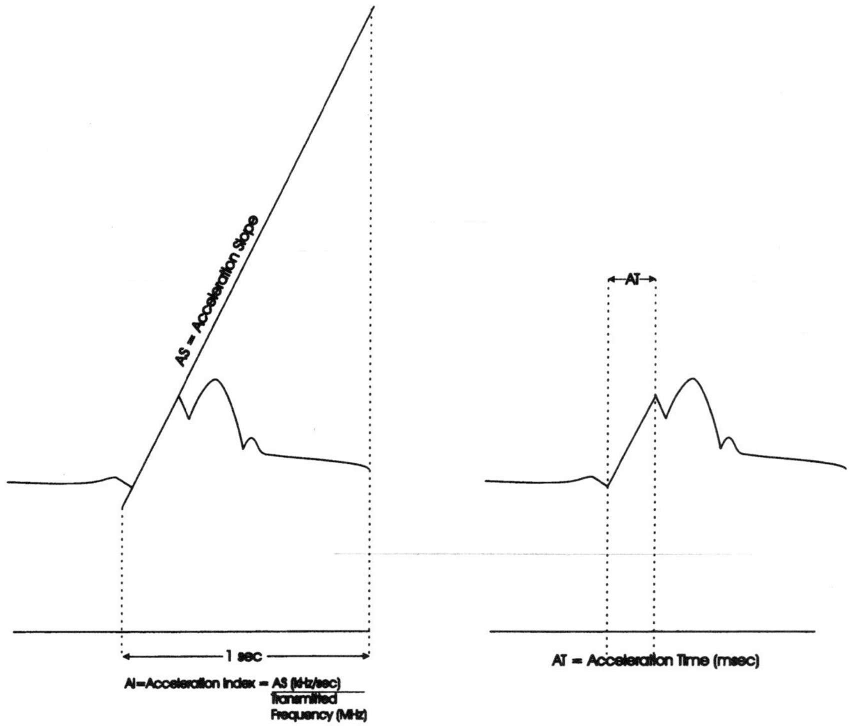

FIGURE.—A waveform showing acceleration index (AI) and acceleration time (AT). (Reprinted by permission of the publisher from Nazzal MMS, Hoballah, JJ, Miller EV, et al: Renal hilar Doppler analysis is of value in the management of patients with renovascular disease. *Am J Surg* 174:164–168. Copyright 1997 by Excerpta Medica, Inc.)

arteriography became nonsignificant. After the operation, RHDU was 86% accurate for AI and 95% accurate for AT.

Conclusions.—In patients with suspected renal artery stenosis, RHDU is a highly accurate procedure that agrees extremely well with arteriography. Problems with this study include the presence of multiple renal arteries, renal artery occlusion, and a high incidence of false-positive results after operation. Renal hilar Doppler US could be useful for noninvasive screening in suspected renal artery stenosis and for postoperative surveillance after renal revascularization.

▶ Remarkably, these authors have concluded that renal artery duplex US has been generally unsatisfactory because of inaccuracies, time required for examination, and a low technical success rate. I think they protest too much. We have found renal artery US quite satisfactory in our vascular laboratory and generally consider that we have an overall 80% accuracy. At any rate, these investigators have examined the use of the RHDU, with insonation of a segmental artery in the renal parenchyma, from which they calculated an AI and an AT. They found a remarkably good sensitivity of 89% and specificity of 92% for the AI and a slightly lesser success for the AT. I note that in recent years there has been an increasing interest in the use of a segmental renal artery insonation in the diagnosis of renovascular hypertension. On balance, however, I am not prepared to give up the renal artery duplex scan, which appears to have worked well for us. The authors must be reminded that they have not prospectively validated this diagnostic test, indeed an essential requirement.

Chronic Mesenteric Ischemia: Use of In Vivo MR Imaging Measurements of Blood Oxygen Saturation in the Superior Mesenteric Vein for Diagnosis

Li KCP, Dalman RL, Ch'en IY, et al (Stanford Univ, Calif; Sunnybrook Med Ctr, Toronto)

Radiology 204:71–77, 1997 3–29

Background.—Chronic mesenteric ischemia can be very difficult to diagnose clinically or by angiography. The percentage of oxygenated hemoglobin (%HbO_2) in the superior mesenteric vein (SMV), as measured by flow-independent T2 MRI, would be expected to decrease in patients with

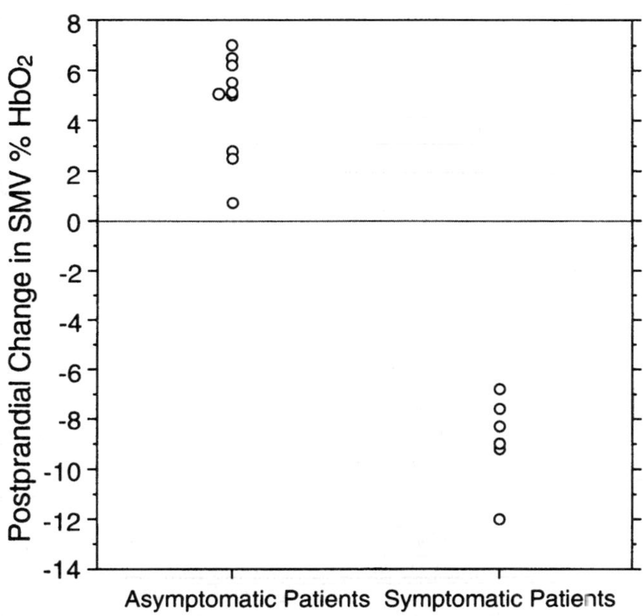

FIGURE 4.—Scatter plot shows comparison of the maximum postprandial change in the superior mesenteric vein (*SMV*) percentage of oxygenated (*%Hbo$_2$*) in 10 patients without symptoms of chronic mesenteric ischemia and 6 patients with symptoms. The SMV %Hbo_2 increased in all patients without symptoms after a standard meal but decreased after a meal in all patients with chronic mesenteric ischemia. (Courtesy of Li KCP, Dalman RL, Ch'en IY, et al: Chronic mesenteric ischemia: Use of in vivo MR imaging measurements of blood oxygen saturation in the superior mesenteric vein for diagnosis. *Radiology* 204:71–77. Copyright 1997, Radiological Society of North America.)

chronic mesenteric ischemia after ingestion of a meal. This hypothesis was tested in dogs and humans with chronic mesenteric ischemia.

Methods.—Gradual stenosis was created in dogs by implanting ameroid rings around the superior mesenteric arteries. Angiography was performed before and after implantation. Before and after a meal, the animals were studied by MR oximetry measurements of $\%HbO_2$ in the SMV, using flow-independent T2 measurements of venous blood.

Also studied were 10 patients with atherosclerosis and 6 with chronic mesenteric ischemia. The patients underwent the same studies, performed after a fasting period of at least 6 hours and at 15, 35, and 45 minutes after ingestion of a liquid nutritional supplement.

Results.—In baseline studies in dogs, postprandial $\%HbO_2$ in the SMV increased by an average of 2.5%. Once hemodynamically significant stenosis of the superior mesenteric artery had developed, postprandial SMV $\%HbO_2$ decreased by an average of 6.3%. The human studies showed a 4.6% increase in postprandial SMV $\%HbO_2$ in the asymptomatic patients, compared with a decrease of 8.8% in the patients with chronic mesenteric ischemia (Fig 4).

Conclusions.—The findings suggest that MR measurement of a reduction in SMV $\%HbO_2$ after a standard meal is an accurate indicator of chronic mesenteric ischemia. In addition to providing a promising diagnostic test, the results give insight into the pathophysiology of chronic mesenteric ischemia.

► I have known for some time that MR is capable of determining oxygen saturation, but it had never occurred to me that MR oximetry may be a valid measure of visceral artery stenosis. I note the postprandial separation in SMV percent hemoglobin saturation between asymptomatic and symptomatic patients was clear-cut and dramatic, with no overlap. Of course, this is preliminary information, and it requires confirmation in many more patients. MR oximetry appears to have the potential to become a useful diagnostic test.

Importance of Diastolic Velocities in the Detection of Celiac Mesenteric Artery Disease by Duplex Ultrasound

Perko MJ, Just S, Schroeder TV (Univ of Copenhagen, Denmark)
J Vasc Surg 26:288–293, 1997 3–30

Introduction.—Ultrasound appears to be a reliable technique for the diagnosis of acute and chronic mesenteric ischemia. However, reports differ as to whether the most accurate duplex scan criterion for mesenteric artery disease is peak systolic velocity (PSV) or diastolic velocity. Many different conditions can affect ultrasound Doppler waveform, particularly PSV. The ability of ultrasound duplex scanning to detect superior mesenteric artery (SMA) and celiac artery (CA) disease was studied.

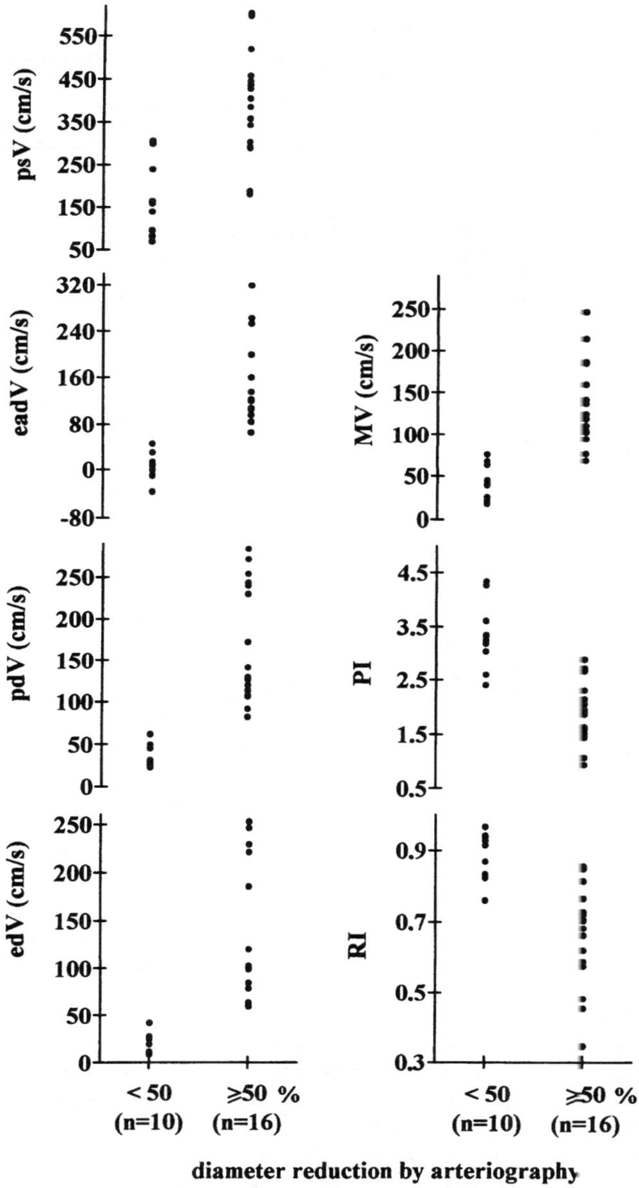

FIGURE 1.—Superior mesenteric artery Doppler variables in 26 patients with ultrasound-detectable forward flow in relation to arteriographically assessed percent of diameter reduction. *Abbreviations: psV*, peak systolic velocity; *eadV*, early diastolic velocity; *pdV*, peak diastolic velocity; *edV*, end diastolic velocity; *MV*, mean velocity; *PI*, pulsatility index; *RI*, resistivity index. (Courtesy of Perko MJ, Just S, Schroeder TV: Importance of diastolic velocities in the detection of celiac mesenteric artery disease by duplex ultrasound. *J Vasc Surg* 26:288–293, 1997.)

Methods.—A total of 39 patients with suspected mesenteric ischemia were studied. All were studied with both duplex scanning and arteriography. The data were analyzed to determine the most sensitive and specific duplex ultrasound findings for SMA and CA occlusion.

Results.—In all patients, duplex scanning provided good visualization of the SMA and CA. A well-visualized vessel with no Doppler signal indicated total occlusion. Stenosis of 50% or greater—as confirmed by arteriography—was signaled by peak diastolic velocities of greater than 70 cm/sec for SMA and 100 cm/sec for CA (Fig 1). In thyrotoxic patients with malabsorption-induced weight loss and abdominal pain, duplex scanning sometimes showed increased blood velocity while arteriography showed a normal SMA. Patients with hyperthyroidism could have had an SMA peak diastolic velocity of greater than 300 cm/sec, with normal diastolic velocities and resistivity indices.

Conclusions.—Superior mesenteric and CA disease are selectively and specifically detected by ultrasound duplex scanning. Increased diastolic velocity is the best indicator of arterial occlusion. In contrast to peak systolic velocity, this criterion can also correctly identify thyrotoxicosis. Duplex ultrasound is recommended as a screening study for patients with suspected mesenteric ischemia, before arteriography.

▶ Our experimental results disagree with those of the authors of this paper. We have found that systolic velocity correlated more closely in our laboratory with visceral artery stenosis.[1] Others besides these authors, however, have also found importance in diastolic flow. I can only conclude that careful attention to either diastolic or systolic flow with proper arteriographic controls and careful attention to detail are capable of producing accurate results in the duplex detection of visceral stenosis. Without question, each vascular laboratory must carefully review the published criteria and determine which works best for them.

Reference

1. Moneta GL, Yeager RA, Dalman R. Duplex ultrasound criteria for diagnosis of splanchnic artery stenosis or occlusion. *J Vasc Surg* 14:511–520, 1991.

Miscellaneous

ECG-Gated Three-dimensional Intravascular Ultrasound: Feasibility and Reproducibility of the Automated Analysis of Coronary Lumen and Atherosclerotic Plaque Dimensions in Humans

von Birgelen C, de Vrey EA, Mintz GS, et al (Erasmus Univ, Rotterdam, The Netherlands; Washington DC Hosp Ctr)
Circulation 96:2944–2952, 1997 3–31

Background.—Although intravascular ultrasound (IVUS) is useful in assessing atherosclerotic plaques, volumetric analysis of the planar image is time consuming. Three-dimensional (3D) image reconstruction systems

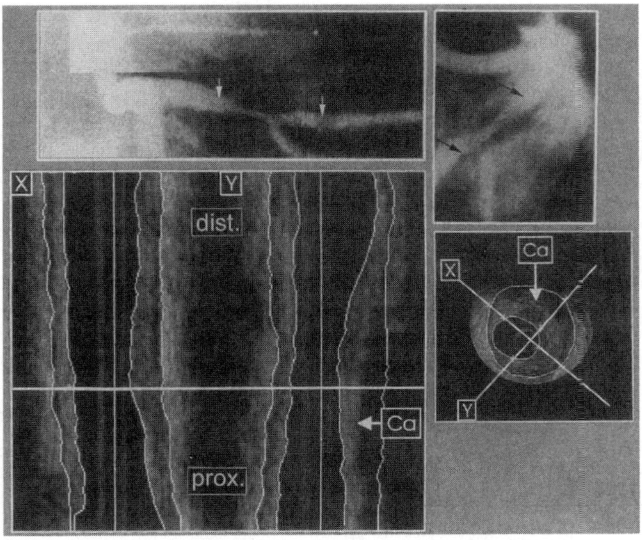

FIGURE 2—Example of automated 3D contour detection analysis in diseased left anterior descending coronary artery. Range of 14.6 mm long IVUS reconstruction and analysis is indicated by *arrowheads* in angiograms (**top**) taken from opposite angiographic projections. Cut planes of 2 reconstructed longitudinal sections (*X, Y*; **lower left**) are indicated on planar IVUS image (**lower right**), depicting calcification (*Ca*) of atherosclerotic plaque. Horizontal cursor on longitudinal sections can be used to scroll from distal (*dist.*) to proximal (*prox.*) through planar images. Thickness of that cursor is artificially increased to improve visibility (true thickness = half a scan line). Three dimensional approach permitted interpretation in longitudinal dimension and facilitated tracing of estimated external vascular contour in acoustic shadowing behind calcium. Angiograms (**top**) and radiographic image of ultrasound catheter during image acquisition (**insert, top left**) illustrate that analyzed arterial segment was relatively straight and showed no more than mild vessel curvatures. As linear 3D analysis systems do not account for vascular curvatures, this premise was important because it limits curve distortion—induced deviation of volumetric measurements. (Courtesy of von Birgelen C, de Vrey EA, Mintz GS, et al. ECG-gated three-dimensional intravascular ultrasound: Feasibility and reproducibility of the automated analysis of coronary lumen and atherosclerotic plaque dimensions in humans. *Circulation* 96:2944–2952, 1997. Reproduced with permission of the American Heart Association.)

help speed analysis, but they cannot reliably detect the external arterial boundary. Furthermore, cyclic changes in vascular dimensions and movements of the IVUS catheter can cause artifacts. These authors developed a system using electrocardiographic (ECG) gating that identifies vascular boundaries of the plaques and avoids cyclic artifacts.

Methods.—Twenty-eight patients (23 men and 5 women, mean age 55.3) underwent cardiac catheterization for diagnostic evaluation (20 patients) or as a follow-up after previous angioplasty (8 patients). Thirty atherosclerotic coronary segments were analyzed by an IVUS catheter transducer in a stationary imaging sheath. The ECG controlled pullback of the IVUS transducer. The range of normal RR intervals was measured, and images that fell outside of the normal RR range were rejected (that is, not saved). Only when a measured RR interval fell within the normal range was the IVUS image stored. Then, the catheter was stepped back 200 μm and the image acquisition process was repeated. The average ECG-gated acquisition time was 3.9 plus or minus 1.5 minutes, with an average of 114

▶ Our radiologists periodically resort to CO_2 angiography, especially in patients with renal disease. I have never favored this, because I have always thought the films were lousy and the procedure potentially dangerous. Nonetheless, occasional patients do have a serious allergic reaction to arteriographic contrast media, and contrast-induced nephrotoxicity is a real phenomenon. This fascinating report described a patient who had livedo reticularis and multiple areas of bowel infarction after CO_2 angiography, followed by death. While the mechanism of CO_2 necrosis is speculative, there is evidence that CO_2 may result in reduction in microvascular blood flow, including vasoconstriction. These authors concluded that the use of CO_2 arteriography should be reduced or avoided in patients who have congestive heart failure. I agree. However, I would extend this to avoidance of CO_2 arteriography in all patients (possibly an example of curmudgeonly over-reaction).

Is Color Duplex Surveillance of Infrainguinal Polytetrafluoroethylene Grafts Worthwhile?

Hoballah JJ, Nazzal MM, Ryan SM, et al (Univ of Iowa, Iowa City)

Am J Surg 174:131–135, 1997 3–35

Introduction.—There is ongoing debate regarding the use of duplex surveillance of infrainguinal prosthetic bypass grafts. Some studies suggest that such follow-up studies have a low yield for the detection of failing bypass grafts, whereas others find it worthwhile. Color duplex surveillance was retrospectively evaluated for use in surveillance of infrainguinal polytetrafluoroethylene (PTFE) bypass grafts.

Methods.—The study included 102 infrainguinal PTFE bypass grafts placed in 95 patients during a 5-year period. Color duplex surveillance was performed 1 month after the operation, then every 3 months for the first year, then every 6 months for the second year, and then annually. The surveillance findings of grafts with different outcomes were 70 primarily patent, 5 revised, and 27 occluded.

Results.—The outcome groups were comparable in mean age, sex, surgical indications, type of initial procedure, and duration of follow-up. A total of 407 surveillance scans were analyzed. Abnormal findings included a focal increase in peak systolic velocity, 3 times that in the adjacent segment and a peak systolic velocity less than 45 cm/sec, indicating low flow. Five primarily patent grafts with abnormal findings on duplex scans showed no angiographic abnormalities. Eight of the revised or occluded grafts had abnormal duplex findings. In the remaining 24 bypass grafts in this group, occlusion occurred without abnormality on the previous duplex examination, which in most cases had been performed within 3 months. Seven of the occluded grafts caused only mild symptoms, necessitating no treatment. Salvage of 16 occluded grafts was attempted; 10 of these had been patent at last follow-up. Duplex surveillance had a sensitivity of 25% and a positive predictive value of 62%.

Conclusions.—For patients with infrainguinal PTFE bypass grafts, duplex surveillance is not effective in detecting impending graft failure, nor in predicting continued graft function. Intervention can improve the patency rate of failing bypass grafts, but intensive surveillance is a low-yield procedure.

▶ Most previous investigators have concluded that duplex surveillance of prosthetic leg grafts is inaccurate. These authors report their experience with insonation of 95 patients with 102 infrainguinal PTFE grafts. They found that 24 bypass grafts occluded without any abnormalities on the latest duplex examination, performed within 3 months of the occlusion. They concluded appropriately that duplex surveillance of infrainguinal PTFE bypass grafts is inadequate for predicting continued bypass patency. I believe that this information is accurate, and at present, I do not see any persuasive indication for duplex surveillance of infrainguinal PTFE grafts. The absence of usefulness of the surveillance suggests that the method of graft failure must be different for prosthetic and vein grafts. High-grade stenosis followed by occlusion is the norm in the vein graft but does not appear to be the norm in the prosthetic graft.

4 Nonatherosclerotic Conditions

Popliteal Artery Compression and Force of Active Plantar Flexion in Young Healthy Volunteers

Hoffman U, Vetter J, Rainoni L, et al (Univ Hosp Zurich, Switzerland)

J Vasc Surg 26:281–287, 1997 4–1

Background.—The finding of popliteal artery compression during plantar flexion has been regarded as specific for popliteal artery entrapment syndrome. However, the provocation maneuver may induce popliteal artery compression even in healthy subjects. The prevalence of popliteal artery occlusion during active plantar flexion was studied in healthy subjects, including a group of highly trained athletes.

Methods.—The study included both limbs of 42 healthy subjects, 18 of whom were highly trained athletes and 24 of whom were normally active subjects. In prone position, each subject performed progressive plantar flexion against a scale, which measured plantar flexion force. The maximum strength (P_{max}) of plantar flexion force was assessed, and the popliteal artery was continuously monitored with color duplex sonography. The level of force necessary to occlude the popliteal artery (P_{occl}) was evaluated.

Results.—Eighty-eight percent of subjects and 77% of limbs showed popliteal artery occlusion during plantar flexion. The prevalences of this finding were similar between athletes and normally active subjects (Table 2). Mean P_{occl} was 45 kg, or 70% of P_{max}. The values of P_{occl} was compa-

TABLE 2.—**A,** Prevalence of Popliteal Artery Occlusion During Active Plantar Flexion in Normally Active Subjects and Athletes

	Normally active	*Athletes*	*Total*
Subjects	24	18	42
Occlusion	20 (83.3%)	17 (94.4%)	37 (38.1%)
Unilateral	5 (25%)	2 (11.8%)	7 (18.9%)
Bilateral	15 (75%)	15 (88.2%)	30 (31.1%)
No occlusion	4 (16.7%)	1 (6.2%)	5 (11.9%)

(Courtesy of Hoffman U, Vetter J, Rainoni L, et al: Popliteal artery compression and force of active plantar flexion in young healthy volunteers. *J Vasc Surg* 26:281–287, 1997.)

rable between athletes and nonathletes. As a percentage of P_{max}, P_{occl} was lower in the athletes; however, the difference arose from 2 extremely low values in a female athlete.

Conclusions.—Active plantar flexion produces positional occlusion of the popliteal artery in a high percentage of healthy young subjects. The force level of active plantar flexion determines the prevalence of this finding. This force level is comparable for athletes and healthy young subjects, who show no difference in the prevalence of popliteal artery occlusion during plantar flexion.

▶ These authors conclusively showed that 88% of healthy individuals, including athletes, can totally occlude their popliteal artery during active foot plantar flexion. In fact, there was little difference between the lower extremities of athletes and those of nonathletes. We are forced to conclude that positional occlusion of the popliteal artery during active plantar flexion is normal, and it most assuredly cannot be used to diagnose the presence of any abnormal condition. The notion that popliteal entrapment or even cystic adventitial disease can be diagnosed by pulse obliteration during plantar flexion simply must be abandoned.

Lymphangiomas in Children: Percutaneous Sclerotherapy With an Alcoholic Solution of Zein

Dubois J, Garel L, Abela A, et al (Hôpital Sainte-Justine, Montréal)

Radiology 204:651–654, 1997 4–2

Background.—Many different treatments have been tried for lymphangiomas in children. Surgery has a high recurrence rate and significant mortality and complications rates. This has led to percutaneous sclerotherapy using various agents. An experience with percutaneous sclerotherapy using an alcoholic solution of zein (Ethibloc) for the treatment of lymphangiomas in children is reported.

Methods.—The experience included 14 children with macrocystic and mixed lymphangiomas. All were treated with percutaneous sclerotherapy using Ethibloc as the sclerosing agent. Ultrasound and/or fluoroscopy was used to guide the percutaneous procedures. The response was assessed by clinical follow-up and serial CT scans.

Results.—Excellent regression was obtained in 64% of lymphangiomas. Four lesions disappeared completely, and 5 regressed to less than 5% of their initial volume. Sclerotherapy produced satisfactory results in the remaining 5 cases. Ethibloc leakage occurred in 10 lymphangiomas, but did not cause any significant sequelae.

Conclusions.—For children with macrocystic and mixed lymphangiomas, percutaneous sclerotherapy with Ethibloc appears to be a safe and effective treatment. The results appear to be better than those obtained with other sclerosants.

► Over the years, various agents have been proposed for injection into lymphangiomas. In recent years, 2 of the more popular have been OK-432[1] and doxycycline.[2] Other proposals for injection include 50% dextrose and bleomycin and triamcinolone. The authors of this article found considerable success with the use of a proprietary substance known as Ethibloc, manufactured by the Ethicon Company of Germany. The message appears to be that significant lymphangiomas in children can be reasonably successfully treated with local injections of a variety of substances. As expected, the injection sclerotherapy of the lesion frequently requires surgical excision, which appears easier after partial regression.

References

1. 1996 Year Book of Vascular Surgery, p 441.
2. 1996 Year Book of Vascular Surgery, p 442.

Interstitial Nd:YAG Photocoagulation for Vascular Malformations and Hemangiomas in Childhood

Clymer MA, Fortune DS, Reinisch L, et al (Vanderbuilt Univ, Nashville, Tenn; Univ of Illinois, Chicago)

Arch Otolaryngol Head Neck Surg 124:431–436, 1998 4–3

Background.—Hemangiomas and vascular malformations cause physical disfigurement and psychological consequences for many affected children. These lesions commonly resolve over time. However, when lesional growth could cause damage to adjacent vital structures—such as the orbit, nose, or tongue—aggressive treatment is needed. The role of interstitial Nd:YAG photocoagulation as an adjunct therapy for treatment-resistant hemangiomas and vascular malformations was evaluated.

Methods.—The prospective, nonrandomized trial included 8 patients with hemangiomas and 2 with vascular malformations of the head and neck. All lesions had failed to respond to other treatments, such as corticosteroid therapy. All patients underwent interstitial laser photocoagulation, with an Nd:YAG fiber introduced into the lesion through a 14-gauge angiocatheter needle. As tissue coagulation progressed, the laser fiber was advanced. The results were assessed in terms of decreased area of the target lesion, amount of laser energy used, and number of treatments required.

Results.—All patients had regression of their hemangiomas or vascular formations over long-term follow-up. The cosmetic results were good, with 20% to 98% reductions in lesion size. At a mean follow-up of 13 months, none of the lesions reexpanded.

Conclusions.—In appropriately selected patients, interstitial photocoagulation is an effective treatment for pediatric hemangiomas and vascular malformations. This adjunct therapy can reduce the size of the lesions while obtaining good cosmetic results.

▶ This information suggests that selected children with vascular malformations including cavernous hemangiomas may expect considerable benefit from lesion treatment with Nd:YAG laser photocoagulation. Laser photocoagulation in this study was used with an interstitial technique in which a fiber was introduced into the lesion with a 14-gauge angiocath needle with the laser fiber being advanced as coagulation proceeded. Significant lesion reduction occurred in all 10 patients, with good cosmetic results. The conclusion appears warranted that interstitial photocoagulation of hemangiomas and vascular malformations represents an effective treatment in selected patients.

Thoracoscopic Upper Thoracic Sympathectomy for Primary Palmar Hyperhidrosis: The Combined Paediatric, Adolescents and Adult Experience

Cohen Z, Levi I, Pinsk I, et al (Ben-Gurion Univ of the Negev, Beer-Sheva, Israel)

Eur J Surg Suppl 580:5–8, 1998 4–4

Background.—The excessive sweating of primary palmar hyperhidrosis causes major psychological, social, and occupational problems for affected patients. Early surgery can avoid many of these problems for children with hyperhidrosis. A 4-year experience with thoracoscopic upper thoracic sympathectomy for patients with primary palmar hyperhidrosis was presented.

Methods.—A total of 223 patients with primary palmar hyperhidrosis were retrospectively studied. There were 135 females and 88 males, and more than 60% were younger than 18 years. The patients underwent a total of 402 thoracoscopic upper thoracoscopic sympathectomy procedures, consisting of ablation of the ganglia and severing of the sympathetic chain at T2 and T3. Sympathectomy was performed on both sides at the same time in 142 patients, on both sides at different times in 37, and on 1 side only in 44.

Results.—Postoperative recovery was uneventful, permitting next-day discharge in 99% of patients. Pneumothorax requiring intercostal drainage resulted in third-day discharge for 3 patients. The procedure resulted in immediate and permanent relief of palmar sweating in 98% of patients, leading to complete satisfaction. Just 4 patients reported dissatisfaction with their results.

Conclusions.—Thoracoscopic upper thoracic sympathectomy can be regarded as the treatment of choice for primary palmar hyperhidrosis. Early surgery can avoid many years of problems for affected children.

► Over the years, I have reached certain conclusions concerning the treatment of upper extremity hyperhidrosis, be it thoracoscopically or with conventional surgery. In the first place, I firmly believe that the first ganglion should not be disturbed at all. The sympathetic pathway should be transected below the first ganglion, with ablation of the second and third ganglia if the hand is the only target. If axillary hyperhidrosis is also present, the T4 ganglion must also be ablated. Postoperatively, one has to inform the patient of compensatory truncal sweating, which almost always occurs, and a peculiar condition known as gustatory hyperhidrosis, during which sweating occurs in response to eating spicy foods. On balance, thoracic sympathectomy, carefully performed, has given durable relief of hyperhidrosis.

Oral Iloprost in the Treatment of Thromboangiitis Obliterans (Buerger's Disease): A Double-blind, Randomised, Placebo-controlled Trial

Verstraete M, for The European TAO Study Group (Centre for Molecular and Vascular Biology, Leuven, Belgium)

Eur J Vasc Endovasc Surg 15:300–307, 1998 4–5

Introduction.—Thromboangiitis obliterans (TAO), or Buerger's disease, is a nonatherosclerotic, inflammatory obliterative disease affecting the small- and medium-sized arteries. The prostacyclin analogue iloprost has given promising results in the treatment of this condition. Iloprost, in 2 different doses, was evaluated for efficacy and tolerability for the treatment of TAO in a placebo-controlled trial.

Methods.—The multicenter trial included 319 patients with TAO, characterized by pain at rest and/or trophic lesions. They were randomly assigned to receive 8 weeks of treatment with iloprost, 100 or 200 μg twice daily, or placebo. They were followed for 6 months for the primary end point of total healing of the most important lesion. Pain relief was assessed as well. The analysis also used a combined end point of survival without major amputation, absence of lesions, absence of rest pain, and absence of analgesic use.

Results.—The iloprost and placebo groups had similar total healing of lesions throughout the study. By the end of follow-up, the rate of pain relief without the need for analgesics was 63% with low-dose iloprost vs. 49% with placebo. Low-dose iloprost also offered a significant advantage in terms of the combined end point: 50% vs. 35%. However, high-dose iloprost did not perform significantly better than placebo in any end point.

Conclusions.—For patients with TAO, low-dose iloprost is more effective than placebo in relieving rest pain without analgesics, and in meeting the combined end point used in this study. However, neither iloprost dose investigated significantly improves total healing of lesions.

► Buerger's disease continues to attract a little attention from vascular surgeons the world over. While a successful surgical bypass can be performed in the occasional patient, this is clearly the exception. In the reported study, iloprost, a prostaglandin analogue, was assessed for its role in wound healing and analgesia in these patients. While it did seem to relieve pain, there was no benefit in wound healing. Too bad. At present, iloprost is not available in the United States.

in patients older than 80 years. Overall, stroke is 5 times more frequent in patients with atrial fibrillation, and is also more severe, with a poorer outcome. At least 6 randomized clinical studies have demonstrated the effectiveness of warfarin in the prevention of stroke in this cohort, with at least a two-thirds reduction in the risk of stroke noted repeatedly. This sobering study indicates that in a broadly based statewide survey, warfarin anticoagulation was dramatically underused in patients with atrial fibrillation. Most of the eligible patients not taking warfarin were also not taking aspirin. It seems to me that when we encounter an elderly patient in atrial fibrillation and not on warfarin we should at least recommend to the primary care physician that warfarin anticoagulation be considered. (See also reference.[1])

Reference

1. 1996 Year Book of Vascular Surgery, p 23.

Vascular Operations

Reoperations, Redo Surgery and Other Interventions Constitute More Than One-third of Vascular Surgery: A Study From Swedvase (the Swedish Vascular Registry)

Bergvist D, for the Swedish Society for Vascular Surgery (Blekinge Hosp, Sweden)

Eur J Vasc Endovasc Surg 14:244–251, 1997 5–5

Background.—Most studies of reoperations and revisionary procedures in vascular surgery have been limited to the immediate postoperative period or to selected procedures. The 30-day incidence of reoperations after vascular surgery was assessed, along with the incidence of later revisionary procedures and other interventions.

Methods.—The study used data from the Swedish Vascular Registry (Swedvase) covering the years 1987 to 1991. It included 8,089 primary operations performed for acute ischemia, elective and emergency aortic aneurysm, intermittent claudication, critical leg ischemia, and carotid artery stenosis. The patients were followed up through the end of 1995 for any subsequent arterial operations.

Results.—A total of 4,927 additional procedures were found. Of these, 24% were done within 30 days, 30% during the remainder of the first year, 14% during the second year, 11% during the third year, and 9% during the fourth year. The overall incidence of additional vascular operations during a 4-year period was 16% to 42%, depending on the indication. Half of the repeated interventions for acute ischemia or emergency aortic aneurysm took place within 30 days. For patients with claudication, critical ischemia, or carotid endarterectomy, the repeated procedures were more likely to occur later during the first year. Four-year freedom from repeated operation was 69%, with a patient survival of 59% and an event-free survival of 39% (Fig 2).

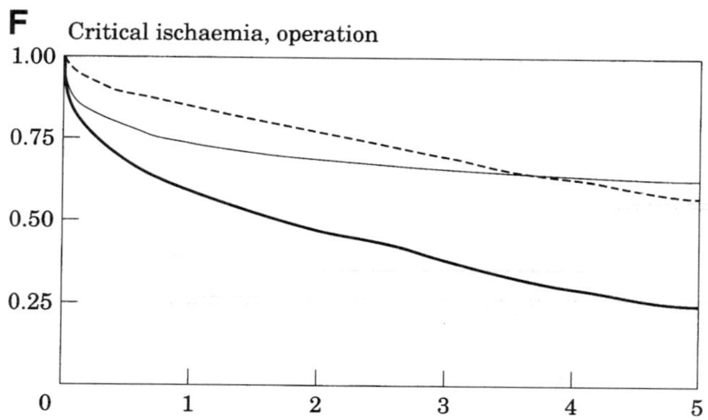

FIGURE 2.—F, survival curves according to Kaplan-Meier, showing proportion without repeated surgery (*thin line*), patient survival (*broken medium line*) and the combination of these 2 into the event-free survival (*heavy line*). (Reprinted from *Eur J Vasc Endovasc Surg*, Vol 14, Oct, Bergqvist D, Elfström J, Hedberg B, et al, Reoperations, redo surgery and other inventions constitute more than one-third of vascular surgery: A study from Swedvase (the Swedish vascular registry, 244–251, copyright 1997, by permission of the publisher WB Saunders Company Limited, London.)

Conclusions.—This study finds a high rate of repeated vascular interventions among patients undergoing vascular surgery. Treatment decisions about patients with vascular disease should consider this risk, as well as the patients' life expectancy. If patient selection is to be improved, more research is needed to find prognostically significant subgroups of patients who are candidates for vascular surgery.

▶ The requirement for reoperation among patients undergoing vascular surgery is legendary. Of 8,000 patients in this study undergoing primary vascular surgery, almost 5,000 follow-up procedures were required during the first 4 years in 41% of the patients. A significant number of these reinterventions were required during the first 30 days after the first operation, and most of the remainder were needed during the first year. There was a lesser requirement for reoperation after the first year. This leads these authors to suggest that the remarkable risk of reintervention in patients undergoing vascular surgery, combined with their limited life expectancy, are important facts that must be considered when making initial treatment decisions. I heartily agree. I am becoming more and more convinced that we have spent the last 40 years in vascular surgery learning what we can do, and that we are going to spend the next period of years learning what we *should* do. I strongly suspect they will not be the same thing.

A Prospective, Randomized Trial Limiting Perioperative Red Blood Cell Transfusions in Vascular Patients

Bush RL, Pevec WC, Holcroft JW (Univ of California, Sacramento)

Am J Surg 174:143–148, 1997 5–6

Background.—Prevention of anemia-induced myocardial ischemia during major arterial reconstructive surgery relies on red blood cell transfusion. The traditional hemoglobin target has been a concentration of above 10 g/dL, but there are no data to support this figure. This randomized trial sought to determine whether vascular surgery patients can tolerate a hemoglobin concentration of 9.0 g/dL.

Methods.—The study included 99 patients undergoing elective aortic or infrainguinal arterial reconstructive surgical procedures. They were randomized to receive 1 of 2 transfusion protocols during surgery: maintenance of hemoglobin level of 10 g/dL (liberal group) or 9 g/dL (restrictive group).

Results.—The mean postoperative hemoglobin level was 11.0 g/dL in the liberal group and 9.8 g/dL in the restrictive group (Fig 1). However, the 2 groups were similar in mortality, cardiac morbidity, and length of hospital stay. Hemodynamic parameters were similar. The restrictive group had lower hemoglobin levels; however, oxygen consumption was similar

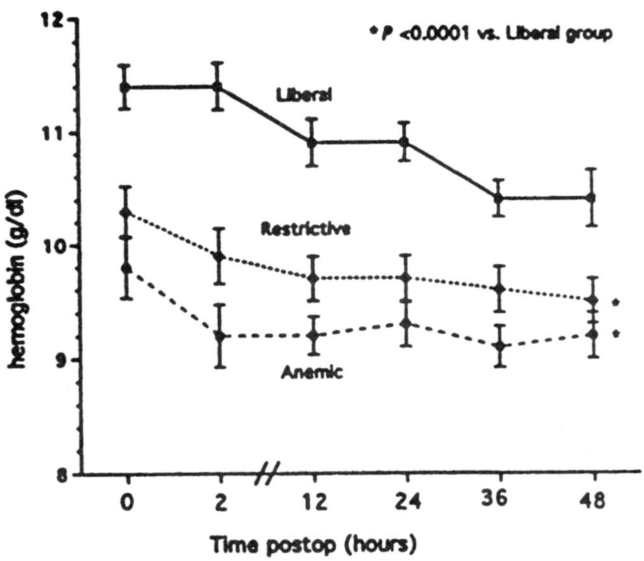

FIGURE 1.—Postoperative hemoglobin levels. The liberal group was transfused to keep hemoglobin levels above 10g/dL. The restrictive group was transfused only for hemoglobin levels below 9 g/dL. The anemic subgroup consisted of patients in the restrictive group in whom the hemoglobin actually dropped below 9/g/dL. Patients with intraoperative uncontrolled hemorrhage or myocardial infarction (n = 3, liberal: n = 2, restrictive) were excluded. (Reprinted by permission of the publisher from Bush RL, Pevec WC, Holcroft JW: A prospective, randomized trial limiting perioperative red blood cell transfusions in vascular patients. AMERICAN JOURNAL OF SURGERY 174:143–148, copyright 1997 by Excerpta Medica Inc.)

TABLE 4.—Blood Use

	Liberal Group*	Anemic Group*	*P* Value
Intraoperative units†	2.4 ± 2.5	1.0 ± 1.4	0.004
Total units‡	3.7 ± 3.5	2.0 ± 1.9	0.01
Cost ($)	920 ± 870	500 ± 470	0.01

*All values are expressed as mean ± standard deviation.
†Intraoperative units are intraoperative units of red blood cells.
‡Total units indicate intraoperative and postoperative.
(Reprinted by permission of the publisher from Bush RL, Pevec WC, Holcroft JW: A prospective, randomized trial limiting perioperative red blood cell transfusions in vascular patients. AMERICAN JOURNAL OF SURGERY 174:143–148, copyright 1997 by Excerpta Medica Inc.)

between groups. The restrictive group had lower transfusion requirements and associated costs (Table 4).

Conclusion.—Patients undergoing major vascular reconstructions can tolerate a hemoglobin concentration of 9 g/dL without adverse clinical consequences. Compensation for the anemia takes place not through increased myocardial work but through increased oxygen extraction in peripheral tissues. A restrictive policy of this type reduces patient exposure to banked blood and transfusion-related costs.

► These authors remarkably point out that the generally accepted dogma of keeping postoperative patients' hemoglobin concentration above 10 g/dL is unsupported by any persuasive data. These authors have examined the hypothesis that vascular patients will satisfactorily tolerate a hemoglobin concentration of 9 g/dL. Despite significant differences in postoperative hemoglobin levels, there were no differences in mortality, cardiac morbidity, or length of stay between the 2 groups. Although oxygen delivery was lower in the group with lower hemoglobin levels, there were no differences in oxygen consumption. Patients did not compensate for anemia by increased myocardial work, but by increasing oxygen extraction in the peripheral tissues. This information may justify keeping postoperative vascular patients' hemoglobin levels slightly lower than we have routinely elected to do.

Perioperative Maintenance of Normothermia Reduces the Incidence of Morbid Cardiac Events: A Randomized Clinical Trial

Frank SM, Fleisher LA, Breslow MJ, et al (Johns Hopkins Med Insts, Baltimore, Md; Vanderbilt Univ, Nashville, Tenn)
JAMA 277:1127–1134, 1997 5–7

Introduction.—Administration of anesthesia, the use of IV fluids, and other factors contribute to development of hypothermia in most surgical patients. Even mild hypothermia (from 0.5°C to 1.2°C below normal core temperature) can trigger sympathetically mediated hypertension and place increased demands on the cardiovascular system. The relationship between body temperature and cardiac morbidity in the perioperative period was assessed among patients receiving routine thermal care vs. those receiving supplemental warming care.

Methods.—The randomized, controlled study enrolled 300 patients during a 3-year period. Those eligible were older than 60 years, were scheduled for peripheral vascular, abdominal, or thoracic surgical procedures and for postoperative admission to the ICU, and had documented coronary artery disease (CAD) or were at high risk for CAD. Patients were also required to have a preoperative tympanic temperature between 36°C and 38°C. Routine thermal care included warming of IV fluids and blood and the use of paper surgical drapes and warmed cotton blankets. The normothermic group had routine care plus an upper- or lower-body forced-air warming cover, with therapy continued through the first 2 hours of postoperative care. Eight body sites were monitored for temperature, and a "blinded" investigator determined morbid cardiac events.

Results.—Hypothermic and normothermic groups were similar in preoperative demographic variables, anesthetic technique, level of invasive hemodynamic monitoring, and intraoperative blood and fluid requirements. Mean core temperature was significantly lower after surgery in the hypothermic group (35.4°C) than in the normothermic group (36.7°C), and remained lower during the early postoperative period. The incidence of perioperative morbid cardiac events was 6.3% in the hypothermic group vs. 1.4% in the normothermic group. Maintenance of normothermia was associated with a reduction in postoperative ventricular tachycardia. In multivariate analysis, hypothermia was an independent predictor of morbid cardiac events (relative risk 2.2).

Conclusions.—Active warming designed to maintain normothermia during the intraoperative and postoperative periods was associated with a decreased incidence of early postoperative morbid cardiac events in patients with cardiac risk factors undergoing noncardiac surgery.

▶ These authors performed a randomized, controlled trial comparing routine thermal care to supplemental warming after major surgery, and determined the relationship of the thermal status of the patient to the relative risk of morbid cardiac events. The mean core temperature after surgery in the group receiving routine thermal care was 35.4°C and 36.7°C in the group receiving supplemental warming. Perioperative morbid cardiac events occurred significantly less frequently in the normothermic group, leading these authors to recommend careful maintenance of normothermia in the perioperative period in patients with cardiac risk factors undergoing major surgery. In recent years there has been a plethora of articles describing numerous adverse effects of hypothermia after surgery. We should all be careful in observing the temperature of our postoperative patients. Abundant evidence indicates the superiority of normothermia over hypothermia.

Prospective Randomized Placebo-controlled Trial of Aprotinin for Elective Aortic Reconstruction

Ranaboldo CJ, Thompson JF, Davies JN, et al (Royal Devon and Exeter Hosp, UK)

Br J Surg 84:1110–1113, 1997 5–8

Background.—Aprotinin is a serine protease antagonist that can reduce blood loss during cardiac surgery and liver transplantation. Previous research has suggested that it may also be useful in reducing bleeding during infrarenal aortic replacement. This hypothesis was tested in a randomized, controlled trial.

Methods.—The study included 136 patients undergoing elective aortic surgery. The first 80 patients were randomized to receive aprotinin (loading dose 2×10^6 kallikrein indicator units followed by 0.5×10^6 kallikrein indicator units/hr) or 0.9% saline in equal volumes. The remaining patients received a doubled infusion dose to achieve plasma levels comparable to those observed in studies of aprotinin for cardiac surgery. During and for the week after surgery, the patients' blood loss, coagulation, and hematologic findings were assessed. The target hemoglobin for blood transfusion was 100 g/L.

Discussion.—Four patients were withdrawn from the study intraoperatively when the planned operation was found to be inappropriate. Thirty-

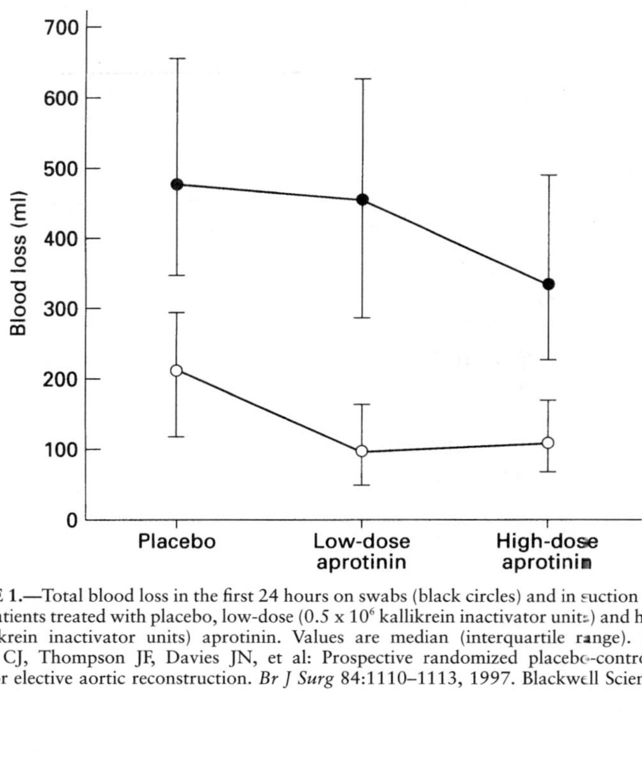

FIGURE 1.—Total blood loss in the first 24 hours on swabs (black circles) and in suction drains (white circles) in patients treated with placebo, low-dose (0.5×10^6 kallikrein inactivator units) and high-dose (1.0×10^6 kallikrein inactivator units) aprotinin. Values are median (interquartile range). (Courtesy of Ranaboldo CJ, Thompson JF, Davies JN, et al: Prospective randomized placebo-controlled trial of aprotinin for elective aortic reconstruction. *Br J Surg* 84:1110–1113, 1997. Blackwell Science Ltd.)

day mortality was 4.5%, with no difference in the complication rate between groups. Median swab-collected blood loss was 379 mL in patients receiving aprotinin, compared with 480 mL in those receiving placebo. Twenty-four-hour blood loss in suction drains was 205 vs. 295 mL, respectively (Fig 1). There were no significant differences in intraoperative blood loss, total blood loss, or transfusion requirements.

Conclusions.—In patients undergoing elective aortic surgery, aprotinin treatment produces a small reduction in blood loss. However, the benefit is insufficient to recommend routine use of aprotinin during aortic reconstruction.

▶ Aprotinin is a bit of a mysterious drug. It has been suggested that it diminishes surgical bleeding by exerting a powerful antifibrinolytic action, as well as by stabilizing platelet membrane glycoproteins. Aprotinin in high doses does appear to reduce bleeding during cardiac surgery. Unfortunately, no significant reduction was found in aortic surgery patients, as measured either by intraoperative or total blood loss or by transfusion requirement. We are forced to conclude from this well-conducted study that the serine protease antagonist aprotinin does not significantly reduce surgical blood loss in patients undergoing infrarenal aortic surgery. Too bad.

Routine Pulmonary Artery Catheterization Does Not Reduce Morbidity and Mortality of Elective Vascular Surgery: Results of a Prospective, Randomized Trial

Bender JS, Smith-Meek MA, Jones CE (Johns Hopkins Univ, Baltimore, Md)
Ann Surg 226:229–237, 1997 5–9

Background.—Although the pulmonary artery catheter is used routinely in patients who are critically ill and during major elective surgery, there are few prospective, randomized studies of the value of the pulmonary artery catheter under such conditions. The effect of preoperative placement of a pulmonary artery catheter with optimization of hemodynamics on outcome after elective vascular surgery were determined.

Methods.—In a tightly controlled, prospective, randomized trial, 104 consecutive patients were randomly assigned to 2 groups. Group 1 had placement of a pulmonary artery catheter on the morning of operation, and group 2 had placement of the catheter only if clinically indicated. In patients in group 1, preestablished end points were maintained before, during, and after operation. Patients in group 2 were given standard care.

Results.—One patient died in each group. In group 1, 13 patients had intraoperative or postoperative complications. In group 2, 7 patients had intraoperative or postoperative complications. More fluid was given to patients in group 1 than in group 2 (Table 6). Overall and surgical ICU

TABLE 6.—Overall Outcome

	Group I (n = 51)	Group II (n = 53)
Operative length (min)	320 ± 13	322 ± 13
Blood loss (mL)	716 ± 84	675 ± 156
Crystalloid (mL)	5137 ± 315*	3789 ± 306
Blood transfused (units)	1.3 ± 0.1	1.8 ± 0.2
FFP transfused (units)	2.3 ± 0.9	2.5 ± 1.5

*$P < 0.003$.
Abbreviation: FFP, fresh frozen plasma.
(Courtesy of Bender JS, Smith-Meek MA, Jones CE: Routine pulmonary artery catheterization does not reduce morbidity and mortality of elective vascular surgery: Results of a prospective, randomized trial. *Ann Surg* 226:229–237, 1997.)

length of stay was similar in both groups. A postoperative pulmonary artery catheter was needed only in 1 patient in group 2.

Discussion.—These results indicate that routine use of a pulmonary artery catheter in patients undergoing elective vascular surgery increases the volume of fluid needed, but does not significantly improve morbidity or mortality, or reduce length of stay or cost. Routine use of the pulmonary artery catheter should be limited to specific clinical situations.

▶ The obvious question is, whoever said it did? These authors have concluded, miraculously, that the routine use of pulmonary artery catheterization in elective vascular surgery considerably increases the volume of fluid administered to patients without demonstrable improvement in mortality or morbidity. I have always been concerned by the typical anesthesiologist who, when a patient has a dip in blood pressure during vascular surgery, promptly responds by the administration of another liter of saline. We then are left with a postoperative patient who looks like a poisoned pup, with about 10–15 liters of saline on board. We then have to worry about getting the saline off before serious pulmonary complications ensue. I will take a savvy anesthesiologist (oxymoron?) over a pulmonary artery catheter any day. In our institution, our anesthesiologists are delighted to routinely delay a vascular case by as much as an hour while they insert a pulmonary artery catheter, which they then appear to have no idea how to use. Just for meanness, I will usually ask them what the cardiac output is at various times during the case, and the typical answer is that something or another is not working properly and they are not able to answer my question. They seem to regard the insertion of the pulmonary artery catheter as more of a therapeutic than a diagnostic exercise. (See also Abstract 5–10.)

Smoking Cessation After Surgery: A Randomized Trial

Simon JA, Solkowitz SN, Carmody TP, et al (Univ of California, San Francisco)

Arch Intern Med 157:1371–1376, 1997 5–14

Background.—Smoking is the most important cause of preventable death in the United States. Although most smokers would like to quit, smoking cessation programs are not very effective. Because most hospitals are smoke free, admissions for surgery may offer a good opportunity for smoking cessation interventions. A perioperative smoking cessation intervention in patients admitted for noncardiac surgery was tested.

Methods.—The randomized, controlled trial included 324 smokers admitted for noncardiac surgery at a VA hospital. The age range was 25 to 82 years; 98% of the patients were men. In the perioperative period, 168 patients underwent a multicomponent smoking cessation intervention designed to increase self-efficacy and coping skills. The intervention included in-hospital counseling, a smoking cessation videotape, self-help literature, nicotine replacement therapy, and 3 months' telephone follow-up. The other 156 patients received only the self-help literature and a brief (10-minute) counseling session. Patient reports of smoking cessation were confirmed by measurement of nicotine levels in serum or saliva.

Results.—The self-reported quit rates were 27% for the intervention group and 13% for the control group. The biochemically confirmed quit rates were 15% and 8%, respectively.

Conclusion.—For patients hospitalized for noncardiac surgery, a perioperative smoking cessation intervention may improve long-term quit rates. Such hospitalizations may provide a "window of opportunity" for smoking cessation in smokers who want to quit.

► This interesting study examines the hypothesis that surgical admissions for smokers present a window of opportunity for patients to successfully stop smoking. Patients who smoke were randomized to either an intensive or a much less intensive smoking intervention program while in the hospital for non-cardiac surgery. At 12 months' follow-up, the intervention group reported a 27% cessation rate and the comparison group reported 13%. Unfortunately, biochemical confirmation indicated that only 15% of the intervention group had really stopped, compared with 8% of the comparison group. Nonetheless, while proving once again that smokers are liars, this is a rather impressive accomplishment after a short period of intervention while patients were in the hospital. I do believe the clear message is that we should use the occasion of surgical hospitalization to diligently attempt to modify our patients' smoking behavior.

Electric Cautery Lowers the Contamination Threshold for Infection of Laparotomies

Soballe PW, Nimbkar NV, Hayward I, et al (Uniformed Services Univ of Health Sciences, Bethesda, Md)

Am J Surg 175:263–266, 1998 5–15

Introduction.—Any modification of surgical technique that could reduce the overall incidence of wound infection would improve quality and reduce costs, for infectious complications significantly increase hospital stay. Researchers hypothesized that electric cautery, which causes more damage than the scalpel, increases the rate of infectious complications.

Methods.—This experimental study used rats randomized to 1 of 3 incisions: cold knife, electric cutting current, or electric coagulating current. Subcutaneous tissue was inoculated with 0.2 mL normal saline containing 0, 10^3, 10^5, 10^7, or 10^9 bacteria. All animals were sacrificed on postoperative day 7 and tissue from the abdominal incision removed for analysis.

Results.—At all levels of bacterial contamination, electric coagulation produced significantly more tissue necrosis and inflammation than the cold knife. Coagulation current caused greater inflammation and necrosis than the cutting current until bacterial contamination reached 10^9. In a comparison of the cutting current with the scalpel, no differences were apparent until contamination reached 10^5. Most wounds had abscesses at higher levels of contamination, whatever the incision method.

Conclusion.—Because electric coagulation current causes more inflammation, necrosis, and abscesses than the scalpel at all bacterial levels, the method should be limited to cases in which there is need for meticulous hemostasis. The indications for electric cutting current are uncertain, for it is less hemostatic, though less destructive, than coagulation cutting.

► Surgical principles are continually rediscovered. The use of a coagulation current for cutting leaves considerable necrotic tissue, the use of a cutting current for cutting leaves less necrotic tissue. By comparison, the use of a scalpel for cutting leaves minimal necrotic tissue. As numerous individuals have observed, there is abundant evidence that the widespread use of electrocautery for cutting does result in an increased rate of wound infection. These authors found that the use of cautery for opening tissue planes makes the tissue more vulnerable to bacterial infection, hardly a revelation.

I must confess that we routinely use electric cautery for the opening of long transmuscular incisions, such as thoracoabdominal, and have yet to recognize any problem with increased infection. I have no doubt that these authors' information is correct; it just does not seem to be particularly relevant.

β-Blocker Dosages and Mortality After Myocardial Infarction: Data From a Large Health Maintenance Organization

Barron HV, Viskin S, Lundstrom RJ, et al (Univ of California, San Francisco; Kaiser Permanente, Oakland, Calif)

Arch Intern Med 158:449–453, 1998 5–16

Introduction.—Long-term β-blocker therapy benefits patients who have had a myocardial infarction, but these agents are underused. Some patients receive dosages considerably less than the dosages found effective in trials, and elderly patients may not be treated at all. A retrospective study examined the association between the dosage of β-blockers prescribed after a myocardial infarction and cardiac mortality.

Methods.—The 1,050 patients included in the study had survived an acute myocardial infarction during January 1990 through December 1992. All had also survived the index hospitalization and were able to be followed from the date of hospital discharge. Follow-up continued through December 1993 or until the date of death. The primary outcome variable was cardiovascular death. Data were obtained on β-blocker use and dosage.

Results.—β-Blocker therapy was prescribed to 37.7% of patients, but almost half of these patients (48.1%) received dosages less than 50% of those determined to be effective in preventing death in large randomized clinical trials. Patients treated with β-blockers tended to be a lower-risk group than those not receiving that therapy. Those given the lower dosage, however, tended to be at higher risk for cardiovascular mortality than those given higher dosages. Nevertheless, the rate of cardiovascular mortality was lower in the low-dosage group than in the higher-dosage group. Patients in the low-dosage group were more likely to have undergone revascularization within the preceding 3 months.

Conclusion.—β-Blocker therapy clearly saves lives when administered after a myocardial infarction, but physicians underuse the therapy. When there is concern that patients may not tolerate the higher dosages used in trials, lower dosages should be considered because of the drug's apparent benefits.

▶ I realize that I include considerable internal medicine and cardiologic information in the YEAR BOOK, which may appear to have limited relevance to vascular surgery. However, it is obvious that many of our vascular patients have cardiac disease and many have had, or are about to have, a myocardial infarction. This information on the use of β-blockers in such patients is potentially quite important. As vascular surgeons, we need considerable knowledge on the treatment of coronary disease, and this includes the use of β-blockers. When we encounter a post–myocardial infarction vascular surgery patient, we should make every effort to have the patient's personal physician begin β-blocker therapy if the patient is not already receiving it. This may seem like interference in the function of the primary physician, but it clearly appears to be in the best interest of our patients.

6 Thoracic Aorta

Intimal Disease

Diagnosis and Management of Patients With Peripheral Macroemboli From Thoracic Aortic Pathology

Lau LS, Blanchard DG, Hye RJ, et al (Univ of California, San Diego)

Ann Vasc Surg 11:348–353, 1997

6–1

Background.—The wide availability of transesophageal echocardiography (TEE) has not only enhanced the evaluation of thoracic aortic disease but also clarified the role of such pathology as a source of peripheral artery emboli. Questions remain about the management of patients with peripheral emboli from thoracic aortic mural thrombus (TAMT). The management of 5 such patients, including the role of anticoagulation therapy, was reported.

Patients.—The experience included 5 patients with peripheral emboli of no identifiable cardiac source. The patients were 4 women and 1 man, aged 56–82 years. Each underwent TEE evaluation of the thoracic aorta. The patients had a total of 8 embolic events originating from TAMT, including emboli to the upper extremities in 4 cases, to the lower extremities in 1, and to the visceral vessels in 1. One patient was initially treated with aortobifemoral bypass; only after he had another embolic event was he found to have TAMT. The other 4 patients were managed with thromboembolectomy. All patients received anticoagulation therapy after TAMT was identified. One patient had an intra-abdominal hemorrhage, necessitating discontinuation of anticoagulants. All patients survived and none required amputation. One patient had recurrent embolization while receiving anticoagulation.

Conclusions.—For patients with arterial emboli of unknown source, TEE is a sensitive diagnostic technique. Although randomized trials of surgery vs. anticoagulation are needed, anticoagulation appears to be effective therapy for patients with peripheral macroemboli from TAMT.

▶ This well-written article extends our database concerning this important disease entity. Peripheral arterial macroemboli typically arise from the heart, infrarenal aortic occlusive disease, or infrarenal aneurysmal disease. A small number arise from arterial sources in the legs. However, 10% to 15% of all embolic sources remain cryptogenic. It is clear that a significant percentage of these cryptogenic emboli arise from a highly diseased thoracic aorta containing mural thrombus.[1, 2] These authors point out that the thoracic embolic source can frequently be diagnosed by TEE. It is interesting to note the upper extremity prevalence of emboli from this source. I do not know whether this represents a real phenomenon or merely a random event, but I suspect it may be real. Of course, once discovered, the problem is how to manage the thoracic aortic pathology. Thoracic aortic endarterectomy in the region of the arch is not particularly attractive. The authors suggest that anticoagulation therapy works well in this patient group, and although unproven may be correct. Overall, the message is that while we are searching for a source of peripheral emboli, we should consider the thoracic aorta and its evaluation by TEE.

References

1. Tunick PA, Perez JI, Kronz NI: Protruding atheromas in the thoracic aorta and systemic embolization. *Ann Intern Med* 115:432–437, 1991.
2. 1997 Year Book of Vascular Surgery, p 227.

Mobile Atheroma of the Aortic Arch Is an Underestimated Source of Embolization

Arko F, Buckley C, Baisden C, et al (Texas A&M Univ, Temple)

Am J Surg 174:737–740, 1997 6–2

Introduction.—Treatment for mobile atheroma in the aortic arch has yet to be defined, although several modalities have been proposed in the literature. They include routine anticoagulation, thrombolysis, endarterectomy, and balloon embolectomy. The patients reported on here had mobile atheroma identified by transesophageal echocardiography (TEE) and were treated with anticoagulation.

Methods.—Fourteen consecutive patients had grade V mobile atheroma and evidence of systemic or peripheral embolization. All underwent TEE when other imaging modalities failed to identify the source of embolization. Once diagnosis was established, patients were anticoagulated with heparin and warfarin. Heparin was discontinued and patients discharged on warfarin once the prothrombin time international ratio was between 2 and 3. Three patients had repeat TEE 6 months later.

Results.—The patients, 8 men and 6 women, had a mean age of 68 years. All have remained anticoagulated and none have had further evidence of systemic embolization since the initiation of therapy during a clinical follow-up ranging from 6 to 30 months. Five patients who had neurologic symptoms have remained symptom free over a mean of 15 months, and 7 patients with lower microembolization and renal insufficiency have remained asymptomatic for a mean of 13.4 months. Follow-up TEE in 3 patients revealed calcified thrombus of the thoracic aorta but no evidence of mobile atheroma.

Conclusion.—Mobile atheroma indicates an increased risk for perioperative stroke in patients undergoing coronary artery bypass surgery. In cases of systemic embolization, patients with generalized atherosclerosis should be screened for the presence of atheroma. Results in this small study support the use of anticoagulant therapy.

▶ Under a misleading title, the authors argue that anticoagulation may terminate embolic events caused by grade V mobile aortic atheroma. At most, this is an interesting observation. The reader should not forget that the exact 95% confidence limits of a zero incidence based on 14 observations is 0% to 23%. Moreover, as also noted by one of the discussants, one cannot avoid speculating on what the natural history would have been. See also Abstract 6–1.

T.V. Schroeder, M.D., D.M.Sc.

Endarterectomy of the Ascending Aorta: An Alternative Method in Patients With Extensively Calcified (Porcelain) Aorta Requiring Aortic Valve Replacement

Shapira OM, Cruz HA, Shemin RJ (Boston Med Ctr)
J Card Surg 12:160–164, 1997 6–3

Background.—Porcelain aorta describes extensive aortic calcification, leading to a rigid tube, as the result of platelike calcification of the intima and media. This uncommon condition causes major technical difficulties. Various techniques have been proposed for the management of porcelain aorta in patients requiring aortic valve replacement. The use of endarterectomy to facilitate aortic valve replacement in patients with porcelain aorta is reported.

Patients.—The patients were 2 elderly women with severe aortic stenosis. Mean aortic valve gradients were 86 and 35 mm Hg, with aortic valve areas of 0.6 and 0.7 cm^2, respectively. Extensive calcification of the aortic root was demonstrated by fluoroscopy. Surgery revealed a porcelain aorta and heavily calcified trileaflet aortic valve in both cases. Both patients underwent endarterectomy of the aortic root. In addition, 1 had endarterectomy of the left main coronary artery ostium and the other had aortic root enlargement with patch aortoplasty. Both patients recovered and were discharged on the fifth day. Both were doing well at follow-up, with normal left ventricular ejection fraction, good aortic valve prosthesis function, and a normal-caliber ascending aorta.

Conclusions.—The authors have had good results with endarterectomy of the ascending aorta in patients with porcelain aorta requiring aortic valve replacement. They describe the technical aspects of this procedure, and discuss the alternative approaches. Though the long-term results are unknown, endarterectomy of the ascending aorta should be considered as an alternative to other more complex operations.

► I include this article to demonstrate the remarkable ability of these cardiothoracic surgeons to perform a circumferential endarterectomy of a "porcelain" ascending aorta. I can only conclude that this disease must be different from what we are used to in other parts of the arterial system. Calcification this extensive in my experience has almost always been transmural, and attempts at endarterectomy have resulted in the remaining tissue being as thin as the proverbial tissue, with many holes and a total inability to withstand arterial pressure. Such is obviously not the case in the ascending aorta, where apparently a routine endarterectomy of extensively calcified media is possible with preservation of adequate adventitia to provide secure closure.

Innominate Artery

Transthoracic Repair of Innominate and Common Carotid Artery Disease: Immediate and Long-term Outcome for 100 Consecutive Surgical Reconstructions

Berguer R, Morasch MD, Kline RA (Wayne State Univ, Detroit)

J Vasc Surg 27:34–42, 1998 6–4

Introduction.—Transthoracic, extra-anatomic cervical, or endovascular repair is used to manage severe occlusive disease of the supra-aortic trunks. Because these lesions are relatively uncommon and difficult to image using noninvasive technology, the natural history of them is not well known. Survival and long-term patency data for direct, transthoracic repair of the supra-aortic trunk reconstruction are limited. A review of supra-aortic trunk reconstructions was conducted.

Methods.—There were 98 patients, ages 24–79 years, who had 8 innominate endarterectomies and 92 bypass procedures based on the thoracic aorta or proximal innominate artery. Four patients had upper extremity ischemia and 83 had cerebrovascular ischemia. No symptoms were seen in 13 patients. In 78 patients, an innominate lesion was bypassed. In 38 patients, the left common carotid artery required reconstruction, and in 9 patients the left subclavian artery required reconstruction. Direct bypass grafting was performed for multiple trunk reconstructions in 35 patients. The approach was via the left thoracotomy in 2 patients, partial sternotomy in 6 patients, and median sternotomy in 92 patients. Concomitant cardiac surgery was performed in 7 patients. Follow-up ranged from 1–184 months, with a mean of 51 months.

Results.—There was a combined stroke/death rate of 16%, with 8 deaths and 8 nonfatal strokes. For supra-aortic trunk reconstruction, the operative mortality rate was 6%, and for supra-aortic trunk reconstruction/cardiac operations, it was 29%. Two asymptomatic graft occlusions, 3 nonfatal myocardial infarctions, 7 significant pulmonary complications, 3 sternal wound infections, and 1 recurrent laryngeal nerve injury were

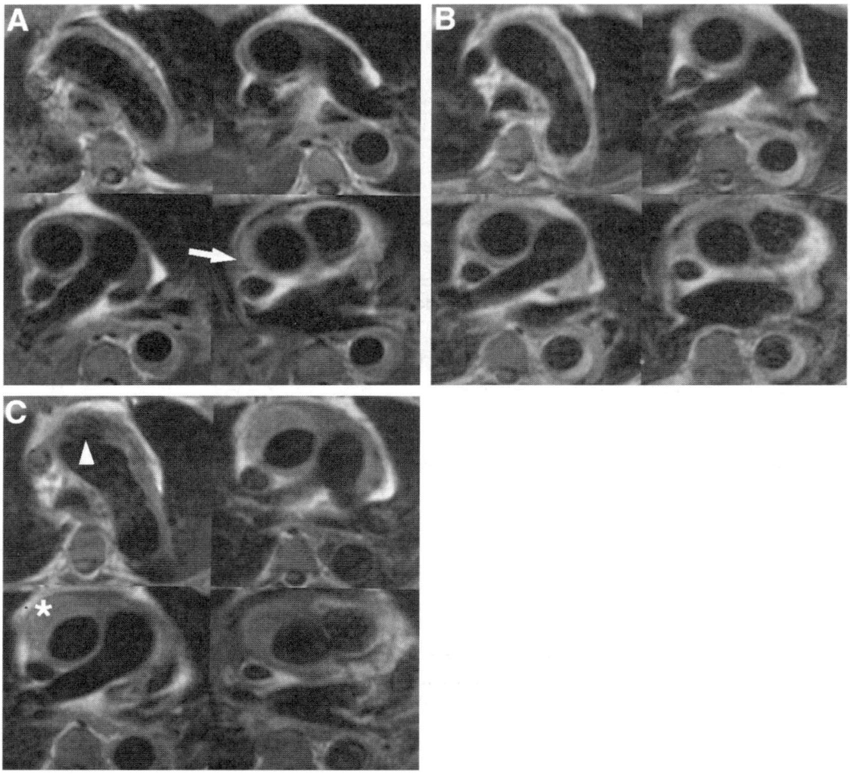

FIGURE 6.—Concurrent communicating dissection and resolution of intramural hematoma. Sequential transaxial T1-weighted SE (minimum RR interval/17) images were obtained (A) 3, (B) 20, and (C) 57 days after the onset of acute symptoms. A, crescentic collection of intermediate signal intensity (*arrow*) involving the descending and ascending portions of the thoracic aorta is consistent with acute type A intramural hematoma. B, images obtained during the early subacute phase show high signal intensity of the intramural hematoma. C, images obtained during the late subacute phase, because of the sudden onset of severe symptoms, demonstrate communicating dissection that is limited to the ascending aorta; the primary tear (*arrowhead*) and false lumen with slow blood flow (*asterisk*) are shown. On the other hand, there are signs of resolution of the intramural hematoma in the descending thoracic aorta; no residual thickening of the aortic wall in this area is noted. (Courtesy of Murray JG, Manisali M, Flamm SD, et al: Intramural hematoma of the thoracic aorta: MR image findings and their prognostic implications. *Radiology* 204:349–355. Copyright 1997, Radiological Society of North America.)

the descending aorta may be followed by MRI to determine complete resolution or impending complications of the hematoma.

▶ Intramural hematoma of the thoracic aorta without penetrating ulcer appears synonymous with aortic dissection without an intimal tear. It appears to be caused by spontaneous rupture of the aortic vasovasorum with propagation of the subintimal hemorrhage. All patients were seen with sudden back or chest pain suggesting aortic dissection. A large majority were hypertensive. Both transesophageal echo and CT scans showed a crescentic mass within the thoracic aorta, representing the contained blood within the wall. Interestingly, 4 of the 5 thoracic intramural hematomas in the ascending aorta eventually developed communication with the aortic lumen, requiring urgent surgery. Only 1 of the patients with descending thoracic aortic hematoma subsequently had communicating aortic dissection requiring grafting. We are slowly learning more about aortic intramural hematomas, as well as penetrating ulcers. It appears that intramural hematoma of the ascending aorta is best treated with surgery, whereas that of the descending aorta is frequently amenable to observation only.

Thoracic Aneurysm

What Is the Appropriate Size Criterion for Resection of Thoracic Aortic Aneurysms?

Coady MA, Rizzo JA, Hammond GL, et al (Yale Univ, New Haven, Conn)
J Thorac Cardiovasc Surg 113:476–491, 1997 6–8

Objective.—Rupture is the most common cause of death in patients with atherosclerotic aneurysms of the ascending aorta. Because the size-rupture correlation does not hold for the thoracic aorta, it is important to understand the risk factors that influence the natural course of the disease to select patients for whom the risk of operation is justified. Criteria for surgical intervention based on a study of 230 patients with thoracic aortic aneurysms were determined.

Methods.—Between October 1985 and March 1996, of the 230 patients (92 female), aged 16–92 years, including 25 patients with Marfan's syndrome, followed at the Yale Center for Thoracic Aortic Disease, 136 were

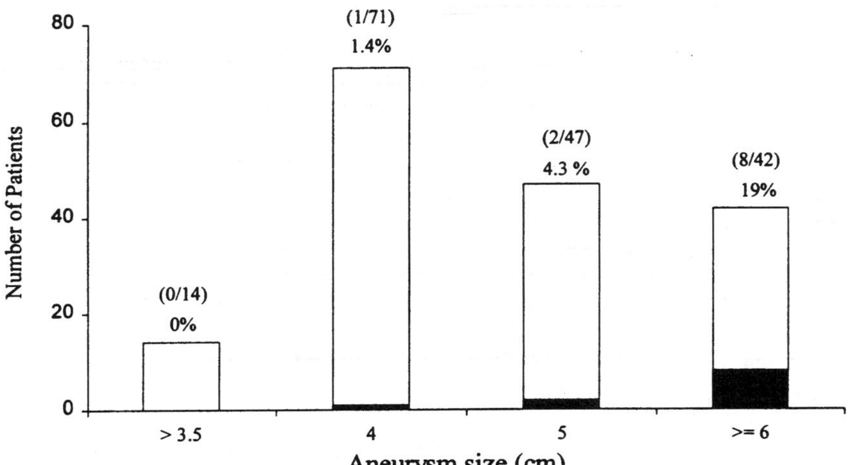

FIGURE 5.—Incidence of rupture as a function of initial aneurysm size. The entire *column* indicates the total number of patients with thoracic aortic aneurysms in each size range. The *black area* indicates the number of patients who incurred a rupture of the aneurysm. (Courtesy of Coady MA, Rizzo JA, Hammon GL, et al: What is the appropriate size criterion for resection of thoracic aortic aneurysms? *J Thorac Cardiovasc Surg* 113:476–491, 1997.)

operated on. There were 67 elective and 69 emergency surgeries. Complication rates and operative mortality were recorded, and 5-year survival estimates were calculated.

Results.—Aneurysms ranged in size from 4.0 to 8.0 cm and averaged 5.2 cm. The estimated annual growth rate was 0.12 cm, with larger aneurysms growing at a greater rate. The growth rate for ascending aortic aneurysms was 0.10 cm and for descending aortic aneurysms was 0.29 cm. The incidence of acute dissection or rupture ranged from 7.1% to 45.2% for aortic sizes from less than 4 cm to greater than 6.0 cm. Similar increases were demonstrated for the incidence of acute dissection alone and rupture alone (Fig 5). Overall, emergency, and nonemergency operative mortality rates were 15.4%, 21.7%, and 9.0%, respectively. One- and 5-year survival for patients with and without aortic dissection were 83% and 46%, and 89% and 71%, respectively. Median sizes at rupture or dissection for ascending and descending arteries were 6.0 and 7.2 cm, respectively. Ascending aneurysms greater than 6.0 cm had a 32.1% increased risk of rupture or dissection (P = 0.005). Descending aneurysms greater than 7.0 cm had a 43.0% increased risk of rupture or dissection (P = 0.006). Criteria for preemptive surgical intervention should be based on size smaller than the median rupture or dissection sizes above.

Conclusions.—Surgical intervention is recommended for descending aneurysms of 6.5 cm and for ascending aneurysms of 5.5 cm.

► A detailed analysis of a significant number of thoracic aortic aneurysms led these authors to recommend 5.5 cm as an acceptable size for elective resection of ascending aortic aneurysms, and 6.5 cm as a reasonable recommendation for resection of descending thoracic aneurysms. While the larger aneurysms had the anticipated increased likelihood of rupture, I am surprised to note that the larger aneurysms also had an increased incidence of dissection. I really have no basis to disagree with these authors' conclusions. However, I do think that waiting for the descending aneurysm to reach 6.5 cm may be a bit late. I am in the camp that believes thoracic aneurysms should be resected at about the same size as infrarenal aortic aneurysms, namely 5.5 cm. In the absence of persuasive evidence to the contrary, I am going to stick with my pig-headed opinion.

Rupture of the Perivisceral Aorta: Atherosclerotic Versus Mycotic Aneurysm

Quiñones-Baldrich WJ, Nene SM, Gelabert HA, et al (Univ of California, Los Angeles)

Ann Vasc Surg 11:331–341, 1997 6–9

Background.—Patients with perivisceral aortic rupture who make it to the hospital often have a contained rupture, permitting preoperative assessment. A 12-year experience with rupture of the perivisceral aorta was analyzed, underscoring the differences between atherosclerotic and mycotic aneurysms (MAs).

Patients.—There were 6 patients with atherosclerotic thoracoabdominal aneurysms (TAAs) that ruptured in the visceral segment of the aorta, and 6 with a ruptured MA. The TAA group had pain in the abdomen, chest, or back developing within 24 hours; those with MA had a 2- to 5-week history of symptoms. None of the TAA group had a history of sepsis, compared with 4 of the MA group. Risk factors for atherosclerosis were similar between the 2 groups. All patients were treated with in situ vascular grafting.

Outcomes.—Operative mortality was 33% in the TAA group vs. no operative mortality in the MA group. There were 2 preoperative cardiac arrests, 1 in a TAA patient who died 5 days after surgery, and 1 in an MA patient who survived. At a mean follow-up of 48 months, 4 TAA patients were alive, 1 with a pseudoaneurysm of the visceral patch-graft anastomosis. All 6 MA patients were alive, none with any signs of graft sepsis or recurrent aneurysm.

Conclusions.—Many patients with aortic rupture in the visceral portion prove to have MA. The clinical presentation and outcomes of such patients are different from those of patients with TAA. Both groups are effectively treated with surgery, although operative mortality is significantly higher in those with ruptured TAA. Patients with ruptured MA treated with in situ prosthetic replacement have low mortality and excellent long-term results.

► This is a very interesting description of 12 patients with a contained rupture of a perivisceral aortic aneurysm encountered over 12 years at the University of California, Los Angeles. Six of these patients had atherosclerotic aneurysm rupture, with symptoms present for less than 24 hours, whereas the remaining 6 had MA rupture, with symptoms present for 2–5 weeks. All patients underwent in situ grafting with the remarkable survival of 10 of 12 patients. Mycotic aneurysms had typical findings on CT, including the absence of aortic wall calcification, and localized saccular-contained ruptures in the presence of a soft tissue mass adjacent to a normal appearing aorta. On balance, this represents an extraordinarily good clinical outcome with a very difficult patient group.

Thoracoabdominal Aneurysm

Renal Failure After Thoracoabdominal Aortic Surgery

Kashyap VS, Cambria RP, Davison JK, et al (Harvard Med School, Boston)
J Vasc Surg 26:949–957, 1997 6–10

Introduction.—A significant and often lethal complication in patients who have had complex aortic surgery is renal failure. The incidence of renal failure varies from 9% to 40% in patients who have thoracoabdominal repair, with a significant increase in the postoperative mortality. There is still debate concerning the optimal intraoperative management to decrease the incidence of postoperative renal failure, with no consensus

TABLE 4.—Stratification of Patients According to Renal Dysfunction

	n (%)
0% to 50% elevation in baseline creatinine level	91 (49.7)
50% to 100% elevation in baseline creatinine level	47 (25.7)
>100% elevation in baseline creatinine level	24 (13.1)
Doubling + creatinine >3.0 mg/dl	16 (8.7)
Dialysis	5 (2.7)

(Courtesy of Kashyap VS, Cambria RP, Davison JK, et al: Renal failure after thoracoabdominal aortic surgery. *J Vasc Surg* 26:949–957, 1997.)

available. The perioperative outcome of patients who had thoracoabdominal surgery was reviewed to identify variables associated with postoperative renal failure.

Methods.—A review of 183 patients who had thoracoabdominal aortic surgery with supraceliac clamping was conducted. In 154 patients, thoracoabdominal aneurysm repair was performed (27% had type I, 11.5% had type II, 30% had type III, and 16% had type IV). Seventeen patients (9%) had suprarenal abdominal aortic aneurysm repair, and 12 patients (6.5%) had visceral/renal revascularization procedures. Thoracoabdominal aortic exposure and clamp-and-sew technique, with renal artery cold perfusion whenever the renal arteries were accessible (79% of patients), were included in intraoperative management.

Results.—Preoperative hypertension was seen in 85 % of patients, diabetes mellitus in 8%, single functioning kidney in 10%, recent intravenous contrast injection in 34%, renal insufficiency in 24%, and emergent operation in 19%. Almost all patients had an elevation in their serum creatinine level, but in half the patients, this elevation was less than 50% from baseline values (Table 4). In 21 patients (11.5%), there was acute renal failure, defined as both a doubling of serum creatinine level and an absolute value greater than 3.0 mg/dL. Five of the patients required hemodialysis. A preoperative creatinine level greater than 1.5 mg/dL and total cross-clamp time greater than 100 minutes were variables associated with this complication. Renal failure significantly increased the operative mortality risk (within 30 days; 8%).

Conclusion.—The risk of early death after thoracoabdominal aortic surgery is greatly increased by renal failure, although renal failure is still uncommon in contemporary practice. Patients with preoperative renal insufficiency are prone to renal failure postoperatively. In the prevention of renal failure after thoracoabdominal aortic surgery, regional hypothermic perfusion and minimal clamp times are important elements.

▶ After TAA resection elevation of serum creatinine to greater than 3 mg/dl occurred in 11.5% of patients, 2.7% of whom required hemodialysis. Predictably, variables associated with postoperative renal failure included a preoperative creatinine level greater than 1.5, and total aortic cross clamp time greater than 100 minutes. These authors believe that cold renal perfusion is desirable, and they were able to use it in 79% of patients. The incidence of renal failure was not apparently improved by partial left heart bypass and distal aortic perfusion. Clearly, this matter is unresolved.

Importance of Intercostal Artery Reattachment During Thoracoabdominal Aortic Aneurysm Repair

Safi HJ, Miller CC III, Carr C, et al (Baylor College of Medicine, Houston)
J Vasc Surg 27:58–68, 1998 6–11

Introduction.—Aortic surgeons continue to be plagued by neurologic complications as a consequence of thoracoabdominal aortic aneurysm repair. A multimethod approach, including reimplantation of intercostal arteries, adjuncts, sequential clamping (Fig 2), and moderate hypothermia, can help avoid neurologic deficits. The influence of selection and management of intercostal arteries T7–T12 on the incidence of neurologic deficit

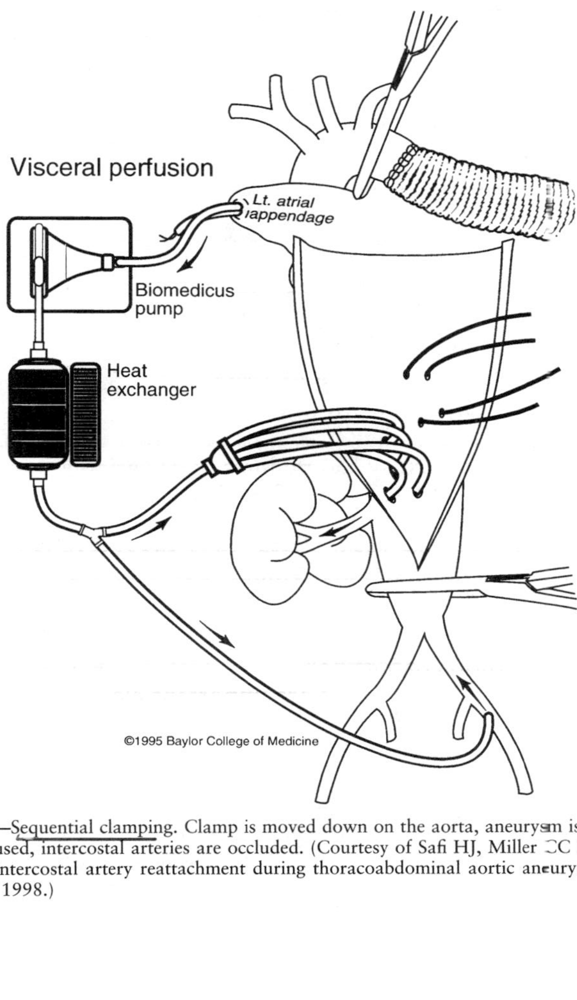

FIGURE 2.—Sequential clamping. Clamp is moved down on the aorta, aneurysm is opened, visceral vessels are perfused, intercostal arteries are occluded. (Courtesy of Safi HJ, Miller CC III, Carr C, et al: Importance of intercostal artery reattachment during thoracoabdominal aortic aneurysm repair. *J Vasc Surg* 27:58–68, 1998.)

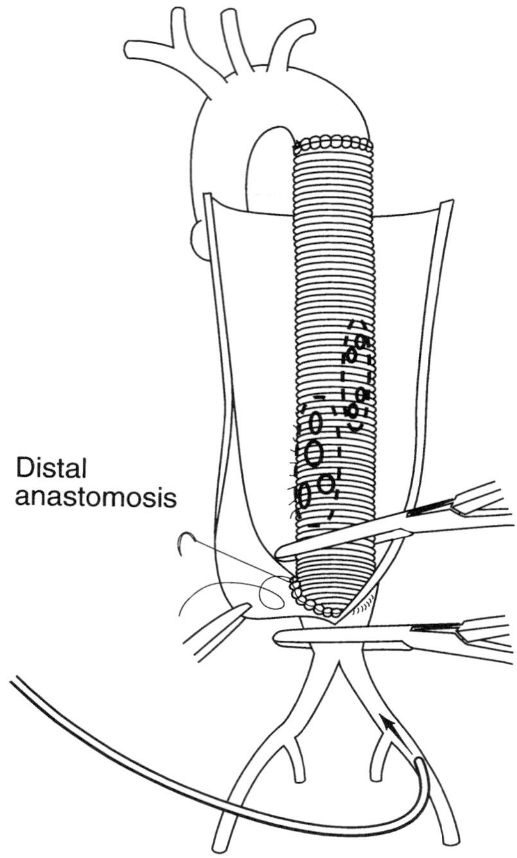

FIGURE 3.—Sequential clamping. Intercostal arteries and visceral vessels have been reattached to graft, and proximal clamp moved down on the graft. Distal anastomosis is completed before withdrawal of clamps. (Courtesy of Safi HJ, Miller CC III, Carr C, et al: Importance of intercostal artery reattachment during thoracoabdominal aortic aneurysm repair. *J Vasc Surg* 27:58–68, 1998.)

was examined by prospectively documenting the arteries occluded, ligated, or reattached during thoracoabdominal aortic aneurysm. The relationship of each artery to previously identified risk factors on the development of neurologic deficits was assessed.

Methods.—There were 343 patients in a 5-year period who had thoracoabdominal aortic aneurysms repaired by 1 surgeon. Of these patients, 264 had Crawford types I (42%), II (44%), and III (14%). In 164 patients (62%), the adjuncts of distal aortic perfusion and cerebrospinal fluid drainage were used. In the majority of patients, cross-clamping was sequential, beginning in the left upper third of the thoracic aorta (Fig 3) Contingency table and multiple logistic regression were used to analyze data.

Results.—In 23 patients (8.7%), early neurologic deficit occurred. In 10 patients (3.8%), late deficit occurred. In 19 of 147 patients (12.9%), neurologic deficit with at least 1 reimplantation and no ligation of arteries T11 or T12 occurred. In 11 of 111 (9.9%) patients, neurologic deficit for occlusion of the same arteries occurred. Neurologic deficit occurred in 3 of 6 patients (50%) for ligation of T11 and T12. In multivariate analysis, reduced late neurologic deficit was significantly associated with reimplantation of intercostal arteries T9 or T10. Modification of the neurologic deficit rate was not associated with any other intercostal artery status. An increased risk of postoperative neurologic deficit was significantly associated with type II aneurysms and acute dissections. There was a protective effect with adjuncts, most often in types II and III. There was 14.1% neurologic deficit in type II with an adjunct, and 35.3% neurologic deficit without an adjunct.

Conclusion.—Highly variable outcomes were seen in patients with patent arteries at the T11/T12 level, depending on whether the arteries were reattached or ligated. When these arteries are patent, reimplantation of thoracic intercostal arteries T11 and T12 is indicated. The risk of late neurologic deficit is lowered with reimplantation of T9 and T10, which decreases the spinal cord's vulnerability to changes in blood and cerebrospinal fluid pressure in the days after surgery. Overall risk is lowered, and adequate time for targeted intercostal artery reimplantation is provided, by adjuncts.

▶ Overall neurologic deficit in this series occurred in 12.5% of patients. These authors are convinced that reimplantation of thoracic intercostal arteries T11 and T12 should be performed when the arteries are patent. Reimplantation of T9 and T10 lowers the risk of late neurologic deficit. Specific adjuncts to which the authors subscribe include Biomedicus pump perfusion of the lower part of the body, spinal fluid drainage, and visceral perfusion. It appears that the 10% to 12% incidence of neurologic deficit may be the minimum we can expect in large series of thoracoabdominal aneurysms. We might not do much better than this.

Impact of Distal Aortic and Visceral Perfusion on Liver Function During Thoracoabdominal and Descending Thoracic Aortic Repair

Safi HJ, Miller CC III, Yawn DH, et al (Baylor College of Medicine, Houston)
J Vasc Surg 27:145–133, 1998 6–12

Introduction.—Interruption of blood flow in the arterial system's central conduit is necessary to repair the thoracoabdominal and descending thoracic aortic aneurysms. But prolonged ischemia and associated end-organ damage is caused by this interruption of circulation. The reduction of insult to the liver during thoracoabdominal and descending thoracic aortic aneurysm repair is a focus of research. During thoracoabdominal and descending thoracic aortic repair, the impact of distal aortic and

Retrograde Aortic and Selective Organ Perfusion During Thoracoabdominal Aortic Aneurysm Repair

Jacobs MJHM, de Mol BAJM, Legemate DA, et al (Academic Med Centre, Amsterdam)

Eur J Vasc Endovasc Surg 14:360–366, 1997 6–15

Introduction.—Renal and intestinal ischemia are major complications of surgery for thoracoabdominal aortic aneurysm (TAAA) A number of different techniques have been tried to preserve the function of visceral organs during cross-clamping. A prospective study of retrograde and selective organ perfusion is reported.

Methods.—The study included 33 consecutive patients undergoing surgical repair of TAAA. Six patients had a history of previous type B dissection. The patients were 30 men and 3 women, mean age 61. The type of TAAA was type I in 35% of patients, type II in 32%, type III in 15%, and type IV in 18%. The patients with type I lesions underwent retrograde aortic perfusion via left atrium femoral artery bypass or partial cardiopul-

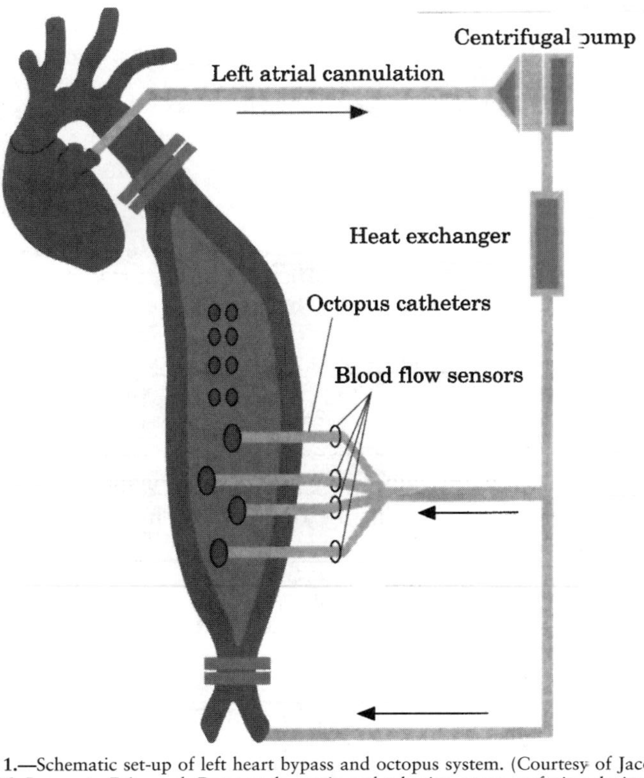

FIGURE 1.—Schematic set-up of left heart bypass and octopus system. (Courtesy of Jacobs MJHM, de Mol BAJM, Legemate DA, et al: Retrograde aortic and selective organ perfusion during thoracoabdominal aortic aneurysm repair. *Eur J Vasc Endovasc Surg* 14:360–366. Copyright 1997. Reprinted by permission of WB Saunders Company Limited, London.)

monary bypass. Those with type II, III, or IV TAAA underwent the same procedure. In addition, after cross-clamping and opening of the abdominal aorta, they underwent selective perfusion of the celiac trunk, superior mesenteric, and both renal arteries with four 9F Pruitt catheters. These were connected in "octopus" fashion to the extracorporeal circulation (Fig 1).

Results.—None of the patients died during the operation. Throughout surgery, flow through each octopus catheter remained at least 60 mL/min. All patients, regardless of cross-clamp time, had uninterrupted urinary output. There was 1 case of renal failure in a patient who had renal insufficiency preoperatively. Overall in-hospital mortality was 15%. The rate of paraplegia was 12%.

Conclusions.—This study demonstrates the safety of retrograde aortic and selective organ perfusion during aortic cross-clamping in patients undergoing TAAA repair. These techniques appear to be effective in preventing renal and intestinal ischemia during the operation. The method of perfusion chosen depends on the type of TAAA present.

▶ Controversy continues to rage as to whether some version of atrial-femoral bypass should be used in patients undergoing thoracoabdominal aneurysm repair. Experienced proponents of the clamp-and-sew technique point out that their results are just as good as results obtained by those who use partial left heart bypass. Certainly a number of surgeons believe that routine atriofemoral bypass should be used, possibly with the addition of octopus catheters into the visceral arteries during the time these vessels are unperfused.

Cerebral Spinal Fluid Drainage and Distal Aortic Perfusion Decrease the Incidence of Neurological Deficit: The Results of 343 Descending and Thoracoabdominal Aortic Aneurysm Repairs

Safi HJ, Campbell MP, Miller CC III, et al (Baylor College of Medicine, Houston)

Eur J Vasc Endovasc Surg 14:118–124, 1997 6–16

Background.—Several techniques have been used to maintain blood supply to the spinal cord during thoracoabdominal aortic aneurysm (TAAA) repair. As adjuncts, both CSF drainage and distal aortic perfusion have improved patient outcomes, but they are not completely sufficient on their own (Fig 1). Their influence on neurologic deficit and death were evaluated in a review of patients operated on for descending aortic aneurysm and TAAA repair.

Patients.—The 5-year experience included 343 patients undergoing this surgery. Aneurysm type was type I in 30% of patients, type II in 34%, type III of IV in 20%, and descending thoracic type in 15%. Twenty percent of patients, managed before 1992 were managed with a simple cross-clamp. Thereafter, adjuncts were used with most patients (54% of the total).

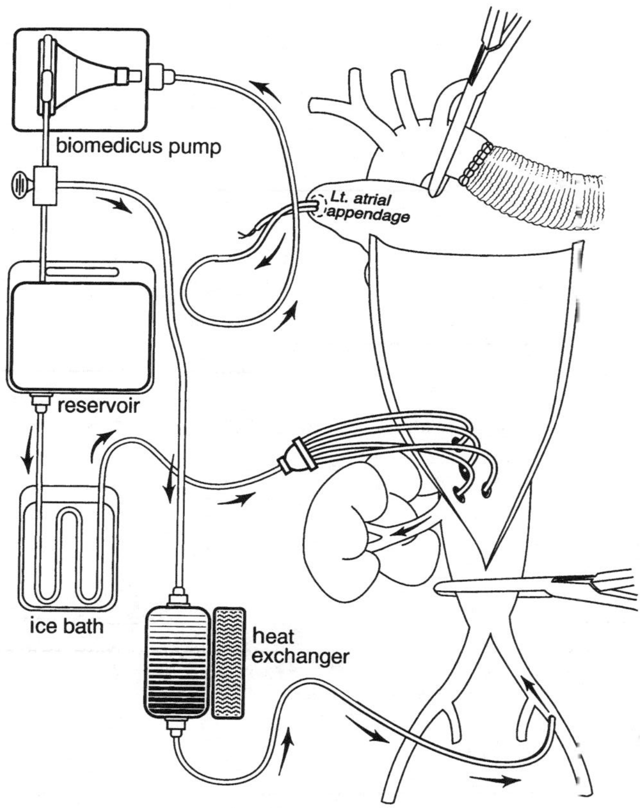

FIGURE 1.—Distal aortic perfusion: blood travels from the left atrial appendage through the pump to the left femoral artery. Visceral perfusion: blood travels through an ice bath before perfusion to the visceral arteries. (Reprinted from Safi HJ, Campbell MP, Miller CC III, et al: Cerebral spinal fluid drainage and distal aortic perfusion decrease the incidence of neurological deficit: The results of 343 descending and thoracoabdominal aortic aneurysm repairs. *Eur J Endovasc Surg* 14:118–124, 1997. By permission of the publisher, WB Saunders Company Limited, London.)

Outcomes.—Neurologic deficit developed in 10% of patients overall. The rate of neurologic deficit was 16% for patients managed with a simple cross-clamp vs. 7% for those managed with adjuncts (odds ratio, 0.36). Among patients with type I or II aneurysm, the incidence of neurologic deficit was 21% with cross-clamping vs. 9% with adjuncts (odds ratio, 0.35). For patients with type II aneurysms, the figures were 41% and 13%, respectively (odds ratio, 0.21). The 30-day mortality rate was 13% when patients whose diagnosis included rupture were included and 10% when those patients were excluded.

Conclusion.—In patients undergoing descending aortic aneurysm and TAAA repair, the adjuncts of CSF drainage and distal aortic perfusion significantly reduce the incidence of neurologic deficit. The benefit is particularly apparent for patients with type II TAAA. Neurologic deficits still pose a major risk to these patients, however.

► These very experienced aneurysm surgeons changed their technique in 1991 for TAAA repair to include routine CSF drainage and distal aortic perfusion. Comparing current results for patients with the new techniques to their own historic controls, they found a reduction in neurologic deficit from 16% to 7% overall. I note that these surgeons also use a visceral perfusion side arm from their bypass apparatus. Although some continue to prefer the cut-and-sew technique without distal perfusion, I believe that the majority opinion is coming down on the side of both distal perfusion, and certainly cerebrospinal fluid drainage. I continue to believe a right axillofem graft constitutes generally adequate distal perfusion.

Observations on Delayed Neurologic Deficit After Thoracoabdominal Aortic Aneurysm Repair

Safi HJ, Miller CC III, Azizzadeh A, et al (Baylor College of Medicine, Houston)

J Vasc Surg 26:616–622, 1997 6–17

Background.—Recent reports have described the delayed development of neurologic deficit in patients undergoing repair of thoracoabdominal aortic aneurysm. A series of 8 patients with this condition and their successful management were described.

Experience.—In all patients undergoing surgery for thoracoabdominal aortic aneurysms, the authors have taken steps to prevent the development of neurologic deficit, including routine CSF drainage and distal aortic perfusion. If possible, reattachment of patent intercostal arteries was performed. Over a 5-year period, 8 patients experienced delayed neurologic complications, which developed from 1 to 14 days after the end of anesthesia. As soon as the condition was recognized, the patients underwent CSF drainage. This was followed by clinical improvement in all patients. On independent classification using a modified Tarlov score, all patients improved by at least 2 points, on a scale of 0 to 5. Tarlov score increased by a mean of 2.4 points from the onset of neurologic deficit to discharge.

Conclusion.—In patients undergoing thoracoabdominal aortic aneurysm repair, delayed neurologic deficit can develop anywhere from 1 day to 2 weeks postoperatively. The outcome is significantly improved by CSF drainage, which should be initiated at the first sign of neurologic deficit.

► This very experienced group from Houston encountered 8 patients in whom delayed paraplegia or paraparesis developed 1–14 days after thoracoabdominal aneurysm repair. All patients had immediate CSF drainage reinstituted upon recognition of symptoms, and significant clinical improvement occurred in all patients, including normalization in 2. Based on this experience, the authors recommend that CSF drainage be immediately reinstituted if signs of delayed neurologic dysfunction develop after thoracoabdominal aneurysm repair. We have had occasion to use this technique in several patients and have also found a gratifying incidence of improvement. I believe the matter is basically settled. If a patient develops delayed lower extremity neurologic symptoms after thoracoabdominal aneurysm repair, immediate reinstitution of CSF drainage appears indicated.

Mesenteric Shunting Decreases Visceral Ischemia During Thoracoabdominal Aneurysm Repair

Cambria RP, Davison JK, Giglia JS, et al (Massachusetts Gen Hosp, Boston; Harvard Med School, Boston)

J Vasc Surg 27:745–749, 1998 6–18

Introduction.—Longer duration of aortic clamp time is associated with major morbidity after thoracoabdominal aneurysm (TAA) repair. The method described here rapidly establishes visceral perfusion immediately after performance of the proximal thoracic aortic anastomosis in TAA repair.

Methods.—The technique was applied in 15 patients over a 4-month period (July to October 1996). All were undergoing type I, II, or III TAA repair with a clamp and sew technique. The prosthesis is prepared by suturing a 10-mm Dacron graft to the aortic graft for subsequent mesenteric shunting. Operative data relative to visceral ischemia in these patients were compared with 15 control patients exactly matched for aneurysm extent and complexity of repair. Controls had been treated in the 9 months before adoption of the mesenteric shunt technique.

Results.—After perfusion was established through the mesenteric shunt, the mean decrease in systolic arterial pressure was 12.5 mm Hg, with a concomitant rise in end-tidal partial pressure of carbon dioxide. The mean time to establishment of visceral perfusion through the shunt was 25.5 minutes, leading to an average decrease in visceral ischemic time of 31.3 minutes. When compared with control patients, those who underwent mesenteric shunting had a significantly decreased (mean, 6.9 mm Hg vs. 21.6 mm Hg) rise in end-tidal carbon dioxide on completion of visceral vessel reconstruction.

Conclusion.—In-line mesenteric shunting during TAA repair is a simple technique, does not require systemic heparin, and can be used with clamp and sew or distal perfusion with sequential clamping operative techniques.

► Although Dr. Cambria espouses the cut and sew technique for TAA repair, he seems to make an exception in providing single-vessel visceral perfusion during anastomosis in an effort to ameliorate the hemodynamic derangements that typically occur with re-establishment of visceral perfusion. Interestingly, no patient had evidence of coagulopathic bleeding. We will have to ask Dr. Cambria to clarify his somewhat conflicting recommendations: Is it cut and sew or single-limb visceral perfusion? (See also Abstract 6–14.)

Cardiac Function is a Risk Factor for Paralysis in Thoracoabdominal Aortic Replacement

Acher CW, Wynn MM, Hoch JR, et al (Univ of Wisconsin, Madison)
J Vasc Surg 27:821–830, 1998 6–19

Introduction.—Patients undergoing thoracoabdominal aortic replacement are at risk for paralysis. Although this risk can be reduced by CSF drainage (CSFD) or hypothermia used together with endorphin receptor blockade, the amount of aorta replaced and clinical presentation continue to be risk factors for paralysis. A prospective study examined additional factors that influence paralysis risk, renal function, and mortality in thoracoabdominal aortic replacement.

Methods.—Study subjects were 217 consecutive patients treated for thoracoabdominal (176) and thoracic (41) aneurysms from 1984 through 1996. Sixty-six (30%) had Crawford type 2 aneurysms. In 150 patients (group A), CSFD and low-dose naloxone (1 µg/kg/hr) were used as adjuncts to reduce the risk of paralysis. The remaining 67 patients (group B) did not receive CSFD and naloxone. No patient had intercostal reimplantation or assisted circulation. Preoperative demographic data and intraoperative physiologic data were used in univariate and multivariate analyses to determine risk factors for paralysis.

Results.—There were 17 deficits in 205 surviving patients: 5 in group A (with 31 expected deficits) and 12 in group B (with 13 expected deficits). There were no deficits in patients with acute or chronic thoracic aneurysms. Eight of the 17 deficit patients awoke with paraplegia and remained paraplegic. Acute presentation, Crawford type 2 aneurysm (Table 3), group B membership, and a decrease in cardiac index with aortic occlusion proved to be significant risk factors for deficit in a multivariate logistic regression model. Group A patients had only 1/40th the risk of paralysis of group B by odds ratio analysis. The overall mortality rate was 9.7%; all but 2 deaths were among patients with acute presentations. The preoperative creatinine level was the single significant predictor of postoperative renal function, and renal function was significantly improved by renal

TABLE 3.—Crawford Type, Clinical Presentation, and Deficits

Type	*Number (%)*	*Elective*	*Acute*	*Dissection*	*Deficit*
CI	35 (16)	21	14	9	3
C2	66 (30)	39	27	13	13
C3	29 (14)	19	10	2	0
C4	46 (21)	32	14	1	1
TA*	41 (19)	16	25	4	0
Total	217 (100)	127	90	29	17

Note: CI, C2, C3, and C4 are Crawford aneurysm types; *Elective*, patients undergoing elective operative treatment; *Acute*, patients with acute clinical presentation; *Dissection*, patients with acute or chronic dissection at presentation; *Deficit*, patients with preoperative paraplegia.

*Patients with Stanford B dissections that were repaired with short thoracic grafts were classified as thoracic aneurysm (*TA*).

(Courtesy of Acher CW, Wynn MM, Hoch JR, et al: Cardiac function is a risk factor for paralysis in thoracoabdominal aortic replacement. *J Vasc Surg* 27:821–830, 1998.)

revascularization. Patients at high risk for death were older, had acute presentation, and had an elevated preoperative creatinine level.

Conclusion.—Use of CSFD and low-dose naloxone significantly reduces the risk of paralysis associated with thoracoabdominal aortic replacement. A decrease in cardiac index with aortic occlusion was identified as a variable that defines a subset of patients at increased risk for paralysis.

► Dr. Acher and his associates have achieved an enviable record of a very low rate of neurologic deficits in patients receiving CSFD and low-dose naloxone without intercostal reimplantation or assisted circulation. In this study, they determined that a decrease in cardiac index with aortic occlusion is a previously unreported variable defining a subset of patients at high risk for paralysis. Interestingly, the actual amount of decrease in cardiac index was only about 6/10 of a liter. The authors speculate that this decrease may reflect the heart's inability to augment collateral blood flow to the spinal cord during cross clamping. Perhaps.

Miscellaneous

Twenty-Year Follow-up of Acute Type A Dissection: The Incidence and Extent of Distal Aortic Disease Using Magnetic Resonance Imaging

Barron DJ, Livesey SA, Brown IW, et al (Southampton Gen Hosp, England)
J Card Surg 12:147–159, 1997 6–20

Introduction.—The commonest catastrophic condition involving the aorta is acute dissection of the ascending aorta, which carries a mortality approaching 90% in the first 72 hours. For acute type A aortic dissection, emergency surgery is now the treatment of choice. By addressing the problem of the persistent distal false lumen, further improvement in survival will be achieved. Because there have been no long-term follow-up studies, the incidence and importance of a distal false lumen have remained difficult to estimate. A review and 20-year follow-up study of patients with acute type A aorta dissection who had surgical treatment were conducted.

Methods.—There were 87 patients who had had surgical repair of type A aortic dissection who were examined 20 years later, with magnetic

TABLE 3.—Site of the Intimal Tear in the 81 of the 87 Patients in Whom the Tear Was Identified

Site of Tear	Number of Cases	Tear Resected	% with Tear Resected
Ascending Aorta	61	59	97
Arch	19	12	63
Arch & Descending	1	0	0
Total	81	71	88

(Courtesy of Barron DJ, Livesey SA, Brown IW, et al: Twenty-year follow-up of acute type A dissection: The incidence and extent of distal aortic disease using magnetic resonance imaging. *J Card Surg* 12:147–159, 1997.)

resonance scanning of the entire aorta. A protocol for long-term management and follow-up was devised, particularly regarding indications for reoperation.

Results.—There was 27.5% early mortality. The 5-year survival was 65%, the 10-year survival 28%, and the 25-year survival 20%. In the last 5 years, early mortality decreased to 18%. Distal aortic disease was the most common cause of late death, accounting for 47% of all late deaths, with a peak incidence at 7–10 years after surgery. Despite 82% of all intimal tears being resected at the time of operation, the incidence of persistent distal false lumen in survivors was 72%. In most patients (76%), the tear was found in the ascending aorta, but the tear was located in the arch in 24% (Table 3). Extension of the repair into the aortic arch, the use of the open technique, or Gelatin-Resorcine-Formal tissue glue did not affect the incidence. A maximum aortic diameter of 6 cm in at least 1 plane on magnetic resonance scanning was reached by 6% of patients with a distal false lumen, and 25% of patients had a diameter which reached 5 cm.

Conclusion.—The choice of surgical technique does not prevent the persistence of a distal false lumen, if dissection has extended beyond the arch at time of presentation. Ideal anatomical and functional assessment of distal aortic disease is given by magnetic resonance scanning, which also provides the surgeon with all the necessary information to plan the timing and indications for further surgery.

► It is indeed remarkable that after resection of a type A aortic dissection (including resection of the intimal tear with grafting) a chronic distal false lumen persisted in 72% of patients and had a distinct propensity to become aneurysmal with time in at least 25%. A significant number of these patients will eventually experience aortic related deaths with the highest incidence being at 7–10 years. It seems prudent to assume that all patients with ascending aortic resection of a type A dissection are at great risk for a persistent patent distal false lumen and the development of distal aneurysms. Careful routine imaging studies appear to be indicated in these patients. Hopefully distal aneurysms will be detected as they develop and appropriate plans developed for elective resection.

Traumatic Aortic Transections: Eight-Year Experience With the "Clamp-Sew" Technique

Sweeney MS, Young DJ, Frazier OH, et al (Univ of Texas-Houston)
Ann Thorac Surg 64:384–389, 1997 6–21

Background.—Mortality is very high for patients with traumatic aortic dissection. There is ongoing controversy regarding the optimal operative approach for this type of injury. An 8-year experience with the "clamp-sew" method for the management of acute traumatic aortic transection is reported.

TABLE 2.—Prevalence of Abdominal Aortic Aneurysms

	CABG (%) (95% CI)	Controls (%) (95% CI)	p*
Overall	18.2	1.4	0.0001
"New" AAA cases	13.0 (8.2–17.8)	1.4 (0–3.4)	0.0001
Female	9.1 (2.1–16.1)	0	—†
Male	15.1 (8.8–21.4)	2.8 (0–6.7)	0.028

*Two-sample t-test.

†As no abdominal aortic aneurysms were found in the control group, statistical analysis was not done.

Abbreviations: AAA, abdominal aortic aneurysm; *CABG*, coronary artery bypass graft; *CI*, confidence interval.

(Courtesy of Bergersen L, Kiernan S, McFarlane G, et al: Prevalence of abdominal aortic aneurysms in patients undergoing coronary artery bypass grafting. *Ann Vasc Surg* 12(2):101–105, 1998.)

that the prevalence of AAA in such patients is higher than that of the general population.

Methods.—Over an 18-month period, patients at the University of Vermont who were older than 50 years and scheduled for elective CABG underwent preoperative US. Controls were a group of patients who also underwent abdominal US but had no history of vascular disease. An aneurysm was defined as a maximal aortic diameter of 3.0 cm or greater. Data were obtained on the patients' medical history, including previous AAA surgery.

Results.—Abdominal US was performed in 192 patients with CABG and 140 controls. Compared with controls, the CABG group was older and had more cardiovascular risk factors. The overall prevalence (including previously repaired AAA and new cases) was 18.2% in the CABG group. The prevalence of new cases in controls was 1.4%, vs. 13.0% for patients. Men were more likely than women to have an AAA (Table 2). Ten patients (5.2%) had an AAA greater than 5.0 cm. Risk factors for AAA in the CABG population were age 65 years or older and smoking.

Conclusion.—The prevalence of AAA was found to be higher in patients undergoing CABG than in a control population. Screening such patients is recommended, especially in the case of older men who smoke.

▶ As we begin to extend more and more screening studies to the general population, it is absolutely essential that we define parameters for selecting that portion of the general population at greatest risk for having the condition in question. As always, a real problem is defining what one means by AAA, in this case any aorta with a maximal diameter equal to or greater than 3.0 cm. Using this casual definition, the overall prevalence of aneurysm in CABG patients was 18%, with about one third of these having an aneurysm greater than 5 cm. This information appears to confirm that patients having had, or about to undergo, CABG are a legitimate screening subset for AAA. I strongly suspect that bean counters of the future will insist upon quantitative data such as these to justify population screening efforts.

Management

What Is the Long-term Outcome for Patients With Very Small Abdominal Aortic Aneurysms?

Watson CJE, Walton J, Shaw E, et al (John Radcliffe Hosp, Oxford, England; Gloucestershire Royal Hosp, Gloucester, England)

Eur J Vasc Endovasc Surg 14:299–304, 1997 7–4

Background.—Most abdominal aortic aneurysms (AAAs) in otherwise healthy older men are small, measuring less than 4 cm. Although surgery is recommended for aneurysms measuring 5.5 cm or larger, the management of smaller aneurysms remains unclear. A population-based screening study assessed the long-term outcomes of patients with AAAs measuring less than 4 cm.

Methods.—The study included 142 patients with AAAs measuring less than 4 cm in anteroposterior dimension at presentation. The patients were followed up by ultrasound every 6 to 12 months. Their outcomes were determined by record review.

Results.—During the 9-year follow-up, aneurysms smaller than 3.0 cm grew at a median rate of 1 mm/yr. This rate increased to 2 mm/yr for aneurysms measuring 3.0 to 3.9 cm, and 3 mm/yr for those measuring 4.0 to 4.9 cm (Fig 5). The threshold value for aneurysm repair increased from 4.0 to 5.5 cm during follow-up. Twenty-three patients underwent surgery; 1 died in the perioperative period, and 3 died later of unrelated causes. Thirty-five patients died with AAA, without surgery. One patient, who refused follow-up, died of a ruptured aneurysm.

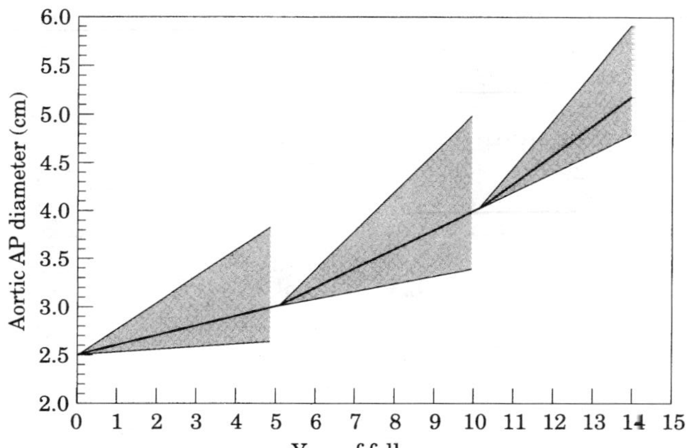

FIGURE 5.—Median aneurysm growth rate. Plot shows the diameter of an imaginary aneurysm growing in each size band according to the median annual growth rates, with the shaded areas between upper and lower quartiles for the band. *Abbreviation: AP*, anteroposterior. (Reprinted from Watson CJE, Walton J, Shaw E, et al: What is the long-term outcome for patients with very small abdominal aortic aneurysms? *Eur J Vasc Endovasc Surg* 14:299–304, copyright 1997, by permission of the publisher, WB Saunders Company Limited, London.)

Conclusion.—Abdominal aortic aneurysms measuring less than 4 cm in diameter have a relatively benign course. The value of early intervention for very small aneurysms is questionable. Risk factors for AAA rupture may include larger aortic diameter and rapid growth rate.

▶ I consider the issue of surgery for small aneurysms a fully developed conundrum. Although there is an extraordinarily limited likelihood of rupture of an aneurysm under 5 or 5.5 cm, the natural history of small aneurysms is to enlarge. The rate of enlargement appears rather modest, on average 2–3 mm per year, but, inevitably, many of these aneurysms will reach a size appropriate for surgery. Thus, when we encounter a patient with a 4-cm aneurysm, should we operate now—or should we wait 3 or 4 years until the aneurysm has grown to 5.5 cm, and the patient is 4 years older and likely represents an increased surgical risk? For now, we have decided to limit our recommendations for aneurysm surgery to those greater than 5.5 cm. As the authors of this article presciently note in their conclusion "patients with small aortic aneurysms may have more to fear from vascular surgeons than from their aneurysms." Perhaps so.

Surgical Treatment of Infected Aortic Aneurysm

Moneta GL, Taylor LM Jr, Yeager RA, et al (Oregon Health Sciences Univ, Portland; Portland Dept of Veteran's Affairs Hosp, Oregon)

Am J Surg 175:396–399, 1998 7–5

Introduction.—Treatment of infected aortic aneurysms involves surgery and is often complicated by patient instability, other coexisting medical conditions, and the need to place prosthetic material in an infected field. Results with surgically treated infected aortic aneurysms over a 20-year period were reviewed (Figure).

Methods.—A retrospective review was conducted of 17 patients who had operations specifically for primary infected aortic aneurysms distal to the left subclavian artery. There were 10 patients with infrarenal infection and 7 with suprarenal infection. The most common condition leading to aortic infections was aortic atherosclerosis, followed by *Salmonella* enteritis (Table 2). Records were obtained of the patient's age, gender, site of the aortic infection, operative and late survival, freedom from late arterial or prosthetic graft infection, conditions thought to have predisposed to the development of aortic infection, signs and symptoms, fever, and complication conditions. Aortic and periaortic tissue débridement and in situ prosthetic or patch graft replacement were done in all patients.

Results.—Abdominal/back pain was found in all patients, 24% were hemodynamically unstable, 71% had leukocytosis, and 88% were febrile. *Staphylococcus aureus* was the most common responsible organism (24%). It was found that all suprarenal infections were caused by gram-positive organisms. Infrarenal infections were treated with preliminary axillofemoral bypass followed by aortic resection. In situ prosthetic graft

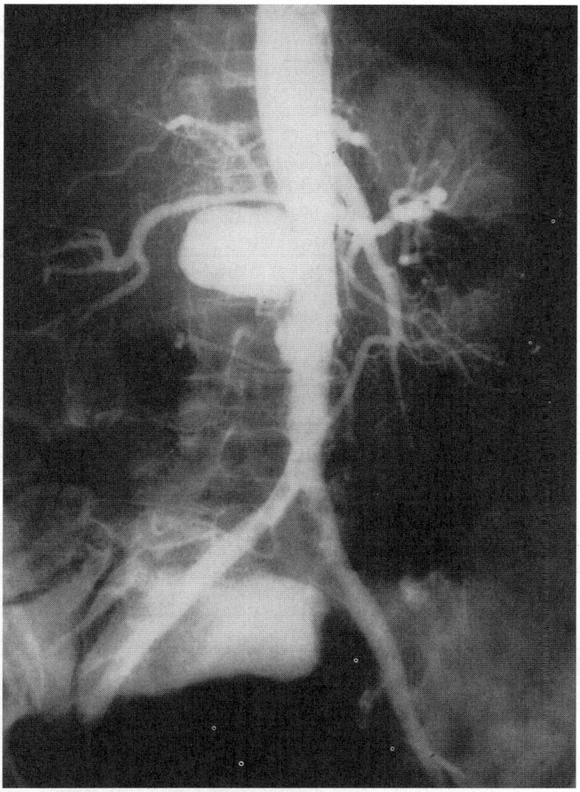

FIGURE.—Typical appearance of an infected aortic aneurysm. Aneurysms such as this are really pseudoaneurysms and represent localized contained rupture of the aorta. (Courtesy of Moneta GL, Taylor LM, Jr, Yeager RA, et al: Surgical treatment of infected aortic aneurysm. *Am J Surg* 175:396–399. Copyright 1998 with permission from Excerpta Medica Inc.)

TABLE 2.—Bacterial Etiology of Infected Aortic Aneurysm in 17 Patients

Organism	Number of Patients
Staphylococcus aureus	5
Salmonella	4
Streptococcus	3
Clostridia	2
Bacteroides	1
Unknown	2

(Courtesy of Moneta GL, Taylor LM Jr, Yeager RA, et al: Surgical treatment of infected aortic aneurysm. *Am J Surg* 175:396–399. Copyright 1998 with permission from Excerpta Medica Inc.)

or patch repairs were used to treat suprarenal infections. Operative survival was 90% for infrarenal infections and 57% for suprarenal infections. Operative deaths occurred in the setting of overwhelming sepsis or severe preopertive hemodynamic instability. No intestinal ischemia, renal failure, or limb loss occurred. In 4 patients, late deaths occurred at 1.3 to 6.3 years postoperatively and were unrelated to aortic repairs. After a median follow-up of 2 years, 9 patients remained alive. No late aortic or graft infections were found.

Conclusion.—Infected aortic aneurysms can be successfully repaired with durable results in the absence of hemodynamic instability and uncontrolled sepsis.

▶ Vascular surgeons are a predictable lot. They invariably embrace things new, different, and exciting while, given a choice, frequently rejecting the solid principles of their background. In the treatment of infected aortic aneurysms, the hot new therapies include in situ grafting, preferably with the use of antibiotic-bonded polyester grafts, aortic homografts, or grafts constructed from the femoral veins. The old idea of complete excision and bypass grafting through a remote field, while acceptable, appears unexciting. In this group of 17 primary aortic infections, 10 were infrarenal and were treated with axillary-bifemoral grafting and aortic excision. Operative survival was 90%. The 7 suprarenal aneurysms were of necessity treated with in situ grafting or patch repair, with an operative survival of 57%. Most of the operative deaths in the suprarenal group occurred in the setting of overwhelming sepsis or severe preoperative hemodynamic instability. In the entire group there was no limb loss, renal failure, or intestinal ischemia. Late deaths were invariably unrelated to aortic repairs. Although not unique, this experience does suggest that we have come a long way in our ability to deal successfully with infected aortic aneurysms, a condition that used to have mortality and limb losses well in excess of 50%.

Long-term Survival and Late Complications After Repair of Ruptured Abdominal Aortic Aneurysms

Cho J-S, Gloviczki P, Martelli E, et al (Mayo Clinic and Mayo Found, Minneapolis, Minn)

J Vasc Surg 27:813–820, 1998 7–6

Introduction.—The hallmark of vascular emergencies is management of the ruptured abdominal aortic aneurysm, and mortality rates are about 50%. Late complications also occur after aortic replacement; these include graft thrombosis, development of para-anastomotic aneurysms, graft-enteric fistulas, and graft infection. One study found that elective repair of abdominal aortic aneurysm prolongs life expectancy. The late outcome in survivors of ruptured abdominal aortic aneurysm was investigated. Survival and late vascular complications in patients who survived elective

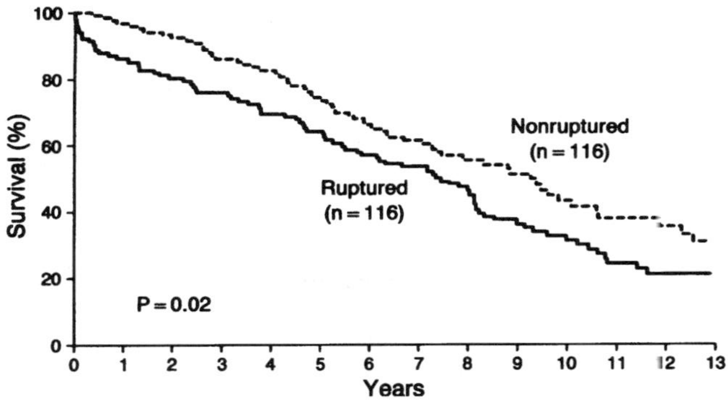

FIGURE 1.—Cumulative survival after repair of ruptured and nonruptured abdominal aortic aneurysm. (Courtesy of Cho J-S, Gloviczki P, Martelli E, et al: Long-term survival and late complications after repair of ruptured abdominal aortic aneurysms. *J Vasc Surg* 813–820, 1998.)

abdominal aneurysm surgery were compared with those in whom ruptured abdominal aortic aneurysms were treated.

Methods.—There were 116 patients (102 men and 14 women, with a mean age of 72.5 years) who had survived repair of ruptured abdominal aortic aneurysms. An equal number of survivors of elective abdominal aortic aneurysm repair, matched for sex, age, surgeon, and date of operation, were compared with those with ruptured abdominal aortic aneurysm to determine survival and complication rates. The age- and sex-matched white population of west–north central United States were also compared for survival.

Results.—Late vascular complications occurred in 17% of patients with ruptured abdominal aortic aneurysm and in 8% of those who underwent elective abdominal aortic aneurysm repair. Para-anastomotic aneurysms occurred more frequently in the ruptured group than in the elective surgery group (17 vs. 8). In the ruptured group, 32 patients (29%) were alive with a medial survival of 9.4 years compared with 53 patients (46%) in the elective surgery group with a medial survival of 8.7 years. For the ruptured group, survival rate at 1 year was 86%; at 5 years it was 64%, and at 10 years it was 33% (Fig 1). For the elective group, survival rates were 97% at 1 year, 74% at 5 years, and 43% at 10 years. The general population had a survival rate of 95% at 1 year, 75% at 5 years, and 52% at 10 years. The most frequent cause of late death in both groups was coronary artery disease. In 3% of the ruptured group and 1% of the elective surgery group, vascular and graft-related complications caused death. Independent prognostic determinants of late survival in the ruptured group were age, cerebrovascular disease, and number of days on mechanical ventilation.

Conclusion.—Late vascular complications after repair of ruptured abdominal aortic aneurysms were higher than after elective repair, and late survival rates were lower. Elective repair of abdominal aortic aneurysms is supported. Aggressive management of ruptured abdominal aortic aneurysms remains justified inasmuch as two thirds of the patients discharged after repair of ruptured aortic aneurysms are alive at 5 years.

▶ We have known for years that survivors of elective infrarenal abdominal aortic aneurysm surgery generally do well but have a survival curve distinctly lower than that for an age-matched population that has never had an aneurysm. Until now we have had no definite information on the long-term survival of patients recovering from ruptured abdominal aortic aneurysm. In this interesting study from the Mayo Clinic, we learn that survival at 1, 5, and 10 years is about 10% lower than that of patients surviving elective aneurysm repair, and 10% to 20% less than that of the general population. Late vascular complications were a bit more frequent in the ruptured group, but not impressively so. On balance, the long-term survival of patients recovering from surgery for a ruptured abdominal aortic aneurysm is surprisingly good and certainly justifies a vigorous approach to this difficult clinical problem.

Ruptured Aortic Aneurysm: The Decision Not to Operate

Hewin DF, Campbell WB (Royal Devon and Exeter Hosp, Wonford, England)
Ann R Coll Surg Engl 80:221–225, 1998 7–7

Introduction.—If left untreated, rupture of an abdominal aortic aneurysm is generally fatal, and the death rate is substantial even with aggressive surgery. According to previous studies, up to 61% of patients with ruptured aortic aneurysms did not reach the hospital, up to 45% had operations, and up to 39% did not have surgical treatment. Before surgery, there is considerable case selection. The views and practices of vascular surgeons in deciding against operations for patients with ruptured aneurysms was documented to inform the debate on this difficult issue and to provide a useful benchmark for any medicolegal activity in this area of practice.

Methods.—Members of the Vascular Surgical Society of Great Britain and Ireland received questionnaires that asked them about their practices and factors influencing the decision not to operate.

Results.—The response rate was 81% with 97% deciding not to operate on selected patients. Seventy-seven percent of the respondents said that age older than 85 was an influence, and 54% said that they seldom or never operate on patients older than 85. Severe neurologic disease was the single most influential factor, with 75% saying that they seldom or never operate. Cardiac disease was an influence for 22%, pulmonary disease for 28%, and renal disease for 21% (Table 3). If two or more of these diseases were present, 74% reported they seldom or never operated. Cardiac arrest influenced 85% of surgeons, loss of consciousness influenced 74%, prolonged hypotension influenced 73%, and long-term nursing care influenced 87%. Hemoglobin level of less than 9 g/dL, absence of a close

TABLE 3—Factors Influencing the Decision Not to Operate

	No influence	*May influence*	*Seldom operate*	*Never operate*
Severe neurological disease	4 (1)	75 (24)	177 (57)	55 (18)
Limiting cardiac disease	21 (7)	218 (71)	66 (21)	4 (1)
Severe pulmonary disease	26 (8)	195 (63)	81 (26)	7 (2)
Renal dysfunction	37 (12)	209 (68)	58 (19)	5 (2)
Two or more of the above	2 (1)	74 (25)	152 (51)	69 (23)
Cardiac arrest	48 (15)	151 (48)	87 (28)	26 (8)
Loss of consciousness	80 (26)	151 (48)	59 (19)	22 (7)
Prolonged hypotension	85 (27)	175 (56)	44 (14)	8 (3)
Haemoglobin < 9g/dl	217 (70)	89 (29)	6 (2)	0 (0)
Long-term care (eg nursing home)	41 (13)	165 (53)	92 (30)	11 (4)
Absence of close caring relative	206 (67)	97 (31)	5 (2)	1 (0)

Values in parentheses are percentages.
(Courtesy of Hewin DF, Campbell WB: Ruptured Aortic Aneurysm: The Decision Not to Operate. *Ann R Coll Surg Engl* 221–225, 1998.)

NO POSTAGE
NECESSARY
IF MAILED
IN THE
UNITED STATES

BUSINESS REPLY MAIL

FIRST-CLASS MAIL PERMIT NO 135 ST LOUIS MO

POSTAGE WILL BE PAID BY ADDRESSEE

SUBSCRIPTION SERVICES
MOSBY, INC.
11830 WESTLINE INDUSTRIAL DRIVE
ST. LOUIS MO 63146-9988

ently dangerous as long as the thrombosed aneurysm was in contact with the pulsating aorta.

Abdominal Aortic Tailoring for Renal, Visceral, and Lower Extremity Malperfusion Resulting From Acute Aortic Dissection

Webb TH, Williams GM (Johns Hopkins Hosp, Baltimore, Md)
J Vasc Surg 26:474–481, 1997 7–11

Background.—There is ongoing debate over the management of ischemic complications resulting from aortic dissection. The role of aortic tailoring in the treatment of acute aortic dissection associated with visceral, renal, or lower extremity ischemia was evaluated.

Methods.—The retrospective study included 7 consecutive patients undergoing abdominal aortic tailoring for the treatment of ischemic complications of acute aortic dissection and a normal-sized aorta. There were 5 men and 2 women with a median age of 68 years. The dissection type was type I in 1 patient and type IIIB in the others.

Results.—The patients survived—with full recovery of mesenteric, renal, and lower extremity function—in all cases. Temporary hemodialysis was required immediately after surgery in 2 patients. At an average follow-up of 19 months, none of the tailored aortic segments showed significant dilation.

Conclusion.—Ischemic complications of acute dissection of a normal-sized aorta can be safely and effectively managed by open abdominal aortic tailoring. Although no significant dilation of the tailored segments is apparent so far, serial imaging studies are needed to confirm the long-term durability of the technique.

► Dr. Williams has had considerable experience with the treatment of aortic dissection and frequently seems to take a course of action contrary to the majority. For malperfusion caused by dissection, he advocates opening of the aorta, excision of the dissection membrane with careful tacking around the orifices of the visceral vessels, followed by closure of the aorta. He reports generally good results in 7 patients with this unusual operation. Interestingly, the authors stated that they considered percutaneous balloon fenestrations, which most of us regard as the treatment of choice for this problem, but found that dissections in these patients were too complex for endovascular techniques. I wonder. Perhaps what they really need is more aggressive interventional radiologists.

Morbidity and Mortality of Reconstructive Surgery of Noninfected False Aneurysms Detected Long After Aortic Prosthetic Reconstruction

Mulder EJ, van Bockel JH, Maas J, et al (Leiden Univ Med Ctr, The Netherlands)

Arch Surg 133:45–49, 1998 7–12

Introduction.—After aortoiliac and aortofemoral reconstruction with a prosthesis, false or anastomotic aneurysms may occur, with a prevalence as high as 29%. The cumulative incidence of false aneurysm increases with time after the primary reconstruction. Little is known about the operative risk and outcome of surgical reconstruction of false aneurysms after aortic reconstruction. The results of operations with false aneurysms after aortoiliac or aortofemoral prosthetic reconstructions were retrospectively reviewed to evaluate the risk and results of surgical repair of false aneurysms at the aortic, iliac, and femoral anastomotic sites.

Methods.—A retrospective review was conducted of 158 surgical procedures in 135 patients with 220 noninfected false aneurysms. The false aneurysms were detected, with yearly surveillance, at a mean interval of 8 years after the initial reconstruction. Sixty percent of patients were asymptomatic. In 25 patients (16%), the operation was performed as an emergency.

Results.—Because of documented rupture in 11 of 18 patients, the mortality rate of patients receiving nonsurgical treatment was very high (61%). Per procedure, the intraoperative death rate was 7.6%, which was higher for emergency (24%) than for elective procedures (4.5%). Patient variables did not significantly influence operative mortality, but operative variables clearly influenced mortality. There was a 17% intraoperative morbidity rate in the patients surviving the operations (26 of 156 patients). The most frequent and serious complication was intraoperative bleeding, which was usually associated with emergency procedures.

Conclusion.—A very high mortality rate occurred with conservative follow-up, and with emergency surgery for a false aneurysm. However, the intraoperative mortality rate of elective reconstruction of a false aneurysm is similar to the intraoperative mortality rate of elective primary aortic reconstruction. After prosthetic aortic reconstruction, a surveillance program with yearly ultrasound studies is recommended for the timely detection and elective repair of all false aneurysms.

▶ This is a maddening article, presenting data in a fashion that makes accurate assessment almost impossible. Clearly, most of these false aneurysms occurred at the aorta-to-graft anastomosis or graft-to-iliac anastomosis. These clearly have a much different prognosis from that of a simple femoral anastomotic aneurysm, which most of us deal with frequently. The extraordinarily high mortality and morbidity rates described with the intraabdominal aneurysms in this series points out the seriousness of the condition, and also suggest that these authors may expect improvement in their own series with increasing experience. Clearly, the femoral anastomotic aneurysms should have been eliminated from this study, as they constitute a distinctly different patient cohort. On balance, I included this article because of the large volume of patients with intra-abdominal false aneurysms. Unfortunately, the obscure method of data reporting must be appreciated by the reader, because it materially detracts from the overall value of the article.

Miscellaneous

Inflammatory Aortic Aneurysms: Regression of Fibrosis After Aneurysm Surgery

Bitsch M, Nørgaard HH, Røder O, et al (Righospitalet, Copenhagen)
Eur J Vasc Endovasc Surg 13:371–374, 1997 7–13

Introduction.—Perianeurysmal fibrosis (PF) is present in up to 15% of patients with abdominal aortic aneurysm (AAA). This condition is sometimes called inflammatory AAA. After the aneurysm is repaired, the PF may regress partially or completely. The course of PF in 21 patients with AAAs was evaluated.

Methods.—The patients were consecutively treated over an 8-year period. Their preoperative and postoperative CT findings were compared. The postoperative scans were done a median of 24 months after surgery. A randomly selected group of 10 patients with AAA without PF were studied for comparison.

Results.—Preoperatively, the PF was thicker than 1 cm in 11 patients and thinner than 1 cm in 10. Seven patients in whom PF was causing ureteral obstruction underwent ureterolysis. The follow-up scans showed complete regression of the PF in 29% of cases, partial regression in 57% (Fig 1), and no change in the remaining 14%. None of the patients had progressive PF or persistent hydronephrosis after surgery. None of the controls had any signs of PF.

Conclusion.—In patients with AAA and associated PF, the fibrosis tends to regress after surgical repair of the AAA. Patients with PF—particularly those with ureteral involvement—should be managed in experienced centers. With successful AAA repair, follow-up is needed only to ensure good renal function.

▶ The behavior of periaortic fibrosis around inflammatory aneurysms after resectional surgery has been the topic of several prior studies. In a small number of patients in Denmark, these authors found complete regression of fibrosis in 29%, partial regression in 57%, and no change in 14%. Progression was not seen. I believe we can accept as proven the observation that a significant number of patients with periaortic fibrosis associated with inflammatory aneurysms can expect significant fibrosis regression after aneurysm surgery. This leads us to be very conservative in the performance of potentially dangerous procedures such as ureterolysis at the same time as aneurysm surgery. Similar findings have been noted by others.[1, 2]

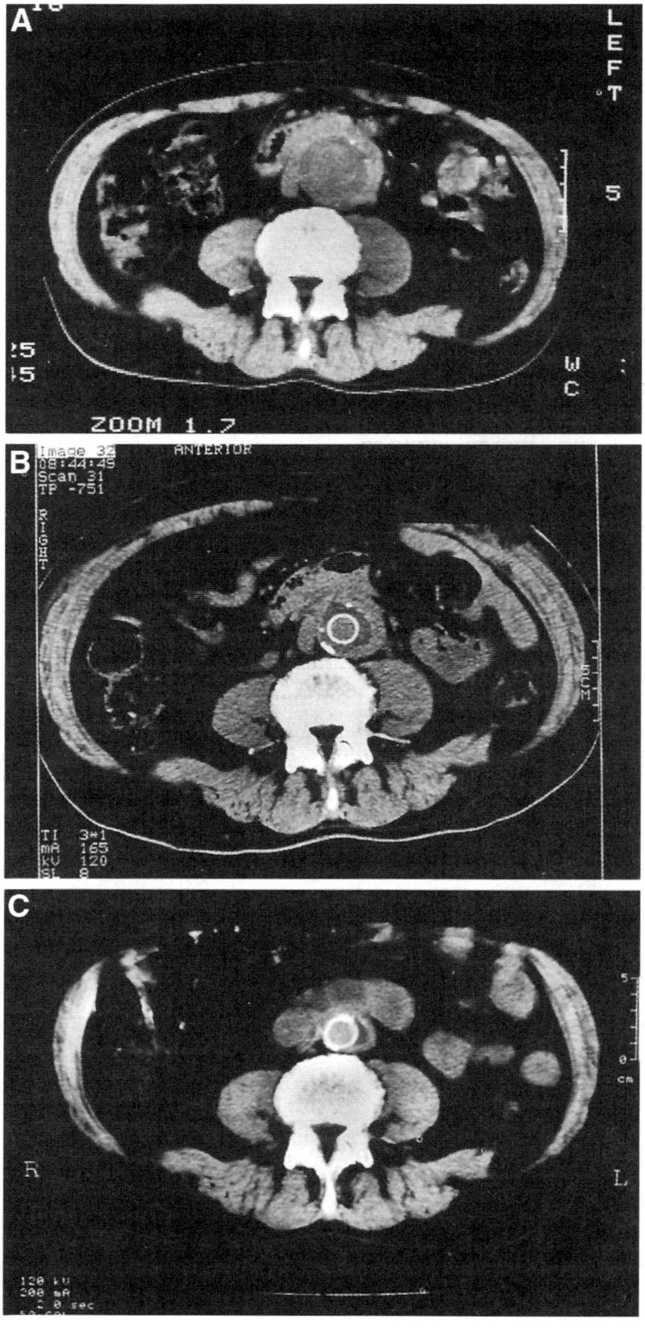
A
LEFT
5
W
C
ZOOM 1.7
B
Image 32
08:44:49
Scan 31
TP -751
ANTERIOR
RIGHT
5CM
TI 3*1
mA 165
kV 120
SL 8
C
5
0
cm
R
L
120 kV
200 mA
2.0 sec

(Continued)

References

1. 1998 YEAR BOOK OF VASCULAR SURGERY, p 260.
2. 1995 YEAR BOOK OF VASCULAR SURGERY, p 189.

A Dynamic View on the Diameter of Abdominal Aortic Aneurysms

Länne T, Sandgren T, Sonesson B (Malmö Univ, Sweden)

Eur J Vasc Endovasc Surg 15:308–312, 1998 7–14

Introduction.—The use of different definitions of abdominal aortic aneurysms causes conflicting results in tracking the incidence and prevalence of the disease. The Society for Vascular Surgery and the International Society for Cardiovascular Surgery define an aneurysm as a 50% dilatation of a normal artery. An increasing diameter with age has been shown, and it is now possible to define the extent of pathologic dilatation with the use of nomograms for the normal diameter on the infrarenal aorta. Abdominal aortic aneurysms between 40 and 50 mm were evaluated to determine whether this new way of defining the aneurysms' size might help in making a decision.

Methods.—In 147 consecutive patients, the anteroposterior diameter of 40- to 55-mm abdominal aortic aneurysms were measured by an echo-tracking ultrasonic technique. Body surface was calculated, and the weight and height were registered. Nomograms were used to define predicted normal aortic diameters, and the diameter increase was defined from the predicted normal aortic size in the individual aneurysms calculate.

Results.—The median abdominal aortic aneurysm diameter was 48 mm, with a range of 40–55 mm. The body surface area was 1.85 m^2 with a range of 1.42–2.37, and the predicted aortic size was 19.4 mm with a range of 15.3–21.6 (Table 1). The spread of data doubled compared with conventional diameter measurements; the calculated increase in size of the individual aneurysm was 2.51, with a range 1.9 to 3.53. In women the median diameter of the abdominal aortic aneurysm was 46.5 mm, and in men it was 48 mm. In women, the body surface area was significantly lower (1.63) than in men (1.89); thus, the predicted normal aortic size was larger in women (16.4 mm) than in men (19.7 mm). In women, the increase in abdominal aortic aneurysm diameter from the predicted size was larger than in men (2.93 vs. 2.46).

FIGURE 1 (cont.)

FIGURE 1.—**A,** male, 64 years. Preoperative CT scan shows a 1-cm-thick perianeurysmal layer of fibrotic tissue, surrounding a 4-cm abdominal aortic aneurysm. Note calcified media central to the fibrotic mass. **B,** Same patient. Three months after implantation of vascular prosthesis, slight reduction of the fibrosis is seen. **C,** same patient 15 months after surgery. Partial regression of the perianeurysmal fibrosis. (Reprinted from Bitsch M, Nørgaard HH, Røder O, et al: Inflammatory aortic aneurysms: Regression of fibrosis after aneurysm surgery. *Eur J Vasc Endovasc Surg* 13:371–374, 1997, by permission of the publisher, WB Saunders Company Limited, London.)

TABLE 1.—Size Evaluation of Abdominal Aortic Aneurysms

Sex	*n*	Age (years)	AAA diameter (mm)	BSA (m^2)	Predicted AO diameter[3]	Predicted AAA size
Males and females	147	72	48	1.85	19.4	2.51
		49–92	40–55	1.42–2.37	14.3–21.6	1.90–3.53
Males	113	72	48	1.89	19.7	2.46
		53–92	40–55	1.47–2.37	18–21.6	1.90–2.94
Females	34	74	46.5	1.63	16.4	2.93
		49–85	40–55	1.42–1.95	14.3–17.8	2.25–3.53
Significance males/females		NS	NS	$p<0.0001$	$p<0.0001$	$p<0.0001$

Patients with abdominal aortic aneurysms, 40–55 mm (median)/range.

(Courtesy of Länne T, Sandgren T, Sonesson B: A dynamic view on the diameter of the abdominal aortic aneurysms. *Eur J Vasc Endovasc Surg* 15:308–312. Copyright 1998 by permission of WB Saunders Company Limited, London.)

Conclusion.—It is now possible to define an aneurysm as a localized dilatation of an artery that exceeds 50% of the expected normal diameter. This may give new information concerning patterns of growth and risk of rupture and may facilitate treatment, especially of smaller aneurysms.

▶ These authors revisit the conundrum of just what constitutes an aneurysm. They refer to a previous study, which they believe permitted them to calculate the anticipated normal aortic size by considering a patient's height, weight, and body surface area.[1] Once one accepts the validity of this measure, one can then measure the aneurysm and calculate the increase over predicted normal. Interestingly, the increase was considerably larger in females than in males because of the reduced body surface area in females. Nonetheless, after dutiful consideration of this abundance of arcane data, it appears that the authors have labored mightily and produced a peanut. They conclude that one may consider an aneurysm as a 50% or more dilatation above the predicted normal. Isn't that about the same thing almost everyone else has said?

Reference

1. Sonesson B, Länne T, Hansen F, et al: Infrarenal aortic diameter in the healthy person. *Eur J Vasc Surg* 8:89–95, 1994.

for all patients. Axillobifemoral bypass may be indicated for patients with a high operative risk, a hostile abdomen, or an infected aorta or synthetic aortic graft. Use of this technique continues to be controversial, and long-term results have been reported to be inferior. Patients who had axillobifemoral bypass procedures in a 10-year period were reviewed to determine whether a planned procedure has more satisfactory results than an emergency operation.

Methods.—Fifty-nine high-risk patients had axillobifemoral bypass to provide palliation of severe aortoiliac occlusive disease. Forty-one patients with a mean age of 71 had elective axillobifemoral bypass. Their indications were limb-threatening ischemia, infected aortic graft, and severe claudication. Eighteen patients with a mean age of 65 had an emergency axillobifemoral bypass, and their indications were acute limb ischemia and aortoduodenal fistula.

Results.—In the group that had the elective procedure, primary patency, limb salvage, and survival were significantly better than in the group that had the emergency procedure. For the elective group, the primary patency at 2 years was 85% vs. 26% for the emergency group (Fig 1). For the elective group, the secondary patency was 90% vs. 69% for the emergency group. For the elective group, limb salvage at 2 years was 86% vs. 53% for the emergency group. For the elective group, 6-month survival without amputation or subsequent revascularization was 53% vs. 11% for the emergency group. For the elective group, 2-year survival was 60% compared with 34% for the emergency group.

Conclusion.—Satisfactory palliation of severe vascular disease in high-risk patients is provided by an axillobifemoral bypass performed electively. The widely disparate clinical results reported in the literature may be explained by the indications for operation and the timing of the operation.

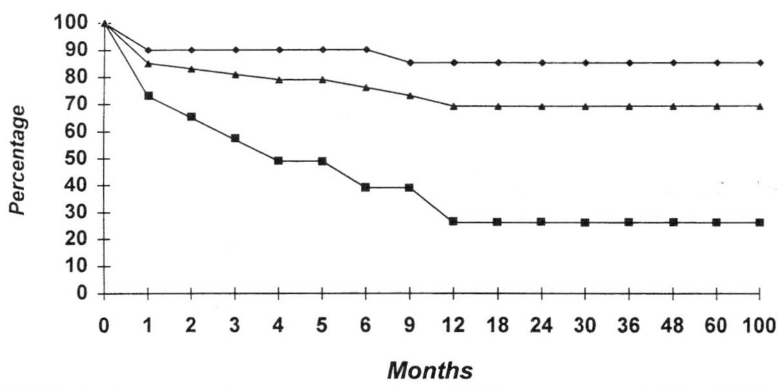

FIGURE 1.—At 2 years, primary patency for elective (85%) vs. emergency (26%) axillobifemoral operations is significant ($P < .002$): *diamond*, elective, *square*, emergency; *triangle*, combined. (Courtesy of Jain KM, O'Brien SP, Munn JS, et al: Axillobifemoral bypass: Elective versus emergent operation. *Ann Vasc Surg* 12:265–269, 1998.)

► Let's consider for a moment the results of elective axillofemoral bypass. Dr. Jain and his associates achieved a 2-year primary patency of 85%. We achieved a 5-year patency of 75%,[1] while the group at Iowa achieved a 3-year primary patency of 80%.[2] This leads me to conclude that, in experienced hands, axillobifemoral bypass grafting is yielding results similar to, if not precisely equal to, aortobifemoral grafting, at least through 5 years. I frankly do not understand the great drop-off in results experienced by Dr. Jain's emergency group. In the first place, the emergency group consisted of only 18 patients, a number that is simply not adequate to permit definitive conclusions. I suspect that, with increasing experience and large numbers, the emergency group will yield exactly the same results as the elective group. This has certainly been true in our experience. Although I am not an evangelist for the axillofemoral graft, I do point out that this can be done with light general anesthesia without invading a body cavity; with a two-team approach, the total time required is about 1 hour. In sick aged patients, this frequently makes a great deal more sense than any attempt to perform aortobifemoral grafting. As must be obvious by now, we are using the axillobifemoral graft much more frequently in recent years than we ever did in the past and are getting patency results equal to those of aortofemoral grafting. At present, however, I am unwilling to extend this procedure to healthy young patients with a prolonged life expectancy, because we simply do not know the behavior of the axillofemoral graft much beyond 5 years.

References

1. 1997 Year Book of Vascular Surgery, p 264.
2. 1997 Year Book of Vascular Surgery, p 326.

Impact of a Clinical Pathway for Elective Infrarenal Aortic Reconstructions

Huber TS, Carlton LM, Harward TRS, et al (Univ of Florida, Gainesville; Gainesville VA Med Ctr, Fla)

Ann Surg 227:691–701, 1998 8–6

Introduction.—In response to the recent changes in the health care market that have emphasized improved patient outcome and cost-effectiveness, clinical pathways have been developed. The impact of clinical pathways on patients undergoing aortic reconstructions is still unclear; yet some reports suggest that the use of clinical pathways during aortic reconstruction is safe and cost-effective. The impact of a clinical pathway for elective infrarenal aortic reconstruction on outcome, resource utilization, and cost was determined.

Methods.—A multidisciplinary group developed a clinical pathway for elective infrarenal aortic reconstructions. An analysis was conducted of the prepathway practice and costs. An efficient, cost-effective practice with specific outcome measures was defined. A retrospective comparison of outcome, resource utilization, and cost (total and direct variable) between

TABLE 3.—Resource Utilization and Cost Analysis for Operative Admission

Parameter	Prepathway (N = 20)	Pathway (N = 45)
Length of stay (days)		
Preoperative	1	0.1 ± 0.5*
Intensive care unit (range)	3.4 ± 3.7 (1–15)	1.8 ± 1.7 (1–10)
Total (range)	12.7 ± 6.4 (7–29)	7.6 ± 2.5 (5–17)*
Hospital cost (S)		
Direct variable cost	9630 ± 5515	5454 ± 1703*
Total cost	21.475 ± 11.947	13.924 ± 4006*

*Significant difference from prepathway at $P < .05$.
(Courtesy of Huber TS, Carlton LM, Harward TRS, et al: Impact of a clinical pathway for elective infrarenal aortic reconstructions. *Ann Surg* 227:691–701, 1998.)

the 45 pathway patients and the 20 prepathway control patients was made to determine the impact of the pathway.

Results.—There were no significant differences between the groups in patient demographics, comorbid conditions, operative indications, or type of reconstruction. The overall complication rate was similar, and there were no operative deaths. The pathway patients had a complication rate of 34%, and the prepathway control group had a complication rate of 35%. Significant decreases in the total length of hospital stay and preoperative length of stay were found in the pathway group, which also showed a trend toward a significant decrease in the length of stay in intensive care for the admission during which the operation was performed. The implementation of the clinical pathway resulted in a 40% reduction in the mean total length of stay for the admission during which the aortic reconstruction was performed (Table 3).

Conclusion.—Resource utilization and hospital costs were dramatically decreased by implementation of a clinical pathway for elective infrarenal aortic reconstructions without affecting the quality of patient care. The costs did not appear to shift to another setting.

▶ I have to admit that my enthusiasm for clinical pathways about equals my enthusiasm for rolling my automobile down a mountain. Having been trained in another era, I will never become accustomed to a nurse coordinator telling me what to do. I do, however, recognize that my provincial attitude is rapidly exiting the mainstream, and I admire Dr. Seeger and his associates at the University of Florida, not only for accepting the clinical pathway concept but for having the gall to publicize it. I am delighted that their implementation of the clinical pathway for elective infrarenal aortic reconstruction appeared to dramatically decrease resource utilization and hospital cost without affecting the quality of patient care. Hooray. Perhaps they will receive a gold star from the bean counters.

9 Visceral Renal Artery Disease

Renal Ischemia

Supraceliac Aortorenal Bypass

Hagino RT, Valentine RJ, Clagett GP (Univ of Texas, Dallas)
J Vasc Surg 26:482–491, 1997 9–1

Background.—In many patients with diffuse atherosclerosis, the aorta and iliac arteries are not suitable inflow sites for renal artery bypass grafting. Supraceliac aortorenal bypass seems like a good alternative in this situation, but has been little studied. Supraceliac aortorenal bypass grafting was studied for efficacy and durability in the management of symptomatic renal artery atherosclerosis.

Patients.—The retrospective study included 27 bypass procedures performed in 17 patients with atherosclerotic renal hypertension over a 10-year period. There were 7 unilateral and 10 bilateral reconstructions (Fig 1). The patients were 9 men and 8 women (mean age, 63 years). Arteriography confirmed the presence of diffuse aortoiliac and visceral atherosclerosis. Eighty-eight percent of celiac axis branches and all infrarenal aortas and common iliac arteries were unusable as donor vessels. Autologous vein grafts were used in all but 1 of the bypass procedures; 63% were done during partial aortic occlusion.

Outcomes.—None of the patients died during surgery or experienced an early occlusion. The complication rate was 24%; the mean follow-up was 28 months. The 5-year primary patency rate was 95% by life table analysis; the assisted primary patency rate was 100%. With surgery, the mean blood pressure decreased from 180/96 to 135/77 mm Hg. The mean number of antihypertensive medications required was halved, from 2.8 to 1.4. Patients who had renal insufficiency before surgery had significantly improved serum creatinine levels. Twenty-nine percent of patients were cured of their hypertension and 53% had significant improvement; in 18%, hypertension was unchanged. Aortic reconstruction was required during follow-up in 24% of patients.

Conclusion.—For patients who need renal artery revascularization, supraceliac aortorenal bypass grafting is a safe procedure that gives lasting

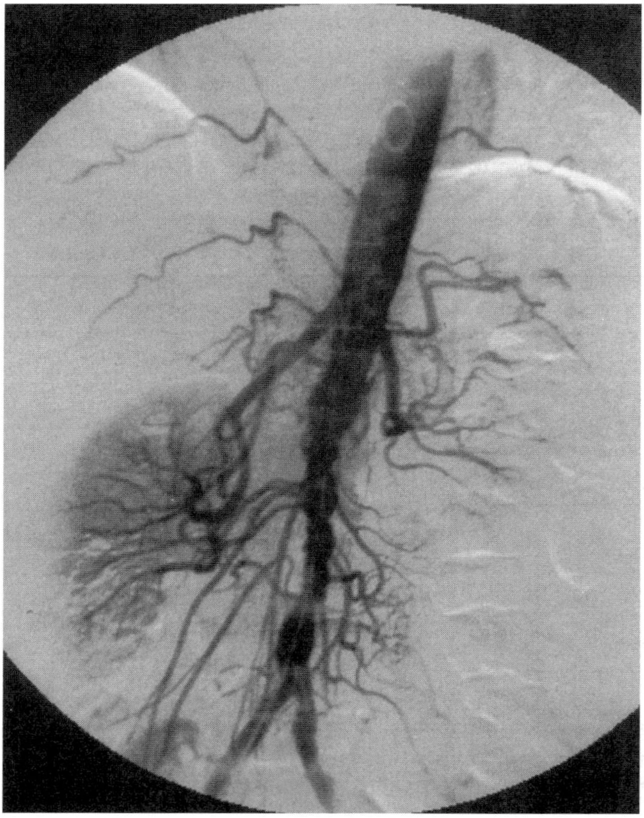

FIGURE 1.—Postoperative angiogram shows bilateral renal artery bypass grafts originating from nondiseased supraceliac aorta. (Courtesy of Hagino RT, Valentine RJ, Clagett GP: Supraceliac aortorenal bypass. *J Vasc Surg* 26:482–491, 1997.)

results. This approach is useful in patients with diffuse infrarenal aortoiliac and visceral artery occlusive disease.

▶ Extra-anatomical renal revascularization has been with us for a number of years. Some of the procedures include hepatic artery to renal bypass, splenic artery to renal bypass, celiac artery to renal bypass, and nonsupraceliac aorta to renal bypass. All of the extra-anatomical bypasses appear to function satisfactorily when carefully performed in well-selected patients.

Renal Artery Repair in African-Americans

Deitch JS, Hansen KJ, Craven TE, et al (Wake Forest Univ, Winston-Salem, NC)

J Vasc Surg 26:465–473, 1997 9–2

Background.—Compared with whites, black patients get hypertension more frequently, more severely, and at a younger age. Blacks are also more likely to have organ damage at any level of hypertension and are believed to have a low prevalence of correctable renovascular hypertension. The results of atherosclerotic renal artery (RA) repair were compared for black and white patients.

Methods.—Of 485 patients undergoing surgical repair of the RA, 28 were blacks and 370 were white patients being treated for atherosclerotic renovascular disease. The black group consisted of 19 women and 9 men with a mean age of 62 years. The white patients were 191 men and 179 women with a mean age of 63 years. The 2 racial groups were compared for preoperative blood pressure and renal function, extent of renal disease, extrarenal atherosclerosis, response to surgical repair, and survival.

Findings.—In the black group, the mean blood pressure was 204/109 mm Hg. Hypertension had been present for an average of 10 years. Eighty-two percent of the patients had ischemic nephropathy, as indicated by a serum creatinine level of greater than 1.3 mg/dL. A total of 45 RA reconstructions were performed in this group, including bilateral procedures in 19 patients. There were 30 RA bypasses, 8 transrenal/transaortic RA endarterectomies, 2 RA reimplantations, and 5 nephrectomies. Combined aortic procedures were performed in 9 patients, 4 with an abdominal aortic aneurysm and 5 with occlusive disease. One patient died of sepsis and multiple-organ failure in the perioperative period.

TABLE 2.—Comparisons of Operative Results Between African-American and White Patients

	African-American (*n* = 28)	White (*n* = 370)	p
Perioperative mortality rate (%)	3.6	3.7	1.0‡
Hypertension response (%)*			
Cured	7	11	0.19†
Improved	63	74	
Unchanged	30	15	
Renal function response (%)*			
(Preoperative SCr ≥ 1.3)			
Improved	59	42	0.12†
Unchanged	41	45	
Worsened	0	13	

*See text for definition.
†χ^2 test.
‡Fisher's exact test.
(Courtesy of Deitch JS, Hansen KJ, Craven TE, et al: Renal artery repair in African-Americans. *J Vasc Surg* 26:465–473, 1997.)

Seventy-four percent of the black patients who survived surgery had a good response in terms of hypertension, including a cure rate of 7%. The mean estimated glomerular filtration rate improved from 34 mL/min/1.73 m^2 before surgery to 42 mL/min/1.73 m^2 after surgery. Fifty-seven percent of the patients with ischemic nephropathy had a greater than 20% reduction in the serum creatinine level. Sixty-eight percent of the black patients had congestive heart failure or left ventricular hypertrophy before surgery, compared with 46% of the white patients. Serum creatinine levels were 2.5 and 2.1 mg/dL, respectively, reflecting more severe renal dysfunction in the black group. The blood pressure and renal function responses to operation were similar for the 2 racial groups, however (Table 2).

Conclusion.—Most black patients undergoing surgical RA repair have a good blood pressure and renal function response—as good as white patients. The results suggest that it is worthwhile to look for RA disease in black patients with hypertension. The authors believe that a significant percentage of these patients have renovascular hypertension.

▶ Hypertension in African Americans appears to be a different disease from that occurring in whites. In the former group, hypertension is more frequent and more severe and occurs at a younger age. Hypertension in African-Americans is associated with a marked increase in cardiovascular morbidity and parenchymal renal disease. It is widely believed that correctable renovascular disease occurs infrequently in African-Americans. During a recent 9-year period, these very experienced renovascular surgeons performed 485 operations for renal artery repair in a patient group consisting of 370 whites and 28 African-Americans. Seventy-four percent of the African-Americans enjoyed a beneficial hypertensive response after surgery, associated with a modest increase in the glomerular filtration rate. These authors appropriately concluded that African-Americans responded the same as whites to renal artery surgery. They further stated that this information supports a vigorous search for renal artery disease in hypertensive African-Americans. Clearly, this racial group should not be eliminated from consideration of renovascular hypertension.

Clinical Evidence of Contralateral Renal Parenchymal Injury in Patients With Unilateral Atherosclerotic Renal Artery Stenosis

Tullis MJ, Zierler RE, Caps MT, et al (Univ of Washington Med Ctr, Seattle)
Ann Vasc Surg 12:122–127, 1998 9–3

Introduction.—Previous studies have shown that with the production of unilateral renovascular hypertension, there is accelerated glomerular sclerosis in the contralateral kidney. In addition, when compared to the stenotic side and the kidneys of patients with essential hypertension, the contralateral kidney in unilateral renovascular hypertension patients has glomerular hypertension and hyperinfiltration. Duplex US has been shown to be an accurate, noninvasive method for the detection of renal artery

TABLE 3.—End-diastolic Ratio and Unilateral Atherosclerotic Renal Artery Stenosis

All unilateral ARAS patients (n = 81)	Renal artery EDR	p
Normal or <60% stenosis	0.27 ± 0.08	0.001
≥60% stenosis	0.30 ± 0.08	
Diabetic unilateral ARAS patients (n = 15)		
Normal or <60% stenosis	0.22 ± 0.08	0.004
≥60% stenosis	0.27 ± 0.08	

Abbreviations: EDR, end-diastolic ratio; *ARAS*, atherosclerotic renal artery stenosis.
(Courtesy of Tullis MJ, Zierler RE, Caps MT, et al: Clinical evidence of contralatera renal parenchymal injury in patients with unilateral atherosclerotic renal artery stenosis. *Ann Vasc Surg* 12:122–127, 1998.)

stenosis, and has been proven useful in the follow-up of atherosclerotic renal artery stenosis and the results of intervention. The flow patterns of renal parenchyma can also be assessed with the end-diastolic ratio. The difference in parenchymal disease, as reflected by duplex measurement of the end-diastolic ratio in patients with unilateral atherosclerotic renal artery stenosis, was assessed.

Methods.—There were 151 patients with atherosclerotic renal artery stenosis who had duplex US and who were prospectively examined. Classifications of renal arteries were: normal, less than 60% stenosis, 60% or greater stenosis, or occluded. Measurements were taken of the renal artery end-diastolic ratio (end-diastolic velocity/peak systolic velocity). As resistance to flow increases, the end-diastolic ratio decreases.

Results.—A unilateral atherosclerotic renal artery stenosis (60% or greater) was found in 81 patients. In the kidney contralateral to the 60% or greater stenosis, the end-diastolic ratio was significantly lower (0.27 ± 0.08 vs. 0.30 ± 0.08) (Table 3). In the subgroup of 15 diabetic patients with a 60% or greater stenosis, the absolute difference in the end-diastolic ratio was even more pronounced (0.22 ± 0.08 vs. 0.27 ± 0.08). There was a trend toward decreasing end-diastolic ratios with time for both the stenotic and nonstenotic sides, but the reductions were not statistically significant (Table 4).

TABLE 4.—Unilateral Atherosclerotic Renal Artery Stenosis End-diastolic Ratio Change Over Time

	Initial renal artery EDR	Final renal artery EDR	p
Normal or <60% stenosis	0.26 ± 0.08	0.25 ± 0.09	0.257
≥60% stenosis	0.30 ± 0.08	0.28 ± 0.08	0.157

Abbreviations: EDR, end-diastolic ratio; *ARAS*, atherosclerotic renal artery stenosis.
(Courtesy of Tullis MJ, Zierler RE, Caps MT, et al: Clinical evidence of contralatera renal parenchymal injury in patients with unilateral atherosclerotic renal artery stenosis. *Ann Vasc Surg* 12:122–127, 1998.)

10 Leg Ischemia

Leg Vein Graft

Long-term Outcome After Early Infrainguinal Graft Failure

Robinson KD, Sato DT, Gregory RT, et al (Eastern Virginia Med School, Norfolk)

J Vasc Surg 26:425–438, 1997 10–1

Background.—In an effort to avoid lower extremity amputation, increasing numbers of patients with recurrent limb ischemia are offered further attempts at revascularization after failure of previous ipsilateral bypass grafts. In some cases, however, aggressive management is unsuccessful, and the patient ultimately loses the limb after undergoing additional operative risk. A retrospective study examined long-term outcome and prognostic factors after early (less than 30 days) infrainguinal graft failure.

Methods.—During the period of review (January 1985 through October 1995), 112 new infrainguinal bypass grafts in 102 patients occluded within 30 days of operation. Indications for surgery were ischemic rest pain (44%), tissue loss (31%), severe lifestyle-limiting claudication (19%), and acute ischemia with rest pain (6%). In 43% of cases, the index procedure was a repeat leg bypass. Patient records were reviewed for limb salvage data, patency, and prognostic risk factors.

Results.—Most of the 112 early graft failures occurred within the first 24 hours after surgery. No further attempts at revascularization were undertaken in 9 lower extremities, 7 of which were amputated within the next month. In the 103 takeback procedures, limb salvage rates were better for patients who underwent surgery for claudication than for those with rest pain or tissue loss. For all takebacks, secondary patency rates were 70% at 1 month (Fig 7) but only 37% at 1 year. Patients with claudication were excluded from limb salvage analysis, leaving 84 threatened limbs. Life-table analysis of the latter group yielded limb salvage rates of 74%, 54%, 40%, and 31% at 1 month, 1 year, 3 years, and 5 years, respectively. Rates of limb salvage and graft patency were significantly lower for patients given anticoagulation medication after the index procedure and for those who had undergone previous ipsilateral leg revascularization. Patients with a single-vessel runoff had a significantly lower limb salvage rate than those with multiple-vessel runoff. The secondary

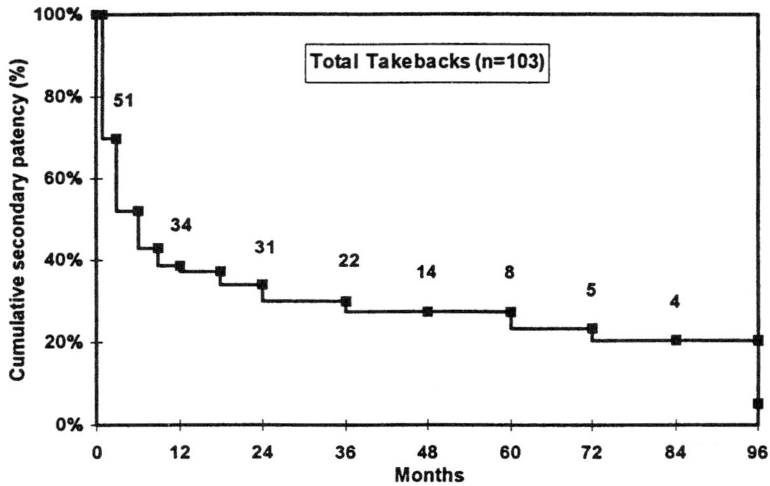

FIGURE 7.—Cumulative secondary patency rate for takeback procedures after early graft failure. (Courtesy of Robinson KD, Sato DT, Gregory RT, et al: Long-term outcome after early infrainguinal graft failure. *J Vasc Surg* 26:425–438, 1997.)

patency rate was better after thrombectomy and revision or complete graft replacement than after thrombectomy alone. Neither limb salvage nor graft patency rates were influenced by age; gender; previous inflow surgery; diabetes; hypertension; smoking; the presence of cardiac, renal, or pulmonary disease; or femoropopliteal vs. femorotibial/femoropedal bypass grafting.

Conclusion.—Although long-term rates of limb salvage and graft patency are poor for patients who have undergone takeback revascularization procedures after early graft failure, a single takeback procedure appears warranted in such cases. Multiple takebacks, however, are generally not advisable.

► These authors ask the haunting question as to just what is the outcome of leg bypass grafts that fail almost immediately and require a takeback to the operating room. In fact, the results are terrible, with limb salvage rates of 54% at 1 year, 40% at 3 years, and 31% at 5 years. The secondary graft patency rates for the takeback procedures were 37%, 27%, and 23% at 1, 3, and 5 years, respectively. The results after multiple takeback procedures were even worse. These authors have concluded that a single takeback procedure is reasonable, but that multiple takeback procedures appear unwarranted. I both agree and disagree with their conclusions. We have a general philosophy in our vascular unit that thrombosed lower extremity bypass grafts should be abandoned. Attempts to salvage a thrombosed graft have simply not been successful across the ages. Perhaps a single thrombectomy within the first few hours after surgery might be indicated, although I am unconvinced. In general, once a graft thromboses, throw it away and get a new one. (See also Abstract 10–5.)

Vein Graft Surveillance: Is Graft Revision Without Angiography Justified and What Criteria Should Be Used?

Idu MM, Buth J, Hop WCJ, et al (Catharina Hosp Eindhoven, The Netherlands; Erasmus Univ, Rotterdam, The Netherlands; Sint Antorius Hosp Nieuwegein, The Netherlands; et al)

J Vasc Surg 27:399–413, 1998 10–2

Introduction.—Follow-up of patients with infrainguinal vein grafts is typically focused on identification of failing grafts. A 3-center, prospective trial was conducted to assess the accuracy of color-flow duplex surveillance parameters in the detection of infrainguinal vein graft stenosis and to determine whether graft revision without angiography is justified.

Methods.—Three hundred patients with autologous vein bypass grafts of the infrainguinal arteries underwent digital subtraction angiography when graft stenosis was suspected. A digital subtraction angiography was also performed in patients with normal grafts to create a control group. These data were used to determine the accuracy of 7 duplex and 3 ankle blood pressure–derived variables. The association between various surveillance criteria and continued graft patency was assessed. The mean follow-up was 20 months (range, 1–40 months).

Results.—The best correlation with angiographic stenoses of 70% or greater was provided by the peak systolic velocity (PSV) on both univariate and multivariate analysis. Sensitivity and specificity were 80% and 84%, respectively, with a PSV ratio cutoff of 3.0. The best combination of efficacy (limitation of the number of unnecessary revisions), safety (minimal number of correctable lesions missed), and reduction of angiograms was obtained by a 2-parameter surveillance algorithm using life-table methods.

The algorithm used a PSV ratio of greater than 2.5 for patients in whom a conservative approach without angiography or revision was appropriate; a PSV ratio of 4.0 or greater for patients in whom vein graft revision without angiography could be scheduled; and PSV ratios between 2.5 and 4.0 in a group of patients in whom angiography was to be performed to determine clinical management, based on stenosis severity. The algorithm had positive and negative predictive values of 93% and 89%, respectively. Use of this algorithm resulted in a decrease in the number of angiograms of 49%, compared with a policy of angiographies in all patients with a PSV ratio of 2.5 and greater.

Conclusion.—The PSV ratio is the best criterion for determining a failing graft. Using a 2-parameter algorithm for vein graft surveillance, the rate of unnecessary revisions and of missed high-grade lesions was acceptably low. The number of angiograms was decreased by one half.

► Only recently has the benefit of a systematic surveillance protocol been shown in a randomized trial, and then only in a single study. Still, it is a generally accepted measure in vein grafts. Most would agree that angiography should be performed only in patients in whom there is a high suspicion of a severe stenosis. Can this prospective, 3-center study, as claimed, contribute toward a decreased use of angiography? I am not sure. The authors' concluding remark, that the PSV ratio best identified a failing graft, is not quite what the data revealed. It is rather that the PSV ratio best identified an angiographic stenosis of 70% or greater. Angiography is considered the gold standard for identifying grafts at risk, but I am curious to see the evidence that this static measure predicts graft failure better than the dynamic information contained in duplex scanning.

T.V. Schroeder, M.D., D.M.Sc.

► Our recent experience indicates duplex alone most assuredly is inadequate to support graft revision. We believe arteriography is essential.[1]

J.M. Porter, M.D.

Reference

1. Landry G, Moneta G, McLafferty R: Duplex imaging alone is not sufficient prior to lower extremity vein graft revision. *J Vasc Surg* 1998. In press.

Antibodies to Cardiolipin May Increase the Risk of Failure of Peripheral Vein Bypasses

Nielsen TG, Nordestgaard BG, von Jessen F, et al (Univ of Copenhagen; Statens Serum Inst, Copenhagen)

Eur J Vasc Endovasc Surg 14:177–184, 1997 10–3

Background.—Most early failures (1 month or less) of peripheral vein bypasses are attributed to technical factors related to the operation, whereas late failures (more than 2 years) usually result from progressive atherosclerotic disease. Graft or anastomotic stenoses cause the majority of failures in the intermediate period between 1 month and 2 years after surgery. Because serologic risk factors may also affect outcome, the association between antibodies to cardiolipin and infrainguinal vein graft patency was assessed in a prospective study.

Methods.—The study group included 103 patients scheduled for elective infrainguinal vein bypass surgery between July 1993 and May 1995. Ninety patients with a median age of 70 years were available for follow-up evaluation. Indications for surgery were rest pain in 33, ischemic ulceration or gangrene in 33, and disabling claudication in 14. The level of the distal anastomosis was above-knee popliteal artery in 8%, below-knee popliteal artery in 25%, and a crural or pedal artery in 68%. Patients were monitored by ankle blood pressure measurements and US duplex scanning of the graft at 1 week; 6 weeks; and 3, 6, 9, and 12 months. Blood samples were collected for biochemical analysis 1 to 3 days before surgery and 6 weeks postoperatively.

Results.—Three patients (4%) died within 30 days of surgery; 15 bypasses thrombosed within 30 days and 10 thrombosed more than 30 days postoperatively. Graft-related stenoses were identified in 21 (34%) of the 62 patients alive with patent bypasses at 30 days. Seven patients (9%) had antibodies to cardiolipin at the preoperative evaluation. The bypasses thrombosed in 4 of these patients within 3 months after surgery; stenoses developed in 2. No new patients had antibodies to cardiolipin at 6 weeks. Of the 5 patients with IgM isotype antibodies to cardiolipin, bypass thrombosis developed in 4 and the fifth had a bypass stenosis at 3 months. Cox regression analysis confirmed that diabetes mellitus and antibodies to cardiolipin each contributed independently in predicting the overall risk of bypass failure. No parameter predicted the risk of events within 30 days of surgery.

Conclusion.—Antibodies to cardiolipin, identified preoperatively in 9% of patients in this series, may be associated with an increased risk of infrainguinal vein bypass failure.

▶ This reported experience differs significantly from our experience.[1] In the first place, we identified anticardiolipin antibodies in a much higher percentage of patients with lower extremity bypass than did these authors, and we found no difference in graft patency between the group with and the group without anticardiolipin antibodies. We have concluded that we are unable to persuasively demonstrate any adverse patency effect of anticardiolipin antibodies. I suspect the number of patients in this study from Denmark is simply too small to permit accurate conclusions. For the present, I shall regard this paper as an aberrancy.

Reference

1. 1998 Year Book of Vascular Surgery, p 290.

Video-assisted Saphenous Vein Harvest: The Evolution of a New Technique

Jordan WD Jr, Voellinger DC, Schroeder PT, et al (Univ of Alabama at Birmingham)

J Vasc Surg 26:405–414, 1997 10–4

Background.—Harvesting of the saphenous vein for lower extremity bypass or coronary artery bypass grafting is associated with serious morbidity in as many as 24% of patients who undergo the traditional method of vein harvest. A new, minimally invasive technique uses laparoscopic equipment to remove the greater saphenous vein (GSV) via small incisions. The outcome was reported for 65 patients who had the GSV harvested by video-assisted techniques.

Methods.—The prospective study included patients who underwent elective lower extremity revascularization with reverse saphenous vein grafts between September 1994 and July 1996. Thirty-one had ischemic ulceration, 23 had rest pain, 11 had claudication, and 3 had popliteal

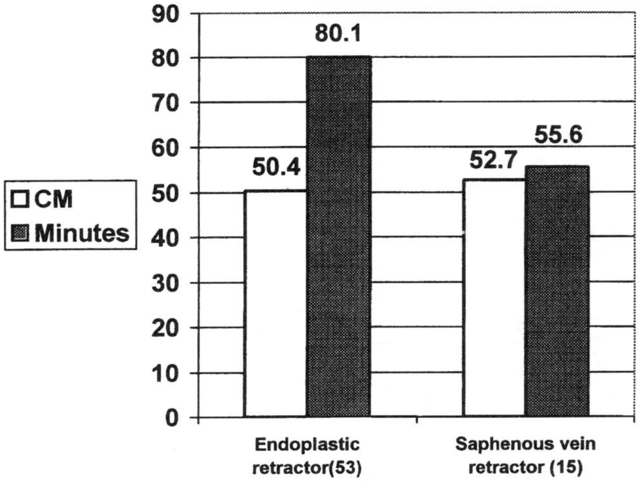

FIGURE 4.—Operating experience using different retractors compared by mean vein lengths removed (*CM*) and average operative time required (*Min*). (Courtesy of Jordan WD Jr, Voellinger DC, Schroeder PT, et al: Video-assisted saphenous vein harvest: The evolution of a new technique. *J Vasc Surg* 26:405–414, 1997.)

aneurysms. After the GSV is exposed through limited incisions, mechanical retraction is maintained with an endoplastic retractor or an endoscopic saphenous vein retractor. The video monitor allows the dissection to be visualized and side branches to be isolated and controlled. Once the vein is removed, arterial bypass grafting is accomplished as a reverse vein graft. Patients were followed up for wound complications, postoperative length of stay, and graft patency.

Results.—The 65 patients had a mean age of 60.5 years; 86% were men. One patient died 2 weeks after hospital discharge, and 4 died during the follow-up (mean, 7.9 months). Sixty-two of 68 grafts have been followed for more than 30 days. Of the 68 operations performed, 52 were to below-knee vessels and 22 included tibial (20) or peroneal (2) vessels. For all patients, the average time required to remove a 45-cm vein segment (the typical length of a groin-to-knee segment) was 60 minutes. When the saphenous vein retractor was used in the latest 15 cases, 55.6 minutes was the average time for removal (Fig 4). The mean postoperative length of stay for all patients was 7.4 days. One patient had bleeding into the leg related to the video-assisted technique, but there were no other significant complications. Three patients (4.4%) were rehospitalized for wound care related to arterial access sites. Patency was confirmed at follow-up in 84% of grafts.

Conclusion.—Postoperative wound complications after GSV harvesting remain a significant problem. The morbidity rate may be improved by shorter, smaller incisions, a technique assisted by laparoscopic surgical techniques. Patients who had the GSV removed by this technique had an improved postoperative wound complication rate and a reduced postoperative hospital stay.

► I have an ambivalent response to this article. I don't like gadgets, and I don't like video-assisted techniques, and I don't like endoscopes. However, I grudgingly admit that some of the most severe problems we encounter in lower extremity bypass surgery are wound-healing problems associated with the GSV harvest incisions. I am impressed that using the technique described here, these authors were able to harvest the vein in about 45 minutes, and they had practically no incidence of significant wound-healing problems related to vein harvest. Unfortunately, at least 2 grafts were injured during graft removal and required operative repair, and 1 of these 2 thrombosed within 5 months. On balance, I suspect there is some merit to the authors' suggestion that laparoscopic technique may represent an improvement in vein harvest. We are actually considering this in our own unit.

Intimal Hyperplasia Following Thrombectomy Versus Thrombolysis in Occluded Vein Grafts

Morasch MD, Zenni GC, Dobrin PB, et al (Loyola Univ, Maywood, Ill; Univ of Utah, Salt Lake City)

Ann Vasc Surg 11:559–564, 1997 10–5

Objective.—Previous reports have detailed the histologic effects of balloon catheter thromboembolectomy in arteries. However, there are few data regarding its effects on arterialized vein grafts. A study was performed in dogs to compare the intimal hyperplasia developing after thrombectomy and thrombolysis in occluded vein grafts.

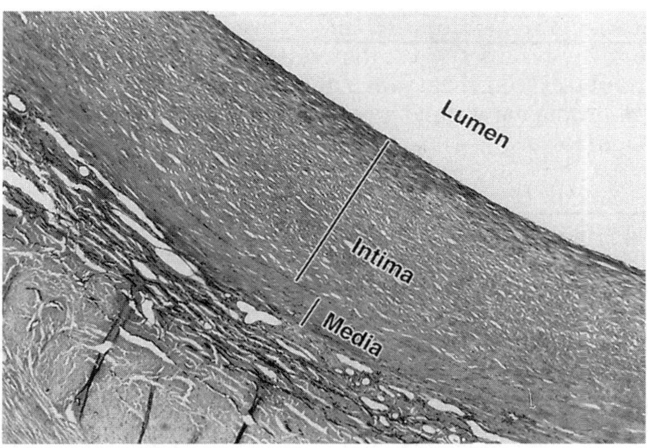

FIGURE 1.—Histologic section showing lumen, intimal hyperplasia, and media in a vein graft following lytic therapy. (Courtesy of Morasch MD, Zenni GC, Dobrin PB, et al: Intimal hyperplasia following thrombectomy versus thrombolysis in occluded vein grafts. *Ann Vasc Surg* 11:559–564, 1997. Reprinted with permission.)

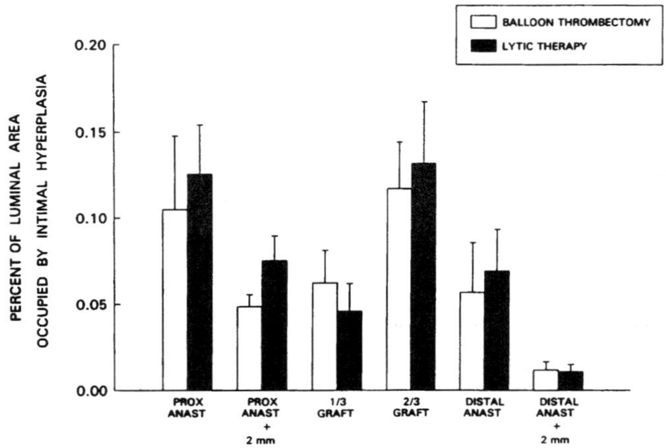

FIGURE 3.—Intimal hyperplasia (means ± SEM) at 6 locations along vein graft. There were no statistically significant differences at any location. (Courtesy of Morasch MD, Zenni GC, Dobrin PB, et al: Intimal hyperplasia following thrombectomy versus thrombolysis in occluded vein grafts. *Ann Vasc Surg* 11:559–564, 1997. Reprinted with permission.)

Methods.—Reversed autogenous vein grafts were placed in dogs, then experimentally occluded. Eleven of 12 dogs operated on survived to undergo graft thrombosis and treatment. Of 21 total grafts, 10 were treated with shear force–controlled balloon catheter thrombectomy and 11 with infusion of urokinase, in an average total dose of 355,833 IU. After 5 weeks, the grafts were excised for histologic evaluation (Fig 1).

Results.—Intimal hyperplasia developed to a similar extent in both treatment groups (Fig 3). There was no significant difference in flow rates between groups.

Conclusions.—This study finds no difference in the intimal hyperplasia response of vein grafts in dogs to balloon thrombectomy versus thrombolytic therapy. The results suggest that vessel wall damage occurring at the time of thrombosis and thrombus adherence to the vessel wall is just as important in producing intimal hyperplasia as are the effects of thrombectomy or thrombolysis.

▶ The implications of this study are potentially significant. For years, we have all accepted that the passage of balloon embolectomy catheters through medium and small arteries is injurious and liable to produce fibrointimal hyperplasia. In fact, the use of a balloon embolectomy catheter is a well-described method for producing intimal hyperplasia in the experimental setting. These investigators have found, surprisingly, that an identical volume of intimal hyperplasia occurs in a formerly thrombosed segment of vein graft following successful thrombolysis with urokinase. They hypothesize, and I suspect correctly, that the presence of thrombus for a period of time causes sufficient damage to the underlying graft wall to induce the hyperplastic process. If this initial observation proves accurate, and I have no reason to doubt it will, this will remove another significant benefit generally

Prosthetic Graft

Myointimal Hyperplasia in Vein Collars for ePTFE Grafts

Tyrrell MR, Wolfe JHN (Kent and Sussex Hosp, Mount Ephraim, England; St Mary's Hosp, London)

Eur J Vasc Endovasc Surg 14:33–36, 1997 10–9

Background.—In patients receiving a prosthetic distal bypass for infrainguinal arterial reconstruction, use of a venous collar at the distal anastomosis significantly reduces the risk of failure. The reasons for intermediate ePTFE graft failure when a venous boot is used are unclear. Understanding these reasons could give useful insight into why the use of a boot improves patency. The reasons for failure of ePTFE/collar grafts were analyzed.

Methods and Findings.—Four anastomoses retrieved after 1–8 months with irreversible occlusion were studied. These grafts showed myointimal hyperplasia at the junction between the ePTFE graft and collar, with relative sparing of the artery. These findings were subsequently corroborated by radiologic studies in 6 patients. Thrombolysis of the occluded graft caused tight stenosis at the level of the ePTFE/vein collar anastomosis, thus leading to failure (Fig 2).

Conclusions.—Analysis of failed ePTFE/collar grafts shows myointimal hyperplasia occurring at the interface between the ePTFE and vein collar, with relative sparing of the recipient artery. The venous boot may protect the recipient artery from occlusion by intimal hyperplasia, leading to improved patency.

► Dr. Wolfe and his associates from St. Mary's have long advocated the use of a modified Miller cuff at the distal end of prosthetic tibial grafts. It is noted that a recent small randomized study appeared to document the superiority of this configuration.[1] Dr. Wolfe has recovered several failed Miller cuff grafts and noted that the fibrointimal hyperplasia that occurred appeared localized to the junction of the prosthesis to the Miller cuff, with the artery appearing relatively spared. Perhaps this is true, but it seems a small consolation if it occurred in a failed graft. (See also Abstracts 10–10 and 10–12.)

Reference

1. Stonebridge PA, Hallett J, Prescott R, Ruckley CV: Randomized trial comparing polytetrafluoroethylene graft patency with and without a Miller cuff. *Br J Surg* 82:555–556, 1995.

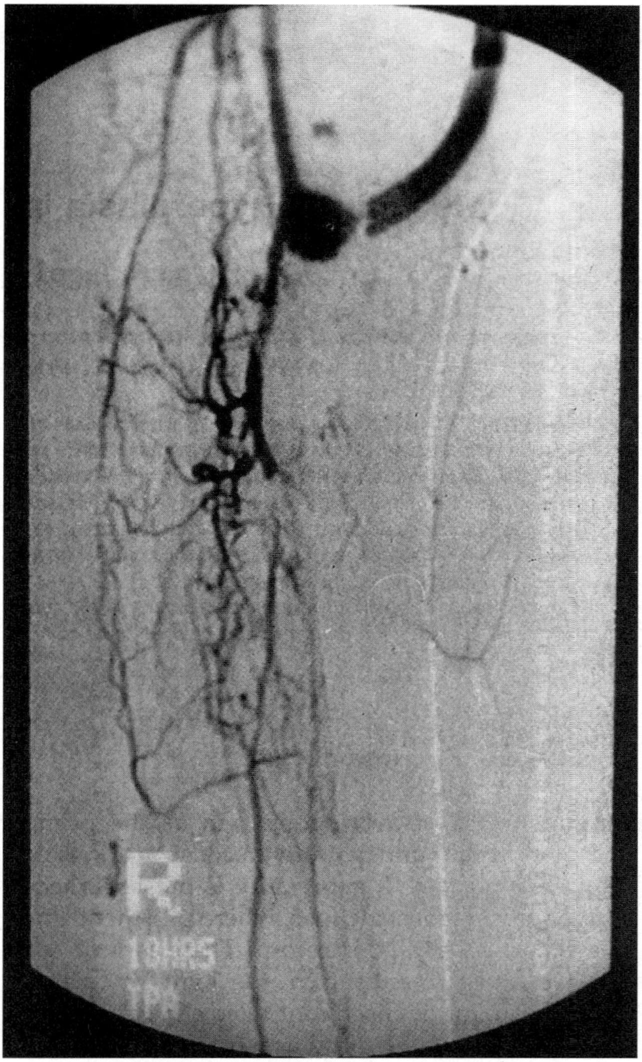

FIGURE 2.—Intra-arterial digital subtraction angiogram showing a tight stenosis at the ePTFE/venous collar anastomosis, following thrombolysis of an occluded graft. (Courtesy of Tyrrell MR, Wolfe JHN: Myointimal hyperplasia in vein collars for ePTFE grafts. *Eur J Vasc Endovasc Surg* 14:33–36. Copyright 1997, by permission of WB Saunders Company Limited, London.)

Prosthetic Bypass With a Distal Vein Patch for Limb Salvage

Neville RF, Attinger C, Sidawy AN (Georgetown Univ, Washington, DC)

Am J Surg 174:173–176, 1997 10–10

Background.—Some patients in need of tibial bypass procedures have no adequate vein for use as a conduit. Patency is reduced in polytetrafluoroethylene (PTFE) bypasses, leading to the addition of venous tissue at the distal anastomosis in the form of cuffs, collars, and boots. The use of a distal vein patch (DVP) interposed between the PTFE and tibial artery was evaluated.

Methods.—During a 3-year period, a PTFE/DVP conduit was used in 25 of 148 tibial bypasses performed (Fig 2). The 24 patients studied were 13 women and 11 men, with a mean age of 67 years. Fifty-seven percent had diabetes, 31% had renal failure, and 83% had high cardiac risk. Surgery was done for limb-threatening ischemia; 58% of patients had rest pain, and 42% had gangrene or a nonhealing ulcer. The reason for lack of adequate vein was previous surgery in 63% of patients, cardiac surgery in 21%, and unsuitability of available vein in 21%. The patients were discharged with Coumadin. The feasibility and graft patency rate of the PTFE/DVP conduit were assessed. The patients were followed up for up to 36 months.

Results.—The origin of the PTFE/DVP bypass was the common femoral artery in 48% of cases, the superficial femoral artery in 11%, and the external iliac artery in patients with previous groin dissection in 41%. The anterior tibial artery was used as the recipient in 7 patients, the posterior tibial artery in 8, and the peroneal artery in 10. On life-table analysis, the cumulative graft patency rate was 91% at 6 months and 78% at 3 years. The limb salvage rate was 91%.

Conclusions.—Good early results were reported with tibial bypass using PTFE/DVP. This conduit offers acceptable patency and limb salvage rates in patients without adequate vein. For such patients, use of a DVP may improve on the results of PTFE bypass to the tibial arteries for limb salvage.

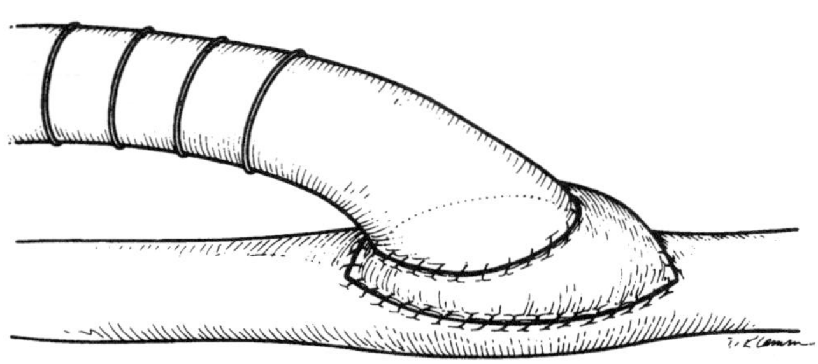

FIGURE 2.—The polytetrafluoroethylene (PTFE) graft is implanted into the vein patch, resulting in a distal vein cuff configuration. (Courtesy of Neville RF, Attinger C, Sidawy AN: Prosthetic bypass with a distal vein patch for limb salvage. *Am J Surg* 174:173–176. Copyright 1997, by Excerpta Medica Inc.)

► Growing evidence suggests that if one must use a prosthetic femorotibial conduit, the addition of a distal vein cuff appears advantageous. The patch that these authors have used is similar to the Miller cuff, and I suppose we should regard it as analogous. I am amazed that they achieved a primary graft patency of 78% at 3 years in this disadvantaged patient group. I do note the patients were maintained after surgery on warfarin anticoagulation. Unfortunately, the lack of any randomized cohort diminishes the impact of this study. However, I will take this as another small piece of evidence that a vein interposition distally in a prosthetic tibial graft is advantageous. (See also Abstract 10–11.)

The Performance of Femoropopliteal Bypasses Using Polytetrafluoroethylene Above the Knee Versus Autogenous Vein Below the Knee

Woratyla SP, Darling RC III, Chang BB, et al (Albany Med College, NY)

Am J Surg 174:169–172, 1997 10–11

Background.—Although results of follow-up data appear to favor autogenous vein over polytetrafluoroethylene (PTFE) for femoropopliteal bypass, some surgeons continue to prefer PTFE. Reasons cited for selection of PTFE include preservation of the autogenous vein for future reconstruction, reduced operating time, and ease of technique. A retrospective study examined the results of femoropopliteal bypasses using PTFE above the knee (AK) vs. autogenous vein below the knee (BK).

Methods.—During a 15-year period (1982 to 1996), 1,313 femoropopliteal arterial reconstructions were performed in 1,187 patients at the study institution. Of these procedures, 438 involved the AK popliteal artery procedure using PTFE and 875 the BK popliteal artery procedure using autogenous vein. In both groups, the main indication for surgery was limb salvage (77% of PTFE procedures and 88% of vein procedures). Patients were followed up for graft patency for a mean of 16 months in the AK/PTFE group and 30 months in the BK/vein group.

Results.—The AK/PTFE and BK/vein groups did not differ significantly in operative mortality rate (3.3% and 1.8%, respectively). Overall limb loss rates were 3.7% in the AK/PTFE group and 3.1% in the BK/vein group, not a significant difference. Primary patency rates at 1, 3, and 5 years were better in the BK/vein group (Table 2) than in the AK/PTFE group. The 2 groups had similarly high 5-year cumulative limb salvage rates (91% for PTFE and 95% for vein). Primary and secondary patency rates relative to the operative indication (claudication or limb salvage) did not differ significantly when groups were compared.

Conclusion.—Patency rates were superior for BK femoropopliteal venous reconstructions than for AK PTFE reconstructions. Use of PTFE should be considered for patients with claudication, a decreased life expectancy, or limited venous conduit, but, in most cases, venous reconstruction offers the optimal long-term result.

TABLE 2.—Primary Secondary Patency

	1 Month	1 Year	2 Years	3 Years	4 Years	5 Years
Primary patency						
AK/PTFE	95%	74%	60%	56%	53%	50%
BK/VEIN	92%	83%	78%	75%	72%	67%
Secondary patency						
AK/PTFE	96%	77%	64%	59%	56%	53%
BK/VEIN	95%	90%	86%	85%	82%	80%

Abbreviations: AK, above knee; *BK*, below knee; *PTFE*, polytetrafluoroethylene.

(Reprinted by permission of the publisher from Woratyla SP, Darling RC III, Chang BB, et al: The performance of femoropopliteal bypasses using polytetrafluoroethylene above the knee versus autogenous vein below the knee. *Am J Surg* 174:169–172. Copyright 1997 by Excerpta Medica Inc.)

▶ These very experienced leg bypass surgeons subjected the preferential use of AK/PTFE to a stringent comparison, namely, to BK autogenous vein. They appeared to have generally equivalent patient groups with limb salvage indications (77% of the PTFE patients, and 88% of the vein group). The 1-, 3-, and 5-year patencies clearly favored the BK vein to the AK/PTFE. Limb salvage rates, however, did not differ. These authors concluded, and very appropriately, that venous reconstruction for femoropopliteal occlusive disease gives better long-term results. They believe, and I agree, that prosthetic reconstruction should be limited to patients who have absolutely no vein conduit or a very decreased life expectancy. Let's face it, the preferential use of PTFE as a lower extremity bypass conduit is a flawed decision with inferior outcome and should not be performed. A more strongly worded opinion to follow.

Randomized Trial Comparing Infrainguinal Polytetrafluoroethylene Bypass Grafting With and Without Vein Interposition Cuff at the Distal Anastomosis

Stonebridge PA, for the Joint Vascular Research Group (Ninewells Hosp, Dundee, Scotland)

J Vasc Surg 26:543–550, 1997 10–12

Background.—The vein cuff developed by Miller is now favored for use with infrainguinal polytetrafluoroethylene (PTFE) bypass grafts. A randomized study was conducted to determine whether a vein cuff improves short-term and medium-term patency and limb salvage rates in patients undergoing femoral–above-knee popliteal artery and femoral–below-knee popliteal artery PTFE bypass procedures.

Methods.—The multicenter trial allocated patients to 1 of 2 groups: the first had an interposition vein cuff constructed at the distal anastomosis as described by Miller, and the second had a direct PTFE-to-artery distal anastomosis constructed. The cuff is created by taking a segment of available vein slightly longer than double the length of the distal arteriotomy. The vein is opened longitudinally, producing a panel that is sewn around the arteriotomy to produce the cuff. The PTFE graft is then sutured

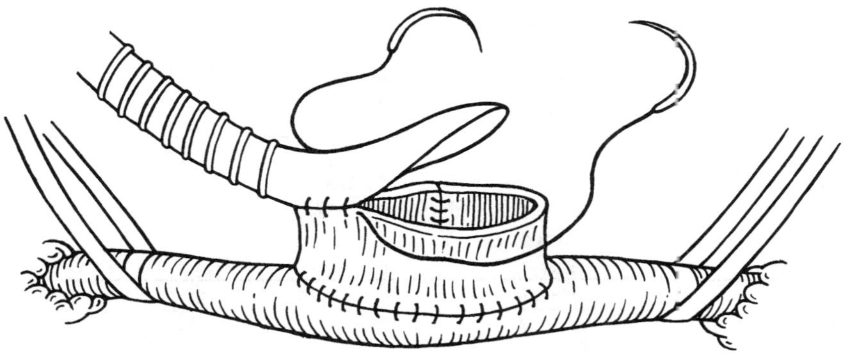

FIGURE 2.—Polytetrafluoroethylene graft is sutured end-to-cuff. (Courtesy of Stonebridge PA, for the Joint Vascular Research Group: Randomized trial comparing infrainguinal polytetrafluoroethylene bypass grafting with and without vein interposition cuff at the distal anastomosis. *J Vasc Surg* 26:543–550, 1997.)

end-to-cuff (Fig 2). Outcome criteria were primary graft patency and limb salvage rates. Patency was assessed by the presence of distal pulses, a persistent significant rise in Doppler pressure, or a patent graft on duplex scan.

Results.—A total of 261 bypass operations were randomized: 133 to vein cuff and 128 to no vein cuff. Twelve-month patency rates were 80%

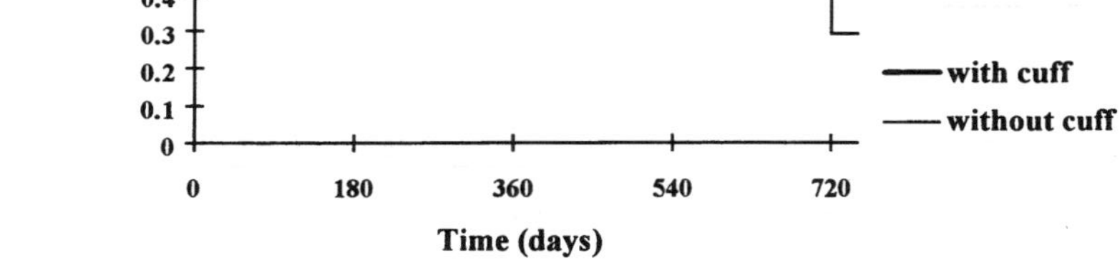

Grafts at risk

Time (months)	0	180	360	540	720
Cuff	48	38	30	25	10
No cuff	47	32	23	17	5

FIGURE 4.—Graft patency data for femoral–below-knee popliteal artery bypass grafts with and without a distal anastomosis vein cuff. (Courtesy of Stonebridge PA, for the Joint Vascular Research Group: Randomized trial comparing infrainguinal polytetrafluoroethylene bypass grafting with and without vein interposition cuff at the distal anastomosis. *J Vasc Surg* 26:543–550, 1997.)

for cuffed and 84% for uncuffed above-knee popliteal artery PTFE bypass grafts. Two-year patency rates in the above-knee procedures were 72% and 70%, respectively, for cuffed and uncuffed groups. Bypass grafts to below-knee popliteal arteries had 12-month patency rates of 80% for the cuffed group and 65% for the uncuffed group; 2-year patency rates were 52% and 29%, respectively (Fig 4). At the end of the follow-up period (median, 617 days), there were 19 major limb amputations and 45 deaths. Differences in limb salvage rates between cuffed and uncuffed groups did not reach statistical significance.

Conclusion.—Use of a distal anastomosis interposition vein cuff did not improve the patency rate of femoral–above-knee popliteal PTFE bypass grafts. There was a statistically significant increase in the patency rate when a cuff was used in femoral–below-knee popliteal PTFE bypass graft procedures.

▶ There is a maddening lack of detail concerning this study. We do not know how many leg graft operations were performed during the period that these 261 prosthetic bypasses were performed, nor do we know the number of patients who were eligible but were not enrolled, nor the reason why they were not. I am also concerned that the trial consisted exclusively of 6-mm PTFE whereas, in my opinion, there is persuasive evidence that 8 mm may be a more successful graft size. At any rate, within the significant limitations of this study, the 1- and 2-year patencies for the 2-graft configurations were identical above the knee and moderately in favor of the cuffed graft configuration below the knee. I really don't know how to interpret this information. For the present, I suppose, if we must use a prosthetic bypass below the knee, we should consider the use of an interposition vein cuff, as described by Miller.[1] Unfortunately, the Taylor patch has not been confirmed by independent studies, and I suppose for the present should be put on the back burner. The authors presented this identical information first to the Vascular Surgery Society of Great Britain and Ireland in 1995.[2] For sending the *Journal of Vascular Surgery* used material 2 years late (and then forgetting to reference the prior work in the *JVS* publication), I proudly present Dr. Stonebridge the much sought-after Camel Dung Award.

References

1. Miller JH, Foreman RK, Ferguson L, et al: Interposition vein cuff for anastomosis of prosthesis to small artery. *Aust N Z J Surg* 54:283–285, 1984.
2. Stonebridge PA, Hallett J, Prescott R, et al: Randomized trial comparing polytetrafluoroethylene graft patency with and without a Miller cuff. *Br J Surg* 82:555–556, 1995.

Leg Bypass Anesthesia

Local Anesthesia for Infrainguinal Arterial Reconstruction

Barkmeier LD, Hood DB, Sumner DS, et al (Southern Illinois Univ, Springfield)

Am J Surg 174:202–204, 1997 10–13

Background.—Several randomized trials suggest no significant difference in cardiac outcome and mortality among patients undergoing regional or general anesthetic techniques for infrainguinal arterial reconstruction. Because patients whose cardiac disease cannot be fully evaluated or treated before urgent limb salvage operation may be at higher risk for perioperative cardiac complications, investigators examined the feasibility and results of local anesthesia in such high-risk patients.

Methods.—Local infiltration anesthesia (0.5% or 1.0% lidocaine) was used during 86 infrainguinal reconstructions performed from January 1994 through August 1996. Supplemental IV sedation was given as needed. The patients were 51 men and 35 women, with a mean age of 67 years; tissue loss was the indication for surgery in 45 cases. Risk factors included coronary artery disease in 69% of patients, diabetes in 47%, and hypertension in 57%; 30% had had a previous myocardial infarction and 48% were smokers. Electrocardiographic monitoring was continued postoperatively in the intermediate care unit or ICU.

Results.—Operations performed included 20 distal graft revisions and 21 femoral-popliteal, 16 femoral-tibial, and 13 popliteal-tibial bypass grafts (Table 1). Autogenous vein was used in all of the femoral-tibial and popliteal-tibial bypass grafts and in 8 of the femoral-popliteal bypass grafts. Two patients, both with known coronary artery disease and recent heart catheterizations, died on postoperative days 2 and 27. Two other patients had nonfatal subendocardial myocardial infarctions. There were no postoperative pneumonias. Most patients tolerated the procedure well with local anesthesia, but 2 required conversion to general anesthesia.

Conclusion.—Selected patients at high risk for cardiac complications may do well with local anesthesia and IV sedation during limb salvage

TABLE 1.—Infrainguinal Procedures

Procedure	No.
Femoral-femoral	7
Femoral-popliteal	21
Above knee (13)	
Below knee (8)	
Femoral tibial	16
Popliteal tibial	13
Distal graft revision ± thrombectomy	20
Pseudoaneurysm repair	9

TABLE 3.—Legs Treated for Limb-Threatening Ischemia During Periods 1 and 2, by Procedure and Result

Treatment	Number of legs Period 1	Number of legs Period 2	% of legs Period 1	% of legs Period 2	Crude relative risk of amputation RR	Crude relative risk of amputation *P*	Relative risk, adjusted for age, sex, diabetes RR	Relative risk, adjusted for age, sex, diabetes *P*
Primary amp	114	79	42	27	*0.45	0.0000	*0.43	0.0000
Secondary amp	51	56	19	20	†0.64	0.06	†0.63	0.05
Successful revasc	104	154	39	53				
Total	269	289	100	100	‡0.51	0.0001	‡*0.49	0.0001

Note: The relative risk of amputation is the odds for legs treated in the second period divided by the odds for legs treated in the first period. Including reoperations and reamputations, 180 revascularizations and 200 amputations were performed during period 1; 254 revascularizations and 156 amputations were performed during period 2.

*Primary amputation vs. successful revascularization (n = 451).

†Secondary amputation vs. successful revascularization (n = 365).

‡Primary or secondary amputation vs. successful revascularization (n =558).

(Reprinted from Karlström L, Bergqvist D: Effects of vascular surgery on amputation rates and mortality. *Eur J Vasc Endovasc Surg* 14:273–283, 1997, by permission of the publisher, WB Saunders Company Limited, London.)

different attitudes toward and rates of vascular surgery—were considered. The analysis included a total of 1,080 vascular procedures and 367 lower-limb amputations.

Findings.—Two hundred sixty-nine lower extremities with limb-threatening ischemia were treated with revascularization or amputation in the first period, increasing to 289 in the second period. There was a 65% increase in the rate of vascular interventions for limb-threatening ischemia from the first to the second period. At the same time, the amputation rate decreased by 23%. The 30-month limb salvage rate increased from 37% to 53%. All of the improvement in amputation resulted from primary amputations. The adjusted risk of amputation for a patient in the second period, relative to the first period, was 0.49. There was no significant difference in mortality rates. The proportion of survivors with an intact leg increased during the second period; for nonsurvivors, this proportion was not significantly different (Table 3).

Conclusion.—The increased use of vascular surgery increases limb salvage rates while reducing amputation rates. Ethical and economic considerations both support the need to identify patients who will respond well to surgical revascularization; the initial treatment choice influences only limb salvage rate, not survival.

▶ The great machine at the Swedish Vascular Registry has labored mightily and produced another thin slice of salami. These authors, remarkably, appear to have proved that a well-applied clinical program of limb salvage surgery actually reduces the number of amputations. Unfortunately, some very sobering information is also included within this article, including a 1-month mortality rate of 14%, and a 48-month mortality rate of 58%. An ancillary observation is that if the patient's revascularized leg remained intact at 3–4 months, it was highly probable that the leg would remain intact for the duration of the patient's life, leading these authors to suggest that 3–4 months of amputation-free survival, from an ethical point of view, appeared to be the lower limit, above which limb salvage surgery was justified. Clearly, these authors and many others are beginning to ask the difficult question—namely, not can we do limb salvage surgery, but should we do limb salvage surgery? The remarkable death rate in patients requiring limb salvage surgery must be taken into account in making recommendations for such surgery.

Foot $TcPO_2$ Response to Lumbar Sympathectomy in Patients With Focal Ischemic Necrosis

Johnson WC, Watkins MT, Baldwin D, et al (Boston Univ)

Ann Vasc Surg 12:70–74, 1998 10–18

Background.—Sympathectomy can be used to treat patients with focal necrotic disease. This report describes a small series of patients who underwent sympathectomy as a primary treatment for persistent small ulcers.

Methods.—All patients who had sympathectomy for superficial foot necrosis of a 1- to 3-cm diameter, with transcutaneous tissue oxygen tension ($TcPO_2$) less than 30 mm Hg, were prospectively assessed. Patients with larger ulcers, with bone or tendon involvement, with wet gangrene, or with lesions suggestive of a neurotrophic origin were excluded. Patients with foot edema, dermatitis, or cellulitis were also excluded. Clinical success was defined as spontaneous healing of focal necrosis or healing of a toe amputation site with no further amputation during the subsequent year. A sensor core temperature of 44°C was used. The upper arm was used for a baseline reading of $TcPO_2$. The response to foot dependency was also examined.

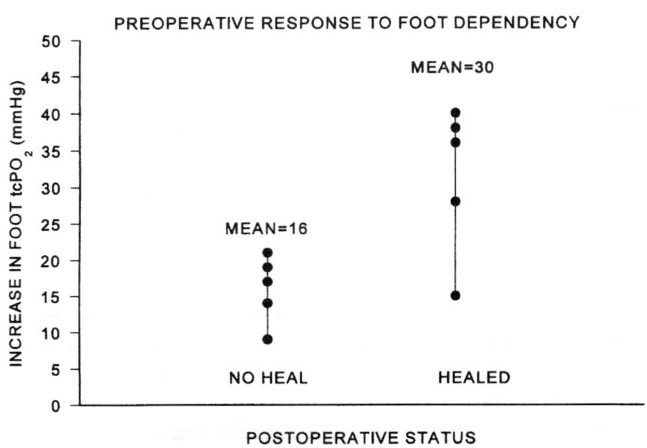

FIGURE 1.—The increase in foot $TcPo_2$ with dependency prior to sympathectomy and patients' healing status after sympathectomy. (Courtesy of Johnson WC, Watkins MT, Baldwin D, et al: Foot $TcPo_2$ response to lumbar sympathectomy in patients with focal ischemic necrosis *Ann Vasc Surg* 12:70–74, 1998.)

Results.—The study group consisted of 10 patients who were available for long-term evaluation. During the first 4–5 days after the procedure, foot $TcPO_2$ increased significantly in all patients. Clinical improvement occurred with an average increase of 29 mm Hg by postoperative day 10. Patients with clinical failure averaged only 5 mm Hg (Fig 1). Preoperative increases of at least 20 mm Hg in response to dependency predicted a favorable response to sympathectomy.

Conclusions.—Sympathectomy provided benefit in half of this small group of patients with focal foot necrosis and low $TcPO_2$. Success was correlated with a preoperative response to foot dependency and a postoperative large improvement in foot $TcPO_2$.

▶ Most of us in vascular surgery have long since lost interest in lumbar sympathectomy and never developed any interest in $TcPO_2$ measurements. These decisions were not arbitrary but were the result of considerable published experience that indicated a monumental lack of utility of these techniques. Without question, there appear to be a few patients with distal limb ischemia who may show benefit, including avoidance of major amputation, in response to lumbar sympathectomy. These patients, on balance, have been so few that most of us have abandoned the operation. Dr. Johnson and his associates tell us herein that an increase in foot $TcPO_2$ with dependency accurately predicts which patients may benefit. Using an increased foot $TcPO_2$ of 20 mm Hg, nonhealing was accurately predicted in 5 of 5 patients, and healing was accurately predicted in 4 of 5 patients. I question the transportability of these data. All patients with edema, dermatitis, and cellulitis of the foot must be excluded, a core temperature of 44°C in the local area is required, and the measured $TcPO_2$ at the site of interest has to be related to a site in the midsternum or upper extremity as a reference. I will require more evidence before accepting this material.

Outcome of Infrainguinal Bypass Surgery for Critical Leg Ischaemia in Patients With Chronic Renal Failure

Peltonen S, Biancari F, Lindgren L, et al (Helsinki Univ)
Eur J Vasc Endovasc Surg 15:122–127, 1998 10–19

Introduction.—Postoperative morbidity and mortality are elevated in patients with chronic renal failure not yet requiring dialysis who need arterial reconstructive procedures for lower limb ischemia. Patients with critical limb ischemia and chronic renal failure were assessed in a longitudinal observational trial to determine the outcome of infrainguinal bypass surgery.

Methods.—The outcome of bypass procedures for critical limb ischemia was compared in 22 patients with moderate renal failure and a serum creatinine level above 150 μmol/L, 10 patients with end-stage renal disease requiring dialysis, and 3 patients with a functioning kidney transplant. Patients underwent 6 femoropopliteal, 14 femorocrural, and 19 femoropedal bypass surgeries.

Results.—Primary patency rates were 97% immediately, 84% at 1 month, and 70% at 1 year after surgery. Limb salvage was 93% and 72% at 1-month and 1-year follow-up, respectively. The patency and leg salvage rates were 81% and 79%, respectively, at 1 year in patients who were not undergoing dialysis. For patients undergoing dialysis, these rates were 47% and 37%, respectively. Fifty-five percent of patients surviving at 1 year had salvaged limbs. No patients in the dialysis group were alive with salvaged legs at 4 months after revascularization. Serum creatinine was the only significant factor in predicting leg salvage and survival.

Conclusion.—The outcome of infrainguinal bypass grafting in patients receiving dialysis is so poor that it is rarely indicated. Leg salvage surgery may be performed with good results in patients with renal failure not requiring dialysis or those with a functioning renal transplant.

▶ Without question, the results of attempted limb salvage in patients receiving dialysis is so poor as to call into question the usefulness of the procedure. In this study, no dialysis patient undergoing surgery for limb salvage was alive 4 months after revascularization. While these results may be a bit extreme, they do point out the problem in this group. I do not believe that an elevated creatinine level without the need for dialysis has much meaning. I do not know what risk a functioning kidney transplant conveys. Clearly, these patients do not do as well as patients who never had end-stage renal disease. However, without question, the worst candidate for a leg graft is a cigarette-smoking diabetic patient with end-stage renal disease. I believe this is the single most difficult patient group that we are called upon to treat in an attempt to save a critically ischemic limb. The results are so universally poor that we are in desperate need of firm guidelines in this area. Perhaps one day they will be forthcoming.

11 Upper Extremity Vascular and Hemoaccess

Hemodialysis Access

Longitudinal Comparison of Dialysis Access Methods: Risk Factors for Failure

Hodges TC, Fillinger MF, Zwolak RM, et al (Dartmouth-Hitchcock Med Ctr, Lebanon, NH)

J Vasc Surg 26:1009–1019, 1997 11–1

Objective.—Attempted salvage of a failed hemodialysis access graft is expensive and seriously affects the already lowered quality of life of hemodialysis patients. Establishing patency and minimizing complications are major goals of dialysis research. Dialysis access patency rates and risk factors for failure were compared for different access methods.

Methods.—All surgically implanted dual-lumen central venous hemodialysis catheter (SIHC), peritoneal dialysis catheter (PDC), arteriovenous fistula (AVF), and prosthetic shunt (PTFE) procedures performed for chronic dialysis at Dartmouth-Hitchcock Medical Center (N.H.) between 1987 and 1996 were retrospectively reviewed. Life table analysis was used to predict primary and secondary patency rates. The influence of age, sex, diabetes, smoking history, and previous access history on patency was evaluated using multivariate proportional hazards regression analysis.

Results.—There were 585 primary procedures (236 PTFEs, 87 AVFs, 112 SIHCs, and 150 PDCs) and 259 secondary procedures (215 PTFEs, 14 AVFs, and 30 PDCs) performed in 350 patients, initially aged 13 to 87. Primary patency rates of AVFs and PTFEs were similar at 1 year and, along with PDCs, were similar after 2 years (Fig 1). Whereas no SIHCs were surgically revised, >90% of PTFEs were revised, the majority with anastomotic patch angioplasty (44%). Secondary patency rates at 1 year were 68% for PDCs, 59% for PTFEs, 46% for AVFs, and 9% for SIHCs. Whereas secondary patency rates for AVFs and PTFEs at 1 year were similar, at 4 years, AVFs had the best patency rates. Primary access failure

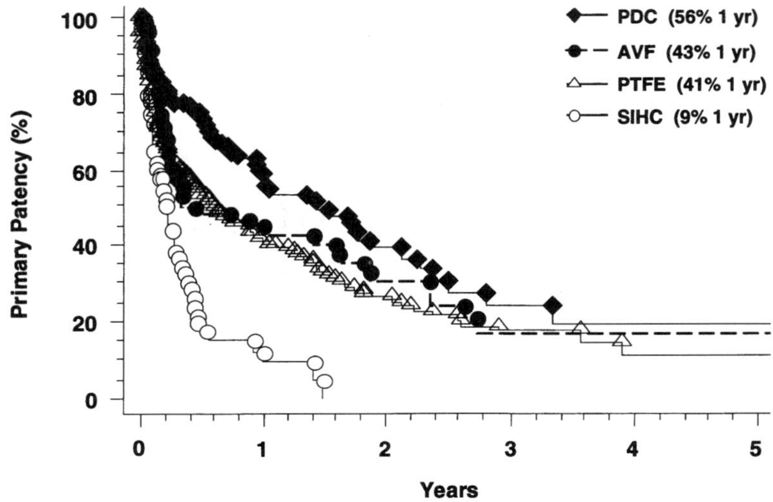

FIGURE 1.—Primary patency life table. Patency is defined as useful access function. One-year primary patency rates are shown in parentheses. Standard error is less than 10% at all times. (Courtesy of Hodges TC, Fillinger MF, Zwolak RM, et al: Longitudinal comparison of dialysis access methods: Risk factors for failure. *J Vasc Surg* 26:1009–1019, 1997).

modes were thrombosis for PTFEs (70%); thrombosis (44%) and failure to mature (31%) for AVFs; inadequate dialysis flow rate (51%) for SIHCs; and infection (37%) and inadequate exchange (34%) for PDCs. Patients were least satisfied with SIHCs and PDCs. The only significant risk factor for failure of a PTFE graft at a new site was prior PTFE failure, and the risk increased with every previous failure. Diabetes mellitus was the only significant risk factor for PDC failure.

Conclusion.—Patency rates for PTFEs and AVFs are similar. AVFs need fewer revisions. The number of PTFE revisions increased with the number of previous failures. PDC failure rates increase in patients with diabetes. SIHCs have the lowest primary patency rates. Patency reporting definitions need to be standardized to make patency data comparable.

► It is hard to know what to take away from the conglomeration of data presented in this article. About the only thing I conclude with certainty is that the surgically implanted dual lumen central venous dialysis catheters produced poor results, and that peritoneal dialysis catheters fared even worse in diabetics. Interestingly, the AVFs and PTFEs performed about equally well (or perhaps poorly). It does appear, however, that abundant data suggest that we should try an autogenous fistula first and reserve the prosthetic for the second or third effort.

Stent-Graft Arteriovenous Fistula: An Endovascular Technique in Hemodialysis Access

Masuda EM, Kistner RL, Eklof B, et al (Univ of Hawaii, Honolulu)

J Endovasc Surg 5:18–23, 1998 11–2

Introduction.—A combined stent-graft device is not used for long-term hemodialysis access. This approach could provide a much needed option for patients undergoing chronic dialysis who have inadequate arm veins or multiple failed fistulas. The feasibility and safety of a new endovascular technique for creating an arteriovenous (AV) fistula using catheter-directed techniques and stents was assessed in 8 patients with a history of multiple failed access procedures or very small arm veins unsuitable for standard vascular access techniques.

Methods.—The device consisted of a balloon-expandable Palmaz stent attached to the designated venous end of a polytetrafluoroethylene graft. The balloon-mounted stent-graft was introduced into the brachial vein through an arteriotomy. It was advanced over a guidewire into the axillary

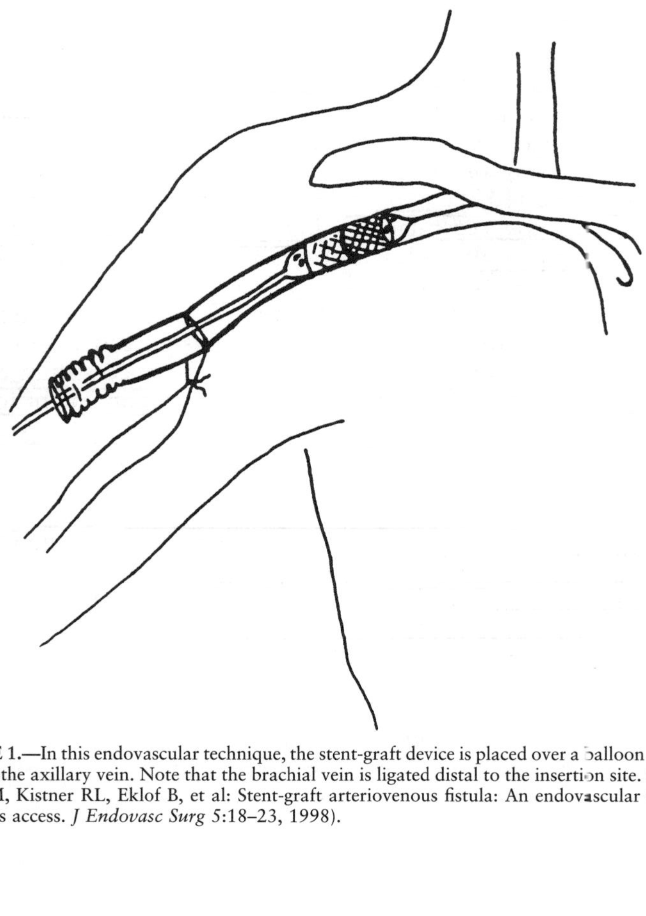

FIGURE 1.—In this endovascular technique, the stent-graft device is placed over a balloon catheter and deployed in the axillary vein. Note that the brachial vein is ligated distal to the insertion site. (Courtesy of Masuda EM, Kistner RL, Eklof B, et al: Stent-graft arteriovenous fistula: An endovascular technique in hemodialysis access. *J Endovasc Surg* 5:18–23, 1998).

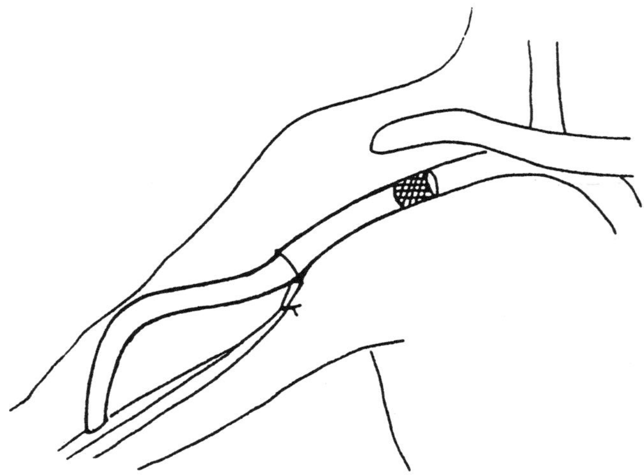

FIGURE 2.—To complete the access pathway, the unstented end of the graft is anastomosed to the brachial artery using standard surgical techniques. (Courtesy of Masuda EM, Kistner RL, Eklof B, et al: Stent-graft arteriovenous fistula: An endovascular technique in hemodialysis access. *J Endovasc Surg* 5:18–23, 1998).

vein where the stent-graft was deployed (Fig 1). The arterial anastomosis was performed in standard surgical fashion, using an end-to-side anastomosis of the graft to the brachial artery (Fig 2).

Results.—Insertion of the stent-graft was successful in all 8 patients. Early failures occurred in 2 patients. In 1 patient, the failure was caused by a steal phenomenon secondary to high flows through the stent-graft, requiring ligation of the fistula. The other stent-graft was placed too peripherally in the upper arm, which caused the stainless steel stent to be crushed by external compression. At 1 year, 3 of the remaining 6 grafts were patent. Two grafts remained functioning at 22 and 13 months.

Conclusion.—Endoluminal stent-grafts may be successfully placed in the axillary vein to create an AV fistula and can remain patent for over 2 years. This approach may be most helpful in patients with very small, unusable arm veins or those with multiple failed AV grafts.

► This study has shown that the technique is feasible. Its value, however, might be questioned, as the patient has to undergo conventional surgery anyway to have the arterial anastomosis performed. I doubt whether the other claimed objective of this study has been achieved, i.e., to find a method to reduce the incidence of venous stenosis. There is no reason to believe that intimal hyperplasia is less prevalent after stent-graft manipulation, compared with conventional surgery. Nor did the results indicate this to be the case, as less than half of the grafts were functioning after 1 year. I admit, though, that the larger dimension of the axillary vein might delay hemodynamically significant stenosis development—in analogy to the pre-

access, it is recommended to all access surgeons as the first choice for treating steal syndrome related to a functioning arteriovenous access. None of the alternate methods for managing steal has achieved the consistent results of the DRIL technique in salvaging a viable extremity and functional arteriovenous access site.

▶ I previously expressed my admiration for the elegant proposal of Dr. Schanzer for dealing with limb steal phenomenon in a patient with a need to maintain dialysis access[1]. We have used this technique a number of times with success. I am pleased to note that the group from the University of Arizona concurs.

Reference

1. 1994 YEAR BOOK OF VASCULAR SURGERY, p 295.

Vascular Access Survival Among Incident Hemodialysis Patients in the United States

Woods JD, Turenne MN, Strawderman RL, et al (Univ of Michigan, Ann Arbor; VA Med Ctr, Ann Arbor, Mich; US Renal Data System, Ann Arbor, Mich)

Am J Kidney Dis 30:50–57, 1997 11–6

Background.—Adequate vascular access is critical for optimal hemodialysis. Vascular access failure causes significant morbidity and cost in patients receiving hemodialysis. The main types of vascular access for chronic hemodialysis are the primary arteriovenous fistula and the polytetrafluoroethylene arteriovenous graft. Both are prone to failure because of thrombosis or infection. Some studies have reported that the failure rate is higher for arteriovenous grafts than for arteriovenous fistulae.

Methods.—Variables that determine survival of the permanent vascular access in use at the beginning of end-stage renal disease were analyzed in a national sample of 784 incident hemodialysis patients insured by Medicare. Claim records were reviewed to identify access failures or revisions in 245 patients with an arteriovenous fistula and in 539 patients with an arteriovenous vascular graft. The effects of age, access type, and peripheral vascular disease on vascular access survival were determined by a proportional hazards analysis of time to first failure or revision, after controlling for sex, race, and cause of end-stage renal disease.

Results.—The risk of access failure was 24% lower in patients with an arteriovenous fistula who were older than 65 years than in patients of the same age with an arteriovenous graft (Table 4). In patients younger than 65 years, the relative risk of access failure for an arteriovenous fistula, but not an arteriovenous graft, varied significantly with age. The relative risk of access failure of an arteriovenous fistula vs. an arteriovenous graft was 67% lower in 40-year-old patients, 54% lower in 50-year-old patients,

TABLE 4.—Relative Risk of Access Failure for Patient Characteristics, Co-Morbid Conditions, and Access Type

Variable	Reference Group	Risk Ratio	Lower 95% CI*	Upper 95% CI*	*P* Value
Fistula (>65 yr)	Graft (>65 yr)	0.76	0.60	0.96	0.02
Age (per 10 yr)	Continuous	0.98	0.90	1.07	0.68
Age/fistula interaction <65 yr (per 10 yr)	Continuous	1.40†	1.09	1.80	<0.01
Peripheral vascular disease	No such history	1.24	1.00	1.54	0.05

*Denotes bound of 95% confidence interval.
†This statistically significant interaction term necessitated description of the risk ratio by age.
(Courtesy of Woods JD, Turenne MN, Strawderman RL, et al: Vascular access survival among incident hemodialysis patients in the United States. *Am J Kidney Dis* 30:50–57, 1997.)

and 24% lower in 65-year-old patients. There was a 24% higher risk of arteriovenous graft or fistula failure associated with a history of peripheral vascular disease.

Discussion.—Reversing the current trend toward greater use of arteriovenous grafts, especially in patients younger than 65 years, may help reduce the morbidity associated with vascular access in patients with end-stage renal disease receiving hemodialysis.

► These authors make a persuasive plea that the use of the arteriovenous (AV) fistulas as the initial dialysis access yields markedly superior results to the use of an AV graft. They present impressive data to support their position. It seems that, at present, a number of dialysis access groups have developed the knee jerk-response of using AV grafts in all dialysis patients. This policy should be re-evaluated. There is persuasive evidence that AV fistulas yield superior results when they can be constructed.

Prophylactic Balloon Angioplasty Fails to Prolong the Patency of Expanded Polytetrafluoroethylene Arteriovenous Grafts: Results of a Prospective Randomized Study

Lumsden AB, MacDonald MJ, Kikeri D, et al (Emory Univ, Atlanta, Ga)
J Vasc Surg 26:382–392, 1997 11–7

Background.—The number of patients in the United States who depend on hemodialysis is growing at about 10% per year. The maintenance of hemodialysis access grafts is an immense social and clinical problem. Because current grafts and graft salvage techniques are inadequate, there has been much interest in minimally invasive, prophylactic catheter techniques for treating stenoses in functioning arteriovenous grafts. Prophylactic balloon angioplasty has been suggested as a means of prolonging assisted primary patency.

Methods.—In a prospective, randomized trial, the results of 32 patients who had percutaneous transluminal angioplasty for graft stenoses greater than 50% were compared to results of 32 control patients who had no

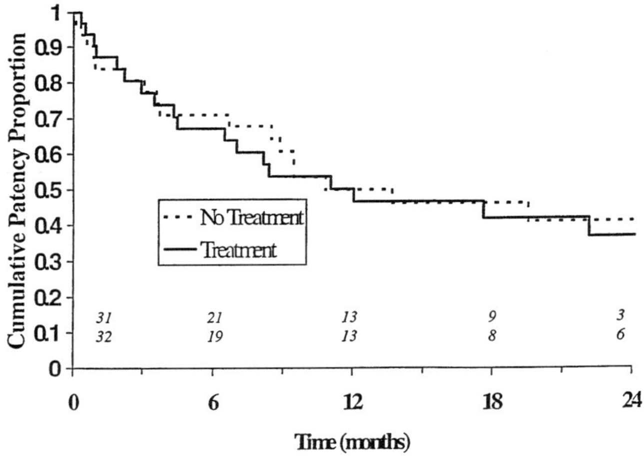

FIGURE 3.—Life table analysis of graft patency data. (Courtesy of Lumsden AB, MacDonald MJ, Kikeri D et al: Prophylatic balloon angioplasty fails to prolong the patency of expanded polytetrafluoroethylene arteriovenous grafts: Results of a prospective randomized study. *J Vasc Surg* 26:382–392, 1997.)

intervention. Stenoses greater than 50% in functioning expanded polytetrafluoroethylene grafts were detected by color flow duplex scanning. After confirmatory angiographic examination, patients with angiographic stenoses greater than 50% were randomly assigned to balloon angioplasty or observation. Duplex scanning was performed every 2 months. Outcome measures were graft thrombosis, graft dysfunction that prevented dialysis, and 6 or more percutaneous transluminal angioplasty procedures in 18 months.

Results.—The patient groups were well matched demographically, but patients in the treatment group had more previous interventions and concurrent central stenoses. The 6-month patency rates were 69% in the treatment group and 70% in the observation group. The 12-month patency rates were 51% in the treatment group and 47% in the observation group (Fig 3). There were no significant differences between groups. There was an 80% confidence limit for detection of a difference greater than 20%.

Discussion.—It is possible that the greater number of patients who had previous intervention in the treatment group adversely affected the outcome. However, these findings indicate that a generic approach of percutaneous transluminal angioplasty for all polytetrafluoroethylene grafts with stenoses greater than 50% does not prolong patency. Therefore, such an approach is not supported.

▶ This small, prospective, randomized study examines the hypothesis that balloon angioplasty of greater than 50% stenoses in a functioning dialysis graft will prolong patency. As expected, the majority of stenoses were in the venous outflow, although a moderate number were in the mid-graft. Absolutely no difference in patency was noted between the patients randomized to angioplasty and those randomized to no treatment. The authors concluded correctly that prophylactic angioplasty of all detected stenoses of 50% or more in a functioning access graft system does not prolong access patency. I agree. (See also Abstract 11–8.)

Balloon Versus Patch Angioplasty as an Adjuvant Treatment to Surgical Thrombectomy of Hemodialysis Grafts

Bitar G, Yang S, Badosa F (Albert Einstein Med Ctr, Philadelphia)

Am J Surg 174:140–142, 1997 11–8

Background.—Transluminal balloon angioplasty has a number of advantages over patch angioplasty as a salvage method for thrombosed hemodialysis grafts. The outcome of 22 balloon angioplasties performed during a 6-month period was compared with that of 22 patch angioplasties performed by the same surgeon during an earlier 2-year period.

Methods.—Patients in both groups were inner city residents with renal failure; most had multiple medical problems. The balloon and patch groups were comparable for average age, gender distribution, average time between graft replacement, and number of times the graft was revised before the balloon or patch procedure. Noncompliant high pressure balloons were used in the balloon angioplasty procedures.

Results.—Primary patencies, defined as function during the period between the procedure and graft thrombosis, were 86% at 1 month, 45% at 3 months, and 17% at 6 months in the patch angioplasty group. In the balloon angioplasty group, primary patencies were 77%, 40%, and 28% at 1 month, 3 months, and 6 months, respectively. Differences between the 2 groups were not statistically significant. Patients who underwent balloon angioplasty required less pain medication than those in the patch group and were discharged on the same day. Patients in the patch angioplasty group were admitted for overnight observation. There were 5 complications in each group; the patch group had more infections and the balloon group had more vein tears.

Conclusion.—With 6 months of follow-up, primary patency was similar after patch angioplasty and balloon angioplasty. Transluminal balloon angioplasty is, thus, recommended for the salvage of dialysis access grafts because it is less invasive than patch angioplasty, has a lower infection rate, requires less operating time, and can better preserve the graft site for future revisions.

► Although these authors noted that balloon angioplasty of the venous stenosis at the upstream site of failed dialysis grafts after thrombectomy appeared as durable as vein patch angioplasty, it is important to note that the results of both were absolutely terrible, with 6-month patency rate of only 28% and 17%, respectively. Using some sort of convoluted logic, these authors come to the conclusion that balloon angioplasty is superior, but I am hard pressed to understand their reasoning. (See also Abstract 11–7.)

Prospective Randomized Comparison of Surgical Versus Endovascular Management of Thrombosed Dialysis Access Grafts

Marston WA, Criado E, Jaques PF, et al (Univ of North Carolina, Chapel Hill)
J Vasc Surg 26:373–381, 1997 11–9

Introduction.—The increasing number of patients receiving long-term dialysis therapy has made preservation of thrombosed hemodialysis shunts a more frequently encountered problem. Salvage of the thrombosed shunt can be accomplished by surgical or endovascular means. The efficacy of these 2 methods was compared prospectively.

Methods.—The 91 patients included in the randomized trial had 115 episodes of polytetrafluoroethylene shunt thrombosis. All shunts were evaluated within 1 week of thrombosis and treated within 48 hours of diagnosis. Endovascular salvage was performed in 59 episodes of shunt thrombosis and surgical salvage in 56. The 2 randomized groups were similar in age, sex, and clinical characteristics. Graft function in the endovascular group was restored with mechanical (82%) or thrombolytic (18%) graft thrombectomy, followed by percutaneous angioplasty. Surgi-

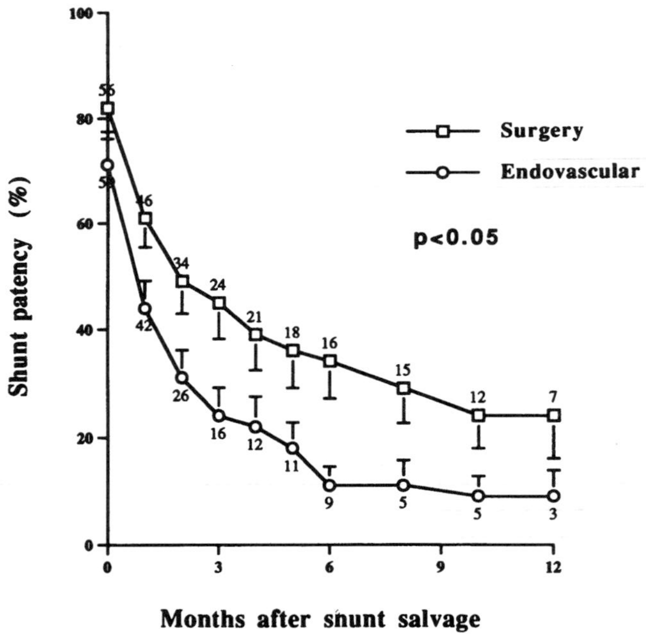

FIGURE 1.—Primary graft patency rate after salvage of thrombosed shunts treated with surgical compared with endovascular techniques. Patency rates are significantly different by log-rank test ($P < 0.05$). (Courtesy of Marston WA, Criado E, Jaques PF, et al: Prospective randomized comparison of surgical versus endovascular management of thrombosed dialysis access grafts. *J Vasc Surg* 26:373–381, 1997.)

cal salvage was attempted with thrombectomy plus graft revision in 78% of shunts and with thrombectomy alone in 22%. Patients were followed up for at least 6 months to compare shunt patency and length of graft function achieved with the 2 methods.

Results.—The initial success rate in restoring graft function was 82% in grafts treated surgically and 71% in those treated with endovascular techniques. In the months after salvage, surgery achieved a significantly better primary graft patency than endovascular therapy (Fig 1). At 12 months, graft patency had been extended in 25% of shunts with surgery, but in only 9% of shunts with endovascular treatment. Patients with venous anastomotic stenosis, the most common cause of shunt thrombosis in both groups (55% overall), had a significantly better patency rate than those with other causes of graft thrombosis. The patency rate was significantly worse in patients with long-segment venous outflow stenosis or occlusion.

Conclusions.—The primary patency rate after graft salvage was found to be significantly better in the surgical group than in the endovascular group. Patency was greatly reduced in both groups, however, at 6 and 12 months after the salvage procedures.

▶ Endovascular repair of thrombosed dialysis fistulas using thrombolysis or graft thrombectomy followed by percutaneous angioplasty has become increasingly popular in recent years. Standard course of therapy consists of thrombectomy plus surgical graft revision in most patients. These authors compared the outcome with these 2 significantly different forms of therapy. No matter which therapy was undertaken the results were terrible, with only 36% of surgically revised grafts functional at 6 months, and 25% at 12 months. The endovascular graft repair fared even worse, with 11% functional at 6 months, and 9% at 12 months. Unfortunately, neither surgical nor endovascular management resulted in long-term function for the majority of shunts after thrombosis, but surgical management appeared superior. I believe their information is precisely correct. The occurrence of shunt thrombosis signals the beginning of a rapid downhill spiral for almost all dialysis grafts.

Cost Efficacy of Duplex Surveillance and Prophylactic Angioplasty of Arteriovenous ePTFE Grafts

Lumsden AB, MacDonald MJ, Kikeri D, et al (Emory Univ, Atlanta, Ga)

Ann Vasc Surg 12:138–142, 1998 11–10

Introduction.—The creation and maintenance of dialysis access accounts for 24% of all hospital expenditures for dialysis patients. Polytetrafluoroethylene grafts' average patency, only 18 months, creates a major clinical problem. A study of chronic hemodialysis patients examined the cost incurred by a program of graft surveillance and prophylactic balloon angioplasty of polytetrafluoroethylene graft stenoses greater than 50% diameter.

Methods.—Patients in a single inner-city dialysis unit were screened for participation. Those found to have a stenosis 50% or greater at color flow duplex imaging underwent angiographic study. Patients confirmed to have such a stenosis by angiography were randomized to observation only or to prophylactic percutaneous transluminal angioplasty (PTA). Ultrasound follow-up was scheduled every 3 months. Patients in the treatment group with recurrent stenosis greater than 50% had repeat PTA. The primary outcome event was functional graft failure. Patient billing records were reviewed for cost calculations.

Results.—Graft patencies were 69% for the treatment group and 70% for the observation group at 6 months; 12-month patencies were 51% and 47%, respectively, not a significant difference. Cost for initial color flow duplex image screening of all patients was $40,440. The overall charge for treating the 32 patients in the treatment arm was $440,834, but this group had no improvement in patency compared with the observation-only group.

Conclusion.—Patients admitted once a year to the hospital for a vascular access procedure incur nearly twice the total annual expenditures of patients not requiring admission. A policy of routine graft surveillance and prophylactic PTA is quite costly, but does not lead to improved graft patency and thus cannot be justified.

▶ Judging from the sheer volume of literature, vascular surgeons are spending considerably more time maintaining patency of access grafts than they may like. This interesting study randomly compared a program of aggressive access graft surveillance, followed by angiography and angioplasty as indicated, to a program of follow-up only. Interestingly, the 6- and 12-month patencies were identical, with an extraordinarily increased cost in the interventional group. Intensive surveillance and endovascular prophylaxis appear futile.

Hand Ischemia

Magnetic Resonance Angiography of the Hand and Wrist: Evaluation of Patients With Severe Ischemic Disease

Kransdorf MJ, Turner-Stepahin S, Merritt WH (St. Mary's Hosp, Richmond, Va; Univ of Virginia, Charlottesville; Med College of Virginia, Richmond)

J Reconstr Microsurg 14:77–81, 1998 11–11

Introduction.—Conventional arteriography is the gold standard for evaluating patients with severe ischemic disease of the hand and wrist. Magnetic resonance imaging is a dependable noninvasive alternative to conventional arteriography. Eleven patients with Raynaud's syndrome and severe ischemic disease of the upper extremity underwent prospective MR evaluation of the wrist and hand.

Methods.—Magnetic resonance angiograms were compared with surgical findings in 7 patients and with conventional arteriography in 4 patients.

Results.—The correlation between MR angiography and surgery and conventional arteriography findings was excellent. For all patients, MR correctly predicted patency or lack of patency of the distal and ulnar arteries and superficial and deep palmar arches. Portions of the palmar arches oriented parallel to the plane were not adequately visualized in 3 of 11 patients. Both conventional and MR angiography were unable to completely visualize common and proper digital arteries.

Conclusion.—Magnetic resonance angiography may be considered a reliable noninvasive method for assessing patients with severe upper-extremity ischemic disease. It accurately reveals peripheral vessels through the level of the palmar arches. Anatomical vascular depiction is adequate in determining patency of the major vessels in the preoperative assessment for reconstructive surgery and sympathectomy.

▶ There is a maddening lack of clinical detail in this article. The authors state that 7 of these 11 patients underwent surgery for treatment of their hand ischemia. I was appropriately curious as to just what surgery was undertaken. Curiously, the article brushes over this and gives no information. We have done a large number of hand arteriograms and routinely use a magnification arteriographic technique with very careful positioning of a catheter in the brachial artery. This has produced absolutely stellar results, in our experience. It seems obvious that MR angiography is capable of delivering results almost as good if one has dedicated personnel. Unfortunately, our MR angiography department is not nearly as good as our interventional radiology group, and for the time being, we shall continue to obtain arteriograms.

Digital Ischemia and Gangrene Due to Red Blood Cell Aggregation Induced by Acquired Dysfibrinogenemia

Kwaan HC, Levin M, Sakurai S, et al (Northwestern Univ, Chicago; Northwestern Univ Technological Inst, Evanston, Ill; Univ of Health Sciences, Chicago)

J Vasc Surg 26:1061–1068, 1997 11–12

Introduction.—Several conditions are associated with microvascular occlusion by red blood cell (RBC) aggregation. The aggregates take the form of rouleaux which may occlude small vessels. In the case reported here, digital ischemia complicated by gangrene was present in a patient with an unusual finding of marked RBC aggregation and rouleaux formation.

Case Report.—A white man, 56 and in good health, had sudden onset of cyanosis and pain in a finger. All fingers and toes became involved over the next 2 days, and 2 fingers showed gangrenous changes. Treatment with heparin, warfarin, prednisone, and va-

TABLE 1.—Residual Lesions

	Total	50–74%	75–99%	OCCL
ICA	6 (3.1%)	1 (0.5%)	3 (1.6%)	2 (1.0%)
ECA	22 (11.5%)	14 (7.3%)	8 (4.2%)	0
CCA	1 (0.5%)	0	0	1 (0.5%)

Abbreviations: *CCA*, common carotid artery; *ECA*, external carotid artery; *ICA*, internal carotid artery.

(Reprinted by permission of the publisher from Ricotta JJ, O'Brien-Irr MS: Completion angiography, Is it really necessary? *AMERICAN JOURNAL OF SURGERY* 174;181–184, copyright 1997 by Excerpta Medica Inc.)

reduce perioperative morbidity and residual disease. Completion imaging is rarely performed in the authors' practice. They examined their carotid registry to determine whether not performing routine completion imaging has had a negative effect on patient outcome.

Methods.—A review was conducted of all cases of carotid endarterectomy performed by 1 vascular surgeon from 1988 to 1996. Persistent residual defects were identified by duplex follow-up. These defects were classified as 50% to 74%, 75% to 99%, and occlusion in the common, internal, and external carotid arteries.

Results.—Duplex follow-up information was available for 192 of the 229 patients. From 1988 to 1996, 8 completion angiograms were performed and 5 arteries were reopened. The combined rate of stroke and death was 3.1%. Duplex follow-up showed residual lesions in 29 patients (15%), but only 3.6% involved the internal or common carotid arteries (Table 1).

Conclusion.—Routine completion imaging is not needed to achieve acceptable morbidity and mortality or to minimize residual problems after carotid endarterectomy. Excellent results can be achieved by strictly adhering to basic principles of complete visualization and removal of all significant plaque, meticulous closure with liberal use of patches, and selective use of imaging.

► Dr. Ricotta's conclusion that routine completion arteriography is not required to achieve acceptable morbidity and mortality after carotid endarterectomy appears precisely correct. I continue to be impressed that the advocates of completion carotid endarterectomy arteriography routinely describe finding an inordinate number of residual defects that "require" carotid reopening and additional surgical manipulation. One can hardly help but be impressed by the observation that the routine arteriography/frequent reopening group seems to experience exactly the same clinical results as the no arteriography/never reopening group. Either the no arteriography group is composed of superior surgeons, or one must conclude that many of the defects repaired by the routine arteriography group do not actually require repair. At any rate, I find no persuasive reason to perform routine arteriography after vascular surgery. We almost never use it. One should keep in mind the old surgical adage: the enemy of good is better.

A Randomized Study on Eversion Versus Standard Carotid Endarterectomy: Study Design and Preliminary Results: The Everest Trial

Cao P, and Collaborators of the EVEREST Study Group (Policlinico Monteluce, Perugia, Italy)

J Vasc Surg 27:595–605, 1998 12–3

Introduction.—Prospective trials comparing eversion and conventional carotid endarterectomy (CEA) have been small and few, making definitive conclusions unavailable. The major perioperative and late complication rates and the durability of eversion CEA were assessed in EVEREST (Eversion Carotid Endarterectomy vs. Standard Trial), a multicentered randomized trial conducted in Italy between October 1994 to March 1997.

Methods.—A total of 1,353 patients with carotid stenosis needing surgical intervention were randomized to receive either standard CEA (675 patients) or eversion CEA (678 patients). Carotid occlusion, major stroke, death, and restenosis rate were primary end points.

Results.—The rate of perioperative major stroke and death were 1.3 for patients in both the eversion and standard CEA groups. Early occlusions were 0.6% and 0.4%, respectively. There were no significant between-group differences in the incidence of perioperative transient ischemic accident, minor stroke, cranial nerve injuries, neck hematoma, myocardial infarction, or surgical defects. Clamping times were 31.7 and 34.5 minutes, respectively, for eversion and standard CEA, a significant difference.

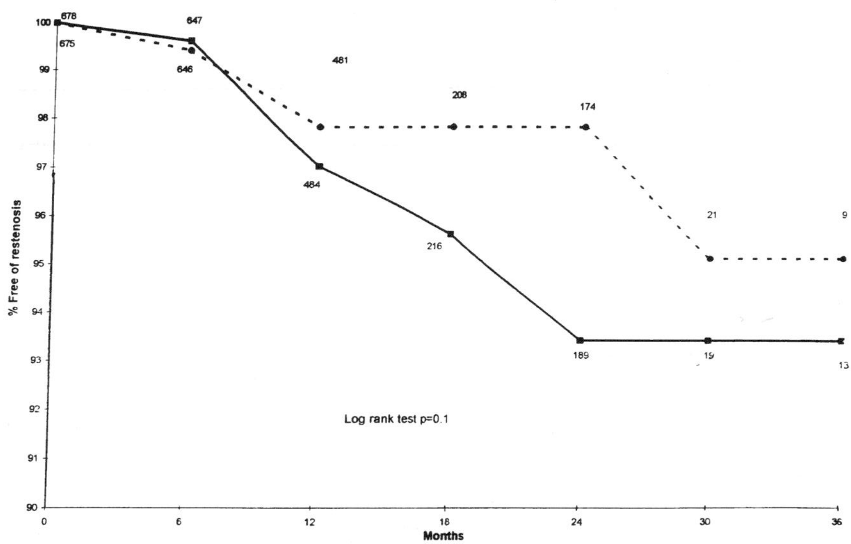

FIGURE 2.—Cumulative percentage of patients free of re-stenosis at 3 years in the eversion (*dotted line*) and standard (*solid line*) groups. (Courtesy of Cao P, and Collaborators of the EVEREST Study Group: A randomization study on eversion versus standard carotid endarterectomy: Study design and preliminary results. The Everest Trial. *J Vasc Surg* 27:595–605, 1998.)

Eleven percent and 16% of patients undergoing eversion and standard procedures, respectively, underwent shunt placement. Thirty-day events were similar in the 2 groups; they were 13.3% in the eversion group and 11.4% in the standard group. The re-stenosis rate at a mean follow-up of 14.9 months (range, 1–38 months) was 2.4% (16 patients) in the eversion group and 4.1% (28 patients) in the standard group, a nonsignificant difference (Fig 2).

Conclusion.—Preliminary findings of the EVEREST Trial indicate that eversion CEA is a safe and quick procedure that yields a low complication rate. There were no significant differences in re-stenosis rates for patients undergoing the 2 procedures in the available follow-up period. Long-term follow-up is needed to determine whether the eversion technique influences the durability of CEA.

▶ This interesting article concludes that eversion CEA and standard CEA with patch yield identical clinical results. Somehow, the concept of eversion CEA reminds me of the old surgical principle: With a little difficulty, there are few things in vascular surgery that cannot be made more difficult. I can see absolutely no reason for performance of an eversion endarterectomy, which, of course, requires reimplantation of the internal carotid artery onto the common carotid artery. I also find, in an increasing number of our current carotid patients, that the plaque seems to go high and sometimes does not stop at all, requiring transection. I really don't know how this would be handled with the eversion technique. At any rate, I am delighted to learn that the eversion technique does not appear to be superior to the standard technique because, even if it were, I would not use it.

Cost Savings Associated With the Nonroutine Use of Carotid Angiography

Garrard CL, Manord JD, Ballinger BA, et al (Alton Ochsner Med Found, New Orleans, La)

Am J Surg 174:650–654, 1997 12–4

Introduction.—Carotid endarterectomy (CEA) is the most frequently performed major peripheral vascular procedure in the United States. Several perioperative components of CEA have been assessed from a cost perspective. The economic impact of performing CEA based only on diagnosis made from duplex scanning was evaluated in 97 consecutive patients treated during 1 calendar year of selective angiography.

Methods.—Patients were assigned to 1 of 2 groups: those with and those without arteriography before surgery. Duplex scans and arteriograms were analyzed to determine their effect on surgical strategy. Hospital charges and physician fees were noted for each patient admission. The groups were compared regarding operative results, complications, and total charges.

Results.—One patient in each group (2%) had an operative stroke. There were 2 notable angiographic complications: 1 stroke and 1 femoral

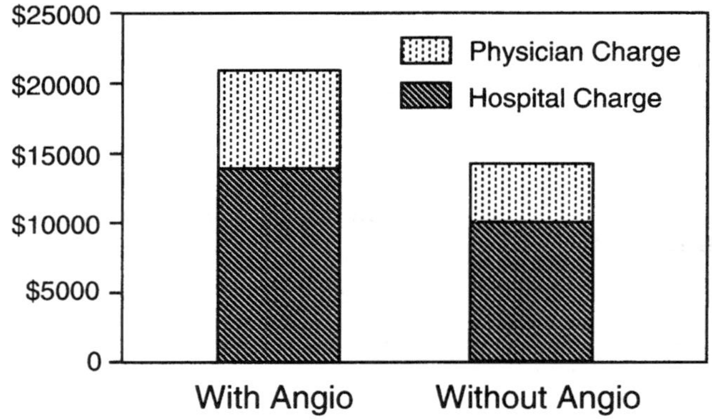

FIGURE 2.—Total hospital and physician charges for patients who underwent carotid endarterectomy with and without an arteriogram. (Reprinted by permission of the publisher from Garrard CL, Manord JD, Ballinger BA, et al: Cost savings associated with the nonroutine use of carotid angiography. *AMERICAN JOURNAL OF SURGERY* 174:650–654, copyright 1997 by Excerpta Medica Inc.)

artery thrombosis. Surgical strategy was changed as the result of 2 arteriograms. Hospital charges for patients who had an arteriogram were significantly higher than for patients who did not ($10,292 vs. $13,906). Physician charges for patients with and without an arteriogram were $6,297 and $3,882, respectively. Total charges for the CEA with and without arteriography were $14,174 and $20,203, respectively (Fig 2). Charges were 43% higher for patients with than without an arteriogram.

Conclusion.—Nonroutine use of carotid angiography was not associated with increased operative risk or postoperative length of stay. Per patient charges were 43% higher in patients who had an arteriogram, compared to those who underwent duplex scanning only.

▶ This study has weak design and insufficient power to prove the authors' first conclusion that avoiding angiography does not increase operative risk. It serves to remind us that even outpatient angiography is expensive and carries a risk of significant complications. In a group of patients, half of whom may be seen with asymptomatic or nonspecific symptoms, advising angiography requires better reasons than the "physician's discretion" reported here. However, we can be certain that comprehensive imaging will be required in some patients, especially those in whom duplex findings are equivocal. The future costs of technologists working to higher standards of precision; upgraded machines; and rigorous quality control in the assessment of inflow, outflow, and plaque morphology must be included in any hypothetical assessment of cost savings. Angiography shows us only the lumen, which makes for an incomplete assessment, but it remains the gold standard for the determination of stenosis.

A.E.B. Giddings, M.D.

Comparison of North American Symptomatic Carotid Endarterectomy Trial and Population-Based Outcomes for Carotid Endarterectomy

Hallett JW Jr, Pietropaoli JA Jr, Ilstrup DM, et al (Mayo Found, Rochester, Minn)

J Vasc Surg 27:845–851, 1998 12–5

Background.—The North American Symptomatic Carotid Endarterectomy Trial (NASCET) has recommended carotid endarterectomy (CEA) for treatment of transient ischemic attacks, nondisabling strokes, and ipsilateral high-grade stenosis in highly selected patients. It is not known whether the results of the NASCET can be achieved in an entire geographically defined population, but it is important to determine whether the NASCET recommendations are to be applied to community-dwelling patients.

Methods.—The medical records of all patients living in Olmsted County, Minnesota, who had undergone CEA for transient ischemic attacks or nondisabling stroke between 1970 and 1995 were reviewed. Survival rates to ipsilateral stroke after CEA were determined for all patients with symptoms. Results were compared with the results of the NASCET.

Results.—In Olmsted County, Minnesota, 297 patients (189 men and 108 women) underwent 322 CEAs. In 254 patients, transient ischemic attacks or nondisabling strokes were the indications for CEA. The other 43 patients had asymptomatic stenosis. Survival without ipsilateral stroke was 97% at 2 years, 93% at 5 years, and 92% at 10 years after CEA for symptomatic lesions. In the NASCET, survival free of ipsilateral stroke was 91% at 2 years. In the current study, survival free of any stroke was 90% at 5 years and 80% at 10 years (Fig 2). The rate of perioperative stroke was 19.2% in patients older than 80 and 2.2% in patients younger than 80 years.

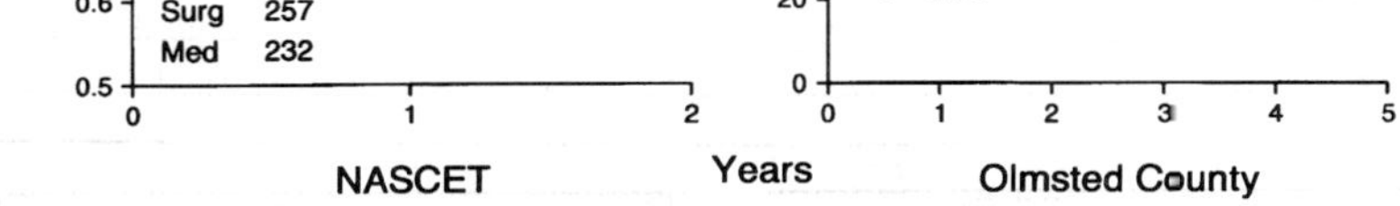

FIGURE 2.—Rates of survival free of any stroke for NASCET and Olmsted County, Minnesota, for 1970 through 1995. Deaths have been censored. The number of patients available for observation was 254 at onset and 80 at 5 years. (Courtesy of Hallett JW Jr, Pietropaoli JA Jr, Ilstrup DM, et al: Comparison of North American Symptomatic Carotid Endarterectomy Trial and population-based outcomes for carotid endarterectomy. *J Vasc Surg* 27:845–851, 1998.)

Discussion.—Early outcome in patients with symptoms after CEA in this population-based study was similar to the early outcome of patients in the NASCET. These findings demonstrate the long-term effectiveness of CEA in preventing stroke when performed by expert surgeons.

► Once again the authors ask the haunting question: Can NASCET results be applied broadly to community patients? Once again the giant salami slicer at the Mayo Clinic has labored mightily and produced a very thin slice of salami concerning the overstudied patient cohort in Olmsted County, Minnesota, this time including those who underwent CEA for symptoms between 1970 and 1995. About the only difference noted in the Mayo Study is that the 30-day postoperative stroke rate for patients older than 80 was, not surprisingly, significantly higher than that for patients younger than 80 years (19.2% vs. 2.2%). This very high 19.2% stroke rate, however, was accounted for by only a small number of patients older than 80, and I am sure it is skewed by the small numbers. On balance, this is another testimonial that the NASCET results are applicable to the real world. I am delighted. (See also Abstract 12–6.)

Variation in Carotid Endarterectomy Mortality in the Medicare Population: Trial Hospitals, Volume, and Patient Characteristics

Wennberg DE, Lucas FL, Birkmeyer JD, et al (Maine Med Ctr, Portland; Maine Med Assessment Found, Augusta; Dartmouth Med School, Hanover, NH, et al)

JAMA 279:1278–1281, 1998 12–6

Background.—Two studies, the North American Symptomatic Carotid Endarterectomy Trial (NASCET) and the Asymptomatic Carotid Atherosclerosis Study (ACAS), have demonstrated the efficacy of carotid endarterectomy (CEA) in reducing the risk of stroke and death in selected patients when the procedure is performed in institutions with demonstrated excellence in the procedure. The 30-day mortality rate was 0.6% in NASCET and 0.1% in ACAS. In the current study, the perioperative (30-day) mortality rate in patients with Medicare insurance who were undergoing CEA in nonfederal facilities was determined.

Methods.—Crude and adjusted perioperative mortality rates were determined in 113,300 patients with Medicare insurance who underwent CEA in 1992 and 1993. Patients underwent CEA in 86 hospitals participating in NASCET (trial hospitals) and 2,613 nonfederal institutions (nontrial hospitals). The nontrial facilities were categorized into high-, average-, or low-volume hospitals according to the average number of CEAs performed annually.

Results.—The perioperative mortality rate was 1.4% in trial hospitals, 1.7% in high-volume nontrial hospitals, 1.9% in average-volume nontrial hospitals, and 2.5% in low-volume nontrial hospitals. Multivariate modeling showed that in trial hospitals the mortality risk reduction was 15%

compared with that in high-volume nontrial hospitals, 25% compared with that in average-volume nontrial hospitals, and 43% compared with that in low-volume nontrial hospitals.

Discussion.—These findings show that, in patients with Medicare insurance, the perioperative mortality rate after CEA is significantly higher than that reported by the trials, even in hospitals participating in randomized studies. Caution is advised in the interpretation of findings from carefully controlled studies of CEA and their application to everyday practice.

▶ These health services research people examined the massive database of 113,000 Medicare patients undergoing CEA in 1992 and 1993 in 2,699 hospitals. They concluded that the perioperative mortality rate was significantly higher in all hospitals than that reported in NASCET and ACAS, curiously including a number of trial hospitals that had participated in the prior studies. They advise caution in transplanting the NASCET and ACAS mortality data to widespread clinical application. I really don't know what to make of this information. The differences are small, although the *P* values are generally significant. The prior abstract indicates that even in Olmsted County, the 30-day mortality rate was a little higher than that reported in NASCET. I conclude that both NASCET and ACAS mortality rates (0.6% and 0.1%) were basically flukes and nonrepresentative of the real world. However, this does not at all change my overall assessment that carotid endarterectomy in selected patients is clearly beneficial.

Indications, Outcomes, and Provider Volumes for Carotid Endarterectomy

Cebul RD, Snow RJ, Pine R, et al (Case Western Reserve Univ, Cleveland, Ohio; Cleveland Clinic Found, Ohio; Peer Review Systems, Inc, Westerville, Ohio)

JAMA 279:1282–1287, 1998 12–7

Introduction.—For reducing subsequent stroke rates among persons at risk, several controlled trials have provided evidence that carotid endarterectomy is superior to best medical therapy. The relative importance of patient selection vs. surgical or institutional proficiency has not been adequately studied because measurements of surgical indications or patients' co-morbid illness have not been adequately made. The use and outcomes of carotid endarterectomy over a 1-year period were profiled. The relationships between surgeon-specific and hospital-specific volumes and 30-day stroke or death rate were examined while controlling for surgical indications and other factors predictive of adverse outcomes.

Methods.—There were 678 charts that were retrospectively reviewed. The patients were non–health maintenance organization Medicare beneficiaries who had carotid endarterectomy in a 1-year period. They were similar to all eligible patients in sociodemographic characteristics and 30-day mortality rates.

Results.—Indications for surgery were asymptomatic carotid stenosis in 24.6% of patients, transient ischemic attack in 43.4%, completed stroke in 9.1%, and nonspecific symptoms in 22.9%. By 30 days postoperatively, 32 patients (4.7%) died or had nonfatal strokes. Rates did not vary by surgeons' volume; they did vary by hospital volume, but the power to detect this difference was limited. Similar indications and distributions of co-morbidities were found among patients at higher- and lower-volume hospitals. Being operated on in a higher-volume hospital conferred a 71% reduction in risk for 30-day stroke or death in analyses controlling for indications, co-morbid conditions, and surgeon's volume.

Conclusion.—Persons who are asymptomatic or have nonspecific symptoms make up almost half (47.5%) of the carotid endarterectomies. It is important to identify patients and providers having the most favorable outcome profiles. Further investigation into the higher rate of adverse outcomes seen in lower-volume hospitals is merited, as it does not appear to be caused by differences in patient selection.

► This large, retrospective study of Medicare beneficiaries having carotid surgery (half for asymptomatic disease or "non-specific" reasons) included 1 year's data. It shows that half of the procedures were done by surgeons performing 21 or less procedures per year at hospitals doing 62 or fewer procedures per year. Numerically, these large datasets have the power to prove that bigger means better, irrespective of the stated indications for operation. If confirmed, this may go some way toward justifying the higher costs of large institutions.

Concentration is certainly required if the volume of work needed to provide good training, meaningful audit, and the expertise to deal with complex problems is to be retained and developed. Experience in other surgical fields suggests that the quality of training, patient selection, and caseload are all important factors in developing competence and that external review is uniquely effective in defining and improving performance.

A.E.B. Giddings, M.D.

Carotid Endarterectomy Does Not Affect Long-term Blood Pressure: Observations From the NASCET

Eliasziw M, for the North American Symptomatic Carotid Endarterectomy Trial (Univ of Western Ontario, London, Canada; John P. Robarts Research Inst, London, Ontario, Canada; Stroke Prevention and Atherosclerosis Research Ctr, London, Ontario, Canada)

Cerebrovasc Dis 8:20–24, 1998 12–8

Purpose.—A study was undertaken to determine how carotid endarterectomy (CEA) affects blood pressure during a 2-year period.

without intervening carotid surgery, while the remainder had either preoperative or simultaneous CEA. The postoperative status of the patient was clearly better in the CEA group. Although this information is interesting, the lack of randomization makes the results uninterpretable as a basis for definitive conclusions. I continue to believe that patients who have high-grade carotid stenosis are generally better treated with preoperative CEA before CABG, or occasionally with simultaneous CABG-CEA, but I cannot prove it. I do note that preoperative CABG is one of the few screening indications approved by the Health Care Financing Administration for carotid screening. Isn't that curious?

Carotid Endarterectomy in Octogenarians: Early Results and Late Outcome

O'Hara PJ, Hertzer NR, Mascha EJ, et al (Cleveland Clinic Found, Ohio)

J Vasc Surg 27:860–871, 1998 12–12

Background.—Large prospective, randomized trials have demonstrated the effectiveness of carotid endarterectomy (CEA) in preventing ischemic stroke in patients with severe internal carotid artery stenoses, both with and without symptoms. In the current study, the safety and efficacy of CEA in octogenarians were determined.

Methods.—An analysis was done of 182 CEAs performed between 1989 and 1995 in 167 patients. There were 98 men and 69 women ranging in age from 80 to 93 years. Of the 182 procedures, 100 were performed for severe asymptomatic stenosis, 48 for hemispheric transient ischemic attacks or amaurosis fugax, 24 for previous stroke, and 10 for vertebrobasilar symptoms. Thirteen procedures were combined with myocardial revascularization, and 5 procedures were carotid reoperations. Nine arteriotomies were repaired primarily and the other 173 were repaired with vein patch angioplasty or synthetic patches. Late information was available for 165 patients; 2 patients were lost to follow-up. The mean follow-up period was 2.7 years.

Results.—Overall, there were 5 early postoperative neurologic events; 3 were strokes and 2 were transient ischemic attacks. Another 15 neurologic events occurred late in the follow-up period; 11 were strokes and 4 were transient ischemic attacks. The 5-year rate of freedom from stroke as estimated by the Kaplan-Meier method was 85%. One patient died of cardiac complications 9 days after CEA. At 5 years, estimated survival was 45% (Fig 1) and estimated stroke-free survival was 42%. Variables that significantly affected survival, as determined by multivariable analysis, were age at operation, abnormal creatinine level, and chronic obstructive pulmonary disease. Factors that were significantly associated with stroke after CEA were presence of chronic obstructive pulmonary disease and a lesser degree of contralateral internal carotid stenosis. The causes of late death were cardiovascular in 16 patients, carcinoma in 6, stroke in 6, miscellaneous in 13, and unknown in 13.

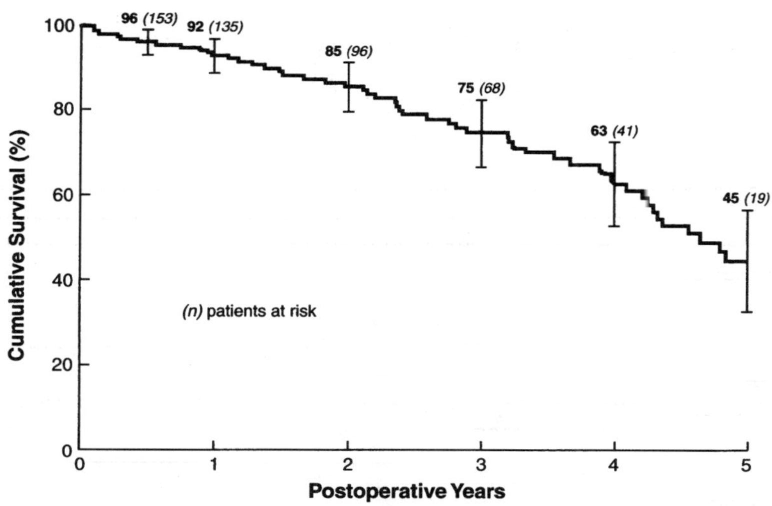

FIGURE 1.—Cumulative survival rate (Kaplan-Meier method) for 167 octogenarians in the entire series who underwent carotid endarterectomy. (Courtesy of O'Hara PJ, Hertzer NR, Mascha EJ, et al: Carotid endarterectomy in octogenarians: Early results and late outcome. *J Vasc Surg* 27:860–871, 1998.)

Discussion.—These results indicate that CEA is safe in selected octogenarians with carotid stenosis and that most of these patients will not experience postoperative stroke. Patients who are otherwise good candidates for CEA should not be excluded because of age alone.

► I have previously stated that the performance of CEA in symptom-free octogenarians makes no sense to me.[1] In this amazing article from the Cleveland Clinic, we learn that of 182 CEAs performed on 167 patients over 80 years of age (mean age, 83), 55% were performed for asymptomatic stenosis. The authors note that the estimated 5-year survival of these patients was 45%, with a 5-year stroke-free survival rate of only 42%. Although I will not quibble with their decision to operate on patients with symptoms, I continue to believe that patients over the age of 80 simply do not live long enough to enjoy sufficient benefits from prophylactic CEA to justify the procedure. I respectfully disagree with the conclusion of the authors who state that "age alone should not exclude otherwise qualified candidates from consideration for CEA," at least insofar as this applies to symptom-free patients. I firmly believe that this remarkable conclusion deserves thoughtful reconsideration, followed by abandonment.

Reference

1. 1998 YEAR BOOK OF VASCULAR SURGERY, p. 338.

Utility of Carotid Duplex in Young Adults With Lower Extremity Atherosclerosis: How Aggressive Should We Be in Screening Young Patients?

Valentine RJ, Hagino RT, Boyd PI, et al (Univ of Texas, Dallas)
Cardiovasc Surg 5:408–413, 1997 12–13

Objective.—Whereas the premature onset of lower extremity atherosclerosis in young adults is associated with rapid progression of disease, the prevalence of carotid atherosclerosis in this subpopulation has not been studied. The prevalence and degree of carotid disease in patients with premature lower extremity atherosclerosis and the relationships between the degree of carotid disease relative to the degree of lower extremity atherosclerosis and progression of lower limb disease are documented.

Methods.—Color Doppler ultrasonography was performed in 76 men (8% black), aged 29 to 49, with premature lower extremity atherosclerosis. The lowest recorded ankle brachial index was recorded for each patient. Patients were followed up on average for 48 months.

Results.—All patients had a high prevalence of risk factors for atherosclerosis. Coronary artery disease was present in 46 (60%) of patients. Mean brachial ankle index was 0.49. During the follow-up period, 6 patients had a TIA, 7 had a hemispheric stroke, 47 required interventions for limb ischemia, and 18 had disease progression. Carotid duplex results revealed advanced or severe disease (60% to 99% stenosis) in 22 patients (29%), moderate disease (40% to 59% stenosis) in 16 patients (21%), mild disease (1% to 39% stenosis) in 18 (24%), and normal carotid arteries in 20 (26%). Medical and smoking histories, ages, disease progression, ankle brachial index, intervention, and death rates were similar for patients with diseased and normal carotid arteries. Transient ischemic attacks developed in 15 patients (27%) with carotid artery symptoms, vs. no patients with normal scans.

Conclusion.—Patients with premature atherosclerosis of the lower extremities have a high incidence of carotid artery atherosclerosis. Advanced asymptomatic disease can be detected using duplex scans.

▶ Several investigators have examined the utility of routine carotid screening in patients who have limb ischemia.[1, 2] Every article with which I am familiar has concluded that patients who have lower extremity ischemia have a significant prevalence of carotid stenosis. This article is no different, finding a high prevalence of carotid occlusion and advanced carotid stenosis. I totally agree with the authors' conclusion that screening carotid duplex scans are indicated in patients with limb ischemia. Unfortunately, the Health Care Financing Administration (HCFA) has specifically disapproved routine screening as an indication for carotid duplex, at least as far as HCFA reimbursement is concerned. I consider this to be a travesty and a complete failure of HCFA to understand tenets of modern health care. Presently, we continue to try very hard to find "approved" indications for carotid duplex in patients who have limb ischemia. Vascular surgeons with an interest in the vascular laboratory must familiarize themselves with the list of approved HCFA indications for carotid duplex.

Reference

1. Marek J, Mills JL, Harvich J, et al: Utility of routine carotid duplex screening in patients who have claudication. *J Vasc Surg* 24:572–579, 1996.
2. Gentile AT, Taylor LM, Moneta GL, et al: Prevalence of asymptomatic carotid stenosis in patients undergoing infrainguinal bypass surgery. *Arch Surg* 130:900–904, 1995.

Multicenter Review of Preoperative Risk Factors for Endarterectomy for Asymptomatic Carotid Artery Stenosis

Goldstein LB, Samsa GP, Matchar DB, et al (Duke Univ, Durham, NC; Durham Dept of Veterans Affairs Med Ctr, NC)

Stroke 29:750–753, 1998 12–14

Background.—The benefit of carotid endarterectomy vs. medical treatment alone depends primarily on surgical risk. There is little information on risk factors of endarterectomy for asymptomatic carotid artery stenosis other than information from randomized controlled trials. The effect of preoperative risk factors on the frequency of postoperative complications in patients undergoing endarterectomy for asymptomatic carotid artery stenosis was examined in a multicenter review.

Methods.—The medical records of a random sample of patients who had carotid endarterectomy at 12 academic medical centers in a 3-year period were reviewed.

Results.—A review was conducted of 1,160 carotid endarterectomy procedures. Of these, 463 were performed for asymptomatic disease. Thirteen patients had postoperative stroke or died, and 3 patients had myocardial infarction. Patients with no symptoms had a lower rate of postoperative stroke or death than patients who had a history of cerebrovascular symptoms in a different vascular distribution; this difference was not significant. No significant differences in these rates were seen to be based on race, history of angina, recent myocardial infarction, chronic obstructive pulmonary disease, hypertension, degree of stenosis in the contralateral or ipsilateral carotid artery, or presence of angiographically determined ulceration, intraluminal thrombus, or siphon stenosis in the ipsilateral vessel. The rate of postoperative stroke or death was higher in women than in men, in patients aged 75 years or older than in those younger than 75, and in patients with a history of congestive heart failure than in those without such history. The risk of stroke or death was also higher in the 16 patients who had carotid endarterectomy plus coronary artery bypass surgery than in those who had endarterectomy alone.

Discussion.—Although the overall risk of postoperative stroke or death in this study was within acceptable guidelines, it was almost twice the risk reported by investigators of the Asymptomatic Carotid Atherosclerosis

Study (ACAS) in clinical trials. High-risk groups in the current study were women, which was supported by the aforementioned study, as well as patients aged 75 years or more, patients with a history of congestive heart failure, and patients who have had endarterectomy for asymptomatic stenosis combined with coronary surgery. If clinicians are aware of these risks and high-risk patient groups, they may be able to make better decisions about a patient's postoperative risk and the potential benefit of surgery.

▶ The authors again ask whether ACAS data can be generalized to the public. Using a complex system, these authors selected a number of carotid endarterectomies performed during the calendar years 1988 to 1990 at 11 of the 12 member hospitals of the Academic Medical Centers Consortium. Postoperative stroke or death occurred in 1.8% of symptom-free patients vs. 4.2% of patients with symptoms. They conclude that the overall risk of postoperative stroke or death was nearly twice that reported by ACAS. Although this is true, I note that the 1.8% is an excellent result, counting the entire population, and I am generally unimpressed with their conclusions.

Epidemiology

Epidemiology of Carotid Endarterectomy Among Medicare Beneficiaries: 1985–1996 Update

Hsia DC, Moscoe LM, Krushat WM (US Department of Health and Human Services; Rockville, Md; US Department of Health and Human Services, Baltimore, Md)

Stroke 29:346–350, 1998 12–15

Introduction.—The annual trend for carotid endarterectomies in the United States has twice changed direction, according to projections from the National Hospital Discharge Survey. The use of the procedure peaked in 1985, out of favor by 1991 and subsequently recovered by 1996. Medical developments pertaining to carotid endarterectomy paralleled these trends. The decline was caused to concerns about the effectiveness of the procedure and proper indications for surgical interventions, but since 1991 controlled trials have affirmed its use in selected patients. Changes in the rate and outcome of carotid endarterectomies among Medicare beneficiaries were reviewed.

Methods.—To calculate carotid endarterectomy frequency, rate, and perioperative mortality by patient demography and hospital characteristics, codes from the *International Classification of Diseases, 9th Revision, Clinical Modification* were analyzed.

Results.—In 1985 there was an initial peak of 61,273 carotid endarterectomies (20.6 per 10,000 Medicare beneficiaries). In 1989 the number of procedures then declined to 46,571 (14.3 per 10,000). In 1996 the number of procedures rose to 108,275 (28.6 per 10,000) (Fig 1). The patients were predominantly male, white, and aged 65–74. Surgery was performed pre-

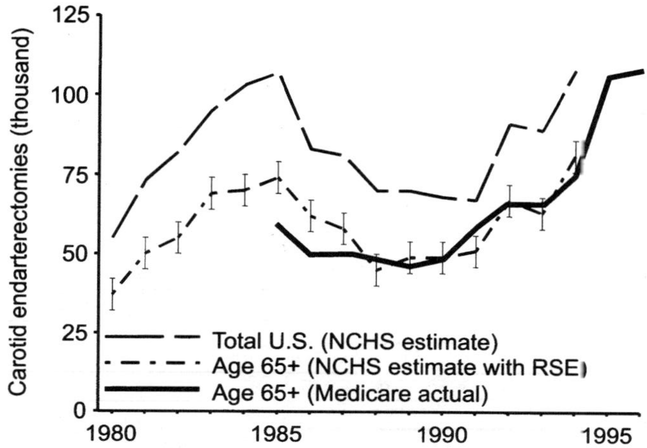

FIGURE 1.—Carotid endarterectomies in short-stay, nonfederal hospitals by patient age, United States 1980–1996. *NCHS*, National Center for Health Statistics; *RSE*, relative standard error. (Courtesy of Hsia DC, Moscie LM, Krushat WM: Epidemiology of carotid endarterectomy among medicare beneficiaries: 1985–1996 update. *Stroke* 29:346–350, 1998.)

dominantly in nonprofit, urban, large, and teaching hospitals. There was a decline in the perioperative mortality from 3% in 1985 to 1.6% in 1996.

Conclusion.—Prompt response to reports from clinical trials were shown by the frequency and rate of carotid endarterectomy. Over time, perioperative mortality improved and converged but did not attain the rates reported by the trials. There was twice the average perioperative mortality among patients 85 and older.

► This large "official" review of Medicare statistics from the Agency for Health Care Policy and Research does indeed produce fascinating information. The number of carotid endarterectomies has again gone up considerably to about 109,000 patients in 1996. Of special interest is the observation that the perioperative mortality declined to 1.6% in 1996, still considerably greater than that reported by the North American Symptomatic Carotid Endarterectomy Trian and the Asymptomatic Carotid Atherosclerosis Study. (See Abstract 12–6.)

Carotid Plaque Morphology Correlates With Presenting Symptomatology

Park AE, McCarthy WJ, Pearce WH, et al (Northwestern Univ, Chicago; Rush-Presbyterian-St. Luke's Med Ctr, Chicago)

J Vasc Surg 27:872–879, 1998 12–16

Objective.—Higher-grade stenosis and transient symptoms correlate with stroke risk in patients undergoing carotid endarterectomy. The biologic basis and the rate of progression of disease are poorly understood.

The relationship between the observed intraoperative gross carotid plaque characteristics and the initial disease parameters of the patient was investigated.

Methods.—Specimens were inspected and plaque characteristics were prospectively recorded during the performance of 1,008 carotid endarterectomies in 880 patients (64.7% men), average age 68.2 years, between July 1, 1982, and July 1, 1996. On the basis of initial symptoms, patients were categorized as transiently ischemic, prior stroke, or without symptoms.

Results.—Whereas the overall incidence of plaque ulceration was 71%, the specific incidence was significantly higher in patients with transient symptoms (77%) and in patients with prior stroke (79%) than in patients with no symptoms (60%). The overall incidence of plaque hemorrhage was 30%, with the prior stroke group having a nonsignificantly higher rate (37%) than the symptom-free group (28%). Intraplaque hemorrhage occurred more frequently in patients with higher-grade stenosis (90% to 99%) than in patients with less than 90% stenosis. The incidence of plaque ulceration was independent of the degree of stenosis.

Conclusion.—The degree of carotid plaque ulceration is significantly correlated with transient ischemia and prior stroke. Intraplaque hemorrhage occurred more frequently in patients with higher-grade stenosis than in patients with lower-grade stenosis.

► There seems little doubt that the presence of visible ulceration on gross examination of the carotid plaque correlates with symptomatic presentations, such as prior stroke, TIA, or amaurosis. Patients with asymptomatic disease tend to have nonulcerated plaques without attached fibrin. I consider the matter settled, and additional repeats of this basic message, while interesting, will not be well received. (See also Abstract 12–19.)

A Review of 100 Consecutive Reconstructions of the Distal Vertebral Artery for Embolic and Hemodynamic Disease

Berguer R, Morasch MD, Kline RA (Wayne State Univ, Detroit)

J Vasc Surg 27:852–859, 1998 12–17

Objective.—Lesions of the vertebral artery (VA) can lead to emboli and infarction of the brain stem. Outcome of distal VA reconstructions at a university-affiliated referral center were reviewed retrospectively.

Methods.—Between 1982 and 1997, 100 consecutive distal VA procedures were performed in 98 patients (33 women), aged 29 to 79 years (Table 3). Comorbid illness included cardiac disease in 39%, hypertension in 55%, diabetes in 20%, peripheral vascular disease in 9%, and chronic pulmonary disease in 5%. Seventeen patients had a confirmed history of stroke. Almost all patients had symptoms, including vertebrobasilar ischemia (n = 89), vertebrobasilar and hemispheric ischemia (n = 7), and hemispheric ischemia (n = 2). Eighteen patients had a fixed neurologic

TABLE 3.—Types of Distal Vertebral Artery Reconstruction

Distal VA Reconstructions	%
Common carotid to distal VA C1-2 bypass	56
External carotid to distal VA C1-2 bypass	6
Internal carotid to distal VA C1-2 bypass	6
Internal carotid to suboccipital VA C1-2 bypass	4
External carotid transposition to distal VA C1-2	18
Occipital artery transposition to distal VA C1-2	5
Distal VA C1-2 transposition to internal carotid	2
Distal VA vein patch angioplasty	1
Carotid to distal VA C1-2 retropharyngeal bypass	1
Laminectomy of atlas	1

(Courtesy of Berguer R, Morasch MD, Kline RA: A review of 100 consecutive reconstructions of the distal vertebral artery for embolic and hemodynamic disease. *J Vasc Surg* 27:852–859, 1998.)

deficit, and 2 symptom-free patients with bilateral internal carotid occlusion and vertebral occlusions underwent operations to provide a single artery for cerebral perfusion before coronary artery bypass surgery. Eighteen patients had symptomatic dynamic bony compression, 14 had VA dissection, and 92 had bilateral flow-impeding VA lesions. At the time of reconstruction, 18 patients also underwent carotid operations and 1 had a subclavian-to-carotid artery transposition. Patients were followed up for an average of 79 months by arteriography, angiography, or direct duplex ultrasonography to study long-term patency.

Results.—Four patients died of perioperative stroke. One patient survived a hemispheric stroke. Sixteen grafts failed, and 2 resulted in a fatal stroke. There were 6 asymptomatic graft occlusions and 8 stenoses. Corrections were attempted in 9 patients. Before the use of routine intraoperative completion imaging, 24% of operations were found to be flawed. After routine imaging was used, only 4% of patients were found to have asymptomatic defects. Concomitantly, perioperative deaths declined from 6% to 2%. Symptoms resolved completely in 71 patients and improved in 16. Ten patients were lost to follow-up. There were 20 late deaths, none from stroke. There were 5 late revisions. At 5 and 10 years, the primary patency rates were 75% and 70% and the secondary patency rates were 84% and 80%, respectively. Median patient survival was 107 months.

Conclusion.—VA reconstruction is an effective and long-lasting stroke-prevention technique. The correctness of reconstitution must be verified with intraoperative arteriography.

▶ A few authors, notably Kieffer from Paris and Berguer from Detroit, have performed a large number of reconstructive procedures on the distal vertebral artery at the level of C2. After 30 years we at Oregon have yet to do our first such operation. I suppose we must be failing to recognize the indications for this procedure. I note that, in the hands of these experienced surgeons, the results appear excellent, basically for the treatment of vertebrobasilar ischemia. We simply do not encounter patients with such severe vertebrobasilar ischemic symptoms, perhaps because of referral peculiari-

13 Grafts and Graft Complications

Autogenous Vein Grafts

Femoropopliteal Bypass: In Situ or Reversed Vein Grafts? Ten-Year Results of a Randomized Prospective Study

Watelet J, Soury P, Menard J-F, et al (Hôpital Charles Nicolle, Rouen, France)

Ann Vasc Surg 11:510–519, 1997 13–1

Objective.—A prospective randomized study compared long-term results in 2 groups that underwent femoropopliteal vein bypass using either in situ or reversed grafts between 1981 and 1985.

Methods.—Fifty in situ vein grafts and 50 reversed vein grafts were randomly performed in 91 patients with chronic (97%) or subacute critical ischemia. Actuarial primary and secondary patencies, survival, and limb salvage rates were calculated. Patients were followed up for 10 to 14 years. The greater saphenous vein was used in 79.6% of procedures.

Results.—Three patients were lost to follow-up. Three patients died during the perioperative period, and 64 died during the follow-up period. As of January 1995, there were 11 patients alive in the in situ graft group and 10 in the reversed graft group, with actuarial survival at 10 years of 30.8% and 29.5%, respectively. There were 7 major amputations in each group despite patencies in 2 of the in situ group and 4 in the reversed bypass group. Actuarial limb salvage at 10 years was 73.% and 74.4%, respectively. During the perioperative period, graft occlusion occurred in 6 grafts in the in situ graft group and 4 in the reversed graft group, with repeat operation establishing temporary patency in 3 grafts and permanent patency in 2 grafts in each group. During the follow-up period, occlusion occurred in 12 in situ grafts and 7 reversed grafts, on average at 17.6 and 41.3 months, respectively. Fourteen of the living patients had patent grafts at the latest follow-up. Lesions developed in 6% of in situ grafts and 8% of reversed grafts. There were 13 repeat operations in 11 patients with in situ grafts and 9 reoperations in 5 patients with reversed grafts, on average at 15.3 and 48.6 months, respectively. Actuarial primary patency rates at 10 years were 41.7% in the in situ graft group and 64.5% in the reversed graft group ($P < 0.05$) (Fig 4). Actuarial secondary patency rates at 10

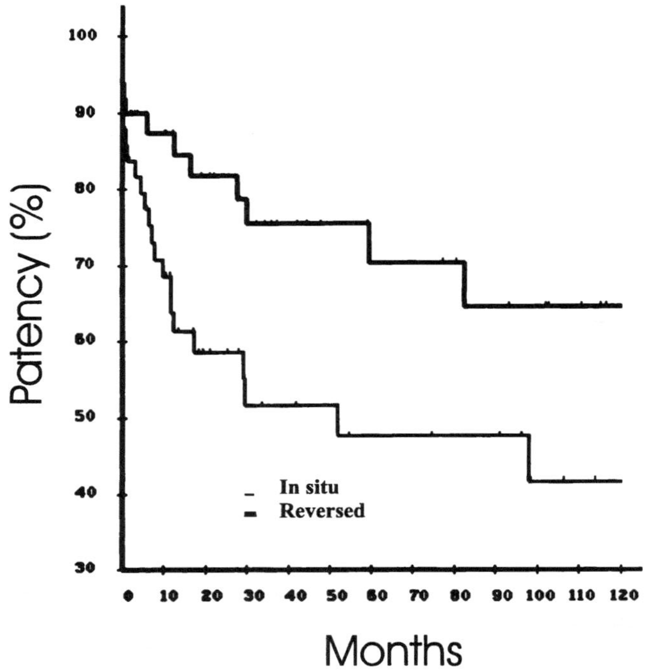

FIGURE 4.—Actuarial primary patency curves (standard deviation <0.09 at 120 months). (Courtesy of Watelet J, Soury P, Menard JF, et al: Femoropopliteal bypass: In situ or reversed vein grafts? Ten-year results of a randomized prospective study. *Ann Vasc Surg* 11:510–519, 1997).

years were 64.8% and 70.2%, respectively. Distal runoff deteriorated in 7 in situ grafts and 6 reversed grafts, and resulted in thrombosis of the bypass and amputation in 2 patients in each group. Actuarial secondary patency at 10 years for the in situ graft group was 37.5% for patients having grafts up to 4 mm and 80.6% for patients having grafts greater than 4 mm. In the reversed graft group, the comparable secondary patency rates were 71.2% and 65.5%, respectively.

Conclusion.—Whereas long-term outcome of femoropopliteal bypass was satisfactory using both procedures, the additional training required to learn the in situ technique and the requirement for valve removal make the reversed graft procedure more desirable.

► This remarkable randomized series followed patients with reversed or in situ grafts for a minimum of 10 years. At 10 years the reversed graft had a higher actuarial primary patency than did the in situ graft. The authors' conclusion that the reversed graft is the procedure of choice for femoropopliteal bypass appears a bit strong. Even I have sufficient charity to recognize the in situ bypass as an acceptable alternative to the reversed vein, although I do have difficulty understanding why anyone would voluntarily choose to use it.

Impact of Inflow Reconstruction on Infrainguinal Bypass

Eagleton MJ, Illig KA, Green RM, et al (Univ of Rochester, NY)
J Vasc Surg 26:928–938, 1997 13–2

Objective.—Results of a study investigating whether multisegmental disease that is severe enough to require an inflow procedure adversely affects infrainguinal graft patency, patient limb salvage, or patient survival rates, compared with patients who have only infrainguinal disease at the time of revascularization, are presented.

Methods.—Preoperative risk factors, indications for operation, graft material, and the sites of distal anastomosis were reviewed for 495 patients who underwent 551 primary infrainguinal revascularization procedures between 1990 and 1995. Where graft failure occurred, the cause was identified. Graft patency was assessed using ankle brachial index, duplex ultrasonography, and arteriography. Patency survival rates were calculated using life table analysis. Prosthetic grafts and saphenous vein grafts were evaluated separately.

Results.—Whereas the 4-year patency rate for revascularization rates with inflow procedures was significantly lower compared with vein grafts from normal inflow sources (41% vs. 54%), primary and secondary patency rates were similar at 4 years (62% vs. 74% and 64% vs. 77%, respectively). For prosthetic infrainguinal grafts with and without inflow procedures the respective primary patency rate (45% vs. 55%), assisted primary patency rate (60% vs. 60%), and secondary patency rate (60% vs. 61%) were similar. The most common failure mode in grafts with inflow procedures was inflow failure (47%). The most common failure in grafts without an inflow procedure was graft failure (32%). One patient in the vein-plus-inflow group and 2 in the vein-only group had complete flow occlusion. Significantly more inflow failures occurred in the vein-plus-inflow group (24%) than in the vein-only group (7%). Significantly more inflow failures occurred in the bypass graft-plus-inflow group (22%) than in the bypass graft-only group (10%). Inflow status did not affect limb salvage and patient survival rates.

Conclusion.—Patency, limb salvage, and patient survival rates did not depend on inflow status. Significantly more inflow failures occurred in those undergoing an inflow procedure, particularly in patients with multisegmental disease. These patients should be followed up carefully to permit intervention before graft occlusion occurs.

▶ I am delighted to learn that lower extremity graft patency is just as good with reconstructed inflow as with inflow that never required reconstruction. Who can argue with the authors' conclusion that lower extremity grafts in patients with reconstructed inflow appear to benefit from postoperative surveillance with special attention to graft inflow?

Failing Grafts

The Increasing Workload Required to Maintain Infrainguinal Bypass Graft Patency

Loftus IM, Reid A, Thompson MM, et al (Leicester Royal Infirmary, England)
Eur J Vasc Endovasc Surg 15:337–341, 1998 13–3

Objective.—Whereas the use of percutaneous transluminal angioplasty has increased treatment options for patients with lower limb ischemia, graft failure still remains a major problem. Graft surveillance programs have been instituted to detect developing lesions before collusion occurs. The workload required to maintain infrainguinal bypass graft patency over a 6-year period was prospectively assessed.

Methods.—Between January 1990 and December 1995, 478 infrainguinal grafts were performed. Patients were followed up to monitor interventions for maintenance of graft patency after the first 30 days.

Results.—There were 131 patients with 144 grafts (30.1%) admitted 330 times for 401 procedures. The number of admissions and interventions increased with time until 1995, when both dropped off. Between 1990 and 1994, the number of surgical interventions increased from 12 to 28, and the number of radiologic interventions increased from 12 to 63, accounting for approximately 70% of the interventions. Patients with more distal grafts had more admissions and interventions (Table 2).

Conclusion.—Workload to maintain bypass patency increased with time and will probably continue to increase. Continued intervention should be part of the vascular service's planning process.

► Our British colleagues have discovered, just as we all have, that the provision of a careful postoperative duplex graft surveillance program results in the need for a large number of interventions to maintain lower extremity graft patency. At the present time, more than 20% of our total lower extremity graft operations are being performed to maintain patency of pre-

TABLE 2.—Details of Procedures Performed on Patients With Infrainguinal Grafts *in situ* for More Than 30 Days

Procedure	Graft AKFPB (n=58)	BKFPB (n=116)	Fem.-distal (n=227)
Angioplasty ± lysis	37	72	163
Revision/distal bypass	11	12	5
Interposition/jump graft	3	6	20
Anastomotic revision	1	8	11
Graft thrombectomy	6	9	11
Amputation	0	5	8
Miscellaneous	0	4	9

Abbreviations: AKFPB, above-knee femoropopliteal bypass. *BKFPB*, below-knee femoropopliteal bypass. (Courtesy of Loftus IM, Reid A, Thompson MM, et al: The increasing workload required to maintain infrainguinal bypass graft patency. *Eur J Vasc Endovasc Surg* 15:337–341.

viously placed grafts. Interestingly, we find almost no use for angioplasty in the maintenance of lower extremity vein grafts. In the reoperations required in this series from Dr. Bell's group in Leicester, radiologic interventions accounted for almost 70% of the workload. I wonder if this may be one of the primary causes of the large number of revisions required, as our experience indicates that the results of interventional radiology in attempting to preserve failing lower extremity grafts are often quite temporary. At any rate, we rarely use interventional radiology in this setting and have no plans to change.

Economising Vein-Graft Surveillance Programs

Idu MM, Buth J, Cuypers P, et al (Erasmus Univ Rotterdam, The Netherlands; Univ Hosp Maastricht, The Netherlands)

Eur J Vasc Endovasc Surg 15:432–438, 1998 13–4

Objective.—Because stenotic lesions develop in approximately 30% of infrainguinal bypass grafts, expensive surveillance testing is required. The effectiveness of reducing the number of patients for continued surveillance by identifying grafts at higher risk of significant stenosis vs. reducing the number of examinations and the duration of the surveillance period to the first 12 months, when the majority of lesions develop, was prospectively evaluated.

Methods.—Duplex surveillance examinations were performed at 6 weeks and at 3, 6, 9, and 12 months after infrainguinal bypass grafting in 300 patients (121 women), aged 33 to 99. If an abnormality was detected, digital subtraction angiography was performed. Percutaneous transluminal angioplasty (PTA) or open surgery was performed if the angiogram revealed stenosis of 70% or more. To identify grafts at high risk of stenosis, grafts were divided into categories based on peak systolic velocity (PSV) ratios calculated at the first duplex scan—PSV ratio less than 1.5 (group 1), PSV ratio 1.5–2.0 (group 2), PSV ratio 2.0–2.5 (group 3), PSV ratio 2.5–3.0 (group 4), and PSV ratio greater than 3.0 (group 5)—and primary patency rates at 12 months were compared with these values. The effect of reducing the duration of the surveillance programs was evaluated by recording the occurrence of primary events and the interval between the event and the first duplex scan.

Results.—Patients with early lesions (groups 2 and 3) did not have significantly different duplex scans than patients without early lesions (group 1). Primary patencies at 12 months for groups 1 to 5 were 63%, 73%, 71%, 38%, and 21%, respectively. The differences between group 4 and groups 1 to 3 and the differences between group 5 and groups 1 to 3 were significant. The sensitivity and specificity of initial PSV ratio for predicting primary 12-month patency for bypass grafts were 54% and 75%; for secondary 12-month patency for groups with a PSV of 3.0 or more and less than 3.0 they were 80% and 92%, respectively. The incidence of *de novo* stenosis dropped off significantly at 6 months (Fig 3).

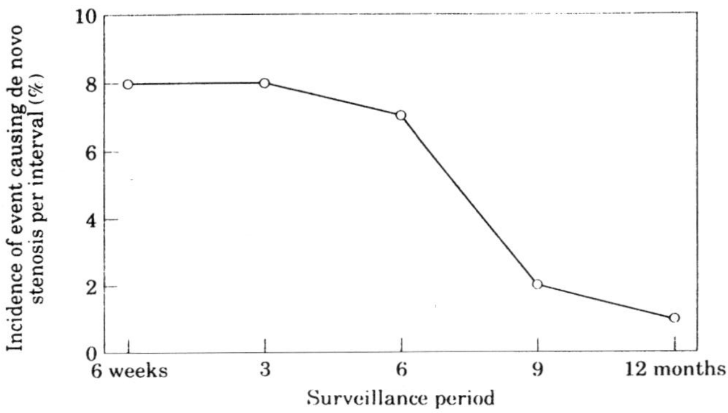

FIGURE 3.—The incidence of event-causing *de novo* stenosis per surveillance interval in previously unrevised grafts during the first postoperative year. (Courtesy of Idu MM, Buth J, Cuypers P, et al: Economising vein-graft surveillance programs. *Eur J Vasc Endovasc Surg* 15:432–438. Copyright 1998. Reprinted by permission of WB Saunders Company Limited, London.)

Conclusion.—The majority of stenotic lesions in infrainguinal bypass grafts occur within the first 6 months after surgery. Therefore, graft surveillance programs can safely be limited to a 6-month period in patients who have a normal bypass.

▶ On the basis of a large personal experience, these authors have concluded that patients who have completely normal lower extremity vein graft surveillance for the first 6 months do not require subsequent surveillance, as only 3% or so of stenoses are observed after this time. Although this is interesting, I note with concern that the 12-month primary patency of their vein grafts was only in the 63% to 73% range, depending on category. This is quite low and quite worrisome. We continue to believe that patients with vein grafts benefit from surveillance every 3 months during the first year, and every 6 months thereafter. About 15% of our graft stenoses have become apparent only after the first 12 months. Although I appreciate the authors' effort to economize the vein graft surveillance requirements, we have no interest in doing so by eliminating duplex surveillance after 6 months.

Selective Use of Duplex Ultrasound to Replace Preoperative Arteriography for Failing Arterial Vein Grafts

Calligaro KD, Syrek JR, Dougherty MJ, et al (Univ of Pennsylvania, Philadelphia)

J Vasc Surg 27:89–95, 1998 13–5

Background.—The diagnosis of failing peripheral arterial bypass grafts (FABs) is generally made from the clinical findings, segmental blood pressures, pressure volume recordings, and duplex ultrasound (DU). The suspected diagnosis is usually confirmed in the radiology suite using preoperative arteriography. This study sought to determine whether DU could be used instead of preoperative arteriography to reduce costs and patient discomfort.

Methods.—The study included 106 FABs treated over a 2-year period. For patients with a focal stenosis identified in the graft or in the inflow or outflow arteries, graft revision was done on the basis of DU only. Criteria were, in the graft, peak systolic velocity of greater than 300 cm/sec, with a ratio of adjacent peak systolic velocities (PSVs) greater than 3.0; and, in the inflow or outflow arteries, uniform graft PSVs of less than 45 cm/sec. Arteriography was frequently performed during surgery to confirm the findings of DU. If DU showed other findings—such as multiple or ill-defined stenosis, diffuse inflow or outflow arterial disease, uniformly low PSVs with no identifiable lesion, or equivocal findings despite the evidence of FABs—preoperative arteriography was performed.

Results.—In 69% of cases, surgical revision was performed on the basis of DU only. Intraoperative arteriography or surgery confirmed the presence of a 75% to 99% diameter stenosis in 91% of stenotic lesions and stenosis of 50% to 74% in 4% of cases. The site of stenosis was incorrectly identified or underdiagnosed in 5% of cases. In 5 cases, DU correctly localized missed arteriovenous fistulas. A wide range of techniques were used to treat the FABs. In 4% of cases, preoperative arteriography might have avoided a significant change in intraoperative strategy.

Conclusions.—Doppler ultrasound appears to be a reliable technique for making decisions about the need for surgical revision of FABS. In about two-thirds of cases, this technique can avoid the morbidity, discomfort, and cost of preoperative arteriography.

▶ There seems to be unanimous agreement that lower extremity autogenous grafts should be followed at frequent intervals with duplex ultrasound to detect impending graft failure, usually manifest as an area of localized increased flow velocity. The typical sequence has been detection of an abnormal area of graft function by duplex, followed by arteriography, followed by graft revision, as dictated by arteriography. In recent years, several investigators have asked the question as to whether a well-performed duplex may replace the need for arteriography before proceeding to graft revision. Based on their experience, these authors give a qualified affirmative answer. I disagree. We have found fully one third additional lesions with arteriography performed after an abnormal duplex.[1] Many of these have required revision. For the time, I continue to believe that the safe method of proceeding with these patients is duplex followed by arteriography followed by surgery. Based on present information, I am unwilling to omit arteriography.

Reference

1. Landry GJ, Moneta GL, Taylor LM, et al: Does color-flow duplex accurately demonstrate lower extremity vein graft stenosis prior to revision? Presented at the 46th Annual Meeting of the International Society for Cardiovascular Surgery, North American Chapter, San Diego, CA, June 7–8, 1998.

The Natural History of "Failing" Arterial Bypass Grafts in a Duplex Surveillance Protocol

Dougherty MJ, Calligaro KD, DeLaurentis DA, et al (Thomas Jefferson Univ, Philadelphia)

Ann Vasc Surg 12:255–259, 1998 13–6

Objective.—Little is known about the natural history of "failing" arterial bypass grafts. The patency of grafts with significant abnormalities on color duplex ultrasonography (CDU) was followed for prolonged periods without intervention.

Methods.—Patients with lower extremity bypass grafts were evaluated by CDU every 3 months for the first year after bypass and every 6 months thereafter. Systolic and diastolic peak velocities were recorded every 10 cm and at any area displaying an abnormality defined as a peak systolic flow velocity (PSFV) greater than 3 times the PSFV in the adjacent graft or a PSFV throughout the graft less than 45 cm/sec.

Results.—Of 572 lower extremity bypass grafts performed between September 20, 1991, and December 20, 1995, 46 grafts in 34 patients demonstrated CDU abnormalities (Table 1). Six (13.0%) grafts showed diffuse slow abnormalities and 35 (76.1%) demonstrated focal abnormalities (PSFV ratio greater than 3). Five grafts (10.7%) showed both abnormalities. No intervention was undertaken for 2 to 50 months, and each patient had an average of 3.6 CDU studies. During the study period, abnormalities regressed in 10 grafts, progressed in 5, and remained unchanged in the rest. Three grafts occluded at 3, 4, and 5 months after the abnormality was first noted, and 2 of these grafts were among 5 that had both focal elevated PSFV ratio and low PSFV throughout the remaining graft. Fourteen grafts were revised at a median of 5 months. The 3 occluded grafts were among 7 with a PSFV ratio greater than 7.0. Occlusion was significantly more likely to occur in grafts with both abnormalities than in grafts with only 1 abnormality.

Conclusion.—Whereas graft patency can be assessed with CDU, current thresholds for prediction of failure may be too sensitive, thereby increasing the morbidity and expense of unneeded surgery or arteriography.

TABLE 1.—Type of Graft Conduit in Patients Followed With Duplex Abnormalities

Graft conduit	*n*	Occluded	Revised
In situ saphenous	9	0	4 (44.4%)
Other saphenous	12	0	6 (50.0%)
Arm veins	4	0	2 (50.0%)
cPTFE	15	2 (13.3%)	2 (13.3%)
Umbilical vein	1	0	0
Composite	5	1 (20.0%)	0
Total	46	3 (6.5%)	14 (30.4%)

(Courtesy of Dougherty MJ, Calligaro KD, DeLaurentis DA, et al: The natural history of "failing" arterial bypass grafts in a duplex surveillance protocol. *Ann Vasc Surg* 12:256–259, 1998.)

outcomes of In situ repair of aortobronchial, aortoesophageal, and aorto-intestinal fistulas using cryopreserved aortic homografts were examined.

Methods.—Between April 1994 and June 1996, 11 patients (1 woman), aged 45–76 years, underwent repair of 5 aortobronchial, 2 aortoesophageal, and 4 aortointestinal fistulas. Five fistulas involved a mycotic aortic aneurysm and 6 involved a prosthetic aortic graft. Eight (73%) patients had emergency surgery. Six (55%) patients had preoperative sepsis.

Results.—There was 1 (9%) operative death after 7 days. The average hospital stay was 42 days, the average stay in intensive care was 6.6 days, the average time on a ventilator was 4.9 days, and the average duration of antibiotic treatment was 38 days. There was 1 reoperation for bleeding on postoperative day 1. There was 1 late reintervention for progressive stenosis of the distal part of the homograft. There have been no other deaths or reinfections after an average follow-up of 14.3 months.

Conclusions.—Although this study was small, the use of cryopreserved aortic homografts provided a safe and simple repair of fistulas and a low operative mortality and infection rate.

▶ For reasons unknown to me, there is a pervasive belief among European vascular surgeons that aortic homografts are especially favored for use in infected arterial fields. These homografts are harvested from heart-beating organ donors, and cryopreserved in liquid nitrogen. While I find no persuasive evidence that this is the superior method of treatment, I do have to admit that anecdotal reports such as this appear exemplary. After a mean follow-up of 14 months, there was no evidence of suture line rupture, reinfection, or anastomotic aneurysms. On balance, I think one must be very careful about going back to the aortic homograft. A careful assessment of this graft revealed general failure in the 1950s and early 1960s because of both aneurysm formation and extreme calcification. At the present time, my choice is the antibiotic-bonded Dacron graft, although there is little information in this area either. I suppose the proper response is to say let's continue with more observations. I am assuredly not ready to accept the cryopreserved aortic homograft as a superior prosthesis for use in an infected field.

Prosthetic Grafts

Use of Antibiotic-bonded Grafts in Vascular Graft Infection

Torsello G, Sandmann W (Univ of Düsseldorf, Germany)

Eur J Vasc Endovasc Surg Suppl A 14:84–87, 1997 13–12

Purpose.—Once a prosthetic vascular graft has become infected, it usually has to be removed. In attempts to develop infection-resistant grafts, bonding of antibacterial substances to vascular prostheses has been tried. An experience with rifampicin-bonded grafts in 12 patients is reported.

Patients.—The experience included 12 patients with vascular infections. All were treated with implantation of rifampicin-soaked grafts. There were 9 men and 3 women; mean age, 70 years. Ten patients underwent implantation of an aortic or iliac graft for occlusive disease. Eight operations were done on an emergency basis.

Outcomes.—One patient with mycotic thoracic aneurysm died of sepsis after 2 months. Two patients died of myocardial infarction 10 and 18 months after the procedure. Mean follow-up was 33 months. At this time, there was 1 recurrence in a patient with late graft infection after aortofemoral bypass grafting with septic bleeding. This infection proved to be caused by *Staphylococcus aureus* resistant to rifampin and oxacillin. The remaining 8 patients remained free of evidence of infection. All had ankle pressure indices of 0.5 to 0.9, with no amputations required. One patient was still alive and free of infection 41/2 years after the original reconstruction.

Conclusions.—This experience supports the results of previous studies suggesting that antibiotic-bonded grafts can be an effective treatment for vascular graft infection. Although more study is required, the problems associated with extra-anatomic reconstructions may lead to increased use of this in situ technique.

▶ There has been increased enthusiasm in recent years for excision and replacement of infected prosthetic grafts with new prosthetic grafts implanted in situ directly in the same field. Most, especially in Europe, favoring such a technique believe that the replacement graft should be bonded to rifampicin. Practically speaking, this means that a Dacron graft which is covered with gelatin is soaked in an appropriately concentrated rifampicin solution for 10–15 minutes before implantation. The rather remarkable series reported herein after a mean follow-up of 33 months found only 1 out of 10 patients with recurrent infection, this being a *Staphylococcus aureus*, which, interestingly, showed resistance to rifampicin. I continue to believe that the best treatment for graft infection is complete graft excision with bypass through a clean extraanatomic field. I do believe that rifampicin soaking of a gelatin-coated Dacron graft is a reasonable second choice if in situ replacement is mandatory.

Heparin-bonded Grafts Induce Platelet Aggregation in the Presence of Heparin-associated Antiplatelet Antibodies

Almeida JI, Liem TK, Silver D (Univ of Missouri-Columbia)
J Vasc Surg 27:896–901, 1998 13–13

Background.—One of the approaches to improving long-term results of distal bypass has been the development of small-diameter prosthetic grafts that are pretreated with antithrombotic compounds, such as heparin. However, the use of a heparin coating has caused problems in other situations; for example, heparin-coated pulmonary artery catheters have led to the development of heparin-induced thrombocytopenia in some patients. Whether such a development would be possible with heparin-bonded grafts (HBGs) was determined.

Methods.—HBGs from different manufacturers were studied: one from company A with an 8-mm diameter (HBGA); and two from company B, one with an 8-mm diameter (HBGB-8) and the other with a 6-mm diameter (HBGB-6). Grafts without heparin coating were also studied as controls. Grafts were cut into segments 1 cm long and incubated for 24 hours in 5 mL of plasma, 10 mL of normal saline, or 10 mL of Ringer's lactate. One milliliter of diluent was assayed for heparin; if heparin was detected, then the sample was incubated another 30 minutes to examine whether the addition of heparin-associated antiplatelet antibodies (HAAbs) induced platelet activation and aggregation.

Findings.—None of the control grafts leaked heparin, whereas all the test grafts did so. Heparin leaching was greatest in plasma, with heparin concentrations of 83.4, 4, and 6.2 U of heparin per milliliter for grafts HBGA, HBGB-8, and HBGB-6, respectively. Heparin leaching was substantially less in saline (10.8, 0, and 0.01 U of heparin per milliliter, respectively) and Ringer's lactate (10.0, and 0.22 U of heparin per milliliter, respectively), but nonetheless evident. After the addition of HAAbs, all HBGs induced platelet aggregation (ranging from 18.3% to 58.5% aggregation), whereas none of the control grafts did so.

Conclusions.—Under physiologic incubation conditions, all HBGs leached heparin into plasma, and all HBGs induced platelet aggregation in the presence of HAAbs. Thus the dissociated heparin from these grafts could lead to the development of heparin-induced thrombocytopenia in patients who have HAAbs. Furthermore, heparin-induced thrombocytopenia could develop even in HAAb-negative patients as a result of long-term exposure to implanted heparin-coated grafts. Thus HBGs should be used with extreme caution.

► This article convinces me that before we develop unbounded enthusiasm for HBGs, we must carefully consider the material presented herein by Dr. Silver and his associates. It is clear that heparin will leach off of the HBG and that sufficient heparin will leach to induce platelet aggregation in patients who have HAAbs. Wouldn't it be awful to have an HBG in place, then have the patient develop heparin-induced thrombocytopenia? I suppose one would have to surgically remove the graft in such a setting, indeed a most unattractive prospect. For the present, it would appear that the use of grafts with heparin bonding should be approached very cautiously.

Prospective Randomized Study of Carbon-impregnated Polytetrafluoroethylene Grafts for Below-Knee Popliteal and Distal Bypass: Results at 2 Years

Bacourt F, and Association Universitaire de Recherche en Chirurgie (Hôpital Américain, Neuilly-sur-Seine, France; Association Universitaire de Recherche en Chirurgie, Bois-Colombes, France)

Ann Vasc Surg 11:596–603, 1997 13–14

Objective.—Whereas carbon-impregnated polytetrafluoroethylene (PTFE) grafts reduce platelet deposition, no comparative studies have investigated whether these grafts achieve better patency than standard grafts do. A prospective randomized multicenter study of bypass grafts compared patency for the carbon-impregnated PTFE graft and standard PTFE grafts and assessed factors contributing to patency of infrainguinal and below-knee prosthetic bypass grafts.

Methods.—Either a carbon-impregnated PTFE graft (n = 81) or a standard PTFE graft (n = 79) was implanted in 160 patients with unsuitable greater saphenous veins in 17 research medical centers in France. There were 83 below-knee femoropopliteal bypass procedures and 77 femorodistal bypass procedures. Patients were followed up for a minimum of 24 months. Primary and secondary patency rates and limb salvage rates were compared.

Results.—The groups were comparable except that the carbon-impregnated PTFE graft group had more members with a greater than 20 pack/years smoking history. During the study 14 patients in the carbon-impregnated PTFE graft group and 10 in the standard PTFE graft group died.

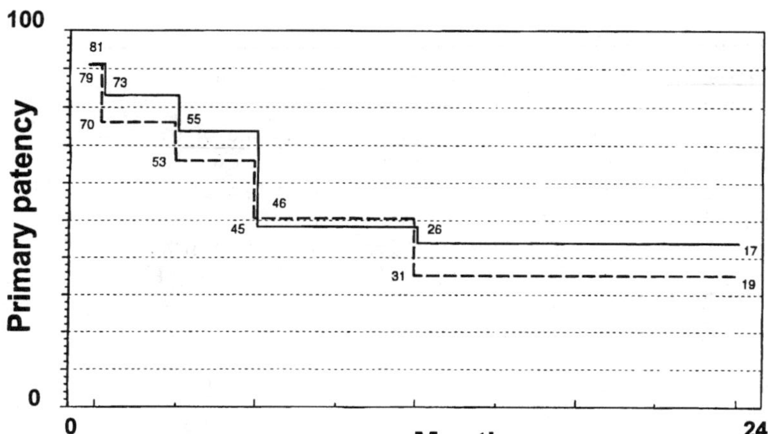

FIGURE 1.—Actuarial primary patency rates (%) at 2 years after below-knee bypass using a carbon-coated PTFE graft (*solid line*) and a standard PTFE graft (*dashed line*) ($P = 0.4$). (Courtesy of Bacourt F, and Association Universitaire de Recherche en Chirurgie: Prospective randomized study of carbon-impregnated polytetrafluoroethylene grafts for below-knee popliteal and distal bypass: Results at 2 years. *Ann Vasc Surg* 11:596–603, 1997).

Occlusion rates were 44.4% in the carbon-impregnated PTFE graft group and 55.5% in the standard PTFE graft group. Actuarial primary patency rates at 2 years were not significantly different (45% and 35%, respectively) (Fig 1). The secondary patency rates at 2 years were almost significantly different (53% and 36%, respectively). The actuarial limb salvage rates at 2 years were 57% and 47%, respectively. Patency was not correlated with diabetic status, number of patent leg arteries, and direct or indirect anastomosis. Patency rates for first and repeat bypass procedures were similar. Patency was correlated ankle-arm pressure difference greater than 0.25 and below-knee femoropopliteal bypass.

Conclusion.—The carbon-impregnated PTFE graft had nonsignificantly higher patency rates than did the standard PTFE graft. Additional research needs to be conducted to determine whether performance differences become significant.

▶ I know little about the role of carbon-impregnated prosthetic grafts, although theoretically their use may result in diminished platelet deposition. This randomized French study indicates that the carbon-impregnated PTFE graft had the same patency as standard PTFE. On the bright side, patency appeared to be no worse.

Albumin-impregnated Prosthetic Graft for Infrarenal Aortic Replacement: Effects on the Incidence and Volume of Perioperative Blood Transfusion

Chakfé N, Beaufigeau M, Nicolini P, et al (Hospices Civils de Strasbourg, France)

Ann Vasc Surg 11:588–595, 1997 13–15

Objective.—Polyester abdominal aortic grafts impregnated with albumin have been in use since 1975. The incidence and volume of blood transfusion and the rate of patency and incidence of infection with this prosthesis were determined in a retrospective review of 290 patients.

Methods.—Abdominal aortic aneurysm (AAA) was present in 218 patients, and occlusive disease of the aortic bifurcation (ODAB) in 72. Patients were followed up for an average of 25.5 months.

Results.—During the postoperative period, 9 patients (3.1%) died, and 39 (13.5%) had complications including colonic ischemia, in 12 patients, postoperative bowel obstruction syndrome in 4, cholecystitis in 1, transient renal insufficiency in 6, acute bladder obstruction in 2, disunion of the surgical wound in 5, recurrent lymphocele in 1, pulmonary insufficiency in 1, and pneumonia in 2. The incidence of preoperative blood transfusions because of AAA and ODAB was 37.2% and 32.3%, respectively, and of postoperative transfusions was 50.0% and 12.9%. The overall incidence of blood transfusion was 36% during the procedure, 22.1% during the postoperative period, and 46.0% during hospitalization. The average number of red cell packs required was 1.4 after elective reconstruction for AAA, 7.0 after emergency reconstruction for AAA, and 1.0 after reconstruction for ODAB. Postoperatively, 279 patients were alive, but 12 of these were lost to follow-up. During follow-up 35 patients died, 12 of cancer, 8 of heart disease, 5 of neurologic events, 4 of pulmonary insufficiency, 3 of gastrointestinal disorders, 2 of renal insufficiency, and 1 after leg amputation because of gangrene. Primary and secondary patency rates calculated using the Kaplan-Meier method were 95.4% and 97.5% at 6 months. There were no graft infections. One patient underwent repeat surgery at 6 months because of false aneurysm.

Conclusion.—Use of albumin-impregnated grafts necessitated a high rate of blood transfusions, suggesting that this method of impregnation does not prevent perioperative blood loss. Patency rates of these grafts are similar to those of other grafts.

▶ I have always considered manufacturers' insistence that vascular surgeons use prosthetic grafts impregnated with anything to be inappropriate and merely an attempt to sell grafts for more money. I despise impregnated prosthetic grafts and categorically refuse to use them. I am delighted to see that this study indicates that use of the impervious graft does not reduce the requirement for blood transfusion. We continue to use exclusively double velour woven Dacron, and have found preclotting to be a monumental nonissue. I wish the manufacturers would take every foreign protein–covered prosthetic graft and incinerate it. A more strongly worded statement to follow.

Long-term In Vivo Alterations of Polyester Vascular Grafts in Humans

Riepe G, Loos J, Imig H, et al (Gen Hosp of Hamburg–Harburg, Germany; Technical Univ Hamburg–Harburg, Germany; Univ of Dortmund, Germany; et al)

Eur J Vasc Endovasc Surg 13:540–548, 1997 13–16

Background.—Polyester vascular grafts, first implanted in humans almost 40 years ago, are now used worldwide for replacement of the aortic and iliac arteries. Although there have been few reports of graft rupture leading to surgical intervention, the potential degradation of polyester fibers after long-term use is a matter of concern. A study of explanted grafts was conducted to examine the chemical and physical aspects of material alteration leading to the failure of polyester vascular grafts.

Methods.—Twenty-nine clinics provided 170 explanted polyester vascular grafts, 65 of which were examined by scanning electron microscopy, infrared spectroscopy, and probe puncture. The examined grafts were implanted between 1971 and 1994. Causes for removal were anastomotic aneurysms (28%), occlusion (18%), graft infection (12%), and rupture of the graft material (11%); 25% were removed post mortem. Most graft infections occurred within a few years of implantation, occlusions between 5 and 10 years, and graft ruptures after 9 years. The peak frequency for the

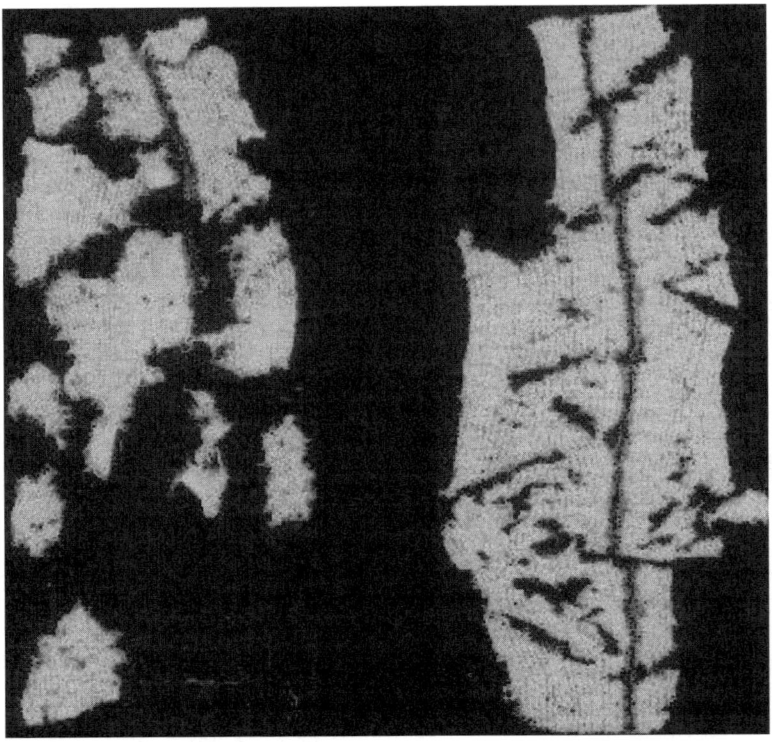

FIGURE 2.—Photo showing the mosaic-like appearance of an 18-year-old dilated femoropopliteal Dacron bypass after enzymatic removal of tissue. (Courtesy of Riepe G, Loos J, Imig H, et al: Long-term in vivo alterations of polyester vascular grafts in humans. *Eur J Vasc Endovasc Surg* 13:540–548, 1997. Copyright 1997. Reprinted by permission of the publisher WB Saunders Company Limited, London.)

occurrence of anastomotic aneurysms (Fig 2) was at approximately 10 years.

Results.—Electron microscopy of filaments often showed a brittle fracture with torsion of the filament. Older grafts exhibited multiple fractures of filaments, accompanied by a general loosening of the textile structure. Probe puncture testing revealed a decrease of maximum bursting strength with duration of implantation. Linear regression analysis showed that, compared with unused grafts, implanted polyester grafts lose 31.4% of their bursting strength at 10 years and 100% by 25–39 years. Chemical examination of explanted grafts demonstrated scission of macromolecular chains and hydrolytic degradation with increasing time of implantation.

Conclusion.—Because degeneration of polyester vascular grafts may occur many years after implantation, vascular surgeons should precisely document the implanted graft material and advise patients of the need for long-term follow-up. The increase of younger vascular patients receiving polyester grafts makes it likely that graft failure will be seen with greater frequency.

► This remarkable study concludes polyester grafts lose 31% of their bursting strength at 10 years, and 100% at 25–39 years. In our practice, we currently have a few patients with Dacron grafts in place for more than 20 years. I have intuitively elected frequent CT scans of these grafts in recent years on the suspicion that no graft lasts forever. To date, I have not detected any generalized graft deterioration, but I do believe that routine imaging is prudent. I am surprised, and not a little bit worried, by the data contained in this paper. It appears that between 25 and 39 years the grafts may simply implode.

Prospective Study of Blunt Aortic Injury: Helical CT Is Diagnostic and Antihypertensive Therapy Reduces Rupture

Fabian TC, Davis KA, Gavant ML, et al (Univ of Tennessee, Memphis)
Ann Surg 227:666–677, 1998 14–3

Introduction.—If aortic rupture occurs in patients with blunt aortic injury (BAI), the result can be immediate death. Conventional chest CT is not effective in recognizing BAI, but helical CT—which offers faster scanning and better resolution—may be useful for this purpose. There is evidence to suggest that antihypertensive medication may help to prevent aortic rupture. Helical CT of the thorax (HCTT) was evaluated for use in the diagnosis of BAI. In addition, β-blockers—with or without nitroprusside—were evaluated for efficacy in the prevention of aortic rupture in BAI.

Methods.—The 4-year prospective study included 494 patients with significant blunt torso trauma. All underwent HCTT. In the first year of the study, aortography was performed in patients whose HCTT scan suggested mediastinal abnormalities. In the latter 3 years, aortography was performed only in patients whose HCTT findings suggested BAI, excluding those with mediastinal hematomas without direct evidence of aortic injury. When aortic injury was suspected, a protocol of IV β-blockers was started, with nitroprusside added if needed to achieve a satisfactory blood pressure. This treatment was evaluated for its ability to prevent rupture before aortic repair or to permit delayed aortic repair in patients with significant associated injuries.

Results.—Seventy-one patients (14%) were given a diagnosis of BAI. Figure 3 shows a severe intimal injury with a large pseudoaneurysm. Helical CT of the thorax had a sensitivity of 100%, a specificity of 83%, accuracy of 86%, a positive predictive value of 50%, and a negative predictive value of 100%. Values for aortography were 92% sensitivity, 99% specificity, 97% accuracy, 97% positive predictive value, and 97%

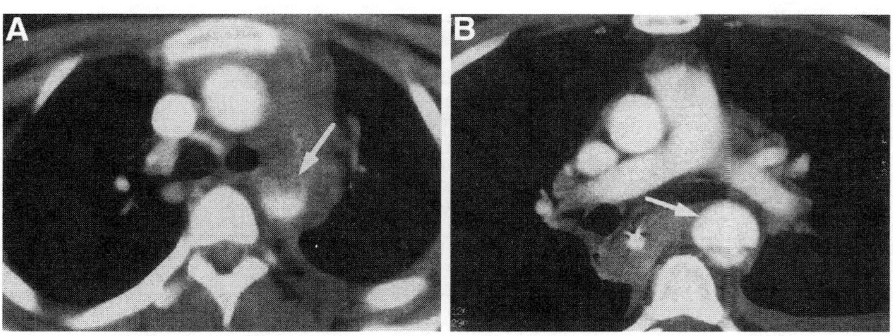

FIGURE 3.—Helical scan demonstrates (**A**) a severe intimal injury (*arrow*) at the carina, distal to the left subclavian artery, and (**B**) a large pseudoaneurysm (*arrow*) at the level of the pulmonary arterial bifurcation, with associated nasogastric tube deviation secondary to a periaortic hematoma. (Courtesy of Fabian TC, Davis KA, Gavant ML, et al: Prospective study of blunt aortic injury: Helical CT is diagnostic and antihypertensive therapy reduces rupture. *Ann Surg* 227:666–677, 1998.)

negative predictive value. There were no cases of spontaneous aortic rupture.

Conclusion.—Patients with blunt torso trauma who have no direct evidence of BAI on HCTT scanning do not need to undergo aortography. If the results of HCTT are indeterminate, aortography can be performed. The use of HCTT for early diagnosis, coupled with antihypertensive treatment for patients with suspected aortic injury, minimizes the risk of aortic rupture and allows aortic repair to be delayed in patients with significant associated injuries.

▶ These authors have had a very large experience with traumatic aortic rupture resulting from the Memphis, Tenn., battlefield campaigns. I am fascinated to learn that contrast-enhanced HCTT is almost as good as aortography in diagnosing thoracic aortic injuries. However, it is important to note that it is not quite as sensitive as aortography, but it does have an absolutely sterling negative predictive value of 100%. Thus, if the HCTT result is negative, no further evaluation is required. Aortography should be reserved for indeterminant or intermediate HCTT scans.

The authors also evaluated the role of β-blockers with and without nitroprusside in preventing rupture before aortic repair and in allowing delayed repair in selected patients. This regimen appeared successful, but interpretation was made almost impossible by lack of randomization. On balance, I believe we can take away from this study the information that a well-done HCTT is extremely helpful in the diagnosis of BAI.

Surgical Indications and Timing of Repair of Traumatic Ruptures of the Thoracic Aorta

Galli R, Pacini D, Di Bartolomeo R, et al (Univ of Bologna, Italy)

Ann Thorac Surg 65:461–464, 1998 14–4

Background.—Up to 90% of patients with acute traumatic rupture of the thoracic aorta caused by a vehicular accident die before they can be transported to a hospital. And even if they survive to reach the hospital, morbidity rates after aortic repair surgery are up to 28%. How can these morbidity rates be improved? These authors report their success with a policy of delaying rupture repair until coexisting injuries have been treated and the patient's condition is stable.

Methods.—Over 16.5 years, 42 patients (32 men and 10 women, mean age 31 years) with acute traumatic rupture of the thoracic aorta were treated. All but 1 patient was involved in a vehicular accident. All but 3 patients had at least 1 concurrent injury, such as skeletal fractures, abdominal organ injuries, neurologic complications, or thoracic lesions. Between 1980 and 1992, 21 patients underwent rupture repair immediately upon diagnosis (group 1). From 1993 to 1996, 21 patients had their rupture repair delayed until other life-threatening conditions were under control (group 2). All patients in group 2 were closely monitored by chest radiographs, computed tomography, and magnetic resonance imaging; in some cases angiography and transesophageal echocardiography were used also. Surgical repair was undertaken in 11 patients in group 2 at an average of 6.9 months (range 1.5–18 months) after injury; the remaining patients in this group are still awaiting repair until timing is optimal.

Findings.—Four patients in group 1 died (3 intraoperative, 1 of sepsis within 30 days), whereas no patients in group 2 died. Furthermore, patients in group 1 experienced substantially more (and more significant) complications, including paraplegia, paraparesis, acute renal failure, laryngeal nerve lesion, coma, and bleeding (morbidity rate 10 of 21, or 47.6%). Only 3 complications, including laryngeal nerve lesion, chylothorax, and pericarditis (morbidity rate 3 of 11, or 27.3%), occurred in the patients in group 2 who had undergone rupture repair.

Conclusions.—Acute rupture of the thoracic aorta is usually associated with other serious injuries, and these injuries are often life threatening. Treating them first allows the patient to gain a stable hemodynamic state, and allows deferral of rupture repair until a more optimal time. Close radiographic monitoring of the patient both before and after repair is crucial to the safety of delaying repair.

▶ It has been observed over the years that a large majority of patients experiencing traumatic transection of the thoracic aorta (almost always from an automobile accident trauma) exsanguinate before treatment can be initiated. For those who do not, elective treatment delay appears possible in the majority. This interesting article suggests that delay of treatment until after a period of intensive medical stabilization results in superior patient outcome. Unfortunately, the study was not randomized, and I fear it likely the immediate and delayed repair groups were not really comparable. Nonetheless, this information is suggestive and should be at least familiar to those caring for patients with traumatic thoracic aortic injuries.

Femoral Pseudoaneurysms in Drug Addicts

Ting ACW, Cheng SWK (Univ of Hong Kong, Pokfulam)

World J Surg 21:783–787, 1997 14–5

Background.—Addicts who habitually inject drugs through the groin are at risk for the development of pseudoaneurysm, a potentially fatal complication caused by inadvertent intra-arterial puncture. The patients reported here were treated with simple ligation of the femoral arteries without revascularization.

Methods.—During a 1-year period (July 1993 to June 1994), 33 drug addicts were treated for 34 infected femoral pseudoaneurysms at the study institution. Their records were reviewed for demographic data, symptoms at admission, duration of symptoms, bacteriology, treatment, associated complications, and outcome. The ankle-brachial pressure index (ABI) was measured the day after surgery.

Results.—Patients were 27 men and 6 women, with a mean age of 40 years. All injected heroin, and more than half had a history of abuse of more than 10 years. Pain and swelling over the groin (mean duration of 6 days) led patients to seek medical attention; 8 reported groin bleeding, and 12 had fever at admission. All but 4 had an elevated white blood cell count, 70% were anemic, and 42% were chronic carriers of hepatitis B. None was HIV-positive. Intraoperative tissue cultures were positive in 85% of cases, with 17 of 29 exhibiting pure growth of methicillin-sensitive *Staphylococcus aureus* (MSSA). Triple ligation of the common femoral, superficial femoral, and profunda femoris arteries was performed in the 24 cases involving the femoral bifurcation. Seven other limbs underwent ligation of the femoral artery alone, and 3 had superficial femoral artery ligation. The external iliac artery also was ligated in 19 limbs for better proximal control. No patient died in the hospital (mean stay of 45 days), and all were discharged with a viable limb. There was no delayed limb loss during a mean follow-up period of 15.5 months, but 29 of 33 patients experienced some degree of intermittent claudication. The mean ABI was 0.57.

Conclusion.—The diagnosis of pseudoaneurysm should be considered in drug addicts with groin swelling and pain. Diagnosis is often obvious and can be made by clinical examination. The antibiotics of choice are systemic agents active against MSSA. Primary ligation and excision of the infected femoral pseudoaneurysm was successful in preserving the limb in these patients.

► An infected femoral pseudoaneurysm resulting from the intra-arterial injection of street drugs represents an especially virulent problem. There is widespread agreement that initial surgery should consist of ligation and excision of the pseudoaneurysm without any vascular repair. If the limb remains markedly ischemic, remote repair through noninfected tissue planes appears to be the only opportunity for limb salvage. Interestingly, a frequently encountered primary organism in this setting appears to be methicillin-resistant *Staphylococcus*. In 33 patients described in this study who were treated with ligation and excision, the mean postoperative ankle brachial index was 0.4. There was no hospital mortality, and all patients were discharged with a viable limb. Most patients suffered some degree of intermittent claudication, but no limb loss was recognized. The message is clear that this particular subset of patients is best treated with ligation and excision, not with primary bypass.[1]

Reference

1. Goldstone J: Invited commentary. *World J Surg* 21:786, 1997.

Treatment of Iatrogenic Femoral Artery Pseudoaneurysm With Percutaneous Thrombin Injection

Liau C-S, Ho F-M, Chen M-F, et al (Natl Taiwan Univ, Taipei; Provincial Tau-Yuen Hosp, Taiwan)

J Vasc Surg 26:18–23, 1997 14–6

Background.—Surgical repair has been the standard method of treatment for pseudoaneurysms of the peripheral arteries, but several nonsurgical approaches were reported in recent years. One approach, which induces thrombosis with intravascular injection of thrombin, has not gained wide acceptance, perhaps because of safety concerns. Five patients with pseudoaneurysms of the femoral artery were monitored to determine the safety and efficacy of percutaneous thrombin injection.

Methods.—The mean age of the 5 study participants was 63 years. Pseudoaneurysm was suspected in all patients by the presence of a painful pulsating mass and vascular bruit at catheterization puncture sites. Diagnosis was confirmed with US in all cases and by angiogram in 1 case. The interval between catheterization and treatment of the pseudoaneurysm was 2 days for 1 patient, 3 days for 3 patients, and 40 days for 1 patient. Patients received local anesthetic with 1% lidocaine before the thrombin

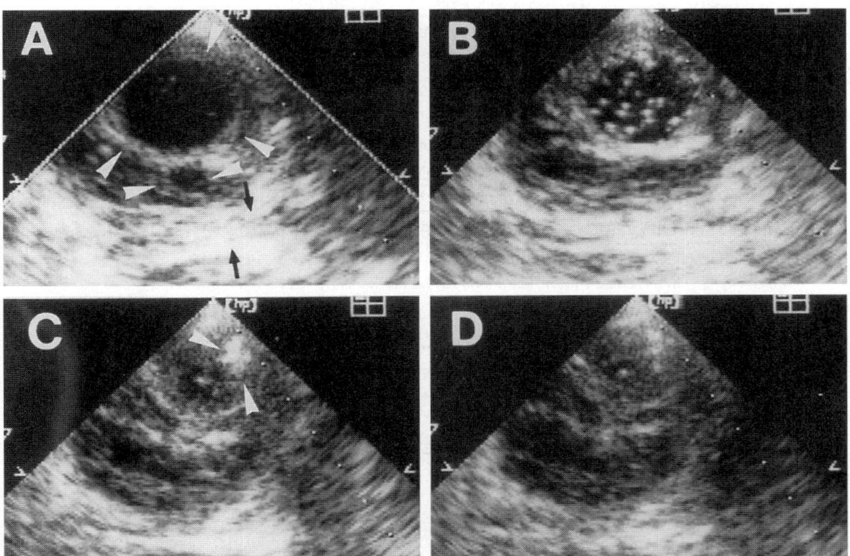

FIGURE 2.—Serial ultrasonograms during percutaneous thrombin treatment of a pseudoaneurysm. **A,** Pseudoaneurysm consisted of 2 chambers (*arrowheads*) and was adjacent and superficial to the femoral arteries (*arrows*). **B,** After injection of saline solution with microbubbles through the catheter, appearance of contrast echoes in the chamber of the pseudoaneurysm confirmed the position of the catheter. **C,** Seconds after thrombin injection, thrombus formation started (*arrowheads*). **D,** Thrombus extended to occupy most portions of the cavity of pseudoaneurysm, and blood flow ceased. (Courtesy of Liau C-S, Ho F-M, Chen M-F, et al: Treatment of iatrogenic femoral artery pseudoaneurysm with percutaneous thrombin injection. *J Vasc Surg* 26:18–23, 1997.)

injection (1,000 units dissolved in normal saline). Under US guidance, an IV catheter was introduced percutaneously into the pseudoaneurysm, and thrombin was injected slowly. Patients were examined with US after the procedure and at clinical follow-up (mean 11.6 months).

Results.—The thrombin injection procedure was successful in all patients, and none experienced an adverse reaction. Thrombus formation was immediately evident under US visualization and was followed by blocking the blood flow from the femoral artery to the pseudoaneurysm (Fig 2). No patient had recurrence of the pseudoaneurysm at follow-up.

Conclusion.—Prolonged firm compression, a technique widely applied in the treatment of pseudoaneurysms, requires a relatively long compression time, often causes pain at the treatment site, and may be followed by a recurrence of the pseudoaneurysm. In comparison, percutaneous thrombin injection is simple, far less time-consuming, does not cause discomfort, and has a high success rate.

▶ Injection of thrombin for treatment of a pseudoaneurysm has been reported sporadically for the past 10 years. Recently, we have had a wave of enthusiasm for ultrasound compression, which seems to work most of the time, but certainly not all of the time. Most recently, we have been informed that, if left alone, most of these iatrogenic pseudoaneurysms will spontaneously thrombose within a relatively short time.[1] These authors injected thrombin directly into femoral artery pseudoaneurysms in 5 patients, achieving a solid thrombotic occlusion of the pseudoaneurysm within a very short time after injection. All procedures were deemed successful, and no recurrences were noted during follow-up periods of 1–28 months. Thrombin injection must be regarded as another acceptable treatment for iatrogenic vascular pseudoaneurysms. However, I must admit that I am most impressed with the recent observation that, if left alone, most of these will spontaneously thrombose without the need for any treatment.

Reference

1. 1998 Year Book of Vascular Surgery, p 408.

Combined Neural–Vascular

Management of Severe Proximal Vascular and Neural Injury of the Upper Extremity

Manord JD, Garrard CL, Kline DG, et al (Ochsner Clinic and Alton Ochsner Med Found, New Orleans, La)

J Vasc Surg 27:43–49, 1998 14–7

Background.—Traumatic injuries of the proximal upper extremity can be treated aggressively or conservatively. Aggressive measures include limb salvage, with the goal of restoring some function; conservative measures include control of hemorrhage without nerve repair, and in some cases

TABLE 2.—Nerve Injuries Grouped According to the Level of Brachial Plexus Injured

Level of injury (n*)	Average disability score Initial	Final	Significance†
Postganglionic			
Spinal nerve avulsions (7)	100	93	NS
Preganglionic			
Root (6)	96	57	$p < 0.01$
Trunk (4)	57	21	$p < 0.01$
Cord (17)	86	48	$p < 0.01$
Nerve (10)	73	46	$p < 0.01$

*44 operatively explored nerve injuries.
†Analysis of variance.
(Courtesy of Manord JD, Garrard CL, Kline DG, et al: Management of severe proximal vascular and neural injury of the upper extremity. *J Vas Surg* 27:43–49, 1998.)

amputation, with the belief that the extremity will no longer be functional. These authors report their experience with limb salvage with revascularization and delayed treatment of neural trauma.

Methods.—Forty-six patients (40 men and 6 women, mean age 27 years) had unilateral traumatic injury of the brachial plexus and at least 1 vessel of the upper extremity or ipsilateral neck. The vascular injuries were treated by primary repair, grafting, or ligation. The neural injuries were followed expectantly, and if the limb showed signs of a potentially reversible deficit, the brachial plexus and extradural roots were examined. Results of clinical examinations, myelography, electromyography, and nerve action potential conduction studies were used to determine whether surgery was appropriate in each case. Disability before and after any treatment was graded on a 100-point functional disability scoring system developed by the American Medical Association (100 points = total limb disability). Patients were studied for a mean of 43 months.

Findings.—Most patients initially had altered pulses (38 patients, or 83%). In the 44 patients who underwent urgent vascular exploration, 37 (86%) had involvement of the subclavian or axillary artery, 43 (93%) had arterial injuries, and 3 (7%) had venous injuries. Vascular repair procedures included grafting, primary repair, or ligation. The most common neurologic disturbance was flail arm (22 patients, or 48%). Of the 44 patients who underwent delayed nerve exploration (30–358 days after injury), all had injuries to the brachial plexus or its terminal components. Nerve repair procedures included nerve grafts, end-to-end repair, and neurolysis. Surgical repair of preganglionic injuries significantly improved the disability score, compared with the score after initial recovery (Table 2). Overall, 40 of 46 patients (86%) experienced objective improvement, with a significant improvement (from 83% initially to 52% after treatment) in disability score. (A disability score of 52% represents stabilizing functions, gross manipulations, and a light load capacity.)

Conclusions.—Aggressive treatment of proximal upper extremity injuries can restore at least limited function in most patients with vascular and neural injuries. Benefits were greatest for those patients with preganglionic nerve injuries. Amputations should be reserved for patients who have extensive nerve avulsions at the level of the spinal cord, who have massive soft tissue loss, or who might not survive limb salvage.

▶ Although I appreciate the intent of the authors, I have reservations about their conclusions. I totally agree with them that the patient should be given the benefit of any doubt if all we have is a functional assessment of arm status. I disagree if we have actual visual evidence of brachial plexus or nerve root disruption. Major plexus or root disruption has, in my experience, never been associated with recovery of substantial upper extremity function. I continue to believe that serious consideration for primary amputation should be given to patients with the most serious neurologic injuries. I subscribe to the belief that prompt upper extremity amputation with maximal attempts at rehabilitation has an infinitely better outlook for the patient than a painfully protracted multi-month recovery period with a neuropraxic extremity which, in the final analysis, has no significant neurologic recovery. These patients are truly crippled for life. This is a complex issue that does not lend itself to easy solutions. Perhaps careful individualization is the best one can recommend.

Aggressive Management of Vascular Injuries of the Thoracic Outlet

Hyre CE, Cikrit DF, Lalka SG, et al (Indiana Univ, Indianapolis)

J Vasc Surg 27:880–885, 1998 14–8

Background.—Some studies have reported that as many as one third of patients with axillary or subclavian vascular trauma die. Mortality rates are worse if the brachial plexus is also injured. The outcomes of thoracic outlet vascular injuries with or without brachial plexus injury were reviewed to determine any prognostic factors.

Methods.—During 10 years, 35 patients (29 men and 6 women, mean age 28 years) were treated for subclavian (n = 18) or axillary (n = 17) vascular injury. Thirty arteries and 16 veins were injured in the 35 patients. The cause of the injury was a gunshot in 19 patients, stabbing in 9, and blunt trauma in 7. Of the 30 patients with arterial injuries, 12 had no pulse, 5 had a diminished pulse, and 13 had a normal pulse. Fifteen patients also had brachial nerve injury (43%), 7 had fractures, and 5 had pneumohemothorax. Angiography was performed in 21 patients and revealed abnormalities in all but 2 patients, including an intimal flap (8 patients), extravasation (5), pseudoaneurysm (3), arteriovenous fistula (2), and arterial occlusion (1). The 46 thoracic outlet vascular trauma injuries were repaired mainly by primary repair (n = 19 injuries) and vein grafting (n = 16).

Findings.—Two of the 35 patients died, resulting in a mortality rate of 6%. One patient died of massive blood loss from a subclavian vein injury, and the other died of an anoxic brain injury and a cerebellar infarct (presumably because of preoperative hypotension). Another patient had

patients with VTE are more likely than the general population to have certain types of cancer.

Methods.—This population-based analysis included 61,998 patients identified from the Swedish Inpatient Register who had VTE diagnosed from 1965 through 1983. Their mean age was 63.9 years, with approximately equal numbers of men and women. Patient records were then cross-referenced with files from the nationwide Cancer Registry. Age- and sex-adjusted cancer incidence rates for these patients were calculated and compared with national incidence rates.

Findings.—At admission for VTE or during the first year thereafter, 2,509 patients received a diagnosis of cancer (standardized incidence ratio [SIR] 3.2). Patients who were aged 65 years or younger had a significantly higher incidence of cancer (SIR 6.7) than patients older than 65 years (SIR 3.9). In particular, patients who had had 2 or more admissions for VTE were at great risk for cancer within the year after the last episode of VTE (SIR 8.2). Standardized incidence ratios were also clearly elevated for certain types of cancer within the first year after a VTE, including cancers of the ovary (11.4), pancreas (7.8), brain (7.6), and liver (6.6), as well as for Hodgkin's lymphoma (7.4) and polycythemia vera (12.9). Beyond the first year after VTE, the risk of cancer declined, with an average SIR of 1.3. Nonetheless, even 10 years or longer after admission for VTE, these patients had an elevated risk for cancer (SIR 1.3).

Conclusions.—Patients with VTE are at an increased risk for a diagnosis of cancer, particularly in the first year after VTE admission. Certain types of cancers (e.g., polycythemia vera, ovarian cancer) are especially more prevalent in these patients. These and other data support the belief that the pathophysiology of VTE and neoplasia are linked.

► These findings are similar to those in the previous paper (Abstract 15–2), although the mechanisms of association are unclear. Similar causes of precancer changes may also predispose to deep venous thrombosis (DVT). Papers from the 1960s showed changes in clotting factors in both early and advanced malignancies. Of no great clinical help.

N. Browse, M.D.

► I both agree and disagree with Professor Browse. One can hardly help being impressed by the dramatic Swedish data describing a greater than 30% increase in cancer in patients with venous thromboembolism. I presently believe a reasonably healthy patient experiencing idiopathic DVT should receive basic cancer screening—including chest x-ray, abdominal CT, carcinoembryonic antigen (CEA), prostate specific antigen (PSA) if male, etc.

J.M. Porter, M.D.

The Risk of a Diagnosis of Cancer After Primary Deep Venous Thrombosis or Pulmonary Embolism

Sørensen HT, Mellemkjær L, Steffensen FH, et al (Univ of Aarhus, Denmark; Inst of Cancer Epidemiology, Copenhagen; Aalborg Hosp, Denmark)

N Engl J Med 338:1169–1173, 1998 15–4

Background.—Controversy exists as to whether there is an association between deep venous thrombosis (DVT) or pulmonary embolism (PE) and the subsequent diagnosis of cancer. Some studies have found no association, whereas others have found as much as a fivefold greater risk of cancer in patients with DVT compared with that in the general population.

Methods.—Patients with DVT (n = 15,348) or PE (n = 11,305) from 1977 through 1992 were identified from the Danish National Registry of Patients. About a third of the patients were younger than 60 years, slightly more than one third were 60–74 years of age, and slightly less than a third were 75 years or older, with approximately equal numbers of men and women. Patient records were then cross-referenced with files from the nationwide Cause of Death Registry and the Cancer Registry. Age- and sex-adjusted cancer incidence rates for these patients were calculated and compared with national incidence rates.

Findings.—Based on general population data, the 15,348 patients with DVT would have been expected to have 1,372 cases of cancer; they actually had 1,737 cases (standardized incidence ratio [SIR] 1.3; 95% confidence interval [CI] 1.21–1.33). Similarly, the 11,305 patients with PE

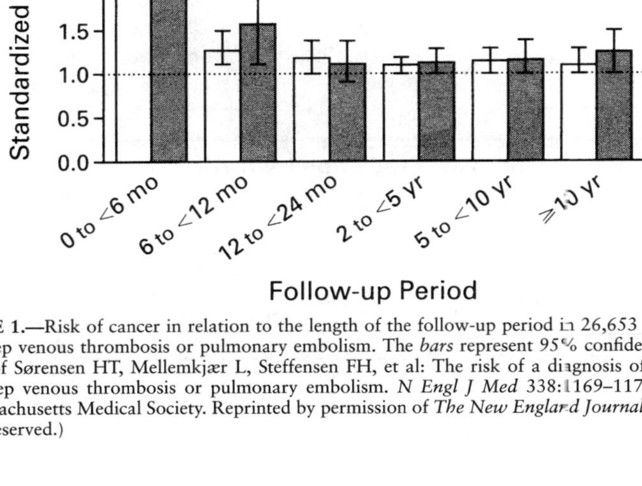

FIGURE 1.—Risk of cancer in relation to the length of the follow-up period in 26,653 patients with primary deep venous thrombosis or pulmonary embolism. The *bars* represent 95% confidence intervals. (Courtesy of Sørensen HT, Mellemkjær L, Steffensen FH, et al: The risk of a diagnosis of cancer after primary deep venous thrombosis or pulmonary embolism. *N Engl J Med* 338:1169–1173. Copyright 1998, Massachusetts Medical Society. Reprinted by permission of *The New England Journal of Medicine*. All rights reserved.)

would have been expected to have 556 cases of cancer; they actually had 730 cases (SIR 1.3; 95% CI 1.22–1.41). The risk of cancer for patients with DVT or PE was substantially greater within 6 months of the thrombotic event (SIR 3.0), then decreased during the follow-up period (Fig 1). During the first year of follow-up, 560 cases of cancer were diagnosed; of these, information about the extent of disease at diagnosis was available in 465 cases. Of these 465 cases, 184 patients had distant metastases (40%), 115 had regional spread of the cancer (25%), and 166 showed no spread (36%). Patients with DVT or PE were more likely to develop cancers of the pancreas, ovary, liver, brain, esophagus, and kidney, as well as non-Hodgkin's lymphoma and leukemia (SIRs ranging from 1.7 to 7.9). However, they were less likely to develop cancers of the stomach, colon, breast, urinary bladder, and rectum, and malignant melanoma (SIRs ranging from 0.3 to 2.1).

Conclusions.—The greatest risk of cancer in a patient with DVT or PE is during the first year of follow-up. Unfortunately, 40% of the patients who did have cancer diagnosed during this period had distant metastases. Furthermore, the types of cancers more common in these patients (pancreas, brain, liver, ovary, etc.) make the prognosis poor. Thus, extensive screening of all patients with DVT or PE is not likely to affect outcome and would not be cost-effective. The most pragmatic approach is to screen only those patients with DVT or PE who show signs or symptoms of cancer.

▶ This very large study confirms what most textbooks say, namely, cancer may be present with DVT or PE, but when it does so it is usually advanced and disseminated. Searching for it rarely helps the patient. Therefore, don't search for cancer in every patient with DVT, rather use clinical judgment. A sensible clinical message.

N. Browse, M.D.

▶ This study from Denmark found a lower risk of cancer than that reported in Abstracts 15–2 and 15–3; however, an increased risk was again noted. The association between idiopathic venous thromboembolism and increased cancer risk appears established beyond reasonable doubt. Unlike Professor Browse, I believe a cancer search is both reasonable and indicated.

J.M. Porter, M.D.

Deep Venous Thrombosis: Prediction by D-Dimer?

Kozman H, Flemmer MC, Rahnama M (Eastern Virginia Med School, Norfolk)

South Med J 90:907–910, 1997 15–5

Objective.—Measurement of D-dimer, a fragment of the cross-linked fibrin molecule released during plasmin-mediated clot lysis, has been suggested as a screening test for deep venous thrombosis (DVT). Whereas the test specificity is low in patients with conditions that elevate D-dimer levels, such as disseminated malignancy, sepsis, disseminated intravascular

TABLE 3.—Specificity, Sensitivity, and Positive and Negative Predictive Value With Various D-Dimer Cutoff Values

D-Dimer Level (ng/mL)	*Specificity*	*Sensitivity*	*PPV*	*NPV*
2,000	59%	100%	50%	100%
3,000	61%	88%	41%	94%
4,000	73%	75%	54%	90%

(Courtesy of Kozman H, Flemmer MC, Rahnama M: Deep venous thrombosis: Prediction by D-dimer? *South Med J* 90:907–910, 1997. Reprinted by permission from the *Southern Medical Journal.*)

coagulation, or inflammatory states, excluding patients with these conditions may help to determine whether a quantitative D-dimer assay might be useful for diagnosing DVT.

Methods.—Between April 1994 and March 1995, 65 patients without inflammatory diseases, infections, or malignant conditions were screened for DVT by venous duplex and duplex Doppler ultrasonography. Serum D-dimer levels were measured.

Results.—Deep venous thrombosis was diagnosed in 16 patients by duplex Doppler ultrasonography. The D-dimer levels for the DVT and non-DVT groups were significantly different, 5,141 ng/mL and 3,024 ng/mL, respectively. Significantly more patients in the DVT group than in the non-DVT group were male (66.6% vs. 39%, respectively), and significantly more patients in the DVT group had experienced surgery and/or trauma (44% vs. 27%, respectively). The sensitivity of the D-dimer screening test increased as the specificity decreased (Table 3).

Conclusion.—Patients with DVT had significantly higher D-dimer levels than did patients without DVT. No patients with D-dimer levels of less than 2,000 ng/mL had DVT.

► I have never known what to make of the D-dimer test in the diagnosis of venous thrombosis. Although this publication accurately notes a high overlap between D-dimer levels in patients with and without venous thrombosis, it also notes that no patient proven to have DVT had a D-dimer less than 2,000 ng/mL. These authors concluded that a D-dimer less than 2000 convincingly excludes the diagnosis of DVT. I am completely unwilling to accept this until independent confirmation is forthcoming. At that time, we will have to carefully review the cost of D-dimer assay vs. the cost of duplex ultrasound for the diagnosis of DVT. (See also Abstract 15–6).

Plasma D-Dimer Measurement in Patients With Suspected DVT: A Means of Avoiding Unnecessary Venography

Khaira HS, Mann J (Good Hope Hosp, Sutton Coldfield, West Midlands, England)

Eur J Vasc Endovasc Surg 15:235–238, 1998 15–6

Background.—Currently, the clinical diagnosis of deep venous thrombosis (DVT) has an accuracy of only about 50%, and thus many patients undergo venography or duplex scanning unnecessarily. A blood test that could screen patients for DVT would be welcome. The usefulness of an immunofiltration assay that detects plasma D-dimers (fibrin-derived fragments in the blood) in screening for DVT was evaluated.

Methods.—Participants were 79 patients (31 men and 48 women, median age 63 years) who were being evaluated for suspected lower limb DVT. All patients provided a blood sample, then underwent venography and/or duplex scanning. Plasma was tested by an immunofiltration test that detects pathologic D-dimer concentrations (NycoCard D-Dimer). The color intensity of the card is compared with a color chart to determine plasma D-dimer levels; plasma D-dimer concentrations of 0.5 mg/L or greater were considered abnormal, and the test was rated positive.

Findings.—Venography and/or duplex scanning identified DVT in 29 patients (37%), with isolated calf vein DVT in 16 patients and additional iliofemoral segment involvement in 13 cases. The duration of symptoms did not correlate with either the plasma D-dimer level or the presence or absence of DVT. The D-dimer test gave only 1 false-negative result, for a sensitivity of 96% and a negative predictive value of 95%. However, D-dimer test results were positive in 28 patients who had DVT, and in 30 patients who did not have DVT, for a positive predictive value of only 48%. Specificity of the D-dimer test was only 40%.

Conclusions.—Except for 1 patient, D-dimer test results were normal in patients without DVT. Thus a negative result on a D-dimer test could be used to screen patients without DVT. This practice would avoid the invasiveness of venography and save time and money for patients and radiographers alike.

▶ The conclusions of this article are about the same as that of the previous article, namely that D-dimer has a high sensitivity for DVT and a low specificity. Thus, it is beset with false-positive results. In fact, the positive predictive value was only 48%, whereas the negative predictive value was 95%. Again, these authors conclude that D-dimer level can be used as an exclusion test for DVT. Perhaps. I wonder how the very small DVT as frequently seen by duplex would check out on the D-dimer test? I require a great deal more information before acceptance of D-dimer as a means to exclude the performance of duplex ultrasonography in the diagnosis of lower extremity DVT. (See also Abstract 15–5.)

Venous Thrombectomy for Iliofemoral Vein Thrombosis: 10-Year Results of a Prospective Randomised Study

Plate G, Eklöf B, Norgren L, et al (Helsingborg, Sweden; Lund Univ, Sweden)
Eur J Vasc Endovasc Surg 14:367–374, 1997 15–7

Objective.—Pulmonary emboli develop in about half of all patients with iliofemoral venous thrombosis. Venous thrombectomy improves venous patency, venous hypertension rates, and valvular competence up to 5 years after surgery. Results of a 10-year follow-up study are reported.

Methods.—Surgical thrombectomy (n = 13) was compared with a temporary arteriovenous fistula and anticoagulation treatment with conventional anticoagulation therapy alone (n = 17) in 30 patients (8 male), ages 15 to 76, followed up for 10 years after acute iliofemoral venous thrombosis. Clinical, morphologic, and physiologic evaluations were performed at follow-up. Patency, outflow capacity, foot volumetry, foot vein pressure, and venous reflux were determined.

Results.—Postthrombotic sequelae were similar between groups (Fig 1). Whereas the surgical group tended to have less severe sequelae (class 0 to 2) and the medical group tended to have more severe sequelae (class 3 to 6), the differences were not significant. Patency was significantly higher in the surgical group than in the medical group (83% vs. 41%). Occlusion of the iliac vein was significantly more common in the medical group than in the surgical group (59% vs. 17%). Venous outflow was nonsignificantly better in the surgical group than in the medical group. Whereas foot volumetry values were similar between groups, severe reflux was slightly more common in the surgical group than in the medical group. Ambulatory venous pressure was slightly lower in the surgical group than in the medical group. Patients in the medical group had more severe pathologic femoral and popliteal reflux than did patients in the surgery group.

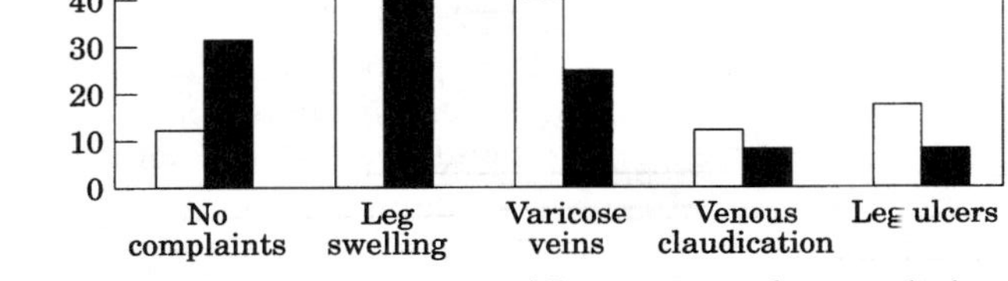

FIGURE 1.—Postthrombotic sequelae at 10-year follow-up. *Open columns*, medical group (n = 17); *black columns*, surgical group (n = 13). (Courtesy of Plate G, Eklöf B, Norgren L, et al: Venous thrombectomy for iliofemoral vein thrombosis: 10-year results of a prospective randomised study. *Eur J Vasc Endovasc Surg* 14:367–374. Copyright 1997. Reprinted by permission of WB Saunders Company Limited, London.)

Conclusion.—Venous thrombectomy appears to improve long-term patency and venous outflow and reduces venous reflux and ambulatory venous pressure, compared with anticoagulation therapy.

► Some people, once they get their teeth into something, simply refuse to let go. The Swedes became convinced decades ago that venous thrombectomy for iliofemoral vein thrombosis was a good thing, and no amount of negative data since that time has persuaded them differently. In their ongoing efforts to convince the rest of us, they present a follow-up group of 30 patients 10 years after iliofemoral venous thrombectomy in one group and medical therapy in the other. Of course, these patients were not randomized, and we have no idea whether the patients were initially comparable or not. A considerable number of patients had been lost to follow-up. Thus, this study is patently invalid from the outset. Although the authors were able to find a few putative benefits in favor of surgery, the overall data were monumentally unconvincing. I continue to have no use for iliofemoral venous thrombectomy, and I doubt if the Swedes are ever going to be able to convince me of the rightness of their position.

Regression of Proximal Deep Venous Thrombosis Is Associated With Fibrinolytic Enhancement

Killewich LA, Macko RF, Cox K, et al (Univ of Maryland, Baltimore)

J Vasc Surg 26:861–868, 1997 15–8

Background.—The mechanism and timing of recanalization after acute deep venous thrombosis (DVT) of the lower limb remain unclear. Activation of the endogenous fibrinolytic system is thought to be responsible for the regression of DVT. The levels of enzymes in the intrinsic fibrinolytic system were compared with the ultrasound morphologic findings in patients with acute DVT.

Methods.—Participants were 19 patients with diagnosed acute DVT. They were followed up with venous duplex ultrasound scanning (VDUS) at intervals from 1 to 36 weeks to evaluate regression of thrombus. At each examination, the extent of thrombus was quantitated in each of 5 major axial venous segments: the common femoral, the superficial femoral, the profunda femoris, the popliteal, and the tibial veins. These data were used to calculate the percentage of residual thrombus. At the same times, serum tissue plasminogen activity (tPA) and plasminogen activator inhibitor (PAI-1) were measured as indicators of endogenous fibrinolytic activity.

Results.—As early as the first or second week, VDUS showed regression of the thrombus. By the 24- to 36-week examination, only 26% of residual thrombus remained. Eighteen patients completed the full 9 months of the study; 56% showed complete resolution of the thrombus. Mean tPA activity increased from 0.60 IU/mL at baseline to 1.31 IU/mL at 1–2 weeks. After remaining high for 8–12 weeks, tPA activity returned to baseline levels at 24–36 weeks. The patients had elevated PAI-1 activity at

TABLE 2.—Residual Thrombus and Fibrinolytic Activity at Each Time Interval

Interval (wk)	*Residual thrombus (%)*	*tPA activity (IU/ml)**	*P*	*PAI-1 activity (AU/ml)**	*P*
Diagnosis	100	0.60 ± 0.07		23.1 ± 1.8	
1 to 2	95	1.31 ± 0.26	0.014	20.0 ± 2.7	0.29
3 to 6	82	1.52 ± 0.48	0.037	18.4 ± 2.5	0.21
8 to 12	60	1.29 ± 0.26	0.038	22.5 ± 1.5	0.77
24 to 36	26	0.68 ± 0.15	0.77	22.4 ± 1.9	0.86

*All values mean ± SEM.

Abbreviations: tPA, tissue plasminogen activator; *PAI-1*, plasminogen activator inhibitor.

(Courtesy Killewich LA, Macko RF, Cox K, et al: Regression of proximal deep venous thrombosis is associated with fibrinolytic enhancement. *J Vasc Surg* 26:861–868, 1997.)

baseline, compared with an age-matched population. There was no subsequent change in PAI-1 level (Table 2). Sixteen percent of patients had thrombus progression. These patients lacked the increase in tPA activity associated with activation of intrinsic fibrinolysis.

Conclusions.—In patients with acute DVT, acute thrombosis appears to regress early, continuing to do so for at least 9 months. The process of DVT regression is associated with increased endogenous fibrinolysis, taking place mainly through increased tPA activity. When thrombus progresses despite antithrombotic therapy, it may represent failure of endogenous fibrinolysis to activate.

► We have all known since the beginning of time that venous thrombi typically regress beginning at about 1 week and proceeding for at least several months, but occasionally for intervals up to 6–8 months. I am hardly surprised to note that tPA activity was elevated during the time of maximal thrombus resolution. The authors noted in the few patients who had progression of thrombus that the anticipated enhancement of tPA activity was not noted. I hereby award these authors a gold star for confirming the obvious.

Early Outcome After Isolated Calf Vein Thrombosis

Meissner MH, Caps MT, Bergelin RO, et al (Univ of Washington, Seattle)
J Vasc Surg 26:749–756, 1997 15–9

Background.—There is debate as to whether isolated calf vein thrombosis (CVT) is associated with development of postthrombotic syndrome. The natural history of CVT was studied in terms of lower extremity symptoms, propagation, recanalization, and valvular incompetence.

Methods.—The 10-year experience included 499 patients with acute deep venous thrombosis (DVT). Fifty-eight patients had thrombosis confined to the calf veins of 1 or both extremities. Twenty-nine patients with isolated CVT, as well as 239 other patients with DVT, were followed up with clinical examination and duplex ultrasonography.

pean countries have an extraordinarily higher prevalence of venous disease than do individuals from North America. This interesting study extends these observations to individuals from Asia and the Pacific Islands finding a very low incidence of idiopathic DVT in these groups compared with North American white individuals. Certainly any attempt to study the epidemiology of venous thrombosis will have to take into account the dramatically different prevalence of DVT in various ethnic groups.

Comparison of Sequential Compression Devices and Foot Pumps for Prophylaxis of Deep Venous Thrombosis in High-risk Trauma Patients

Spain DA, Bergamini TM, Hoffmann JF, et al (Univ of Louisville, Ky; Veteran Affairs Med Ctr, Louisville, Ky)

Am Surg 64:522–525, 1998 15–13

Background.—The risks of deep venous thrombosis (DVT) and subsequent pulmonary embolism (PE) are increased in patients with multiple trauma. Approaches to aggressive DVT and PE prophylaxis in these patients include compression devices, subcutaneous heparin, and vena cava filters. Heparin can cause bleeding complications in trauma patients, and while vena cava filters can prevent PE, they do not prevent the underlying DVT. Thus sequential pneumatic compression devices (SCDs) are often used in high-risk patients, unless they have lower extremity or soft-tissue injuries that preclude their use. In such cases, foot pumps may be of benefit. The results of SCDs and foot pumps in the prophylaxis of DVT in high-risk blunt trauma patients were evaluated.

Methods.—Chart review identified 184 high-risk blunt trauma patients who survived more than 48 hours and who received DVT prophylaxis with compression devices. About two thirds of the patients (118, or 64%) received thigh-high SCDs. The remaining one third (66, or 36%) of patients received foot pumps because they had lower extremity fractures that precluded the use of SCDs. Demographic, injury, and illness pattern data were collected for all patients and compared between the SCD and foot pump groups.

Findings.—At enrollment, the patients with foot pumps were significantly more likely to have lower extremity fractures (as expected; 65% vs. 26%), chest injuries (61% vs. 26%), and pelvic fractures (59% vs. 25%) than the patients with SCDs. Patients with SCDs had more severe head injuries (Glasgow Coma Scale 10.5 vs. 7.9), although the 2 groups did not differ with respect to the incidence of head injuries. Only 10 of the 154 patients had a DVT (5.4%), and the incidence of DVT did not differ significantly between the 2 groups. Two patients with foot pumps had a nonfatal PE, and 1 patient with an SCD had a nonfatal PE. There were no device-related complications, and the SCD and foot pump failure rates were 7% and 3%, respectively.

Conclusions.—Foot pumps and SCDs were effective in preventing DVT and PE in these high-risk trauma patients. In particular, foot pumps were effective in patients in whom lower extremity fracture precluded the use of SCDs.

▶ I have been fascinated by the repeated observation that intermittent compression of the plantar venous plexus appears to provide effective prophylaxis against DVT in various patient groups.[1] In this fascinating study from the University of Louisville Trauma Center, the foot pump appeared at least as effective as the full lower extremity sequential compression devices in DVT prophylaxis. They were used exclusively in high-risk trauma patients in whom lower extremity fractures precluded the use of sequential compressive devices, thus, if anything, prejudicing the study against the foot pump. On balance, the intermittent compression of the plantar venous plexus for DVT prophylaxis appeared quite effective. (See also Abstract 16–14.)

Reference

1. 1997 Year Book of Vascular Surgery, p 403.

Upper Extremity Versus Lower Extremity Deep Venous Thrombosis

Hingorani A, Ascher E, Hanson J, et al (Maimonides Med Ctr, Brooklyn, NY)

Am J Surg 174:214–217, 1997 15–14

Background.—No consensus has been reached on the treatment of upper extremity deep vein thrombosis (UEDVT), a disease considered more benign than lower extremity deep vein thrombosis (LEDVT). At the study institution, however, a substantial number of patients with UEDVT were diagnosed with pulmonary embolus, and nearly half died within 6 months. The records of 52 patients with UEDVT were reviewed to determine the impact of this condition on pulmonary embolism and mortality.

Methods.—Between January 1994 and June 1995, 430 patients with LEDVT and 52 with UEDVT were seen at Maimonides Medical Center, in Brooklyn. Ventilation–perfusion scans were used to confirm a clinically suspected diagnosis of pulmonary embolism. Medical problems in the UEDVT group were assessed by calculating APACHE (Acute Physiology, Age, Chronic Health Evaluation) III scores; 52 randomly selected patients with LEDVT also had APACHE III scores calculated using data obtained from medical records.

Results.—Patients with UEDVT were 36 women and 16 men with a mean age of 66 years. The LEDVT group included 241 women and 189 men with a mean age of 62 years. Pulmonary embolism was documented in 9 (17%) patients with UEDVT and in 33 (8%) of those with LEDVT. Within 6 months of the diagnosis of deep vein thrombosis, 25 (48%) patients in the UEDVT group and 14 (13%) patients in the LEDVT group had died. In both groups, treatment for deep vein thrombosis had consisted of systemic anticoagulation, with placement of a superior vena cava filter when anticoagulation failed or the patient had a contraindication to anticoagulants. APACHE III scores were higher in patients with UEDVT than they were in those with LEDVT (mean 42 vs. 33), a factor which may have contributed to the higher mortality in patients with UEDVT.

Conclusion.—Compared with earlier reports, this report found UEDVT to be a more benign condition than LEDVT. Both the incidence of pulmonary embolism and 6-month mortality were significantly higher in patients with UEDVT than they were in those with LEDVT.

► These authors have concluded that upper extremity DVT is associated with a higher morbidity and mortality than lower extremity DVT. They further concluded that upper extremity DVT has been an underrecognized predictor of morbidity and mortality. Although dealing with relatively small numbers, I suppose their data are correct. Unfortunately, they do not give the causes of death for these patients, a majority of which, I suspect, were unrelated to the occurrence of venous thrombosis or pulmonary embolism. Nonetheless, I believe one can confidently conclude that upper extremity DVT should be regarded as at least as serious a threat as lower extremity DVT in terms of risk of pulmonary embolism and perhaps should be regarded as an even greater threat as a predictor of near-term mortality.

Noninvasive Diagnosis

Noninvasive Venous Testing in the Diagnosis of Pulmonary Embolism: The Impact on Decisionmaking

Lipski DA, Shepard AD, McCarthy BD, et al (Henry Ford Hosp, Detroit)
J Vasc Surg 26:757–763, 1997 15–15

Background.—Pulmonary arteriography is the preferred method for diagnosing pulmonary embolism, although it is invasive, expensive, and associated with complications. Ventilation/perfusion lung scanning is less invasive and cheaper but is also less accurate. Lower extremity noninvasive venous testing is a newer approach. It identifies deep venous thrombosis (DVT) and uses the presence of DVT as a marker for pulmonary embolism and an indication for anticoagulation medication. Noninvasive venous testing has no risks, is highly accurate for diagnosing acute proximal DVT, and is relatively inexpensive. The value of this technique in the diagnosis and treatment of pulmonary embolism was described.

Methods.—Noninvasive venous testing was performed in 450 patients. Medical records were reviewed for the rate of positive results, the amount of new information provided by noninvasive venous testing, and any changes in management that were based solely on the results of noninvasive venous testing.

Results.—Of the 450 patients, 41 had DVT. The rate of DVT detected by noninvasive venous testing in patients who were not evaluated by ventilation/perfusion scanning was 8%. The rate of DVT detected by noninvasive venous testing in patients with a high-probability ventilation/perfusion scan before noninvasive venous testing was 39%. In this group, no treatment decisions were based on a positive noninvasive venous testing result, and only 2 treatment decisions were based on a negative result. The prevalence of DVT detected by noninvasive venous testing in patients with a negative diagnostic result of ventilation/perfusion scanning (low or very low probability or normal) before noninvasive venous testing was 2%. Overall, only 2.5% of changes in treatment decisions were based on noninvasive venous testing. In the other patients, treatment was based on results of ventilation/perfusion scanning or pulmonary arteriography.

Discussion.—These findings indicate that the results of noninvasive venous testing are usually negative for acute DVT in patients with suspected pulmonary embolism. Treatment decisions are nearly always based on results of ventilation/perfusion scanning or pulmonary arteriography, not noninvasive venous testing. The value of noninvasive venous testing for identifying DVT in these patients is limited. Its value in diagnosing pulmonary embolism may improve with a more selective approach.

▶ The appropriate role of noninvasive venous testing in patients suspected of pulmonary embolism remains problematic. In many vascular laboratories, primary care physicians routinely do noninvasive venous DVT testing in virtually all patients whom they suspect of having pulmonary embolism. This interesting study confirmed that only 9% of patients suspected of having pulmonary embolism actually have DVT by noninvasive venous testing, ranging from about 45% in patients with high-probability VQ scan, to about 6% to 7% in patients with low-probability VQ scans. On balance, the performance of lower extremity noninvasive venous testing for DVT appeared to add little to therapeutic decision making in patients suspected of pulmonary embolism. I believe that this is a precisely accurate conclusion, and I seriously question the wisdom or necessity for the currently widespread practice of routinely using lower extremity noninvasive venous testing in patients suspected of having pulmonary embolism. The information is simply of no value.

Screening for Asymptomatic Deep Vein Thrombosis in Surgical Intensive Care Patients

Harris LM, Curl GR, Booth FV, et al (State Univ of New York, Buffalo; Buffalo Gen Hosp, NY)

J Vasc Surg 26:764–769, 1997 15–16

Introduction.—Up to 10% of all deaths in U.S. hospitals are accounted for by deep vein thrombosis and pulmonary emboli. Duplex scanning has emerged as the gold standard for detection of deep vein thrombosis because the clinical diagnosis of deep vein thrombosis (DVT) is so inaccurate, yet more than one half of patients with typical symptoms do not have deep vein thrombosis. However, routine duplex screening for DVT is labor intensive and costly. To identify high-risk groups that would benefit from duplex screening and to identify low-risk patients on whom pneumatic compression devices could be placed without screening studies, patients in a surgical ICU population were reviewed.

Methods.—There were 294 patients with an anticipated length of stay greater than 36 hours who were admitted to a surgical ICU to determine the prevalence of risk factors for asymptomatic proximal DVT over a 24-month period. Multilineal regression, *t* tests, and χ^2 analysis were used to analyze data on risk factors, demographics, and operative data.

Results.—In the 294 patients, there was a 7.5% prevalence of major DVT. Multifactorial analysis revealed an association between DVT and APACHE II scores (14.5±6.24 vs. 10.3±3.15) and emergent procedures (45.5% vs. 23.2%). Univariate analysis revealed significance for age. To limit screening by 30% while achieving a 95.5% sensitivity for identification of proximal DVT, the presence of any one of the 3 risk factors identified could be used: Apache II score of 12 or more; emergent procedures; or age 65 years or older.

Conclusion.—A very low risk for DVT (1.1%) is indicated by an absence of all 3 risk factors. Because of a high prevalence of asymptomatic disease, screening of surgical ICU patients is indicated. Active therapy, not prophylaxis, is required for patients with proximal DVT. By using the above risk factors as a filter for duplex screening, costs and resources may be contained.

▶ We have learned in recent years that DVT is prevalent in both trauma units and medical ICUs, and we now learn, hardly to anyone's surprise, that such is also the case in surgical ICUs. Overall, 7.5% of patients studied had DVT, with this being more frequent in patients with higher APACHE II scores, emergent procedures, and older age. The authors concluded that DVT screening of surgical ICU patients was indicated because of the high prevalence of asymptomatic DVT, and that duplex screening of high-risk patients admitted to the surgical ICU should be routine. Because their policy is to use sequential pneumatic compression devices on everyone, they wish to avoid this in patients who already have DVT because of theoretical harm. They may be correct, but I am unaware of any persuasive evidence supporting this position.

Screening for Major Deep Vein Thrombosis in Seriously Injured Patients: A Prospective Study

Satiani B, Falcone R, Shook L, et al (Grant Med Ctr, Columbus, Ohio)
Ann Vasc Surg 11:626–629, 1997 15–17

Objective.—Deep vein thrombosis (DVT) is a risk in severely injured patients. Whether routine screening is cost-effective is unknown. The efficacy of routine noninvasive surveillance in seriously injured trauma patients receiving prophylaxis for DVT and its cost-effectiveness were investigated.

Methods.—Venous duplex scanning (VDS) was performed in 148 patients with multiple trauma (45 female; 295 limbs), average age 36.5, with an anticipated hospital stay of more than 4 days, and an injury severity score (ISS) greater than 10. Contrast venography was performed when duplex scanning results were abnormal. Scans were obtained on days 2 through 5, 11, and 30 after admission. Compression and/or subcutaneous heparin was provided to 99% of patients, who were monitored by trauma room nurses.

Results.—Of 272 VDS performed, scans in 8 limbs (2.7%) in 6 patients were abnormal and 28 were indeterminate and were repeated in most cases. In 6 of the 8 limbs with abnormal scans, contrast venography revealed DVT. Four of these patients had symptoms. Two patients with a pulmonary embolism had a normal VDS.

Conclusion.—Because 272 VDS, performed at a cost of $111,520, detected DVT in only 8 limbs (2.7%) of 6 patients, 4 without symptoms, the routine use of VDS in severely injured patients is not cost-effective.

► Numerous articles in recent years have purported to describe the incidence of DVT in trauma patients. Unfortunately, the results have varied so widely that it is difficult for one to come away with any definitive conclusions. In this interesting study, either sequential lower extremity pneumatic compression or subcutaneous heparin was used for prophylaxis in 99% of trauma patients. In this selected group, DVT was found in only 6 patients, with most being asymptomatic. The authors concluded (and I suspect accurately) that trauma center patients receiving aggressive DVT prophylaxis do not require routine screening by duplex ultrasound. The question is just how many trauma center patients are ineligible for either lower extremity compressive stockings or heparin. Of course, based on the information in Abstract 15–13, we now think we know that intermittent compression of the plantar venous plexus appears to be equally as effective as sequential leg pneumatic compression.

Ultrasonographic Screening Before Hospital Discharge for Deep Venous Thrombosis After Arthroplasty: The Post-Arthroplasty Screening Study

Robinson KS, Anderson DR, Gross M, et al (Dalhousie Univ, Halifax, Nova Scotia, Canada; McMaster Univ, Hamilton, Ont, Canada)

Ann Intern Med 127:439–445, 1997 15–18

Background.—Despite the use of antithrombotic prophylaxis, asymptomatic deep venous thrombosis (DVT) develops in many patients after joint arthroplasty. The clinical significance of these thrombi and the value of screening tests for their detection are uncertain. A randomized, controlled trial investigated the value of US screening for DVT after arthroplasty and the rates of symptomatic venous thromboembolic and major bleeding complications during the 90 days after hospital discharge.

TABLE 2.—Asymptomatic and Symptomatic Events in the Screening Compression Ultrasonography and Sham Ultrasonography Groups

Variable	Patients Undergoing Screening Compression Ultrasonography			Patients Undergoing Sham Ultrasonography		
	Total Patients	Patients Undergoing Hip Arthroplasty	Patients Undergoing Knee Arthroplasty	Total Patients	Patients Undergoing Hip Arthroplasty	Patients Undergoing Knee Arthroplasty
Patients, *n*	518	257	261	506	249	257
Asymptomatic screening events, *n (%)**	13 (2.5)	7 (2.7)	6 (2.3)	–	–	–
Symptomatic events after randomization, *n (%)*						
Proximal deep venous thrombosis	4 (0.8)	3 (1.2)	1 (0.4)	3 (0.6)	2 (0.8)	1 (0.4)
Nonfatal pulmonary embolism	0	0	0	2 (0.4)	1 (0.4)	1 (0.4)
Fatal pulmonary embolism	0	0	0	0	0	0
Major bleeding episode†	1 (0.2)	1 (0.2)	0	–	–	–
Total symptomatic events	5 (1.0)	4 (1.6)	1 (0.4)	5 (1.0)	3 (1.2)	2 (0.8)

*All asymptomatic events were proximal deep venous thromboses.

†In patients receiving anticoagulants to treat asymptomatic deep venous thrombosis, major bleeding was a primary outcome event.

(Courtesy of Robinson KS, Anderson DR, Gross M, et al: Ultrasonographic screening before hospital discharge for deep venous thrombosis after arthroplasty: The post-arthroplasty screening study. *Ann Intern Med* 127:439–445, 1997.)

Methods.—The trial was conducted at a tertiary care hospital between July 1993 and December 1995. During this period, 1,284 patients underwent total hip or knee arthroplasty; 1,024 of these patients met eligibility criteria and completed study enrollment. Randomization was to bilateral compression US or a sham procedure to be performed before hospital discharge. Patients diagnosed with asymptomatic DVT received standard anticoagulant therapy after discharge; others were treated with warfarin until the time of discharge.

Results.—Asymptomatic proximal deep venous thrombosis was detected in 13 of the 518 patients (2.5%) randomized to screening US. Another 4 patients in the group were later diagnosed with symptomatic proximal DVT, and 1 patient who was treated for asymptomatic DVT experienced major bleeding. The total outcome event rate of the screened group was thus 1.0%. The 506 patients assigned to the sham US group also had a total event rate of 1.0%; 2 had nonfatal pulmonary embolism, and 3 were diagnosed with symptomatic proximal DVT (Table 2).

Conclusion.—Screening compression US performed before hospital discharge to identify asymptomatic proximal DVT did not reduce the rate of subsequent symptomatic thromboembolic complications in patients who underwent total hip or knee arthroplasty. Warfarin prophylaxis during hospitalization appears to be adequate for prevention of symptomatic DVT or pulmonary embolism after hospital discharge.

▶ This paper concludes, interestingly, that in patients undergoing total hip or knee arthroplasty there is a very low incidence of new venous thrombosis after hospital discharge. I must say, at the present time I am confused. Persuasive evidence cited in the 1998 YEAR BOOK OF VASCULAR SURGERY clearly indicated there was a significant incidence of DVT after hospital discharge and continued prophylaxis for a considerable period of time was desirable.[1] Presently, I suppose the only conclusion is that we must regard this matter as unresolved and await additional information.

Reference

1. 1998 YEAR BOOK OF VASCULAR SURGERY, pp 416 and 418.

Emboli Observed With Use of Transesophageal Echocardiography Immediately After Tourniquet Release During Total Knee Arthroplasty With Cement

Berman AT, Parmet JL, Harding SP, et al (Allegheny Univ Hosps, Philadelphia)
J Bone Joint Surg Am 80-A:389–396, 1998 15–19

Background.—No one is sure why the release of a tourniquet after total joint arthroplasty causes hemodynamic collapse. However, thrombi have been found in the central circulation in these instances. Transesophageal echocardiography was used to examine the relationship between tourni-

16 Chronic Venous and Lymphatic Disease

Venous Reflux

Clinical and Haemodynamic Sequelae of Deep Venous Thrombosis: Retrospective Evaluation After 7–13 Years

Janssen MCH, Haenen JH, van Asten WNJC, et al (Univ Hosp Nijmegen, The Netherlands)

Clin Sci (Colch) 93:7–12, 1997 16–1

Background.—Many patients who have had an episode of deep venous thrombosis (DVT) subsequently experience post-thrombotic syndrome (PTS). The reported incidence of PTS and other complications after DVT varies considerably, however, and few studies have included hemodynamic findings. Eighty-one patients with venographically confirmed lower extremity DVT were examined clinically and underwent vascular testing to determine the long-term sequelae of DVT.

Methods.—The patients, 54 men and 27 women with a mean age of 52, were examined at periods ranging from 7 to 13 years (mean 10 years) after a first acute DVT of the leg. All were treated initially with intravenous heparin and oral anticoagulants and were advised to wear graduated compression stockings. At follow-up the patients were asked about the presence of subjective signs of PTS, such as restless legs, cramps, and heaviness. They were examined for objective criteria of PST, including varicosis, ulceration, and edema. Investigators who were unaware of the initial venographic findings classified PTS on a scale of 0 to 6. Patients were also assessed for venous outflow resistance and calf muscle pump function (CMP), using the supine venous pump function test (SVPT).

Results.—Only 20 patients (25%) were asymptomatic at a mean of 10 years after their episode of DVT. Recurrent DVT had developed in 9 patients (11%). Post-thrombotic syndrome was classified as mild in 34 (42%), moderate in 25 (31%), and severe in 2 (2%). More than half (57%) had an abnormal CMP. Fifty-three percent were still wearing compression stockings. Both clinical PTS (Fig 1) and hemodynamic findings were related to the initial site of the thrombosis. Calf muscle pump

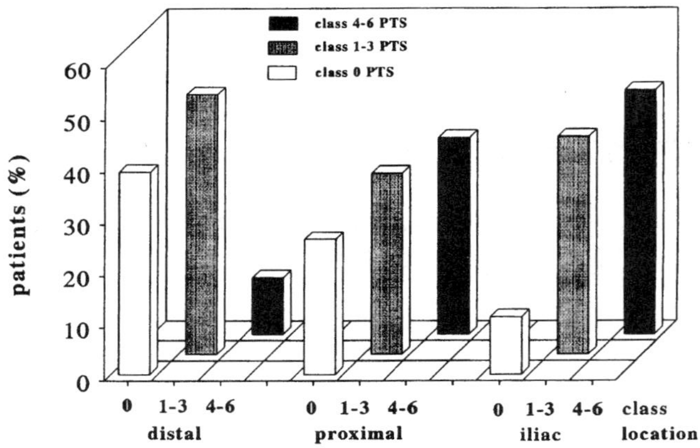

FIGURE 1.—Relation between location of initial DVT (distal, proximal, iliac) and clinical class PTS. Class 0 = no signs of PTS. Class 1–3 = mild signs of PTS (corona phlebectatica, edema). Class 4 = moderate signs of PTS (pigmentation, lipodermatosclerosis, atrophy blanche). Class 5–6 = severe signs of PTS (ulceration). Because only 2 patients developed ulceration class 4–6 are analyzed together. (Courtesy of Janssen MCH, Haenen JH, van Asten WNJC, et al: Clinical and hemodynamic sequelae of deep venous thrombosis: Retrospective evaluation after 7–13 years. *Clin Sci (Colch)* 93:7–12, 1997.)

function and the difference in CMP between the post-thrombotic and non-thrombotic leg were significantly related to PTS class.

Conclusion.—The findings in these patients confirm that long-term sequelae typical of PTS occur frequently after DVT. Although only 2 of 81 patients had an ulcer, almost one-third (31%) had moderate PTS. Even after distal DVT, the incidence of moderate DVT was 11%. The SVPT was useful in detecting a decreased CMP.

▶ This study once again confirms that a large majority of patients who experience deep vein thrombosis remain continually symptomatic for years after the thrombotic event. Hemodynamic abnormalities were demonstrated in a majority of the patients 7–13 years after the DVT episode. What we do not know is whether these abnormalities resulted exclusively from the initial deep vein thrombosis or whether over the years these patients likely experienced recurrent episodes of venous thrombosis, some of which may have involved the proximal veins. For the time being, we should regard venous thrombosis as a recurrent disease and one prone to cause chronic symptoms.

Variability and Reliability of Air Plethysmographic Measurements for the Evaluation of Chronic Venous Disease

Yang D, Vandongen YK, Stacey MC (Univ of Western Australia, Fremantle)
J Vasc Surg 26:638–642, 1997 16–2

Background.—Air plethysmography (APG) has been widely used to evaluate patients with chronic venous insufficiency and to assess the effects of treatment. Because there are few reports on the reliability of APG data, patients with recently healed venous ulcers were recruited for a study designed to determine the variation in different measuring parameters, the test-retest reliability of the APG method, and its accuracy in monitoring changes in limbs with chronic venous disease.

Methods.—Patients were 12 men and 5 women with an average age of 73.2. The APG machine used consisted of a tubular, polyvinyl chloride air cuff that enclosed the leg from knee to ankle; a pressure transducer; a cuff-inflator pump; an amplifier; and a recorder. The cuff was inflated to a pressure of 6 mm Hg. Tests were performed on 2 occasions, 1 to 6 weeks apart, and 3 tests were performed at each visit. (Three patients had 10 tests at 1 visit.) Coefficients of variation were calculated for repeated measurements and test-retest reliability.

Results.—For the majority of parameters of APG, the coefficients of variation (CV) for the repeated measurements ranged from 7.5% to 27%. Differences between the means of 3 tests and the means of 10 tests were less than 10%. Although there were some differences between test and retest measurements for all of the APG parameters, when the CV method of error was used to evaluate differences, most measuring parameters had approximately 10% variation. Exceptions were the time taken to achieve 90% venous filling after exercise and the venous filling index after exercise, which had variations of 15.6% and 29.8%, respectively.

Conclusion.—The evaluation of calf pump function and venous reflux with APG yields variations in both repeated measurements and in test-retest measures. Because variations were found within patients and on retesting patients on different days, it appears unlikely that this technique can detect small changes in measured parameters. Clinicians should be aware of the inherent variation of APG measurements when the measurements are used to evaluate treatment outcome.

► Overall, we have found the air plethysmographic methodology too inconsistent and nonreproducible to be of any consistent value in clinical testing for venous insufficiency. I am convinced a great deal of the variability lies in the imperfect fit of the plethysmographic bag to the calf. I am pleased that these authors have objectively confirmed some of the problems that we have routinely experienced with this device. (See also Abstract 3–20.)

Where Does Venous Reflux Start?

Labropoulos N, Giannoukas AD, Delis K, et al (Loyola Univ, Maywood, Ill; St Mary's, London; St Bartholomew's Hosp, London)

J Vasc Surg 26:736–742, 1997 16–3

Introduction.—The identification of reflux in patients who are asymptomatic and in the early stages of primary chronic venous disease would enhance understanding about the development of this disorder. Patients with prominent or varicose veins and aysmptomatic volunteers were evaluated by color flow duplex imaging to determine the origin of lower limb primary venous reflux.

Methods.—Forty age- and sex-matched volunteers with no symptoms (age, 15–35 years; 80 limbs, group A), 20 volunteers with prominent but nonvaricose veins (age, 19–32 years; 26 limbs, group B) and 50 patients with varicose veins (age, 17–34 years; 64 limbs, group C) underwent color flow duplex imaging. Patients stood for evaluation of all proximal veins and were seated for evaluation of all distal veins.

Results.—The prevalence of reflux in group A, group B, and group C was 14% (11 of 80), 77% (31 of 40), and 87% (87 of 100), respectively. Reflux was confined to the superficial veins alone in 80% of limbs from all 3 groups. Deep venous reflux or combined patterns of reflux were rare, even in group C. Reflux was observed in all segments of the saphenous veins and their tributaries. The most frequent sites of reflux in 125 limbs with superficial venous incompetence were the below-knee segment of the greater saphenous vein (68%), the above-knee segment of the greater saphenous vein (55%), and the saphenofemoral junction (32%). Non-saphenous reflux was uncommon (2 patients, 2.4%). Reflux in the lesser saphenous vein was observed in 21 patients (17%) from all 3 groups. All patients with involvement of both greater and lesser saphenous veins (8, 6.4%) were from group C. The incidence of multisegmental reflux was significantly higher in group C than group A or group B (95%, 18%, and 54%, respectively). The prevalence of distal reflux was similar for all 3 groups.

Conclusions.—Primary venous reflux may occur in any lower leg superficial or deep veins. Below-knee veins are frequently involved in individuals who are asymptomatic and in those with prominent or varicose veins. Reflux seems to be a local or multifocal process in addition to, or separate from, a retrograde process.

▶ It appears that most people with prominent veins and almost all people with varicose veins have reflux, and in a large majority of these individuals the reflux is confined to the superficial veins alone. More and more in recent years we are being informed that a significant amount of venous reflux in symptomatic patients appears to be either confined to the superficial veins or has major prominence in the superficial veins. Thus, selective removal of superficial veins may have a very favorable impact upon chronic venous insufficiency problems, if the patients are carefully selected using duplex. I believe this to have been a significant step forward in our understanding both of venous pathophysiology and selection of treatment.

Late Clinical and Hemodynamic Sequelae of Isolated Calf Vein Thrombosis

McLafferty RB, Moneta GL, Passman MA, et al (Oregon Health Sciences Univ, Portland)

J Vasc Surg 27:50–57, 1998 16–4

Background.—Though isolated calf vein thrombosis (ICVT) is common, little is known about its long-term clinical and hemodynamic sequelae. Late clinical symptoms and vascular laboratory abnormalities were reported.

Methods.—A total of 146 patients had ICVT, documented by color flow duplex scanning, between 1989 and 1994. Thirty-seven patients were reassessed after a mean of 3.4 years. A control group of 37 patients with no history of venous disease underwent the same clinical and hemodynamic assessments for comparison.

Findings.—In the ICVT group, venous recovery time was abnormal in 23% of the extremities with ICVT and in 9% of extremities without ICVT. None of the control group extremities had an abnormal venous recovery time. Duplex valve closure time was abnormal in 1 or more venous segments in 26% of extremities with ICVT and in 6% of control extremities. Thirty-five percent of patients with ICVT had reticular veins; 27%, varicose veins; 5.4%, edema; 2.7%, pigmentation and ulcer; 35%, mild discomfort; and 2.7%, severe pain. All symptoms attributable to ICVT were mild, except in 1 patient who had severe pain and no physical or hemodynamic vascular abnormalities at follow-up (Table 4).

Conclusions.—At a mean of 3.4 years after ICVT, about one third of the patients had mild to moderate venous valvular insufficiency, but mostly in

TABLE 4.—Number (%) of Venous Segments With Abnormal Duplex Valve Closure Times in Patients With Isolated Calf Vein Thrombosis and in Control Participants

Vein segment	*Patients with ICVT* — *Lower extremities with ICVT (n = 38)*	*Patients with ICVT* — *Lower extremities without ICVT (n = 34)*	*Control lower extremities (n = 34)*
Common femoral	2 (5)	2 (6)	2 (6)
Popliteal	4 (11)	5 (15)	0 (0)
Posterior tibial	2 (5)	3 (9)	0 (0)
Greater saphenous	4 (11)	1 (3)	1 (3)
Lesser saphenous	2 (5)	2 (6)	0 (0)
Total	14 (7)*	13 (8)*	3 (1.7)

*P less than or equal to 0.05 when compared with control participants.

(Courtesy of McLafferty RB, Moneta GL, Passman MA, et al: Late clinical and hemodynamic sequelae of isolated calf vein thrombosis. *J Vasc Surg* 27:50–57, 1998.)

segments uninvolved with ICVT. Few patients had significant clinical symptoms attributable to venous disease.

▶ This article describes an interesting study confirming the variability and unpredictability of symptoms and signs after isolated calf vein thrombosis. The finding that 38% of patients had mild symptoms is similar to the findings in studies based upon phlebography and fibrinogen uptake tests. It is unfortunate that the control group was not studied twice at a 3–4 year interval. How many of these participants would have developed symptoms? We don't understand what has to go wrong with the calf veins to produce symptoms. Venous recovery time and duplex valve closure time don't help much. Much longer and more detailed studies are required.

N. Browse, M.D.

Duplex Ultrasound in the Hemodynamic Evaluation of the Late Sequelae of Deep Venous Thrombosis

Haenen JH, Janssen MCH, van Langen H, et al (Univ Hosp, Nijmegen, The Netherlands)

J Vasc Surg 27:472–478, 1998 16–5

Background.—Persistent venous abnormalities occur after the development of acute deep venous thrombosis (DVT), resulting in postthrombotic syndrome. The use of duplex US to assess long-term hemodynamic outcomes of DVT was reported.

Methods.—Seventy-two patients were studied 7–13 years after DVT had been diagnosed by phlebography. A total of 1212 segments of vein were reassessed with duplex US to detect reflux and obstruction and evaluate flow. Initially, 611 segments were thrombosed, and 601 were open. Reversed flow in 31 healthy persons was also measured to define reflux.

Findings.—Eleven percent of the patients had normal duplex findings in all veins. Forty-six percent of the patients had reflux, 8% had at least 1 noncompressible vein segment, and 35% had both reflux and noncompressibility. Seventy-three percent of segments without initial thrombosis and 46% with initial thrombosis were normal in the proximal vein. The frequency of reflux and noncompressibility was significantly greater in initially thombosed proximal vein segments than in vein segments without initial thrombosis. Seventeen percent of 720 vein segments distal to the knee were not traceable. A significantly greater percentage of initially thrombosed vein segments were untraceable. In the distal vein segments, reflux and noncompressibility did not differ significantly between vein segments with and without initial thrombosis. Flow was observed in 99% of the previously thrombosed proximal and distal segments (Table 2).

Conclusions.—Most of the patients still had venous abnormalities 7–13 years after receiving an initial diagnosis of DVT. Reflux was the most common finding. Significantly more abnormalities occurred in initially

TABLE 2.—Outcome for All Veins in Each Patient, Measured With Duplex Scanning 7–13 Years After Initial Episode of Deep Venous Thrombosis

Location of thrombosis at initial phlebography	*No. of patients*	*Outcome with duplex scanning* Normal	Reflux	NC	Reflux and NC
Proximal	12	0	8 (67%)	0	4 (33%)
Proximal and distal	44	2 (5%)	17 (39%)	6 (14%)	19 (43%)
Distal	16	6 (38%)	8 (50%)	0	2 (12%)
Total	72	8 (11%)	33 (46%)	6 (8%)	25 (35%)

Abbreviation: NC, noncompressible.
(Courtesy of Haenen JH, Janssen MCH, van Langen H, et al: Duplex ultrasound in the hemodynamic evaluation of the late sequelae of deep venous thrombosis. *J Vasc Surg* 27:472–478, 1998.)

thrombosed segments. The abnormalities were found in the proximal and distal vein segments, though less often in the latter.

▶ This article describes a long-term study (7–13 years) using duplex after initial diagnosis with phlebography and states that the veins that were thrombosed remain abnormal, with either reflux or total occlusion. Surprise, surprise! No clinical correlations are presented (to be the subject of a later article). A restatement of the theoretically obvious and clinically well-known.

N. Browse, M.D.

▶ Perhaps deserving of an honorable mention Camel Dung Award (CDA)!

J M. Porter, M.D.

Saphenectomy in the Presence of Chronic Venous Obstruction

Raju S, Easterwood L, Fountain T, et al (Univ of Mississippi, Jackson)
Surgery 123:637–644, 1998 16–6

Background.—Authorities have long thought that excising secondary saphenous varices associated with deep venous obstruction would compromise its collateral contribution. Recent advances in functional assessment of venous obstruction make it possible to test this hypothesis.

Methods.—Saphenectomy was performed in 51 limbs without morphologic or functional obstruction, and in 64 limbs with various grades of venous obstruction. The latter group had significant deep venous obstruction on ascending venography. Evaluation of obstruction was based on the arm/foot venous pressure differential method, outflow fraction measures, and outflow resistance determinations.

Findings.—Both groups of patients tolerated saphenectomy well. Outcomes did not differ according to objective tests for obstruction. Improvement in reflux and calf venous pump function was comparable. Five of 7 limbs with preoperative grade III or IV venous obstruction showed signif-

nonoperative treatment in most patients. I have found elastic compression therapy most useful, but unfortunately it is often of limited benefit.

Treatment of Venous Malformations by Direct Injection With Ethanol

Shireman PK, McCarthy WJ, Yao JST, et al (Northwestern Univ, Chicago)

J Vasc Surg 26:838–844, 1997 16–10

Background.—Venous malformations can be discrete or extensive, and surgical removal of larger lesions can be difficult. Lesions that are not completely removed tend to recur. There have been reports that direct puncture of the lesions and injection of a sclerosing agent, such as ethanol, has been effective. Ethanol causes necrosis of vessel walls with sludging of red blood cells and thrombosis, which leads to production of intimal fibrosis related to the protein denaturing and hydroscopic properties of the ethanol.

Methods.—Twelve patients with venous malformations were evaluated with MRI before treatment. The mean patient age was 37 years. Seven of the patients had a total of 19 previous surgical excisions. All 12 patients had symptoms, including bleeding, pain, swelling, and limited ability to exercise. The venous malformations were in the lower extremities in 7

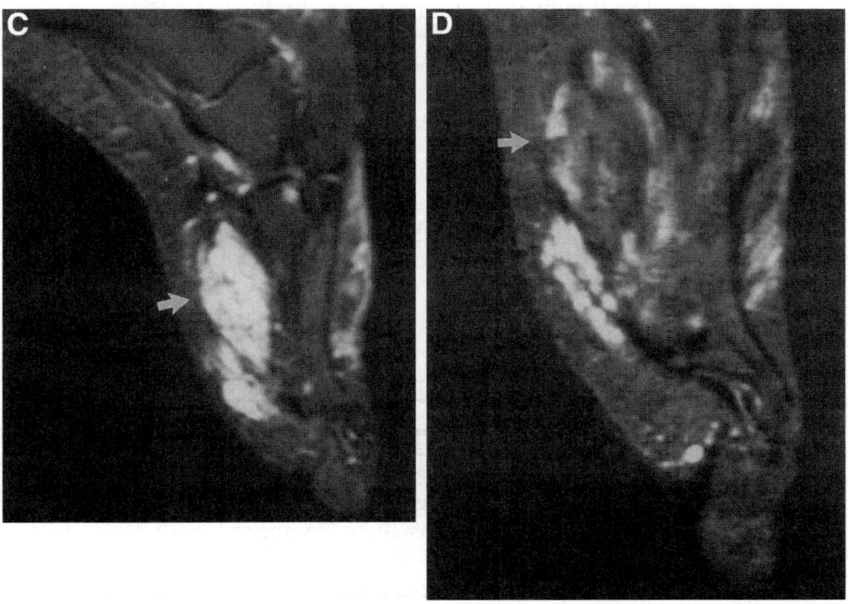

FIGURE 1.—Various imaging methods in a patient with venous malformation of the left foot. C, venous malformation between the fourth and fifth metatarsals as a hyperintense (white) signal on this T_2 MR scan (*arrow*); D, T_2 MR scan shows the same area as C 1 month after direct injection of ethanol into the lesion (*arrow*). Notice the greatly decreased size of the venous malformation, as well as the residual soft-tissue swelling from the procedure. (Courtesy of Shireman PK, McCarthy WJ, Yao JST, et al: Treatment of venous malformations by direct injection with ethanol. *J Vasc Surg* 26:838–844, 1997.)

patients, upper extremities in 3 patients, and flank and buttocks in 2 patients.

Results.—Thirty injection procedures were performed in the 12 patients; 6 patients required just 1 procedure, 3 patients required 2, 2 patients required 3, and 1 patient required 12. Eleven patients had general anesthesia. Blood loss was minimal and 28 procedures were technically successful. About half of the treated venous malformations had skin ulceration, all of which healed with local wound care. In 6 patients, focal venous malformations were injected, and 5 patients had resolution after a single treatment (Fig 1C, D). At a mean of 10 months, all 6 patients were asymptomatic. In 5 patients, extensive venous malformations were injected for discrete, symptomatic areas. Regression was seen in all lesions, and 4 of the 5 patients were asymptomatic at a mean of 23 months. However, multiple treatments were needed as additional areas became problematic.

Discussion.—These results indicate that ethanol sclerosis is a safe and effective adjunct to the management of venous malformations. Ethanol injection is well tolerated and can be used to treat a very localized area without an incision. Extensive lesions may be palliated as symptoms occur.

▶ In recent years, we are coming to depend more and more on the percutaneous injection of noxious substances to induce thrombosis, both in pseudoaneurysms as well as in venous malformations, as described here. Although our experience is limited, it has been generally favorable, and I agree with these authors that ethanol may be the injectate of choice in dealing with venous malformations.

Presentation and Management of Venous Aneurysms

Gillespie DL, Villavicencio JL, Gallagher C, et al (Walter Reed Army Med Ctr, Washington, DC; Uniformed Services Univ of the Health Sciences, Bethesda, Md)

J Vasc Surg 26:845–852, 1997 16–11

Background.—Venous aneurysms can occur in most major veins and may be misdiagnosed as soft-tissue masses or inguinal or femoral hernias. Venous aneurysms of the deep system have been associated with deep venous thrombosis and pulmonary embolism.

Methods.—A retrospective review was conducted of the authors' experience with venous aneurysms during a 22-year period. The presentation and management of these aneurysms were compared with those in the literature.

Results.—There were 39 venous aneurysms treated in 30 patients (14 men and 16 women). The patients were between 3 and 75 years of age. Thirty aneurysms were in the lower extremities, 4 were in the upper extremities, and 5 were in the internal jugular vein. Of the aneurysms in the lower extremities, 57% were in the deep system. Symptoms included a

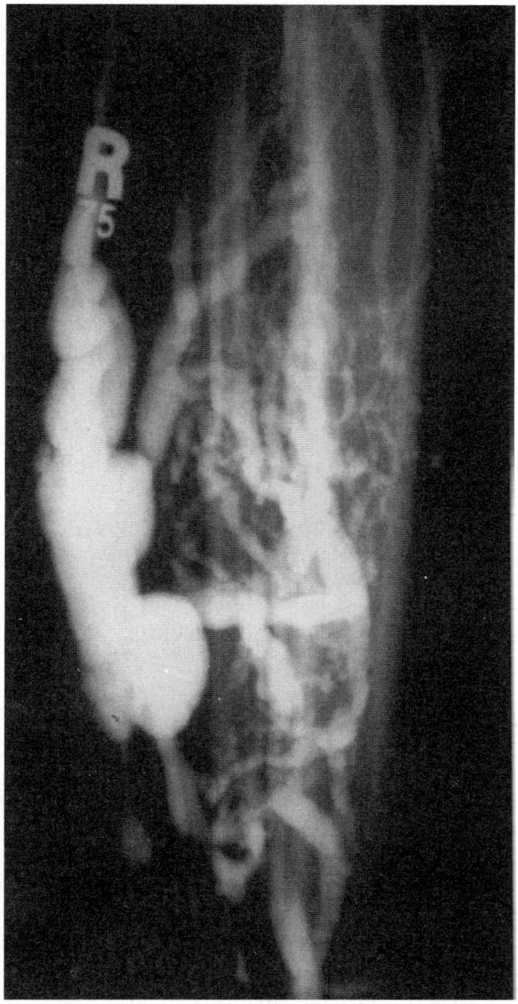

FIGURE 2.—Large venous aneurysm of the calf in a young patient with Klippel-Trenaunay syndrome. These anomalies are frequent in vascular malformations involving the venous system and explain the high incidence of thromboembolism in most series. (Courtesy of Gillespie DL, Villavicencio JL, Gallagher C, et al: Presentation and management of venous aneurysms. *J Vasc Surg* 26:845–852, 1997.)

mass (75% of patients) associated with pain (67% of patients) and swelling (42% of patients). Six patients had thromboembolism, 3 had deep venous thrombosis, and 3 had pulmonary embolism. Seven patients had Klippel-Trenaunay syndrome and aneurysms of the deep venous system (Fig 2). Of 9 patients with aneurysms of the superficial venous system, 8 had a misdiagnosis. Diagnosis was made by phlebography, color flow duplex scanning, continuous-wave Doppler scanning, or MRI. The size of the aneurysms was 1.7 cm to 6.0 cm. Tangential excision was performed in 5 aneurysms and total excision was performed in 23. Seven aneurysms were managed by observation.

Discussion.—Venous aneurysms are unusual vascular malformations that occur at any age. They occur in males and females equally. Most patients report a painful mass of the extremity. Diagnosis is usually made by radiologic examination. Superficial venous aneurysms of the inguinal area are usually misdiagnosed. Thromboembolism is more common in aneurysms of the deep system. In most cases, surgical management is recommended because of potential morbidity.

► Most venous aneurysms are located in the lower extremities. The real hazard with these lesions is their propensity to undergo partial thrombosis and serve as a nidus for pulmonary embolism. In general, significant venous aneurysms should be treated surgically when discovered, usually by tangential excision with preservation of venous patency. Most affected patients present with a painful mass of the extremity, and this eventually leads to the correct diagnosis.

Vein Reconstruction

Venous Reconstructions Using the Superficial Femoral–Popliteal Vein

Hagino RT, Bengtson TD, Fosdick DA, et al (Univ of Texas, Dallas; Dallas Presbyterian Hosp)

J Vasc Surg 26:829–837, 1997 16–12

Background.—In major venous reconstruction, it is difficult to obtain nonthrombogenic, large-caliber conduits that will remain patent in the low-pressure, low-velocity venous system. Large-diameter polytetrafluoroethylene prostheses are often recommended for venous bypass grafting. Reported patency rates of such prostheses at 5.5 to 60 months are 50% to 100%, although acceptable graft longevity requires external supporting rings, proximal arteriovenous fistulas, chronic anticoagulation, antiplatelet therapy, or a combination of these. The autologous spiral vein graft made from greater saphenous vein has excellent patency, but the technique can be lengthy and difficult, and the greater saphenous vein may not be of sufficient quality or length. The feasibility of venous reconstruction with the superficial femoral–popliteal vein was determined.

Methods.—Major venous reconstruction using the superficial femoral–popliteal vein was performed in 7 patients. A retrospective review was conducted of all medical records. Graft patency was established with noninvasive testing and invasive contrast studies. The patients were between 6 and 64 years of age.

Results.—Three central venous reconstructions (Fig 1) and 4 peripheral major venous reconstructions were performed. The superficial femoral–popliteal vein grafts provided an excellent size match. The grafts were of adequate length without enlargement by paneling or spiraling techniques. Postoperative anticoagulation medication was not required. There were no early graft failures. At a mean of 20 months, patency was documented by

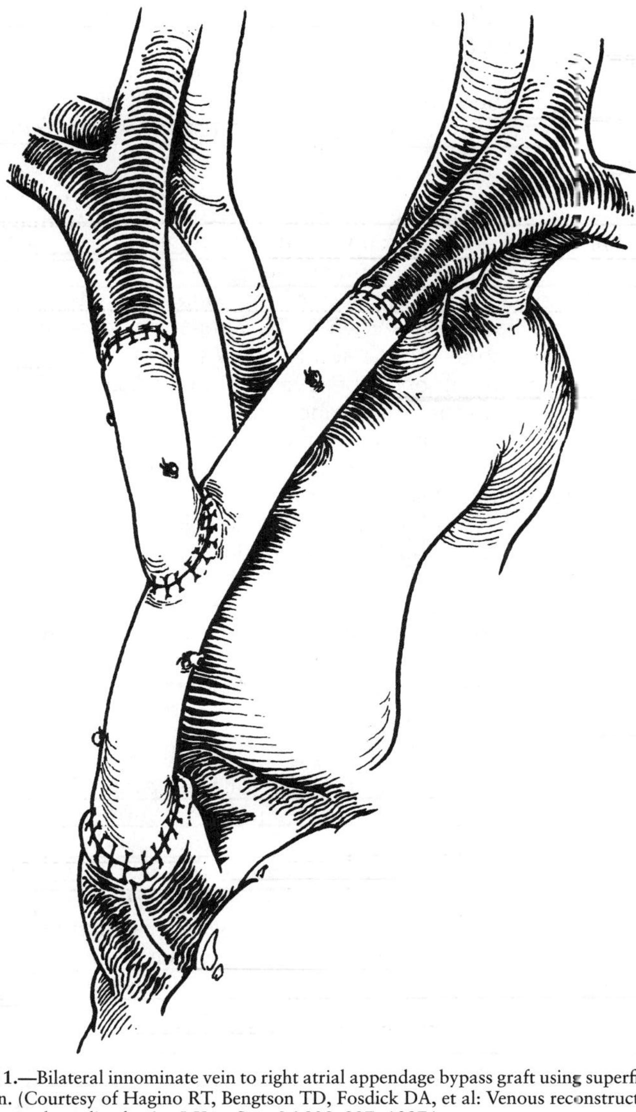

FIGURE 1.—Bilateral innominate vein to right atrial appendage bypass graft using superficial femoral–popliteal vein. (Courtesy of Hagino RT, Bengtson TD, Fosdick DA, et al: Venous reconstruction using the superficial femoral–popliteal vein. *J Vasc Surg* 26:829–837, 1997.)

duplex ultrasound, venogram, or both in all patients. There have been no cases of venous thromboembolism, and only minimal lower extremity venous morbidity has occurred.

Discussion.—Patients who have obstructive iliofemoral venous disease and postphlebitic changes from chronic deep venous thrombosis in the axial veins of the lower limb may have severe donor limb morbidity after the superficial femoral–popliteal vein is removed. Therefore, removing this vein in patients with chronic lower extremity venous insufficiency is not recommended. In selected patients who need large-caliber conduits for venous reconstruction, the superficial femoral–popliteal vein graft is versatile and durable. The superficial femoral–popliteal vein is an excellent conduit for major venous reconstruction because of its size and availability.

► I have to admit that once the group in Dallas gets their teeth into a good idea, they hang on like a snapping turtle. The potential usefulness of the superficial femoral vein (now known as the femoral vein) for reconstruction was demonstrated years ago by Dr. Schulman and associates in New York. Recently, this vein has been shown to be applicable for arterial grafting, especially in infected areas. These authors now show that the vein is useful in major venous reconstructions. I believe of all the indicated uses, this may ultimately turn out to be the most important. We know that large-diameter prosthetics generally do not give durable results when used in venous reconstruction. We also know, through increased experience, that careful harvesting of the femoral vein does not result in major morbidity for most patients. In today's world, if I had to perform a major venous reconstruction, I believe the femoral vein would be my conduit of choice.

Iliac Vein Reconstructions to Treat Acute and Chronic Venous Occlusive Disease

Alimi YS, DiMauro P, Fabre D, et al (Hôpital Nord, Marseille, France)
J Vasc Surg 25:673–681, 1997 16–13

Background.—Replacement of the inferior vena cava (IVC) or the iliac veins with externally supported expanded polytetrafluoroethylene (ePTFE) grafts and distal arteriovenous (AV) fistulas yielded good results in several experimental studies, but the long-term patency of such grafts is unknown. This study reports intermediate-term outcome in 8 consecutive patients treated over a period of 38 months for iliac vein obstruction.

Methods.—The patients, 6 men and 2 women with a mean age of 45.6, underwent venous bypass grafting for the reconstruction of iliac veins. Four had acute and 4 had chronic vein obstruction. In the acute group, reinforced ePTFE grafts were used to treat obstruction caused by May-Thurner syndrome (1 patient), compression of the left common iliac vein by the left internal iliac artery (2 patients), and accidental ligation of the left external iliac vein during cystectomy (1 patient). Causes of chronic obstruction were left iliac deep venous thrombosis (DVT) (2 patients), left and right iliac IVC/DVT (1 patient), and trauma-related right common femoral and external iliac DVT (1 patient). Definitive AV fistulas were created in 5 patients and temporary AV fistulas in 3 (Fig 1D).

Results.—There were no early deaths, and no patient had evidence of pulmonary embolism during the first 30 days after surgery. Fistulographic examination performed systematically before discharge demonstrated pa-

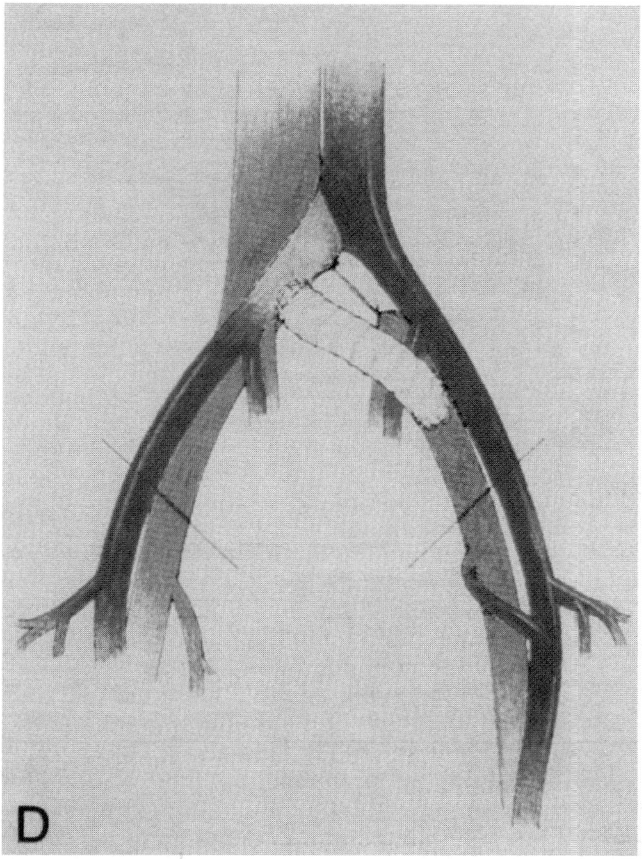

FIGURE 1.—D, Scheme of bypass and of temporary arteriovenous fistula created with last centimeters of great saphenous vein, implanted in superficial femoral artery. (Courtesy of Alimi YS, DiMauro P, Fabre D, et al: Iliac vein reconstructions to treat acute and chronic venous occlusive disease. *J Vasc Surg* 25:673–681, 1997.)

tency in 7 of 8 grafts. Five patients required secondary surgical procedures. During a mean follow-up period of 19.5 months, 1 patient had died of an unknown cause (without evidence of pulmonary embolism). One patient with a patent graft was totally asymptomatic when lost to follow-up at 11 months. Twenty-three months after reconstruction, a patient in the chronic obstruction group underwent thrombectomy of the graft and resection of the AV fistula after a false aneurysm on the graft implantation of the AV fistula occurred. All 7 patients with a patent graft are currently taking warfarin.

Conclusion.—Patients who underwent direct reconstruction of iliac vein obstruction with a large-diameter, reinforced ePTFE graft associated with a temporary or definitive distal AV fistula had good intermediate-term results. The procedure is recommended for cases of permanent compression of iliac veins or for selected cases of symptomatic benign iliac vein obstruction.

▶ Although these authors state that prosthetic bypass in the iliac-femoral region for treatment of a variety of chronic iliac vein occlusions provides durable results, I have my doubts. If I felt absolutely compelled to recommend some treatment for chronic iliac venous occlusion, perhaps I would try the unconventional treatment recommended by Dr. Dake from Stanford, namely urokinase followed by venous angioplasty and stents. On the other hand, I would probably choose to perform venous bypass using the superficial femoral vein (see Abstract 16–12). On balance, I am not convinced the use of prosthetic bypasses ever produces durable results.

Miscellaneous

Hemodynamic Evaluation of Foot Venous Compression Devices

Ricci MA, Fisk P, Knight S, et al (Univ of Vermont, Burlington)
J Vasc Surg 26:803–808, 1997 16–14

Introduction.—For prophylaxis of deep venous thrombosis, intermittent pneumatic compression has been proved to be a safe and effective method. Application of devices to the calf or thigh is often precluded by major trauma, and there is a need for application of a device to the foot. A unique venous structure and physiologic mechanism is found in the foot. Four different compressive devices were used to evaluate the venous hemodynamic change produced and were compared with a commonly used calf intermittent pneumatic compression device. Whether calf-only devices would produce more pronounced alterations in the venous hemodynamics was investigated.

Methods.—There were 27 volunteers who had each device applied followed by duplex scanning to determine the venous hemodynamics at the common femoral vein and at the popliteal vein. Measurements were taken of resting peak systolic velocity; maximum venous velocity during device activation; acceleration, the slope of the line from resting systolic velocity to maximum venous velocity; and return time from maximum venous velocity back to resting systolic velocity. Two commercially available foot devices were evaluated, foot compressive device 1 and foot compressive device 2; an experimental mechanical foot device; an experimental pneumatic foot device; and a calf-only intermittent pneumatic compression device.

Results.—In the common femoral vein, the resting peak systolic velocity was higher than in the popliteal vein. At either the popliteal vein or common femoral vein, the initial resting systolic velocity was not statistically significant between the 5 experimental groups, but the resting systolic velocity was higher in the common femoral vein than in the calf. With the foot compressive device 2 and the calf-only intermittent pneumatic compression device, maximum venous velocity was significantly higher at the popliteal vein level, but this difference decreased at the common femoral

17 Portal Hypertension

Experimental, Clinical, and Metabolic Results of Side-to-Side Portacaval Shunt for Intractable Cirrhotic Ascites

Orloff MJ, Orloff MS, Orloff SL, et al (Univ of California, San Diego)

J Am Coll Surg 184:557–570, 1997 17–1

Background.—Approximately 10% of patients with ascites from cirrhosis fail to respond to medical therapy, and mortality in such cases is high. Intractable cirrhotic ascites appears to be initiated by sinusoidal hypertension resulting from hepatic venous outflow obstruction. Treatment involves the use of portal-systemic shunts to decompress the liver, achieving sinusoidal decompression by shunting splanchnic blood away from the liver and by improving the outflow of hepatic blood. Outcome is reported for a group of patients with cirrhosis and truly intractable ascites who underwent side-to-side portacaval shunt.

Methods.—Studies in patients were preceded by experiments in dogs with hepatic outflow obstruction and massive ascites produced by direct ligation of the hepatic veins. Animal studies measured the effect of portacaval shunts on ascites, thoracic duct lymph flow, and aldosterone secretion. Patients had a mean age of 47.3; 75% were men and 91% were alcoholic. Ascites had failed to respond to intensive medical therapy for 5 to 24 months. A postshunt pressure gradient between the portal vein and inferior vena cava (IVC) was required and obtained in all patients. Postoperative monitoring included serial measurements of cardiovascular, pulmonary, and hepatic and renal function; fluid, electrolyte, and acid-base balance; and blood count and blood coagulation. Patients and their families were counseled at length about dietary requirements and abstinence from alcohol. Follow-up continued monthly for 1 year, then every 3 months.

Results.—Experimental studies showed end-to-side portacaval shunts to be much less effective than side-to-side portacaval shunts. In the clinical study, patients who underwent side-to-side portacaval shunt had a significant reduction in mean portal vein-IVC pressure gradient from 282 mm saline to 4 mm. Ascites was permanently relieved in all patients, and none required diuretic therapy. Thirty-day mortality was 6%; long-term survival was 75% at 5 years, 74% at 10 years, and 73% at 15 years (Fig 1). Terminal ascites developed in 2 patients who died of hepatoma and 1 who died of heart failure. Most patients (91%) abstained from alcohol during

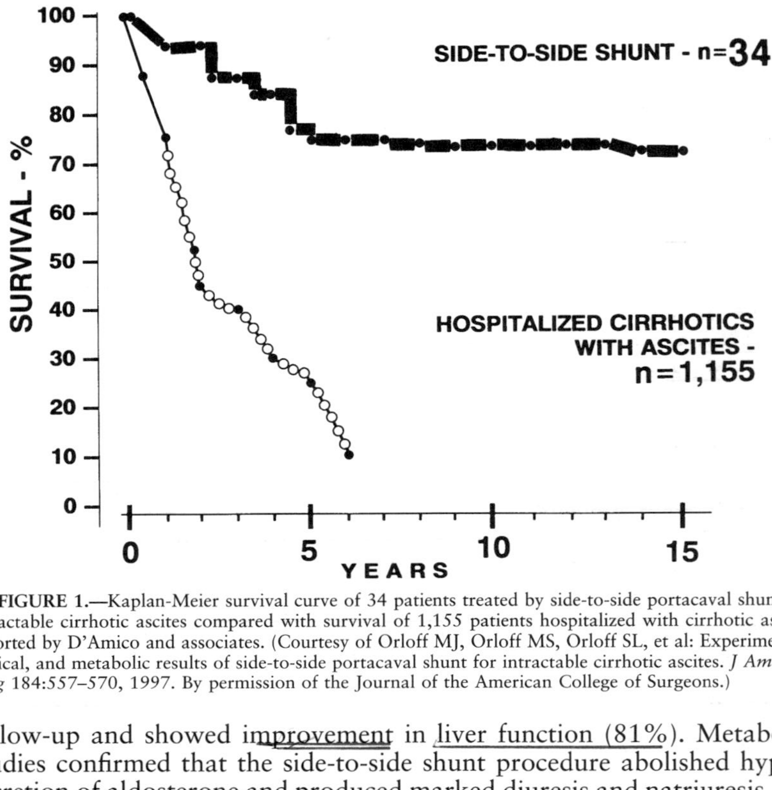

FIGURE 1.—Kaplan-Meier survival curve of 34 patients treated by side-to-side portacaval shunt for intractable cirrhotic ascites compared with survival of 1,155 patients hospitalized with cirrhotic ascites reported by D'Amico and associates. (Courtesy of Orloff MJ, Orloff MS, Orloff SL, et al: Experimental, clinical, and metabolic results of side-to-side portacaval shunt for intractable cirrhotic ascites. *J Am Coll Surg* 184:557–570, 1997. By permission of the Journal of the American College of Surgeons.)

follow-up and showed improvement in liver function (81%). Metabolic studies confirmed that the side-to-side shunt procedure abolished hypersecretion of aldosterone and produced marked diuresis and natriuresis. All patients had a permanently patent portacaval anastomosis.

Conclusion.—With careful patient selection, education, and life-long follow-up, side-to-side portacaval shunt offers an effective treatment of intractable cirrhotic ascites. Operative mortality was low, and long-term survival was higher than previously reported in such cases.

► One of the most serious complications of portal hypertension is intractable ascites refractory to medical therapy, occurring in about 10% of patients with cirrhotic ascites. Patients with intractable cirrhotic ascites have an extraordinarily high mortality rate, ranging from 20% to 50% at 1 year. The family Orloff performed side-to-side portacaval shunts in 34 such patients, with permanent relief of ascites in all. Five-year survival was a remarkable 75%. It seems clear that the side-to-side portacaval shunt is established as effective therapy in this difficult patient group, and remarkable survival can be achieved when combined with a dedicated program of patient care and education.

Endoscopic Sclerotherapy Compared With Percutaneous Transjugular Intrahepatic Portosystemic Shunt After Initial Sclerotherapy in Patients With Acute Variceal Hemorrhage

Cello JP, Ring EJ, Olcott EW, et al (San Francisco Gen Hosp; Univ of California, San Francisco; Stanford Univ, Calif; et al)

Ann Intern Med 126:858–865, 1997 17–2

Background.—Endoscopic sclerotherapy became the preferred treatment for acute variceal hemorrhage during the past 15 years, but its status in the long-term care of patients with bleeding varices has been questioned. Newer techniques, such as band ligation and pharmacologic agents, are also selected over surgical shunting. In a recent study, however, surgical portacaval shunting was associated with a significantly reduced need for rehospitalization for recurrent variceal hemorrhage compared with sclerotherapy. The efficacy of these 2 treatment methods was assessed in a randomized, controlled trial.

Methods.—Study participants were 49 adults hospitalized at 3 teaching hospitals from November 1991 to December 1995. All received endoscopic sclerotherapy at the time of diagnosis. Twenty-five were assigned to sclerotherapy and 24 to transjugular intrahepatic portosystemic shunt (TIPS), a nonsurgical procedure in which an expandable metal prosthesis is used to connect an intrahepatic portal vein with an adjacent hepatic vein. These therapies were compared for their success in preventing recurrent variceal hemorrhage.

Results.—The 2 groups were similar in pretreatment clinical and laboratory variables, except that the TIPS group had a worse Child-Pugh score and higher blood transfusion requirements before randomization. Mean

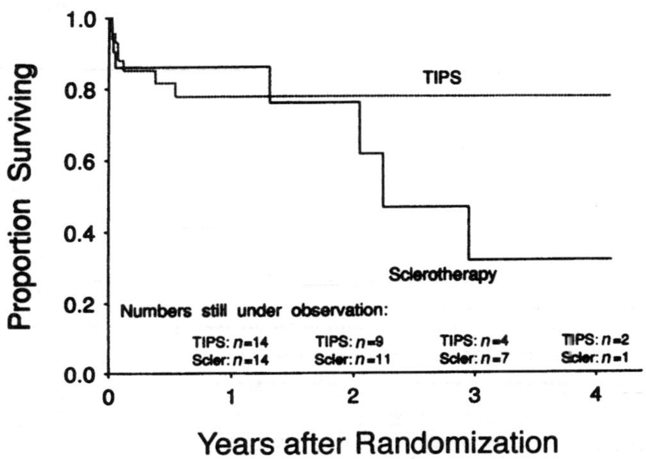

FIGURE.—Adjusted survival curves for patients randomly assigned to transjugular intrahepatic portosystemic shunt (TIPS) or sclerotherapy. (Courtesy of Cello JP, Ring EJ, Olcott EW, et al: Endoscopic sclerotherapy compared with percutaneous transjugular intrahepatic portosystemic shunt after initial sclerotherapy in patients with acute variceal hemorrhage. *Ann Intern Med* 126:858–865, 1997.)

follow-up was 567 days in the sclerotherapy group and 575 days in the TIPS group. Varices were obliterated more reliably in the TIPS group, and patients who underwent TIPS were significantly less likely to rebleed from esophageal varices than patients receiving sclerotherapy (3 of 24 vs. 12 of 25, respectively). The other follow-up measures, including index hospitalization survival, duration of hospitalization for variceal bleeding, blood transfusion needs after randomization, and total health care costs, did not differ significantly between groups. After 2 years there was a trend toward improved survival with TIPS (Figure).

Conclusion.—Although TIPS was more effective than sclerotherapy in obliterating esophageal varices and reducing rebleeding events, morbidity and health care costs did not differ significantly between the 2 therapies. There was slightly better survival in patients treated with TIPS.

▶ Although a few benefits appear to favor the TIPS group, the critical variable of survival was statistically the same in the 2 groups. These authors concluded, and I believe appropriately, from this well-conducted prospective, randomized study, that TIPS was more effective than sclerotherapy in obliterating varices and reducing rebleeding events; however, TIPS did not decrease morbidity after randomization or decrease health care cost. Any increase in survival attributable to TIPS was not statistically significant. It seems, in most medical centers in America, portal hypertensive patients have been taken away from vascular surgery and are now shared between the general surgeons and the radiologists. Who can complain about this? (See also Abstract 17–3.)

Transjugular Intrahepatic Portosystemic Shunts Compared With Endoscopic Sclerotherapy for the Prevention of Recurrent Variceal Hemorrhage: A Randomized, Controlled Trial

Sanyal AJ, Freedman AM, Luketic VA, et al (Med College of Virginia, Richmond)

Ann Intern Med 126:849–857, 1997 17–3

Introduction.—For patients with recurrent variceal hemorrhage, transjugular intrahepatic portosystemic shunts (TIPS) help avoid the risks associated with anesthesia and major surgery by functioning like side-to-side portacaval shunts. The efficacy of TIPS has not been compared with other treatments in controlled trials. The efficacy and safety of TIPS was prospectively compared with endoscopic sclerotherapy for the prevention of recurrent variceal hemorrhage in a randomized, controlled trial.

Methods.—One hundred patients with cirrhosis were assessed at a mean of 10 days after an episode of acute variceal bleeding. Twenty patients had to be excluded: 6 because of portal venous thrombosis, 3 because of hepatoma, 6 because of florid alcoholic hepatitis, and 5 refused to give consent. Forty-one patients underwent TIPS and 39 underwent sclerotherapy by freehand injections of 5% Na morrhuate at 2- to 3-week intervals.

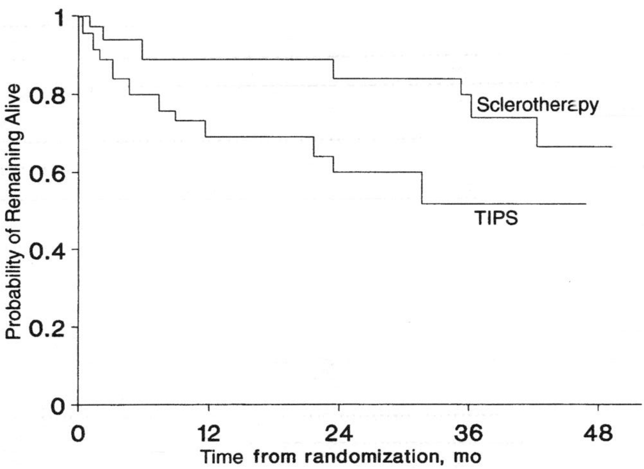

FIGURE 3.—Kaplan-Meier analysis of the risk for death, plotted as the probability of remaining alive over time. Patients in the sclerotherapy group had a definite survival advantage over those in the transjugular intrahepatic portosystemic shunts (TIPS) group (P = 0.03). (Courtesy of Sanyal AJ, Freeman AM, Luketic VA, et al: Transjugular intrahepatic portosystemic shunts compared with endoscopic sclerotherapy for the prevention of recurrent variceal hemorrhage: A randomized, controlled trial. *Ann Intern Med* 126:849–857, 1997).

Patients were followed up for rebleeding and survival (primary end points), and complications and rates of rehospitalization (secondary end points). Patients receiving sclerotherapy who rebled from varices were offered TIPS.

Results.—At a mean of 1,000 days, recurrent gastrointestinal bleeding resulted from variceal hemorrhage for 9 patients in the TIPS group and 8 patients in the sclerotherapy group; from portal gastropathy for 1 patient in each group; and from gastric lipoma for 1 patient in the sclerotherapy group. Mortality was significantly higher in the TIPS group than in the sclerotherapy group (Fig 3). Causes of death were variceal bleeding for 5 patients in the TIPS group and 3 patients in the sclerotherapy group, sepsis (3 and 2 patients, respectively), liver failure (2 patients in each group), hepatoma (1 and 0 patients, respectively), and hemoperitoneum (1 and 0 patients, respectively). The most common complication in the TIPS group was encephalopathy (12 patients), whereas in the sclerotherapy group, the most common complication was pain (10 patients). There were no between-group differences in rates of rehospitalization.

Conclusions.—Long-term incidence of rebleeding was similar for patients in the TIPS and sclerotherapy groups. Survival was significantly better for patients in the sclerotherapy group compared with those in the TIPS group.

▶ This carefully conducted prospective, randomized trial compared the efficacy and safety of TIPS with that of repeated endoscopic sclerotherapy for the prevention of late variceal rebleeding in stable patients who survived an episode of esophageal variceal bleeding. With a follow-up of almost 3 years, both therapies were about equally successful in preventing rebleeding; however, sclerotherapy appeared to be superior to TIPS with respect to patient survival. The more we learn about portal hypertension, the more it becomes obvious that the less we do to these patients, the better off they seem to be. For the present, it appears that we should give sclerotherapy a generous trial before considering either TIPS or portal decompressive surgery. (See also Abstract 17–2).

Shunt Surgery During the Era of Liver Transplantation

Rikkers LF, Jin G, Langnas AN, et al (Univ of Nebraska Med Ctr, Omaha)
Ann Surg 226:51–57, 1997 17–4

Background.—For many years, surgical shunts were the only method to control variceal bleeding permanently. More recently, liver transplantation and other therapies have reduced the number of shunt operations being performed. This article reviews the use of shunts in managing bleeding caused by portal hypertension.

Methods.—Over 10 years, 71 patients with chronic liver disease received surgical shunts. Forty-four patients were considered good candidates for a potential future transplant because of good functional reserve (group 1). The remaining 27 patients were not good candidates because of either age, uncontrolled alcoholism, cardiopulmonary disease, mental re-

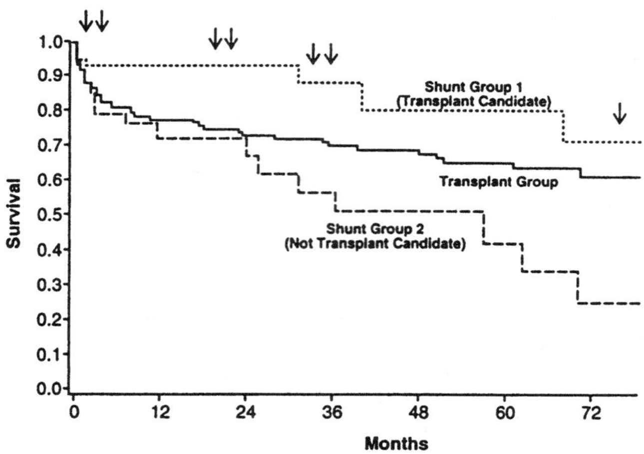

FIGURE 1.—Kaplan-Meier survival analysis of shunt group 1 (*dotted line*), transplant group (*continuous line*). and shunt group 2 (*broken line*). The *vertical lines* on the shunt group 1 curve indicate when patients from that group underwent liver transplantation. Survival of shunt group 1 is significantly different from that of the transplant group ($P = 0.003$) and shunt group 2 ($P = 0.018$) at 1 year (log-rank test). At 5 years, the shunt group 1 and transplant group curves are no longer different, but both are significantly different from the shunt group 2 curve ($P = 0.006$ and $P = 0.029$, respectively). (Courtesy of Rikkers LF, Jin G, Langnas AN, et al: Shunt surgery during the era of liver transplantation. *Ann Surg Oncol* 226:51–57, 1997. Copyright © the Society of Surgical Oncology.)

tardation, or refusal to receive blood transfusion (group 2). A separate group of 180 patients, who had a history of variceal bleeding and who received a liver transplant soon after referral, were also studied. Mean follow-up for group 1, group 2, and the transplant group was 33 ± 30, 33 ± 31, and 37 ± 29 months, respectively.

Findings.—Not surprisingly, the transplant group had more advanced liver disease, and thus significantly higher operative mortality (within 30 days of surgery) rates than either group 1 or group 2 (19% vs. 5% or 7%, respectively). However, by 1 year after surgery, survival in group 1 was significantly superior to that in group 2 or in the transplant group (Fig 1). By 5 years after surgery, survival in group 1 was no longer significantly different from that in the transplant group, but survival in group 2 was significantly worse compared to that in the other groups. Eight patients in group 1 have died, with 3 deaths attributable to hepatic failure; but 7 patients in this group received a liver transplant, and 6 of these patients are still alive. Sixteen patients in group 2 have died, with 9 deaths attributable to hepatic failure.

Conclusions.—Shunts remain a viable option as a bridge to liver transplantation in patients with a good hepatic reserve. Shunts can also improve survival in patients who are not good candidates for transplantation.

► Any attempt to accurately assess the role of shunt surgery in cirrhotic variceal bleeders in the era of liver transplantation is ultimately dependent upon the individual centers' indications for transplantation. More and more, liver transplantation strikes me as a solution in search of a problem. We now find transplantation recommended for advanced alcoholism in patients who continue to drink or have only been abstinent for a very short time, patients with advanced liver cancer, etc. Only a few years ago, these indications would have been accepted by no one as appropriate. Within the limits of one's own philosophy concerning the propriety of liver transplant for alcoholic cirrhosis, these authors conclude that shunt surgery may serve as an excellent long-term bridge to transplantation in selected patients with portal hypertension. This article mandates careful study.

Computed Radiography of the Chest in Patients With Paraesophageal Varices: Diagnostic Accuracy and Characteristic Findings

Lee SJ, Lee KS, Kim SA, et al (Sung Kyun Kwan Univ, Seoul, South Korea)
AJR 170:1527–1531, 1998 17–5

Introduction.—The rate of reported visibility of paraesophageal varices on chest radiography ranges from 5% to 8%. One hundred consecutive patients with portal hypertension underwent computed radiography of the chest to determine its accuracy in detecting CT-diagnosed paraesophageal varices and to describe characteristic radiographic observations.

Methods.—All patients had clinical and radiologic evidence of portal hypertension. Patients underwent computed radiographs of the chest and

percutaneous transluminal, restenosis after, probucol and multivitamins in prevention of, 7
patch, *vs.* balloon, as adjuvant treatment to surgical thrombectomy of hemodialysis grafts, 349
percutaneous transluminal
alone or with primary stenting in femoropopliteal obstructions, 144
carotid, hemodynamic cerebral ischemia and microembolic signals detected during, 140
carotid, with stent placement, carotid endarterectomy for progressive carotid stenosis after, 141
for claudication, intermittent, 134
coronary *(see* Angioplasty, coronary, percutaneous transluminal *above)*
failure to prolong patency of ePTFE arteriovenous grafts, 347
prophylactic, for arteriovenous ePTFE grafts, cost efficacy of, 351
for stenosis, infrainguinal graft-related, 393
for stenosis, "short," of failing vein grafts, 146
stenting with, *vs.* endarterectomy for carotid artery stenosis, cost of, 139
vs. patch angioplasty as adjuvant treatment to surgical thrombectomy of hemodialysis grafts, 349
subintimal, of infrapopliteal occlusions in critically ischemic limbs, 135
Angiotensin
-converting enzyme inhibition, effect on endothelial function in insulin-dependent diabetes mellitus, 57
Ankle
-brachial index, ability to detect lower extremity atherosclerotic disease progression, 174
Antibiotic
-bonded grafts for vascular graft infection, 398
-treated cryopreserved aortic allografts, in situ replacement for vascular graft infection (in dog), 396
Antibody(ies)
antiplatelet, heparin-associated, heparin-bonded grafts induce platelet aggregation in presence of, 399
to cardiolipin and failure of peripheral vein bypasses, 310
Chlamydia pneumoniae, elevated, and cardiovascular events in survivors of myocardial infarction, 38
Anticoagulation
oral
for carotid artery dissections, traumatic, from blunt softball injuries, 410
long-term, effect on bone mass in patients with previous hemispheric infarction and nonrheumatic atrial fibrillation, 49
after popliteal artery trauma improves limb salvage, 407
therapy
for atheroma of aortic arch, mobile, 236
for patients with peripheral macroemboli from thoracic aortic pathology, 235
vs. antiplatelet therapy after coronary stent placement for myocardial infarction, outcome of, 43
Antihypertensive
therapy reduces rupture after blunt aortic injury, 411
Antimicrobial
prophylaxis in vascular surgery, duration of, 229
Antiplatelet
antibodies, heparin-associated, heparin-bonded grafts induce platelet aggregation in presence of, 399
vs. anticoagulation therapy after coronary stent placement for myocardial infarction, outcome of, 43
Antisense
basic fibroblast growth factor gene transfer reduces early intimal thickening after femoral artery injury (in rabbit), 100
Antithrombin
-independent inhibitors, thrombin inactivation by, 47
Aorta
abdominal
rupture, spontaneous nonaneurysmal, case reports, 292
surgery, retroperitoneal closure after, Preclude Pericardial Membrane for, 289
tailoring, for renal, visceral, and lower extremity malperfusion after acute aortic dissection, 283
allograft, cryopreserved
in situ repair of aortobronchial, aorotoesophageal, and aortoenteric fistulae with, 397
in situ replacement for vascular graft infection (in dog), 396

aneurysm (*see* Aneurysm, aortic)
arch, mobile atheroma of, as underestimated source of embolization, 236
ascending, endarterectomy of, 237
atherosclerosis causing infected aortic aneurysm, 272
dissection, acute
  abdominal aortic tailoring for renal, visceral, and lower extremity malperfusion after, 283
  type A, 20-year follow-up, 263
grafts, prosthetic, infection, in situ arterial allografts for, 395
infrarenal
  atherosclerotic, nonaneurysmal, rupture of, 291
  diameter, relationship to age, gender, race, and body size, 267
  reconstruction, elective, impact of clinical pathway for, 295
  replacement, albumin-impregnated prosthetic graft for, 402
  residual, natural history after infrarenal abdominal aortic aneurysm repair, 278
injury, blunt, 411
intra-aortic balloon pump counterpulsation, prolonged, implications for vascular surgeon with, 331
mega, reversed elephant trunk procedure for, 265
perfusion
  distal, during aortic aneurysm repairs, effect on incidence of neurologic deficit, 258
  distal, impact on liver function during thoracoabdominal and descending thoracic aortic repair, 251
  retrograde, during thoracoabdominal aortic aneurysm repair, 257
perivisceral, rupture of, 246
reconstruction
  elective, aprotinin in, 223
  prosthetic, aneurysms after, noninfected false, morbidity and mortality of reconstructive surgery for, 284
smooth muscle cells, protein kinase C isoforms in, 96
surgery
  colitis after, *Clostridium difficile,* 290
  lung injury after, acute, 82
thoracic, 235
  descending, repair, impact of distal aortic and visceral perfusion on liver function during, 251
  hematoma of, intramural, fate of, 241
  hematoma of, intramural, MRI of, 243
  intimal disease of, 235
  pathology, diagnosis and management of patients with peripheral macroemboli from, 235
  rupture of, traumatic, surgical indications and timing of repair of, 412
thoracoabdominal
  repair, impact of distal aortic and visceral perfusion on liver function during, 251
  replacement, cardiac function as risk factor for paralysis in, 262
  surgery, renal failure after, 247
transections, traumatic, clamp-sew technique for, 264
Aortitis
  abdominal aneurysmal, in Behçet's disease, endovascular treatment of, 130
Aortobifemoral
  bypass, laparoscopic, 147
Aortobronchial
  fistulae, in situ repair with cryopreserved aortic homografts, 397
Aortoenteric
  fistulae, in situ repair with cryopreserved aortic homografts, 397
Aortoesophageal
  fistulae, in situ repair with cryopreserved aortic homografts, 397
Aortoiliac
  aneurysm, anastomotic, noninfected, endovascular graft for, 123
  disease, 289
    occlusive, angiography of, CT *vs.* intra-arterial digital subtraction, 190
Aortorenal
  bypass, supraceliac, 297
Apolipoprotein(a)
  induces monocyte chemotactic activity in vascular endothelial cells, 103
Aprotinin
  in aortic reconstruction, elective, 223
Arteriography
  (*See also* Angiography)
  carbon dioxide, livedo reticularis, rhabdomyolysis, massive intestinal infarction, and death after, 203
  magnetic resonance, in distal lower extremity revascularization, 202

preoperative, for failing grafts, selective use of duplex ultrasound to replace, 390
vs. ultrasound, color duplex, for imaging infrapopliteal arterial lesions, 165
Arterioles
coronary, integrin signaling transduces shear stress–dependent vasodilation of, 104
Arteriovenous
fistula
for hemodialysis access, survival of, in U.S., 346
stent-graft, 339
graft, hemodialysis (*see* Hemodialysis, access, graft)
Arteritis
temporal, diagnosis with color duplex ultrasound, 158
Artery(ies)
allograft, in situ, for aortic prosthetic infection, 395
blood pressure, segmental, in lower extremity arterial evaluation, 170
carotid (*see* Carotid, artery)
celiac, disease, detection by duplex ultrasound, importance of diastolic velocities in, 196
cerebral (*see* Cerebral, artery)
coronary (*see* Coronary, artery)
distal
lower extremity, evaluation with two-dimensional MR digital subtraction angiography, 168
reconstruction for embolic and hemodynamic disease, 378
endothelial dysfunction, hyperhomocysteinemia as risk factor for, 68
enlargement, flow-induced, inhibited by suppression of nitric oxide synthase activity, 79
femoral (*see* Femoral, artery)
femoropopliteal, obstructions, balloon angioplasty with primary stenting *vs.* angioplasty alone in, 144
graft, autogenous, for carotid artery replacement during operation for neck malignancy, 368
iliac
aneurysm, noninfected anastomotic, endovascular graft for, 123
dissection after bifurcated AneuRx graft for abdominal aortic aneurysm, 127
infrainguinal, reconstruction, local anesthesia for, 327
infrapopliteal, lesions, imaging with color duplex ultrasound *vs.* arteriography, 165
innominate (*see* Innominate, artery)
intercostal, reattachment during thoracoabdominal aortic aneurysm repair, importance of, 249
intra-arterial thrombolysis, limitations of, 149
lower extremity
disease, with renal artery atherosclerosis, 302
evaluation, segmental arterial blood pressures in, 170
mesenteric
disease, detection by duplex ultrasound, importance of diastolic velocities in, 196
resistance, nitric oxide production in, flow-dependent, direct in vivo measurement of (in dog), 83
occlusion
proximal, upper limb, combined treatment approach with endovascular stents, 138
thrombotic, dissolution by ultrasound and dodecafluoropentane emulsion, 117
occlusive disease, magnetic resonance spectroscopy in, dynamic phosphorus-31, 87
peripheral, biochemical composition of, as examined with near-infrared Raman spectroscopy, 89
popliteal (*see* Popliteal, artery)
pulmonary artery catheterization
routine, effect on morbidity and mortality of elective vascular surgery, 224
utility of hemodynamic measurements acquired by, 226
renal (*see* Renal, artery)
smooth muscle cells, heparin inhibits thrombin-induced mitogen-activated protein kinase signaling in (in baboon), 50
stenosis, multiple, in vitro evaluation using three-dimensional power Doppler angiography, 172
tibial, anterior, optimal methods for autogenous bypass to, 318
trauma, 407
neointimal hyperplasia after, inhibition of leukocyte and platelet adhesion reduces (in rabbit), 45
walls, lower extremity, detection of *Chlamydia pneumoniae* in atherosclerotic plaques in, 31

Arthroplasty
  hip, total, thrombosis after, deep venous, detection with technetium-99m-labeled tissue plasminogen activator, 180
  knee, total
    with cement, tourniquet release during, transesophageal echocardiography for emboli immediately after, 444
    thrombosis after, deep venous, detection with technetium-99m-labeled tissue plasminogen activator, 180
  thrombosis after, deep venous, ultrasound screening before hospital discharge for, 442
Ascites
  cirrhotic, retractable, results of side-to-side portacaval shunt for, 477
Asians
  incidence of idiopathic deep venous thrombosis and secondary thromboembolism in, 435
Aspirin
  early use in acute ischemic stroke, 42
  /ticlopidine after coronary stent placement for myocardial infarction, 44
Atheroma
  mobile, of aortic arch, as underestimated source of embolization, 236
Atherosclerosis
  aneurysm in perivisceral aorta due to, rupture of, 246
  aortic
    infected aortic aneurysm due to, 272
    infrarenal, nonaneurysmal, rupture of, 291
  carotid
    Chlamydia pneumoniae, cytomegalovirus, and herpes simplex virus in, 32
    Chlamydia pneumoniae infection in, distribution of, 34
    insulin and, serum, 56
    mast cell distribution, activation, and phenotype in, 116
    plaques in, echolucency of computerized ultrasound images of, association with increased levels of triglyceride-rich lipoproteins and increased plaque lipid content, 160
    risk of, and body iron stores, 19
  changes in carotid artery bulb as measured by B-mode ultrasound, association with extent of coronary atherosclerosis, 12
  coronary
    dilator responses of epicardial coronary arteries in, effects of conjugated estrogens and tamoxifen on (in monkey), 60
    extent of, association with atherosclerotic changes in carotid artery bulb as measured by B-mode ultrasound, 12
    plaques in, ultrasound of, ECG-gated 3D intravascular, 198
    progression, role of cholesteryl ester transfer protein gene variant in, 22
  development accelerated by *Chlamydia pneumoniae* infection, prevention with azithromycin (in rabbit), 36
  intracranial, stenosis from, natural history by serial angiography, 382
  lower extremity
    progression of, ability of ankle-brachial index to detect, 174
    in young adults, carotid duplex in, 374
  mesenteric ischemia due to, chronic, surgical therapy results for, 304
  plaques in lower extremity artery walls, detection of *Chlamydia pneumoniae* in, 31
  progression and smoking, 15
  renal artery
    carotid and lower extremity arterial disease and, 302
    stenosis due to, hemodynamically significant, MR angiographic features of, 191
    stenosis due to, unilateral, contralateral renal parenchymal injury with, 300
Atrial
  fibrillation
    nonrheumatic, and previous hemispheric infarction, long-term oral anticoagulation reduces bone mass in patients with, 49
    patients, warfarin use in, 217
Aurintricarboxylic acid
  inhibition of leukocyte and platelet adhesion reduces neointimal hyperplasia after arterial injury (in rabbit), 45
Axillobifemoral
  bypass, elective *vs.* emergent, 293

Azathioprine
  for saphenous vein allograft bypass surgery, 394
Azithromycin
  for *Chlamydia pneumoniae* prevents development of atherosclerosis (in rabbit), 36
  in myocardial infarction survivors, and elevated *Chlamydia pneumoniae* antibodies and cardiovascular events, 38

B

Bacterial
  etiology of infected aortic aneurysms, 273
Balloon
  angioplasty (*see* Angioplasty, percutaneous transluminal)
  pump counterpulsation, intra-aortic, prolonged, implications for vascular surgeon with, 331
  thrombectomy in occluded vein grafts, intimal hyperplasia after (in dog), 314
Basic fibroblast growth factor (*see* Fibroblast, growth factor, basic)
Behçet's disease
  aortitis in, abdominal aneurysmal, endovascular treatment of, 130
Beta-blockers
  aortic rupture after blunt injury reduced by, 411
  dosages, and mortality after myocardial infarction, 233
Beta-carotene
  supplements, effect on incidence of major coronary events in men with previous myocardial infarction, 17
Biochemical
  composition of peripheral arteries examined with near-infrared Raman spectroscopy, 89
  markers of exercise-induced inflammatory response, effect of exercise training for intermittent claudication on, 26
Biology
  vascular, 92
Blacks
  renal artery repair in, 299
Blood
  cell, red
    aggregation induced by acquired dysfibrinogenemia causing digital ischemia and gangrene, 353
    transfusions, perioperative, limiting in vascular patients, 220
  flow-induced arterial enlargement inhibited by suppression of nitric oxide synthase activity (in rat), 79
  oxygen saturation in superior mesenteric vein, in vivo MR imaging measurements for diagnosis of chronic mesenteric ischemia, 195
  pressure
    arterial, segmental, in lower extremity arterial evaluation, 170
    long-term, carotid endarterectomy does not affect, 366
  velocity, middle cerebral artery, during carotid endarterectomy with Javid *vs.* Pruitt-Inahara shunt, 153
  viscosity and elevated carotid intima-media thickness in men and women, 14
Body
  iron stores
    risk of carotid atherosclerosis and, 19
    risk of myocardial infarction and, in men, 21
  size related to infrarenal aortic diameter, 267
Bone
  mass in patients with previous hemispheric infarction and nonrheumatic atrial fibrillation, long-term oral anticoagulation reduces, 49
Bowel
  ischemia after endovascular *vs.* open abdominal aortic aneurysm repair, 133
Brachial
  -ankle index, ability to detect lower extremity atherosclerotic disease progression, 174
  plexus injury with vascular injuries of thoracic outlet, aggressive management of, 418
Brain
  damage, ischemic, after middle cerebral artery occlusion, effect of CP101,606 on volume of (in cat), 69
  edema, cytotoxic, after middle cerebral artery occlusion, effect of CP101,606 on (in cat), 69
  infarct size, effect of ZD9379 on (in rat), 70
Buerger's disease
  iloprost in, 211

Buttocks
  venous malformations in, direct injection of ethanol for, 464
Bypass
  aortobifemoral, laparoscopic, 147
  aortorenal, supraceliac, 297
  autogenous, to anterior tibial artery, optimal methods for, 318
  axillobifemoral, elective *vs.* emergent, 293
  coronary
    aneurysms in patients undergoing, abdominal aortic, 269
    carotid stenosis in patients undergoing, high-grade, prophylactic endarterectomy for, 371
    myocardial infarction and cardiac mortality rate after, 10
    in patients with ischemic cardiomyopathy and residual myocardial viability, improved outcome after, 5
    in vascular patients, 214
  distal, below-knee, carbon-impregnated polytetrafluoroethylene grafts for, 2-year results, 401
  femoropopliteal
    polytetrafluoroethylene, above knee, performance of, *vs.* autogenous vein below knee, 323
    with reversed or in situ vein grafts, 10-year results, 385
  grafts, infrainguinal polytetrafluoroethylene, color duplex surveillance of, 205
  infrainguinal
    for critical leg ischemia with chronic renal failure, outcome of, 335
    graft patency, increasing workload required to maintain, 388
    impact of inflow reconstruction on, 387
  leg, anesthesia for, 327
  popliteal, below-knee, carbon-impregnated polytetrafluoroethylene grafts for, 2-year results, 401
  prosthetic, with distal vein patch for limb salvage, 322
  saphenous vein allograft, surgery, immunosuppression for, 394
  vein, peripheral, failure, and antibodies to cardiolipin, 310

C

Calf
  vein thrombosis, isolated
    early outcome after, 431
    sequelae of, late clinical and hemodynamic, 455
Cancer
  diagnosis risk after primary deep venous thrombosis or pulmonary embolism, 425
  thromboembolism and, venous, 422, 423
Carbon
  dioxide arteriography, livedo reticularis, rhabdomyolysis, massive intestinal infarction, and death after, 203
  -impregnated polytetrafluoroethylene grafts for below-knee popliteal and distal bypass, 2-year results, 401
Cardiac (*see* Heart)
Cardiolipin
  antibodies to, and failure of peripheral vein bypasses, 310
Cardiomyopathy
  ischemic, and residual myocardial viability, improved outcome after coronary bypass surgery in patients with, 5
Cardiovascular
  disease, prevalent, in non–insulin-dependent diabetes mellitus, and metabolic control, 55
  events and elevated *Chlamydia pneumoniae* antibodies in survivors of myocardial infarction, 38
  risk factor in end-stage renal disease, adverse hyperhomocysteinemia as, 65
β-Carotene
  supplements, effect on incidence of major coronary events in men with previous myocardial infarction, 17
Carotid
  angiography, cost savings associated with nonroutine use of, 361
  angioplasty, percutaneous transluminal
    hemodynamic cerebral ischemia and microembolic signals detected during, 140
    with stent placement, carotid endarterectomy for progressive carotid stenosis after, 141
  artery
    atherosclerosis (*see* Atherosclerosis, carotid)

bulb, atherosclerotic changes measured by B-mode ultrasound in, association with extent of coronary atherosclerosis, 12
common, disease, transthoracic repair of, outcome, 238
common, intima-media thickness, and risk of stroke and myocardial infarction, 11
disease, 357
disease, epidemiology, 376
disease, with renal artery atherosclerosis, 302
internal, traumatic dissections due to blunt softball injuries, 409
intima-media thickness, elevated, and blood viscosity in men and women, 14
plaque morphology correlates with presenting symptomatology, 377
plaques, lipid-rich, echolucent appearance on ultrasound B-mode images, and association with intraplaque hemorrhage, 383
resection and replacement with autogenous arterial graft during operation for neck malignancy, 368
stenosis, after endarterectomy, duplex imaging predicts, 155
stenosis, asymptomatic, moderate, natural history and management of, 369
stenosis, asymptomatic, preoperative risk factors for endarterectomy for, 375
stenosis, comparison of hemodynamic cerebral ischemia and microembolic signals detected during carotid endarterectomy and carotid angioplasty for, 140
stenosis, cost of balloon angioplasty and stenting *vs.* endarterectomy for, 139
stenosis, high-grade, in patients undergoing coronary bypass, prophylactic endarterectomy in, 371
stenosis, of 70%–99%, predictive ability of duplex ultrasound for, 154
stenosis, progressive, after angioplasty and stent placement, endarterectomy for, 141
stenosis, symptomatic, recently, endarterectomy for, 380
stenosis, ultrasound of, power Doppler, 157
atherosclerosis risk and body iron stores, 19
duplex in young adults with lower extremity atherosclerosis, 374
endarterectomy (*see* Endarterectomy, carotid)

Catheterization
femoral venous, incidence of deep venous thrombosis after, 433
pulmonary artery
routine, effect on morbidity and mortality of elective vascular surgery, 224
utility of hemodynamic measurements acquired by, 226

Cautery
electric, contamination threshold for infection of laparotomies lowered by (in rat), 232

CD-44
expression in vein grafts, effect of hypercholesterolemia on (in rabbit), 24

Celiac
artery disease detection by duplex ultrasound, importance of diastolic velocities in, 196

Cell(s)
adhesion molecule-1, vascular, increase in chronic venous disease, 108
endothelial (*see* Endothelium, cell)
mast
in dermal microcirculation in chronic venous insufficiency, 474
distribution, activation, and phenotype in carotid atherosclerosis, 1[illegible]6
red
aggregation induced by acquired dysfibrinogenemia causing digital ischemia and gangrene, 353
transfusions, perioperative, limiting in vascular patients, 220
smooth muscle (*see* Smooth muscle, cells)

Cement
knee arthroplasty with, total, tourniquet release during, transesophageal echocardiography for emboli immediately after, 444

Cephalosporin
prophylaxis, prolonged, for aortic surgery, *Clostridium difficile* colitis after, 290

Cerebral
artery, middle

blood velocity, during carotid endarterectomy with Javid *vs.* Pruitt-Inahara shunt, 153
occlusion, effect of CP101,606 on volume of ischemic brain damage and cytotoxic brain edema after (in cat), 69
occlusion, effect of ZD9379 on number of spreading depressions and infarct size after (in rat), 70
infarction (*see* Stroke)
intracerebral hemorrhage after t-PA in ischemic stroke, 73
ischemia
hemodynamic, detection during carotid endarterectomy and carotid angioplasty, 140
valvular strands and, 163
Cerebrospinal
fluid drainage
during aortic aneurysm repairs, effect on incidence of neurologic deficit, 258
for neurologic deficit, delayed, after thoracoabdominal aneurysm repair, 260
in prevention of paralysis in thoracoabdominal aortic replacement, 262
Cerebrovascular
disease, 357
epidemiology, 376
Chemotactic
activity, monocyte, in vascular endothelial cells, apolipoprotein(a) induces, 103
Chest
radiography, computed, in paraesophageal varices, 483
Children
hemangiomas in, interstitial Nd:YAG photocoagulation for, 209
Klippel-Trénaunay syndrome in, spectrum and management of, 461
lymphangiomas in, percutaneous sclerotherapy with alcoholic solution of zein for, 208
palmar hyperhidrosis in, primary, thoracoscopic upper thoracic sympathectomy for, 210
vascular malformations in, interstitial Nd:YAG photocoagulation for, 209
Chlamydia pneumoniae
antibodies, elevated, and cardiovascular events in survivors of myocardial infarction, 38
in atherosclerosis, carotid artery, 32
detection in atherosclerotic plaques in lower extremity artery walls, 31
infection
atherosclerosis development accelerated by, prevention with azithromycin (in rabbit), 36
in atherosclerotic carotid artery, distribution of, 34
viable, endovascular presence in coronary artery disease, 35
Cholesteryl
ester transfer protein gene, common variant of, role in progression of coronary atherosclerosis, 22
Cigarette
smoking
atherosclerosis progression and, 15
cessation after surgery, 231
Circulating
mediators, lung and leg microvascular permeability to, and acute lung injury after aortic surgery, 82
Cirrhotic
ascites, intractable, results of side-to-side portacaval shunt for, 477
Clamp and sew technique
for aortic transections, traumatic, 264
thoracoabdominal aneurysm repair with, 255
Claudication, 25
assessment of, noninvasive, near infrared spectroscopy for, 28
distance is poorly estimated and inappropriately measured, 25
evaluation, treadmill testing for, 176
intermittent
angioplasty for, percutaneous transluminal, 134
exercise therapy for, 228
exercise training for, 26
patients, gait characteristics of, 30
Clavulanate
/ticarcillin prophylaxis in vascular surgery, duration of, 230
Clinical pathway
for elective infrarenal aortic reconstructions, impact of, 295
Clostridium difficile
colitis after aortic surgery, 290
Clot
dissolution by ultrasound and dodecafluoropentane emulsion, 117
CO_2
arteriography, livedo reticularis, rhabdomyolysis, massive intestinal infarction, and death after, 203

upper
aneurysm in, venous, presentation and management of, 464
arterial occlusions, proximal, combined treatment approach with endovascular stents, 138
hemoaccess, 337
injury, severe proximal vascular and neural, management of, 416
thrombosis, deep venous, *vs.* lower extremity thrombosis, 438
vascular access, 337
venous malformations in, direct injection of ethanol for, 464
venous obstruction, central, interventional radiology in management of, 143

F

Factor
V Leiden and peripheral vascular disease, 52
Fatty acids
augment endothelium-dependent dilation in hand veins by cyclooxygenase-dependent mechanism, 101
Femoral
artery
injury, early intimal thickening after, antisense basic fibroblast growth factor gene transfer reduces (in rabbit), 100
ligation for pseudoaneurysm in drug addicts, 413
pseudoaneurysm (*see* Pseudoaneurysm, femoral)
superficial, as carotid artery replacement during operation for neck malignancy, 368
walls, atherosclerotic plaques in, detection of *Chlamydia pneumoniae* in, 31
vein catheterization, incidence of deep venous thrombosis after, 433
Femorocrural
reconstruction, duplex assessment of run-off before, 167
Femorodistal
bypass, below-knee, carbon-impregnated polytetrafluoroethylene grafts for, 2-year results, 401
Femoropopliteal
artery obstructions, balloon angioplasty with primary stenting *vs.* angioplasty alone in, 144
bypass
below-knee, carbon-impregnated polytetrafluoroethylene grafts for, 2-year results, 401
polytetrafluoroethylene, above knee, performance of, *vs.* autogenous vein below knee, 323
with reversed or in situ vein grafts, 10-year results, 385
vein, superficial, venous reconstructions using, 466
Fever
postoperative, after abdominal aortic aneurysm repair
endovascular and open, 133
infrarenal, by Stentor system, 121
Fibrillation
atrial
nonrheumatic, and previous hemispheric infarction, long-term oral anticoagulation reduces bone mass in patients with, 49
warfarin use in patients with, 217
Fibrin
degradation products, soluble, thrombin binds to, 47
Fibrinolytic
effects of intermittent pneumatic compression, 112
enhancement and regression of proximal deep venous thrombosis, 430
Fibroblast
growth, dermal, reduced in chronic venous ulcers, stimulation with growth factors, 107
growth factor
acidic, angiogenic potential of (in rat), 1
basic, antisense, gene transfer, effect on early intimal thickening after femoral artery injury (in rabbit), 100
basic, dermal fibroblast growth in chronic venous ulcers stimulated by, 107
basic, extracellular matrix–, inactivation by photodynamic therapy, 102
Fibrosis
regression after surgery for inflammatory aortic aneurysms, 285
Fistula
aortobronchial, in situ repair with cryopreserved aortic homografts, 397

aortoenteric, in situ repair with cryopreserved aortic homografts, 397
aortoesophageal, in situ repair with cryopreserved aortic homografts, 397
arteriovenous
for hemodialysis access, survival of, in U.S., 346
stent-graft, 339
Flank
venous malformations in, direct injection of ethanol for, 464
Flexion
plantar, active, force of, and popliteal artery compression, 207
Foeldi technique
for lymphedema of extremities, 472
Folate
intake and risk of coronary heart disease in women, 64
plasma, related to total plasma homocysteine and methylenetetrahydrofolate reductase gene variant, and myocardial infarction in young women, 63
Foot
pumps *vs.* sequential compression devices for prophylaxis of deep venous thrombosis in high-risk trauma patients, 437
$TcPO_2$ response to lumbar sympathectomy for focal ischemic necrosis, 334
venous compression devices, hemodynamic evaluation of, 470
Forearm
hemodialysis access, linear, comparison of two ePTFE grafts for, 343
vein transposition in, for autogenous hemodialysis access, 341
Fradafiban
platelet aggregation inhibited by, 40

G

Gadolinium
-enhanced magnetic resonance venography, "bull's-eye" sign determines thrombus presence and age on, 185
Gait
characteristics of patients with claudication, 30
Gangrene
digital, due to red cell aggregation induced by acquired dysfibrinogenemia, 353
Gaseous
microemboli detected by transcranial Doppler ultrasound, oxygen inhalation differentiates nongaseous microemboli from, 162
Gender
infrarenal aortic diameter and, 267
Gene(s)
cholesteryl ester transfer protein, common variant of, role in progression of coronary atherosclerosis, 22
expression of novel components of extracellular matrix in vein grafts, effect of hypercholesterolemia on (in rabbit), 23
methylenetetrahydrofolate reductase, variant, related to plasma total homocysteine and plasma folate, and myocardial infarction in young women, 63
transfer, antisense basic fibroblast growth factor, effect on early intimal thickening after femoral artery injury (in rabbit), 100
vascular endothelial growth factor, intramuscular injection for acute limb ischemia (in rabbit), 3
Glycine
site antagonist ZD9379, effect on number of spreading depressions and infarct size after middle cerebral artery occlusion (in rat), 70
Goretex
vs. Impra graft for linear forearm hemodialysis access, 343
Graft, 385
allograft (*see* Allograft)
antibiotic-bonded, for vascular graft infection, 398
arterial, autogenous, for carotid artery replacement during operation for neck malignancy, 368
arteriovenous, ePTFE, patency, prophylactic balloon angioplasty fails to prolong, 347
complications, 385
endovascular, 119
for aneurysm, aortic, abdominal, postoperative fever, bowel ischemia, and cytokine response to, 133
for aneurysm, aortic, endoleak after (in dog), 121

for aneurysm, aortoiliac anastomotic, noninfected, 123
modular bifurcation, for abdominal aortic aneurysm, 127
transfemoral, for aneurysm management, CT angiographic imaging of abdominal aortic aneurysms for, 124
failing, 388
natural history in duplex surveillance protocol, 392
hemodialysis (*see* Hemodialysis, access, graft)
heparin-bonded, platelet aggregation in presence of heparin-associated antiplatelet antibodies induced by, 399
homograft (*see* Allograft)
infection
allografts for, in situ cryopreserved aortic (in dog), 396
antibiotic-bonded grafts for, 398
infrainguinal
polytetrafluoroethylene, color duplex surveillance of, 205
polytetrafluoroethylene, with vein interposition cuff at distal anastomosis, 324
-related stenoses, percutaneous angioplasty for, 393
should autogenous vein be spared for future operations? 316
polyester, long-term in vivo alterations in, 403
polytetrafluoroethylene
carbon-impregnated, for below-knee popliteal and distal bypass, 2-year results, 401
expanded, for linear forearm hemodialysis access, comparison of two, 343
expanded, myointimal hyperplasia in vein collars for, 320
prosthetic, 320, 398
albumin-impregnated, for infrarenal aortic replacement, 402
aortic, infected, in situ arterial allografts for, 395
stent- (*see* Stent, -graft)
vein
endothelium-dependent relaxation in, effect of topical vascular endothelial growth factor on (in rabbit), 2
extracellular matrix components in, novel, hypercholesterolemia alters gene expression of (in rabbit), 23
failing, selective use of duplex ultrasound to replace preoperative arteriography for, 390
failing, "short" stenosis of, balloon angioplasty for, 146
hyperplasia, intimal, effect of topical vascular endothelial factor on (in rabbit), 2
hyperplasia in, intimal, local effects of nitric oxide supplementation and suppression on development of (in rabbit), 77
infrainguinal, failure, and antibodies to cardiolipin, 310
infrainguinal, failure, long-term outcome after, 307
infrainguinal, surveillance, 309
leg, 307
leg, surveillance, 309
nitric oxide synthase expression in, inducible, 75
occluded, intimal hyperplasia after thrombectomy *vs.* thrombolysis in (in dog), 313
saphenous, dilatation by nitric oxide, 76
saphenous, in legs, effect of ticlopidine on long-term patency of, 315
surveillance programs, economizing, 389
vascular endothelial growth factor expression in (in dog), 98
for vascular injuries of thoracic outlet, 418
Groin
wound infection after bifurcated AneuRx graft for abdominal aortic aneurysm, 127
Growth
factor
fibroblast (*see* Fibroblast, growth factor)
platelet-derived, and extracellular matrix proteins provide synergistic stimulus for vascular smooth muscle cell migration, 92
stimulation of dermal fibroblast growth in chronic venous ulcers, 107
transforming growth factor-β1 in dermal microcirculation in chronic venous insufficiency, 474
vascular endothelial (*see* Vascular, endothelial growth factor)

H

Hand
- ischemia, 352
  - severe, magnetic resonance angiography of, 352
- veins, fatty acids augment endothelium-dependent dilation in, 101

Healing
- ulcer, after subfascial endoscopy for perforating veins of lower leg, 460

Heart, 5
- complications in major vascular surgery, importance of preoperative 12-lead ECG in predicting, 213
- disease, coronary
  - (*See also* Coronary, artery disease)
  - risk in women, relation to folate and vitamin B_6 intake, 64
- events, morbid, perioperative maintenance of normothermia reduces incidence of, 221
- failure
  - congestive, and renal insufficiency, carbon dioxide arteriography in patient with, livedo reticularis, rhabdomyolysis, massive intestinal infarction, and death after, 203
  - congestive, as risk factor for endarterectomy for asymptomatic carotid stenosis, 375
  - after myocardial infarction, effect of ramipril on, follow-up study, 18
- function as risk factor for paralysis in thoracoabdominal aortic replacement, 262
- mortality rate after bypass surgery or angioplasty, 10

Heat
- shock protein expression, enhancement after transient ischemia in preconditioned spinal cord (in rabbit), 71

Hemangioma
- photocoagulation for, interstitial Nd:YAG, in children, 209

Hematoma
- intramural, 241
  - of aorta, thoracic, fate of, 241
  - of aorta, thoracic, MRI of, 243

Hemoaccess
- upper extremity, 337

Hemodialysis
- access, 337
  - autogenous, vein transposition in forearm for, 341
  - endovascular technique in, 339
  - forearm, linear, comparison of two ePTFE grafts for, 343
  - graft, arteriovenous, PTFE, cost efficacy of duplex surveillance and prophylactic angioplasty of, 351
  - graft, arteriovenous, PTFE, patency, prophylactic balloon angioplasty fails to prolong, 347
  - graft, survival of, in U.S., 346
  - graft, thrombectomy of, surgical, balloon *vs.* patch angioplasty as adjuvant treatment to, 349
  - graft, thrombosed, surgical *vs.* endovascular management of, 350
  - in ischemic steal syndrome, distal revascularization-interval ligation for maintenance of, 344
  - survival of, in U.S., 346
- patients, hyperhomocysteinemia as adverse cardiovascular risk factor in, 65

Hemodynamic
- cerebral ischemia detected during carotid endarterectomy and carotid angioplasty, 140
- disease, distal vertebral artery reconstruction for, 378
- evaluation
  - of foot venous compression devices, 470
  - of late sequelae of deep venous thrombosis, duplex ultrasound in, 456
- measurements acquired by pulmonary artery catheterization, utility of, 226
- sequelae
  - late, of isolated calf vein thrombosis, 455
  - long-term, of deep venous thrombosis, 451

Hemodynamically
- significant atherosclerotic renal artery stenosis, MR angiographic features of, 191

Hemorrhage
- intracerebral, after t-PA in ischemic stroke, 73
- intraplaque, association with lipid-rich carotid artery plaque echolucency on ultrasound B-mode images, 383
- variceal
  - acute, sclerotherapy in, endoscopic, *vs.* transjugular intrahepatic portosystemic shunt for, 479

recurrent, endoscopic sclerotherapy *vs.* transjugular intrahepatic portosystemic shunt for prevention of, 480

Heparin
- angiogenic potential of (in rat), 1
- -associated antiplatelet antibodies, heparin-bonded grafts induce platelet aggregation in presence of, 399
- for atheroma of aortic arch, mobile, 236
- -bonded grafts induce platelet aggregation in presence of heparin-associated antiplatelet antibodies, 399
- -coated femoral vein catheters and incidence of deep venous thrombosis, 433
- inhibits thrombin-induced mitogen-activated protein kinase signaling in arterial smooth muscle cells (in baboon), 50
- IV, for traumatic carotid artery dissections from blunt softball injuries, 410
- low-molecular-weight
  - in thromboembolism, venous, 447
  - *vs.* unfractionated, for coronary artery disease, unstable, 53
  - *vs.* unfractionated, for pulmonary embolism, acute, 448
- after popliteal artery trauma improves limb salvage, 408

Herpes
- simplex virus in atherosclerosis of carotid artery, 32

Hip
- replacement, total, deep venous thrombosis after
  - detection with technetium-99m-labeled tissue plasminogen activator, 180
  - ultrasound screening before hospital discharge for, 443

Hispanics
- incidence of idiopathic deep venous thrombosis and secondary thromboembolism in, 435

Homocysteine, 61
- plasma
  - mortality of coronary artery disease and, 61
  - total, related to plasma folate and methylenetetrahydrofolate reductase gene variant, and myocardial infarction in young women, 63

Homograft (*see* Allograft)

Hospital(s)
- discharge, ultrasound screening for deep venous thrombosis after arthroplasty before, 442
- trial, carotid endarterectomy mortality in Medicare population in, 364
- volume and carotid endarterectomy mortality in Medicare population, 364

Hyaluronic acid
- synthase expression in vein grafts, effect of hypercholesterolemia on (in rabbit), 23

Hypercholesterolemia
- alters gene expression of novel components of extracellular matrix in vein grafts (in rabbit), 23
- in postmenopausal women, estrogen replacement and pravastatin for, 58

Hyperglycemia
- -induced defective migration in cultured endothelial cells, nitric oxide mediation of, 85

Hyperhidrosis
- primary palmar, thoracoscopic upper thoracic sympathectomy for, 210

Hyperhomocysteinemia
- as adverse cardiovascular risk factor in end-stage renal disease, 65
- history of venous thromboembolism and, prothrombin fragment F1+2 levels in patients with, 67
- as risk factor for arterial endothelial dysfunction, 68

Hyperinsulinemia
- carotid atherosclerosis and, 56

Hyperplasia
- intimal
  - after thrombectomy *vs.* thrombolysis in occluded vein grafts (in dog), 313
  - vein graft, development of, local effects of nitric oxide supplementation and suppression on (in rabbit), 77
  - vein graft, effect of vascular endothelial factor on, topical (in rabbit), 2
- myointimal, in vein collars for ePTFE grafts, 320
- neointimal, after arterial injury, inhibition of leukocyte and platelet adhesion reduces (in rabbit), 45

Hypertension
- portal, 477

Hypertrophy
  limb, in Klippel-Trénaunay syndrome, 461
Hypoinsulinemia
  carotid atherosclerosis and, 56

I

Iliac
  artery
    aneurysm, noninfected anastomotic, endovascular graft for, 123
    dissection after bifurcated AneuRx graft for abdominal aortic aneurysm, 127
Iliofemoral
  vein thrombosis, venous thrombectomy for, 429
Iloprost
  in thromboangiitis obliterans, 211
Imaging
  magnetic resonance (*see* Magnetic resonance imaging)
  vascular, 151
  venous, 178
Immunocytochemical
  detection of *Chlamydia pneumoniae* in atherosclerotic plaques in lower extremity artery walls, 31
Immunosuppression
  for saphenous vein allograft bypass surgery, 394
Impra
  vs. Goretex graft for linear forearm hemodialysis access, 343
Indium-111
  labeled transferrin, lung and leg microvascular permeability to, and acute lung injury after aortic surgery, 82
Infarct
  brain, size, effect of ZD9379 on (in rat), 70
Infarction
  cerebral (*see* Stroke)
  intestinal, massive, after carbon dioxide arteriography, 203
  myocardial (*see* Myocardial, infarction)
Infection
  aortic aneurysm, surgical treatment of, 272
  aortic prosthetic, in situ arterial allografts for, 395
  graft
    allografts for, in situ cryopreserved aortic (in dog), 396
    antibiotic-bonded grafts for, 398
  of laparotomies, electric cautery lowers contamination threshold for (in rat), 232
  wound, groin, after bifurcated AneuRx graft for abdominal aortic aneurysm, 127
Inflammatory
  aortic aneurysms, 285
  mediators, circulating, lung and leg microvascular permeability to, and acute lung injury after aortic surgery, 82
  response, exercise-induced, biochemical markers of, effect of exercise training for intermittent claudication on, 26
Inflow reconstruction
  impact on infrainguinal bypass, 387
Infragenicular
  smooth muscle cells, proliferation and extracellular matrix production by, effect of interleukin-1β on, 95
Infrainguinal
  arterial reconstruction, local anesthesia for, 327
  bypass
    graft patency, increasing workload required to maintain, 388
    impact of inflow reconstruction on, 387
    surgery for critical leg ischemia with chronic renal failure, outcome of, 335
    surveillance programs, economizing, 389
  graft
    polytetrafluoroethylene, color duplex surveillance of, 205
    polytetrafluoroethylene, with vein interposition cuff at distal anastomosis, 324
    vein, failure, long-term outcome after, 307
Infrapopliteal
  artery lesions, imaging with color duplex ultrasound *vs.* arteriography, 165
  occlusions in critically ischemic limbs, subintimal angioplasty for, 135
Infrared
  near-infrared spectroscopy (*see* Spectroscopy, near-infrared)
Infrarenal
  abdominal aneurysm
    endovascular treatment by Stentor system, 120
    repair, natural history of residual infrarenal aorta after, 278

aorta (*see* Aorta, infrarenal)
Injury
arterial, neointimal hyperplasia after, inhibition of leukocyte and platelet adhesion reduces (in rabbit), 45
femoral artery, early intimal thickening after, antisense basic fibroblast growth factor gene transfer reduces (in rabbit), 100
lung
acute, after aortic surgery, 82
ischemia/reperfusion of lower extremities causing, role of nitric oxide and tumor necrosis factor in (in rat), 80
renal parenchymal, contralateral, with unilateral atherosclerotic renal artery stenosis, 300
Innominate
artery, 238
disease, occlusive, central reconstructive techniques for, 240
disease, transthoracic repair of, outcome, 238
Insulin
-dependent diabetes mellitus, endothelial function in, effect of angiotensin-converting enzyme inhibition on, 57
serum, and carotid atherosclerosis, 56
Integrin
signaling transduces shear stress–dependent vasodilation of coronary arterioles, 104
Intensive care
patients, surgical, screening for asymptomatic deep vein thrombosis in, 440
Intercostal
artery reattachment during thoracoabdominal aortic aneurysm repair, importance of, 249
Interleukin
-1β
dermal fibroblast growth in chronic venous ulcers stimulated by, 107
effect on proliferation and extracellular matrix production by infragenicular smooth muscle cells, 95
-8 levels and acute lung injury after aortic surgery, 83
Intestinal
infarction, massive, after carbon dioxide arteriography, 203
Intimal
hyperplasia (*see* Hyperplasia, intimal)
Intra-aortic
balloon pump counterpulsation, prolonged, implications for vascular surgeon with, 331
Intra-arterial
thrombolysis, limitations of, 149
Intracerebral
hemorrhage after t-PA in ischemic stroke, 73
Intracoronary
radiation therapy after percutaneous transluminal angioplasty, long-term angiographic and clinical outcome after, 6
Intracranial
atherosclerosis, stenosis from, natural history by serial angiography, 382
Intrahepatic
portosystemic shunt, transjugular, *vs.* endoscopic sclerotherapy for variceal hemorrhage
acute, 479
for prevention of recurrent hemorrhage, 480
Intraluminal
thrombus, effect on abdominal aortic aneurysm wall stress, 114
Intramural
hematoma (*see* Hematoma, intramural)
Intravascular
ultrasound, ECG-gated 3D, of coronary atherosclerotic plaques, 198
Iron
stores, body
risk of carotid atherosclerosis and, 19
risk of myocardial infarction and, in men, 21
Ischemia
bowel, after endovascular *vs.* open abdominal aortic aneurysm repair, 133
brain damage due to, after middle cerebral artery occlusion, effect of CP101,606 on volume of (in cat), 69
cardiomyopathy due to, and residual myocardial viability, improved outcome after coronary bypass surgery in patients with, 5
cerebral
hemodynamic, detection during carotid endarterectomy and carotid angioplasty, 140
valvular strands and, 163
colonic
after endovascular treatment of infrarenal abdominal aneurysms by Stentor system, 121

fatal, after stent graft for aortic aneurysm, 132
during coronary angioplasty, phentolamine prevents adaptation to, 8
digital, due to red cell aggregation induced by acquired dysfibrinogenemia, 353
hand, 352
  severe, magnetic resonance angiography of, 352
leg, 307
  critical, with chronic renal failure, outcome of infrainguinal bypass for, 335
limb
  acute, intramuscular injection of vascular endothelial growth factor gene for (in rabbit), 3
  critical, diagnosis, skin perfusion pressure measurement in, 329
  critical, subintimal angioplasty of infrapopliteal occlusions in, 135
  lower, limitations of intra-arterial thrombolysis for, 149
mesenteric, chronic
  MRI measurements of blood oxygen saturation in superior mesenteric vein for diagnosis, in vivo, 195
  surgical therapy results for, 304
necrosis due to, focal, foot $TcPO_2$ response to lumbar sympathectomy for, 334
perioperative, in major vascular surgery, importance of preoperative 12-lead ECG in predicting, 213
renal, 297
/reperfusion of lower extremities causing lung injury, role of nitric oxide and tumor necrosis factor in (in rat), 80
steal syndrome, distal revascularization-interval ligation for limb salvage and maintenance of dialysis access in, 344
stroke due to, acute, early aspirin use in, 42
transient
  carotid plaque morphology correlates with, 378
  in preconditioned spinal cord, enhancement of heat shock protein expression after (in rabbit), 71
visceral, 304
  during thoracoabdominal aneurysm repair, mesenteric shunting decreases, 261
wrist, severe, magnetic resonance angiography of, 352

J

Javid shunt
  carotid endarterectomy with, middle cerebral artery blood velocity, embolization, and neurologic outcome during, 153
Jugular
  vein, internal, aneurysm in, presentation and management of, 464
Juxtarenal
  placement of covered stent-grafts for abdominal aortic aneurysms, 119

K

Kidney (*see* Renal)
Klippel-Trénaunay syndrome
  spectrum and management of, 461
  venous aneurysms in, presentation and management of, 465
Knee
  below-knee popliteal and distal bypass, carbon-impregnated polytetrafluoroethylene grafts for, 2-year results, 401
  femoropopliteal bypass with polytetrafluoroethylene above, performance of, 323
  replacement, total
    with cement, tourniquet release during, transesophageal echocardiography for emboli immediately after, 444
    thrombosis after, deep venous, detection with technetium-99m-labeled tissue plasminogen activator, 180
    thrombosis after, deep venous, ultrasound screening before hospital discharge for, 443

L

Laboratory
  vascular, 151
Laparoscopic
  aortic aneurysm repair, abdominal, 279
  aortobifemoral bypass, 147
Laparotomies
  infection of, electric cautery lowers contamination threshold for (in rat), 232

Plantar
  flexion, active, force of, and popliteal artery compression, 207
Plaque
  atherosclerotic
    carotid, lipid content increase in, echolucency of computerized ultrasound images associated with, 160
    coronary, ultrasound of, ECG-gated 3D intravascular, 198
    in lower extremity artery walls, detection of *Chlamydia pneumoniae* in, 31
  carotid
    lipid-rich, echolucent appearance on ultrasound B-mode images and association with intraplaque hemorrhage, 383
    morphology, correlation with presenting symptomatology, 377
Plasminogen
  activator, tissue
    serum, increased activity, and regression of proximal deep venous thrombosis, 430
    in stroke, ischemic, intracerebral hemorrhage after, 73
    technetium-99m-labeled, detection of postoperative deep venous thrombosis with, 178
Platelet
  adhesion inhibition reduces neointimal hyperplasia after arterial injury (in rabbit), 45
  aggregation
    fradafiban and lefradafiban inhibition of, 40
    in presence of heparin-associated antiplatelet antibodies induced by heparin-bonded grafts, 399
  -derived growth factor and extracellular matrix proteins provide synergistic stimulus for vascular smooth muscle cell migration, 92
Plethysmography
  air
    in diagnosis of chronic venous insufficiency, 181
    in venous disease, chronic, variability and reliability of, 452
Pneumatic
  compression
    devices, sequential, *vs.* foot pumps for prophylaxis of deep venous thrombosis in high-risk trauma patients, 437
    intermittent, fibrinolytic effects of, 112
Polycythemia
  vera and venous thromboembolism, 424
Polyester
  -covered nitinol stent-grafts, juxtarenal placement for abdominal aortic aneurysms, 119
  graft, long-term in vivo alterations in, 403
Polymerase chain reaction
  detection of *Chlamydia pneumoniae* in atherosclerotic plaques in lower extremity artery walls, 31
Polytetrafluoroethylene
  bypass, femoropopliteal, above knee, performance of, *vs.* autogenous vein below knee, 323
  graft
    carbon-impregnated, for below-knee popliteal and distal bypass, 2-year results, 401
    hemodialysis (*see* Hemodialysis, graft)
    iliac vein, in venous occlusive disease, 468
    infrainguinal, color duplex surveillance of, 205
    infrainguinal, stenosis in, percutaneous angioplasty for, 393
    infrainguinal, with vein interposition cuff at distal anastomosis, 324
    vein collars for, myointimal hyperplasia in, 320
    with vein patch, distal, for limb salvage, 322
  pericardial membrane for retroperitoneal closure after abdominal aortic surgery, 289
Popliteal
  artery
    compression and force of active plantar flexion, 207
    trauma, anticoagulation and intraoperative thrombolysis improves limb salvage after, 407
    walls, atherosclerotic plaques in, detection of *Chlamydia pneumoniae* in, 31
  bypass, below-knee, carbon-impregnated polytetrafluoroethylene grafts for, 2-year results, 401
  femoropopliteal (*see* Femoropopliteal)
Porcelain
  aorta, endarterectomy of ascending aorta for, 237

Portacaval
  shunt, side-to-side, for intractable cirrhotic ascites, results of, 477
Portal
  hypertension, 477
Portosystemic
  shunt, transjugular intrahepatic, *vs.* endoscopic sclerotherapy for variceal hemorrhage
    acute, 479
    for prevention of recurrent hemorrhage, 480
Port-wine stains
  in Klippel-Trénaunay syndrome, 461
Postmenopausal women
  estrogen replacement therapy in, duration in relation to risk of myocardial infarction, 216
  hypercholesterolemia in, estrogen replacement and pravastatin for, 58
Postoperative
  thrombosis, deep venous, detection with technetium-99m-labeled tissue plasminogen activator, 178
pp60$^{c\text{-}src}$
  activation, role in vascular smooth muscle cell migration, 94
Pravastatin
  alone or combined with estrogen replacement for hypercholesterolemia in postmenopausal women, 58
  for coronary atherosclerosis, and TaqIB, 23
Preclude Pericardial Membrane
  for retroperitoneal closure after abdominal aortic surgery, 289
Preconditioned
  spinal cord, enhancement of heat shock protein expression after transient ischemia in (in rabbit), 71
Probucol
  in prevention of restenosis after coronary angioplasty, 7
Prostate
  cancer and venous thromboembolism, 422
Prosthetic
  aortic reconstruction, aneurysms after, noninfected false, morbidity and mortality of reconstructive surgery for, 284
  bypass with distal vein patch for limb salvage, 322
  graft, 320, 398
    albumin-impregnated, for infrarenal aortic replacement, 402
    aortic, infection, in situ arterial allografts for, 395
Protein(s)
  amyloid A, serum, as marker of exercise-induced inflammatory response, effect of exercise training for intermittent claudication on, 26
  C resistance, activated, and peripheral vascular disease, 52
  cholesteryl ester transfer protein gene variant, role in progression of coronary atherosclerosis, 22
  C-reactive
    as marker of exercise-induced inflammatory response, effect of exercise training for intermittent claudication on, 26
    plasma, and risk of developing peripheral vascular disease, 97
  extracellular matrix, and platelet-derived growth factor provide synergistic stimulus for vascular smooth muscle cell migration, 92
  heat shock, enhanced expression after transient ischemia in preconditioned spinal cord (in rabbit), 71
  kinase
    C isoforms in aortic smooth muscle cells, 96
    mitogen-activated, activation of, smooth muscle cell migration and proliferation mediated by, 93
    signaling in arterial smooth muscle cells, thrombin-induced mitogen-activated, heparin inhibits (in baboon), 50
Prothrombin
  fragment F1+2 levels in patients with hyperhomocysteinemia and history of venous thromboembolism, 67
Provider
  volumes for carotid endarterectomy, 365
Pruitt-Inahara shunt
  carotid endarterectomy with, middle cerebral artery blood velocity, embolization, and neurologic outcome during, 153
Pseudoaneurysm
  femoral
    in drug addicts, 413
    iatrogenic, percutaneous thrombin injection for, 415
    rupture, delayed, after successful compression therapy, 175

PTFE (*see* Polytetrafluoroethylene)
Pulmonary
  (*See also* Lung)
  angiography in acute major pulmonary embolism, 446
  artery catheterization
    routine, effect on morbidity and mortality of elective vascular surgery, 224
    utility of hemodynamic measurements acquired by, 226
  complications of endovascular treatment of infrarenal abdominal aneurysms by Stentor system, 121
  embolism (*see* Embolism, pulmonary)
Pump
  counterpulsation, intra-aortic balloon, prolonged, implications for vascular surgeon with, 331
  foot, *vs.* sequential compression device for prophylaxis of deep venous thrombosis in high-risk trauma patients, 437

R

R15.7
  inhibition of leukocyte and platelet adhesion reduces neointimal hyperplasia after arterial injury (in rabbit), 45
Race
  infrarenal aortic diameter and, 267
Radiography
  computed, chest, in paraesophageal varices, 483
Radiology
  in combined approach to treatment of proximal arterial occlusions of upper limb with endovascular stents, 138
  interventional, in management of upper extremity central venous obstruction, 143
Radiotherapy
  intracoronary, after percutaneous transluminal angioplasty, long-term angiographic and clinical outcome after, 6
Raman spectroscopy
  biochemical composition of peripheral arteries examined with, 89
Ramipril
  effect on heart failure after myocardial infarction, follow-up study, 18
Reconstruction
  aortic
    elective, aprotinin in, 223
    infrarenal, elective, impact of clinical pathway for, 295
  arterial
    infrainguinal, local anesthesia for, 327
    vertebral, distal, for embolic and hemodynamic disease, 378
  femorocrural, duplex assessment of run-off before, 167
  inflow, impact on infrainguinal bypass, 387
  surgery of aneurysms, noninfected false, detected long after aortic prosthetic reconstruction, morbidity and mortality of, 284
  vascular
    central, for innominate artery occlusive disease, 240
    lower extremity, based on color duplex imaging alone, 164
  vein, 466
    femoral-popliteal vein in, superficial, 466
    iliac, in venous occlusive disease, 468
Red cell
  aggregation induced by acquired dysfibrinogenemia causing digital ischemia and gangrene, 353
  transfusions, perioperative, limiting in vascular patients, 220
Red wine
  effect on endothelium-dependent relaxation (in rabbit), 86
Redo surgery
  after vascular surgery, 218
Reflux
  venous, 451
    origin of, 453
    after thrombosis, deep venous, duplex ultrasound in evaluation of, 456
Renal
  artery
    atherosclerosis, with carotid and lower extremity arterial disease, 302
    disease, visceral, 297
    repair, failed, consequence of, 303
    repair, in African-Americans, 299
    stenosis, atherosclerotic, hemodynamically significant, MR angiographic features of, 191
    stenosis, atherosclerotic unilateral, clinical evidence of contralateral renal parenchymal injury with, 300
  disease, end-stage, hyperhomocysteinemia as adverse cardiovascular risk factor in, 65
  failure

chronic, and critical leg ischemia, outcome of infrainguinal bypass for, 335
after thoracoabdominal aortic surgery, 247
hilar Doppler analysis in management of renovascular disease, 193
insufficiency and congestive heart failure, carbon dioxide arteriography in patient with, livedo reticularis, rhabdomyolysis, massive intestinal infarction, and death after, 203
ischemia, 297
malperfusion after acute aortic dissection, abdominal aortic tailoring for, 283
parenchymal injury, contralateral, with unilateral atherosclerotic renal artery stenosis, 300

Renovascular
disease management, renal hilar Doppler analysis in, 193

Reoperations
after vascular surgery, 218

Reperfusion
of lower extremities causing lung injury, role of nitric oxide and tumor necrosis factor in (in rat), 80

Resource
utilization, impact of clinical pathway for elective infrarenal aortic reconstructions on, 295

Restenosis
after angioplasty, percutaneous transluminal coronary, probucol and multivitamins in prevention of, 7

Retired men
nonsmoking, effects of walking on mortality among, 227

Retroperitoneal
closure after abdominal aortic surgery, Preclude Pericardial Membrane for, 289

Revascularization
distal revascularization-interval ligation for limb salvage and maintenance of dialysis access in ischemic steal syndrome, 344
lower limb
distal, MR arteriography in, 202
in high-risk patients, local anesthesia for, 328

Reviparin sodium
in venous thromboembolism, 448

Rhabdomyolysis
after arteriography, carbon dioxide, 203

Rifampicin
-bonded grafts for vascular graft infection, 398

Run-off
duplex assessment before femorocrural reconstruction, 167

Rupture
aneurysm, aortic
abdominal, associated with high-attenuating crescent sign, 188
abdominal, repair of, long-term survival and late complications after, 274
decision not to operate, 276
aorta
abdominal, spontaneous nonaneurysmal, case reports, 292
after blunt injury, antihypertensive therapy reduces, 411
infrarenal, nonaneurysmal atherosclerotic, 291
perivisceral, 246
thoracic, traumatic, surgical indications and timing of repair of, 412
pseudoaneurysm, femoral artery, delayed, after successful compression therapy, 175

S

Salmonella
enteritis causing infected aortic aneurysm, 272

Saphenectomy
in presence of chronic vein obstruction, 457

Saphenous vein
allograft bypass surgery, immunosuppression for, 394
bypass grafts in legs, effect of ticlopidine on long-term patency of, 315
graft, dilatation by nitric oxide, 76
harvest, video-assisted, 311
infrainguinal bypass using, should vein be spared for future operations? 316
normal, collagen subtype pattern in, 471
thrombophlebitis as deceptively benign disease, 434
varicose, collagen subtype pattern in, 471

Scan
lung, in acute major pulmonary embolism, 446

Sciatic
  vein, persistent, in Klippel-Trénaunay syndrome, 461
Scintigraphy
  thallium-201, of residual myocardial viability and outcome after coronary bypass surgery for ischemic cardiomyopathy, 5
Sclerotherapy
  endoscopic, *vs.* transjugular intrahepatic portosystemic shunt for variceal hemorrhage
    acute, 479
    for prevention of recurrent hemorrhage, 480
  percutaneous, with alcoholic solution of zein for lymphangiomas, in children, 208
Shear stress
  –dependent vasodilation of coronary arterioles transduced by integrin signaling, 104
Shunt
  Javid, carotid endarterectomy with, middle cerebral artery blood velocity, embolization, and neurologic outcome during, 153
  portacaval, side to-side, for intractable cirrhotic ascites, results of, 477
  portosystemic, transjugular intrahepatic, *vs.* endoscopic sclerotherapy for variceal hemorrhage
    acute, 479
    for prevention of recurrent hemorrhage, 480
  Pruitt-Inahara, carotid endarterectomy with, middle cerebral artery blood velocity, embolization, and neurologic outcome during, 153
  surgery during era of liver transplantation, 482
Shunting
  mesenteric, decreases visceral ischemia during thoracoabdominal aneurysm repair, 261
Skin
  perfusion pressure measurement in diagnosis of critical limb ischemia, 329
Smoking
  atherosclerosis progression and, 15
  cessation after surgery, 231
Smooth muscle
  cells
    aortic, protein kinase C isoforms in, 96
  arterial, heparin inhibits thrombin-induced mitogen-activated protein kinase signaling in (in baboon), 50
  vascular, infrageniculár, proliferation and extracellular matrix production by, effect of interleukin-1β on, 95
  vascular, migration, platelet-derived growth factor and extracellular matrix proteins provide synergistic stimulus for, 92
  vascular, migration, role of pp60$^{c\text{-}src}$ activation in, 94
  vascular, migration and proliferation mediated by activation of mitogen-activated protein kinase, 93
S-nitroso-N-acetylpenicillamine
  effect on development of intimal hyperplasia in vein grafts (in rabbit), 77–78
Sodium
  morrhuate in endoscopic sclerotherapy for prevention of recurrent variceal hemorrhage, 480
Softball
  injuries, blunt, causing traumatic internal carotid artery dissections, 409
Spectroscopy, 87
  magnetic resonance, dynamic phosphorus-31, in arterial occlusive disease, 87
  near-infrared
    in claudication, 28
    Raman, biochemical composition of peripheral arteries examined with, 89
    of venous insufficiency in primary varicose veins, 182
Spinal
  cord, preconditioned, enhancement of heat shock protein expression after transient ischemia in (in rabbit), 71
Stains
  port-wine, in Klippel-Trénaunay syndrome, 461
Staphylococcus aureus
  infection
    of aortic aneurysm, 272
    methicillin-resistant, of femoral pseudoaneurysm in drug addicts, 414
Stenosis
  arterial, multiple, in vitro evaluation using three-dimensional power Doppler angiography, 172
  carotid artery (*see* Carotid, artery, stenosis)

infrainguinal graft-related, percutaneous angioplasty for, 393
from intracranial atherosclerosis, natural history by serial angiography, 382
renal artery, atherosclerotic
hemodynamically significant, MR angiographic features of, 191
unilateral, clinical evidence of contralateral renal parenchymal injury with, 300
restenosis after angioplasty, percutaneous transluminal coronary, probucol and multivitamins in prevention of, 7
short, of failing vein grafts, balloon angioplasty for, 146
Stent
coronary, placement for myocardial infarction, outcome with antiplatelet *vs.* anticoagulant therapy after, 43
endovascular, in combined approach to treatment of proximal arterial occlusions of upper limb, 138
-graft
for aortic aneurysm, fatal colonic ischemia after, 132
arteriovenous fistula, 339
covered, juxtarenal placement for abdominal aortic aneurysms, 119
placement with carotid angioplasty, carotid endarterectomy for progressive carotid stenosis after, 141
Stenting
with balloon angioplasty *vs.* endarterectomy for carotid artery stenosis, cost of, 139
primary, with balloon angioplasty, *vs.* angioplasty alone in femoropopliteal obstructions, 144
Stentor system
endovascular treatment of infrarenal abdominal aneurysms by, 120
Strands
valvular, and cerebral ischemia, 163
Stress
shear stress–dependent vasodilation of coronary arterioles transduced by integrin signaling, 104
Stroke
hemispheric, previous, and nonrheumatic atrial fibrillation, long-term oral anticoagulation reduces bone mass in patients with, 49
ischemic
acute, aspirin use in, early, 42
acute, thrombolytic therapy for, systematic review of evidence on, 74
plasminogen activator for, tissue, intracerebral hemorrhage after, 73
perioperative
does prophylactic carotid endarterectomy in patients with high-grade stenosis undergoing coronary bypass decrease? 371
microembolus detection by transcranial Doppler in identification of patients at high risk of, 151
prevention in atrial fibrillation patients, warfarin for, 217
prior, carotid plaque morphology correlates with, 378
risk and common carotid intima-media thickness, 11
Subfascial
endoscopic perforating vein surgery (*see* Perforating vein, surgery, subfascial endoscopic)
Subintimal
angioplasty of infrapopliteal occlusions in critically ischemic limbs, 135
Supraceliac
aortorenal bypass, 297
Surgeon
vascular, implications of prolonged intra-aortic balloon pump counterpulsation for, 331
Surgery
smoking cessation after, 231
Surgical
intensive care patients, screening for asymptomatic deep vein thrombosis in, 440
Sympathectomy
lumbar, for focal ischemic necrosis, foot $TcPO_2$ response to, 334
thoracic, thoracoscopic upper, for primary palmar hyperhidrosis, 210

T

Tamoxifen
effect on dilator responses of atherosclerotic epicardial coronary arteries (in monkey), 60
TaqIB
role in progression of coronary atherosclerosis, 22

TcPO$_2$
  foot, response to lumbar sympathectomy for focal ischemic necrosis, 334
Technetium
  -99m tissue plasminogen activator, detection of postoperative deep venous thrombosis with, 178
Temporal
  arteritis, diagnosis with color duplex ultrasound, 158
Thallium 201
  scintigraphy of residual myocardial viability and outcome after coronary bypass surgery for ischemic cardiomyopathy, 5
Thoracic
  aorta (*see* Aorta, thoracic)
  outlet vascular injuries, aggressive management of, 418
  sympathectomy, thoracoscopic upper, for primary palmar hyperhidrosis, 210
Thoracoabdominal
  aorta (*see* Aorta, thoracoabdominal)
Thoracoscopic
  upper thoracic sympathectomy for primary palmar hyperhidrosis, 210
Thrombectomy
  in occluded vein grafts, intimal hyperplasia after (in dog), 313
  surgical, of hemodialysis grafts, balloon *vs.* patch angioplasty as adjuvant treatment for, 349
  venous, for iliofemoral vein thrombosis, 429
Thrombi
  intraluminal, effect on abdominal aortic aneurysm wall stress, 114
  presence and age, "bull's eye" sign on gadolinium-enhanced MR venography determines, 185
  venous, deep, lower extremity, origin in acute venous thrombosis, 421
Thrombin
  binds to soluble fibrin degradation products, 47
  -induced mitogen-activated protein kinase signaling in arterial smooth muscle cells inhibited by heparin (in baboon), 50
  injection, percutaneous, for iatrogenic femoral pseudoaneurysm, 415
Thromboangiitis
  obliterans, iloprost in, 211
Thrombocytopenia
  transitory, after endovascular treatment of infrarenal abdominal aneurysms by Stentor system, 121
Thromboembolism
  venous
    cancer and, 422, 423
    heparin in, low-molecular-weight, 447
    history of, and hyperhomocysteinemia, prothrombin fragment F1+2 levels in patients with, 67
    secondary, and ethnicity, 435
Thrombolysis
  intra-arterial, limitations of, 149
  intraoperative, improves limb salvage after popliteal artery trauma, 407
  in occluded vein grafts, intimal hyperplasia after (in dog), 313
  in pulmonary embolism, acute major, 446
  for stroke, acute ischemic, systematic review of evidence on, 74
Thrombophlebitis
  saphenous vein, as deceptively benign disease, 434
Thrombosis
  chronic, endothelial cell adaptation to (in dog), 46
  graft, dialysis access, surgical *vs.* endovascular management of, 350
  venous, 421
    calf, isolated, outcome after, early, 431
    calf, isolated, sequelae of, late clinical and hemodynamic, 455
    deep *(see below)*
    diagnosis, noninvasive, 439
    iliofemoral, venous thrombectomy for, 429
  venous, deep, 421
    after arthroplasty, ultrasound screening before hospital discharge for, 442
    asymptomatic, screening surgical intensive care patients for, 440
    idiopathic, and ethnicity, 435
    incidence after femoral venous catheterization, 433
    lower extremity, origin of thrombi in, 421
    major, screening in seriously injured patients for, 44[illegible]
    postoperative, detection with technetium-99m-labeled tissue plasminogen activator, 178
    prediction by D-dimer, 426, 428

primary, risk of cancer diagnosis after, 425
prophylaxis in high-risk trauma patients, sequential compression devices *vs.* foot pumps for, 437
proximal, regression associated with fibrinolytic enhancement, 430
sequelae of, late, duplex ultrasound in hemodynamic evaluation of, 456
sequelae of, long-term clinical and hemodynamic, 451
symptoms of, unilateral, venous duplex scanning for, 186
upper extremity *vs.* lower extremity, 438
Thrombotic
arterial occlusion, dissolution by ultrasound and dodecafluoropentane emulsion, 117
Thrombus (*see* Thrombi)
Tibial
artery, anterior, optimal methods for autogenous bypass to, 318
bypass, prosthetic, with distal vein patch for limb salvage, 322
Ticarcillin
/clavulanate prophylaxis in vascular surgery, duration of, 230
Ticlopidine
/aspirin after coronary stent placement for myocardial infarction, 44
effect on long-term patency of saphenous vein bypass grafts in legs, 315
Tissue
oxygen tension, transcutaneous, foot, response to lumbar sympathectomy for focal ischemic necrosis, 334
plasminogen activator (*see* Plasminogen, activator, tissue)
α-Tocopherol
supplements, effect on incidence of major coronary events in men with previous myocardial infarction, 17
Tomography
computed (*see* Computed tomography)
Tourniquet
release during total knee arthroplasty with cement, transesophageal echocardiography for emboli immediately after, 444
t-PA (*see* Plasminogen, activator, tissue)
Training
exercise, for intermittent claudication, 26
Transcranial
Doppler (*see* Ultrasound, Doppler, transcranial)
Transcutaneous
tissue oxygen tension, foot, response to lumbar sympathectomy for focal ischemic necrosis, 334
Transferrin
indium-111 labeled, lung and leg microvascular permeability to, and acute lung injury after aortic surgery, 82
Transforming growth factor-β1
in dermal microcirculation in chronic venous insufficiency, 474
Transfusion
perioperative, incidence and volume, effects of albumin-impregnated prosthetic graft for infrarenal aortic replacement on, 402
red cell, perioperative, limiting in vascular patients, 220
Transjugular
intrahepatic portosystemic shunt *vs.* endoscopic sclerotherapy for variceal hemorrhage
acute, 479
for prevention of recurrent hemorrhage, 480
Transluminal
angioplasty, percutaneous (*see* Angioplasty, percutaneous transluminal)
Transplantation
liver, shunt surgery during era of, 482
Transthoracic
repair of innominate and common carotid artery disease, outcome, 238
Trauma
aortic, blunt, 411
aortic rupture due to, thoracic, surgical indications and timing of repair of, 412
aortic transections due to, clamp-sew technique for, 264
arterial, 407
popliteal, anticoagulation and intraoperative thrombolysis improves limb salvage after, 407
brachial plexus, with vascular injuries of thoracic outlet, aggressive management of, 418
carotid artery dissections due to, from blunt softball injuries, 409
neural-vascular, combined, 416
lower extremity, management of, 416
patients

Statement of Purpose

The YEAR BOOK Service

The YEAR BOOK series was devised in 1901 by practicing health professionals who observed that the literature of medicine and related disciplines had become so voluminous that no one individual could read and place in perspective every potential advance in a major specialty. In the final decade of the 20th century, this recognition is more acutely true than it was in 1901.

More than merely a series of books, YEAR BOOK volumes are the tangible results of a unique service designed to accomplish the following:

- to *survey* a wide range of journals of proven value
- to *select* from those journals papers representing significant advances and statements of important clinical principles
- to provide *abstracts* of those articles that are readable, convenient summaries of their key points
- to provide *commentary* about those articles to place them in perspective

These publications grow out of a unique process that calls on the talents of outstanding authorities in clinical and fundamental disciplines, trained literature specialists, and professional writers, all supported by the resources of Mosby, the world's preeminent publisher for the health professions.

The Literature Base

Mosby and its editors survey approximately 500 journals published worldwide, covering the full range of the health professions. On an annual basis, the publisher examines usage patterns and polls its expert authorities to add new journals to the literature base and to delete journals that are no longer useful as potential YEAR BOOK sources.

The Literature Survey

The publisher's team of literature specialists, all of whom are trained and experienced health professionals, examines every original, peer-reviewed article in each journal issue. More than 250,000 articles per year are scanned systematically, including title, text, illustrations, tables, and references. Each scan is compared, article by article, to the search strategies that the publisher has developed in consultation with the 270 outside experts who form the pool of YEAR BOOK editors. A given article may be reviewed by any number of editors, from one to a dozen or more, regardless of the discipline for which the paper was originally published. In turn, each editor who receives the article reviews it to determine whether the article should be included in the YEAR BOOK. This decision is based on the article's inherent quality, its probable usefulness to readers of that YEAR BOOK, and the editor's goal to represent a balanced picture of a given field in each volume of the YEAR BOOK. In addition, the editor indicates when to include figures and tables from the article to help the YEAR BOOK reader better understand the information.

Of the quarter million articles scanned each year, only 5% are selected for detailed analysis within the YEAR BOOK series, thereby assuring readers of the high value of every selection.

The Abstract

The publisher's abstracting staff is headed by a seasoned medical professional and includes individuals with training in the life sciences, medicine, and other areas, plus extensive experience in writing for the health professions and related industries. Each selected article is assigned to a specific writer on this abstracting staff. The abstracter, guided in many cases by notations supplied by the expert editor, writes a structured, condensed summary designed so that the reader can rapidly acquire the essential information contained in the article.

The Commentary

The YEAR BOOK editorial boards, sometimes assisted by guest commentators, write comments that place each article in perspective for the reader. This provides the reader with the equivalent of a personal consultation with a leading international authority—an opportunity to better understand the value of the article and to benefit from the authority's thought processes in assessing the article.

Additional Editorial Features

The editorial boards of each YEAR BOOK organize the abstracts and comments to provide a logical and satisfying sequence of information. To enhance the organization, editors also provide introductions to sections or individual chapters, comments linking a number of abstracts, citations to additional literature, and other features.

The published YEAR BOOK contains enhanced bibliographic citations for each selected article, including extended listings of multiple authors and identification of author affiliations. Each YEAR BOOK contains a Table of Contents specific to that year's volume. From year to year, the Table of Contents for a given YEAR BOOK will vary depending on developments within the field.

Every YEAR BOOK contains a list of the journals from which papers have been selected. This list represents a subset of approximately 500 journals surveyed by the publisher and occasionally reflects a particularly pertinent article from a journal that is not surveyed on a routine basis.

Finally, each volume contains a comprehensive subject index and an index to authors of each selected paper.

The 1999 Year Book Series

Year Book of Allergy, Asthma, and Clinical Immunology: Drs. Rosenwasser, Boguniewicz, Borish, Routes, Spahn, and Weber

Year Book of Anesthesiology and Pain Management®: Drs. Tinker, Abram, Chestnut, Roizen, Rothenberg, and Wood

Year Book of Cardiology®: Drs. Schlant, Collins, Gersh, Graham, Kaplan, and Waldo

Year Book of Chiropractic®: Dr. Lawrence

Year Book of Critical Care Medicine®: Drs. Parrillo, Balk, Calvin, Franklin, and Shapiro

Year Book of Dentistry®: Drs. Meskin, Berry, Jeffcoat, Leinfelder, Roser, Summitt, and Zakariasen

Year Book of Dermatology and Dermatologic Surgery™: Drs. Thiers and Lang

Year Book of Diagnostic Radiology®: Drs. Osborn, Dalinka, Groskin, Maynard, Pentecost, Ros, Smirniotopoulos, and Young

Year Book of Emergency Medicine®: Drs. Wagner, Dronen, Davidson, King, Niemann, and Hamilton

Year Book of Endocrinology®: Drs. Bagdade, Braverman, Horton, Kannan, Landsberg, Molitch, Morley, Odell, Poehlman, Rogol, and Fitzpatrick

Year Book of Family Practice®: Drs. Berg, Bowman, Davidson, Dexter, and Scherger

Year Book of Gastroenterology: Drs. Aliperti and Fleshman

Year Book of Hand Surgery®: Drs. Amadio and Hentz

Year Book of Medicine®: Drs. Klahr, Frishman, Malawista, Mandell, Jett, Young, Barkin, and Bagdade

Year Book of Neonatal and Perinatal Medicine®: Drs. Fanaroff, Maisels, and Stevenson

Year Book of Nephrology, Hypertension, and Mineral Metabolism: Drs. Schwab, Bennett, Emmett, Hostetter, and Moe

Year Book of Neurology and Neurosurgery®: Drs. Bradley and Gibbs

Year Book of Nuclear Medicine®: Drs. Gottschalk, Blaufox, Coleman, Strauss, and Zubal

Year Book of Obstetrics, Gynecology, and Women's Health: Drs. Mishell, Herbst, and Kirschbaum

Year Book of Oncology®: Drs. Ozols, Eisenberg, Glatstein, Loehrer, and Urba

Year Book of Ophthalmology®: Drs. Wilson, Augsburger, Cohen, Eagle, Grossman, Laibson, Maguire, Nelson, Penne, Rapuano, Sergott, Spaeth, Tipperman, Ms. Gosfield, and Ms. Salmon

Year Book of Orthopedics®: Drs. Morrey, Beauchamp, Currier, Tolo, Trigg, and Swiontkowski

Year Book of Otolaryngology–Head and Neck Surgery®: Drs. Paparella, Holt, and Otto

Year Book of Pathology and Laboratory Medicine®: Drs. Raab, Cohen, Dabbs, Olson, and Stanley

Year Book of Pediatrics®: Dr. Stockman

Year Book of Plastic, Reconstructive, and Aesthetic Surgery®: Drs. Miller, Bartlett, Garner, McKinney, Ruberg, Salisbury, and Smith

Year Book of Psychiatry and Applied Mental Health®: Drs. Talbott, Ballenger, Frances, Lydiard, Meltzer, Jensen, and Tasman

Year Book of Pulmonary Disease®: Drs. Jett, Castro, Maurer, Peters, Phillips, and Ryu

Year Book of Rheumatology, Arthritis, and Musculoskeletal Disease™: Drs. Panush, Hadler, Hellman, LeRoy, Pisetsky, and Simon

Year Book of Sports Medicine®: Drs. Shephard, Drinkwater, Eichner, Torg, Alexander, and Mr. George

Year Book of Surgery®: Drs. Copeland, Bland, Deitch, Eberlein, Howard, Luce, Seeger, Souba, and Sugarbaker

Year Book of Urology®: Drs. Andriole and Coplen

Year Book of Vascular Surgery®: Dr. Porter

Journals Represented

Mosby and its editors survey approximately 500 journals for its abstract and commentary publications. From these journals, the editors select the articles to be abstracted. Journals represented in this YEAR BOOK are listed below.

Academic Emergency Medicine
American Journal of Emergency Medicine
American Journal of Kidney Diseases
American Journal of Medicine
American Journal of Roentgenology
American Journal of Surgery
American Surgeon
Annals of Internal Medicine
Annals of Surgery
Annals of Thoracic Surgery
Annals of Vascular Surgery
Annals of the Royal College of Surgeons of England
Archives of Internal Medicine
Archives of Otolaryngology Head and Neck Surgery
Archives of Physical Medicine and Rehabilitation
Archives of Surgery
British Journal of Surgery
Cardiovascular Surgery
Cardiovascular and Interventional Radiology
Cerebrovascular Diseases
Circulation
Circulation Research
Clinical Radiology
Clinical Science
European Journal of Surgery
European Journal of Vascular and Endovascular Surgery
Hypertension
Investigative Radiology
Israel Journal of Medical Sciences
Journal of Bone and Joint Surgery (American Volume)
Journal of Cardiac Surgery
Journal of Cardiovascular Surgery
Journal of Clinical Investigation
Journal of Computer Assisted Tomography
Journal of Endovascular Surgery
Journal of Neurosurgery
Journal of Nuclear Medicine
Journal of Pathology
Journal of Reconstructive Microsurgery
Journal of Surgical Research
Journal of Thoracic and Cardiovascular Surgery
Journal of Vascular Surgery
Journal of the American College of Cardiology
Journal of the American College of Surgeons
Journal of the American Medical Association
Lancet

Mayo Clinic Proceedings
Medical Journal of Australia
New England Journal of Medicine
Radiology
Southern Medical Journal
Stroke
Surgery
Thorax
Thrombosis and Haemostasis
World Journal of Surgery

Standard Abbreviations

The following terms are abbreviated in this edition: acquired immunodeficiency syndrome (AIDS), cardiopulmonary resuscitation (CPR), central nervous system (CNS), cerebrospinal fluid (CSF), computed tomography (CT), deoxyribonucleic acid (DNA), electrocardiography (ECG), health maintenance organization (HMO), human immunodeficiency virus (HIV), intensive care unit (ICU), intramuscular (IM), intravenous (IV), magnetic resonance (MR) imaging (MRI), and ribonucleic acid (RNA).

Note

The Year Book of Vascular Surgery® is a literature survey service providing abstracts of articles published in the professional literature. Every effort is made to assure the accuracy of the information presented in these pages. Neither the editors nor the publisher of the Year Book of Vascular Surgery® can be responsible for errors in the original materials. The editors' comments are their own opinions. Mention of specific products within this publication does not constitute endorsement.

To facilitate the use of the Year Book of Vascular Surgery® as a reference tool, all illustrations and tables included in this publication are now identified as they appear in the original article. This change is meant to help the reader recognize that any illustration or table appearing in the Year Book of Vascular Surgery® may be only one of many in the original article. For this reason, figure and table numbers will often appear to be out of sequence within the Year Book of Vascular Surgery®.

Introduction

Each year I attempt to keep you dear readers informed as to the current status of our national transition to managed care. A significant majority of Americans now receive their health care through the managed care model in one form or another. Until recently, everything had been rosy for the companies. They were making huge profits, their stocks had rise to dizzying heights, they paid their CEOs millions, and they underwent mega–million dollar mergers on a regular basis. But reality seems to be catching up with these for-profit health care companies. Without question, they made their initial dizzying profits by eliminating some genuine waste in the system, but primarily by denying certain types of health care. Now the waste is eliminated and, unfortunately for them, legislative bodies, especially the U.S. Congress, are beginning to severely restrict their ability to limit care. Many of the HMOs in this country that were so profitable in the past are now losing money hand over fist, their stock values have declined to unimaginably low levels, and many appear to be on the verge of bankruptcy. It seems that financial survival for many of these companies will require raising health premium charges just as high as the private system was raising them in the past. Too bad.

As for our assigned topic, vascular surgery, there have been no breakthroughs in the past year, but as always there have been areas of significant progress. One of the areas that has attracted the most attention is that of therapeutic angiogenesis. Led by Dr. Isner and his group in Boston, a number of investigators have been attempting to stimulate the growth of new blood vessels in ischemic limbs by the injection of growth factors, primarily acidic fibroblast growth factor and vascular endothelial growth factor. Presently, I find this work difficult to assess. The investigators are absolutely confident they have produced a myriad of tiny new blood vessels in the ischemic areas, but what is visible on the radiographs they have published shows vessels so small that, in my opinion, I doubt they could carry any significant blood flow. Of course, they claim benefit, but to date these are uncontrolled studies. The time has come to mount a proper prospective, randomized, controlled study in which one group gets the real growth factor, the other group gets a placebo, and exactly the same observations are made on both groups after the treatment. Until that is done, I will have a healthy doubt about the benefits of therapeutic angiogenesis.

There continues to be a groundswell of interest in the use of therapeutic radiation with angioplasty to reduce posttreatment fibrointimal hyperplasia. To date, the irradiation has been catheter-delivered for a matter of a few minutes directly after the angioplasty. Several comparative studies have shown that the irradiated arteries greater than 6 months posttreatment show considerably wider lumens and less occlusive disease than do the nonirradiated arteries. I am certain arterial irradiation is going to be with us for the next period of years and will soon be applied to arteries other than the coronary.

During the past year, another remarkable megatrial funded by the NIH was published, examining patients with coronary disease eligible for either CABG or PTCA, with randomization between the two treatments. A significant survival benefit at 5 years was present in the patients randomized to CABG, but almost the entire difference between the two groups resided in diabetic patients, who fared much better with CABG. As you will recall, based on prior studies, the NIH issued a clinic alert several years ago pointing out that diabetic patients fared poorly with PTCA compared with nondiabetic patients.

The results from another major trial published this past year, unfortunately, were negative. A large group of people received antioxidants, including α-tocopherol or β-carotene supplements, that were supposed to have a protective effect by reducing low-density lipoprotein cholesterol oxidation. The trial was conducted primarily to investigate the effect of these drug supplements on lung cancer, but a secondary end point was an investigation of cardiovascular disease. Unfortunately, the findings were not only negative, but the risk of fatal coronary disease was actually increased in the groups receiving β-carotene or the combination of α-tocopherol and β-carotene. To date, the clinical use of antioxidants has been a major disappointment. It is always sad when a well-conceived trial comes a cropper.

An area of increasing interest is the association between body iron stores and the risk of myocardial infarction. While no one knows the mechanism, it appears that excess iron facilitates lipid peroxidation and lipoprotein modificatons. I suspect there will be large control led trials of iron reduction in patients at risk for myocardial infarction in the near future. An interesting study by Dr. Jack Collin and associates at Oxford University deserves comment. We make many therapeutic decisions for our patients with claudication based upon the patients' assessments of how far they can walk. The Oxford group has done a number of studies and found that patients' statements have little or no relationship to actuality. These investigators further note that reliance on the treadmill as a substitute for real-terrain walking results in considerable distortion. In all likelihood, the patients' real walking distances are considerably greater than what they report.

Without question, one of the most exciting areas in the past year has been the further disclosure of the close association between atherosclerotic plaque and *Chlamydia pneumoniae*. Investigators have found anti-chlamydial antibody, chlamydial mRNA, or actual living *Chamydia* in about three fourths of atherosclerotic plaques taken from patients. We, of course, do not know whether the *Chlamydia* is a fellow traveler or perhaps an important causation of the atherosclerosis. One small trial administered an anti-chlamydial antibiotic, azithromycin, to one group of patients with atherosclerosis and a placebo to the other group and noted that the incidence of "adverse cardiovascular events" was much lower in the group receiving antibiotics. Will it not be wonderful if it turns out that atherosclerosis, like many peptic ulcers, is bacteria-dependent and susceptible to treatment by antibiotics? This may be the breakthrough of the century.

this gene product than nonischemic muscle. As stated in other commentaries, however, I continue to have reservations about the new tiny blood vessels presented as proof of angiogenesis. On balance, I have no idea whether this entire therapeutic approach is ever going to be of any clinical value. I inherently believe it will not, but I have been wrong before. One has only to recall my initial negative response to the first issue of Microsoft stock.

Cardiac/Lipids

Improved Outcome After Coronary Bypass Surgery in Patients With Ischemic Cardiomyopathy and Residual Myocardial Viability

Pagley PR, Beller GA, Watson DD, et al (Univ of Virginia, Charlottesville)

Circulation 96:793–800, 1997 1–4

Background.—For patients with coronary artery disease and large areas of asynergy, residual myocardial viability has been linked to improvement of ventricular function after coronary bypass surgery. However, how viability affects clinical outcome remains unclear. This study compared the outcomes of bypass surgery in patients with poor ventricular function and predominantly viable vs. less viable myocardium.

Methods.—The retrospective study included 70 patients with multivessel coronary artery disease and left ventricular ejection fraction <40%. Before surgery, each patient underwent quantitative thallium 201 scintigraphy. On blinded review of the scans, each segment was scored in terms of defect magnitude. A viability index was constructed by adding the segmental viability scores and dividing them by the number of segments seen. The study hypothesis was that greater myocardial viability would be related to better postoperative outcome.

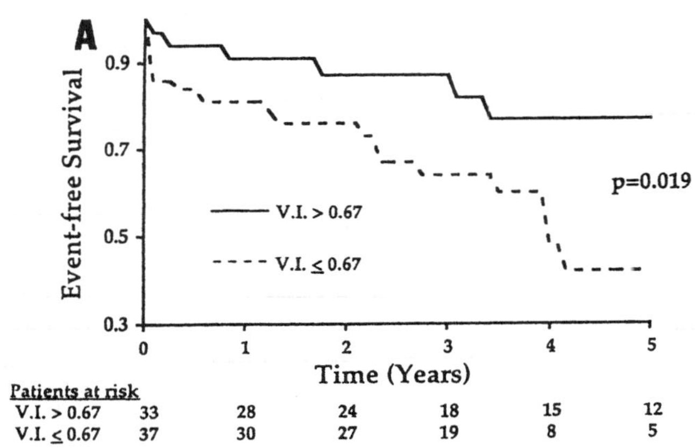

FIGURE 2.—Kaplan-Meier survival analysis demonstrating survival free from cardiac events (cardiac death or heart transplantation). Comparison of event-free survival among patients in group 1 (viability index >0.67; *solid line*) and group 2 (viability index ≤0.67; *broken line*). (Courtesy of Pagley PR, Beller GA, Watson DD, et al: Improved outcome after coronary bypass surgery in patients with ischemic cardiomyopathy and residual myocardial variability. *Circulation* 96:793–800, 1997.)

Results.—There was a significant association between viability index and 3-year survival. This was so regardless of of age, ejection fraction, and number of coronary vessels involved. Thirty-three patients had a viability index >0.67 (group 1), and 37 had a viability index of ≤0.67 (group 2). The 2 groups were comparable in age, comorbidity, and extent of coronary artery disease by group 1, 6 patients died of cardiac causes and none required heart transplantation. In group 2, 15 patients died of cardiac causes, and 2 required heart transplantation. The survival difference was significant on Kaplan-Meier analysis (Fig 2).

Conclusions.—For patients with low ejection fraction and multivessel coronary artery disease, greater myocardial viability on preoperative ^{201}Tl scintigraphy is associated with better outcomes of coronary artery bypass grafting. Thus resting ^{201}Tl scintigraphy could be useful in identifying those patients most likely to benefit from surgical revascularization.

► In our elderly vascular surgery population, we frequently encounter patients with severe congestive heart failure. I have always been uncertain as to the benefits of coronary bypass in specifically improving heart failure in this cohort. Remarkably, these authors conclude that ^{201}T1 cardiac scintigraphy allowed calculation of a cardiac viability index that was significantly related to 3-year survival free of cardiac events after coronary bypass surgery. Thus, it appears that we now have an objective test allowing us to predict just which heart failure patients may benefit from coronary bypass. This may be important information.

Long-term Angiographic and Clinical Outcome After Percutaneous Transluminal Coronary Angioplasty and Intracoronary Radiation Therapy in Humans

Condado JA, Waksman R, Gurdiel O, et al (Emory Univ, Atlanta, Ga)
Circulation 96:727–732, 1997 1–5

Background.—Studies of restenosis in animals have found that ionizing radiation can significantly reduce neointimal formation. Clinical studies of endovascular radiation in restenosed stented femoral arteries have shown low restenosis rates with long-term follow-up. Intracoronary radiation therapy (ICRT) was studied for the prevention of coronary artery restenosis after percutaneous transluminal coronary angioplasty (PTCA).

Methods.—The study included 21 patients with unstable angina undergoing PTCA on a total of 22 coronary arteries. An iridium 192 source wire, as a high-energy γ-emitter, was hand delivered to the angioplasty site for ICRT. The patients were examined by angiography at 24 hours, 30 to 60 days, and 6 months. The ICRT was assessed for feasibility, safety, and effectiveness.

Results.—Successful angioplasty was achieved in 86% of arteries. The source wire was successfully placed in all arteries. The 24-hour angiograms revealed early late loss of luminal diameter, from 1.92 to 1.40 mm. At 30 to 60 days, 2 arteries had become completely occluded, 1 had developed a pseudoaneurysm, and 2 had become significantly dilated at the treatment site. The 20 remaining arteries were still patent at 6 months; their mean luminal diameter was 1.65 mm. Late luminal loss was calculated at 0.27 mm, with a late loss index of 0.19. At 1 year, 1 patient had a myocardial infarction, 3 required repeat angioplasty to the same site, and 7 had continued angina.

Conclusions.—This study demonstrates that ICRT is feasible in patients undergoing PTCA. The complication rate is acceptable. The findings suggest that ICRT may inhibit late luminal loss by inhibiting neointima formation or by promoting favorable remodeling. However, without randomized trials, no conclusions can be made about efficacy.

► As these authors note, prevention of restenosis after coronary angioplasty remains the greatest therapeutic challenge facing interventional cardiology. As the authors modestly state, this study describes the first human trial of intracoronary radiation therapy after angioplasty. The mean irradiation treatment time, catheter delivered, was 580 seconds. At greater than 6 months' follow-up, repeat coronary angiography showed 20 of 22 arteries remained patent, with minimal luminal diameter loss. Realistically, these are very preliminary results and demonstrate only that intracoronary radiation therapy after coronary intervention is feasible, certainly not that it is proven successful. Large-scale prospective, randomized trials will be required for that determination. A small randomized trial is described in the 1998 YEAR BOOK.[1]

Reference

1. 1998 YEAR BOOK OF VASCULAR SURGERY, p 6.

Probucol and Multivitamins in the Prevention of Restenosis After Coronary Angioplasty

Tardif J-C, for the Multivitamins and Probucol Study Group (Univ of Montreal)
N Engl J Med 337:365–372, 1997 1–6

Background.—Oxidizing metabolites produced at the site of coronary angioplasty can cause chain reactions that may result in restenosis. Previous studies have suggested that antioxidants may prevent restenosis after angioplasty. Whether drugs with antioxidant properties reduce the incidence and severity of restenosis after angioplasty was determined.

Methods.—A total of 317 patients were enrolled in the double-blind, randomized study. One month before angioplasty, the patients were assigned to placebo, 500 mg of probucol, multivitamins (30,000 IU of β-carotene, 500 mg of vitamin C, and 700 IU of vitamin E), or probucol plus multivitamins. Treatments were taken twice a day for 4 weeks before and for 6 months after angioplasty. Twelve hours before angioplasty, the groups received additional doses of the treatments to which they had been assigned.

Findings.—Six months after angioplasty, the mean decrease in luminal diameter was 0.12 mm in the probucol group, 0.22 mm in the combined-treatment group, 0.33 mm in the multivitamin group, and 0.38 mm in the placebo group. Restenosis rates per segment were 20.7%, 28.9%, 40.3%, and 38.9%, respectively. The respective rates of repeated angioplasty were 11.2%, 16.2%, 24.4%, and 26.6%.

Conclusions.—The antioxidant probucol effectively decreases the rate of restenosis after balloon coronary angioplasty. It is unclear why multivitamins do not prevent restenosis, because they are also antioxidants.

▶ I continue to include a number of cardiologic reports on coronary angioplasty restenosis, because I feel it likely that those data provide important clues to both peripheral arterial and vein graft stenosis. This study compared the effects of placebo, the antioxidant probucol, as well as vitamin E, vitamin C, and β-carotene on restenosis. The only agent effective was probucol, which reduced restenosis by a remarkable 50%. Of course, it is totally unknown whether it was the antioxidant properties of this agent resulting in the benefit, or some unsuspected other pharmacologic property. It is well known, for example, that probucol has well-defined lipid-lowering properties. The information appears conclusive, however, that whatever the role probucol may play, β-carotene, vitamin E, and vitamin C do not appear to have any defined role in the prevention of restenosis. Too bad! More good theories shot to hell.

Phentolamine Prevents Adaptation to Ischemia During Coronary Angioplasty: Role of α-Adrenergic Receptors in Ischemic Preconditioning

Tomai F, Crea F, Gaspardone A, et al (Università di Roma Tor Vergata, Rome; Università Cattolica del Sacro Cuore, Rome)

Circulation 96:2171–2177, 1997 1–7

Background.—α-Adrenergic receptors appear to play a role in ischemic preconditioning, experimental studies suggest. However, their involvement in preconditioning among humans is unknown. The α-adrenergic receptor antagonist phentolamine was used to examine the role of α-adrenergic receptors in ischemic preconditioning in humans.

Methods.—Eighteen consecutive patients undergoing elective coronary angioplasty for an isolated obstructive lesion of the left anterior descending coronary artery were studied. They were randomly assigned to receive either IV phentolamine or placebo during the procedure. After the first 2 balloon inflations, the patients' intracoronary ECG readings and cardiac pain were assessed. A Doppler guidewire was used to measure average peak velocity in the contralateral coronary artery during occlusion as a measure of collateral recruitment.

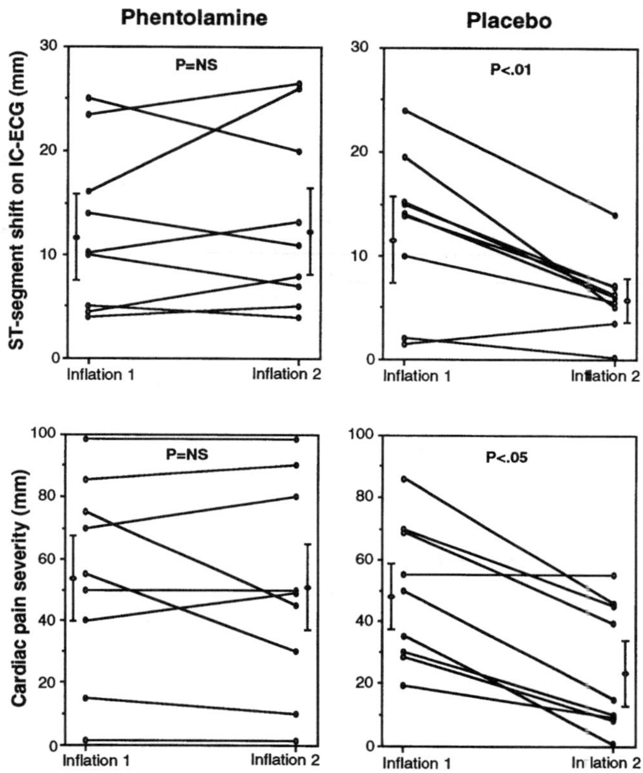

FIGURE 2.—Values of ST-segment shifts on the intracoronary ECG (*IC-ECG*) and of cardiac pain severity at the end of the first and second balloon inflations in the 2 groups of patients. In phentolamine-treated patients, ST-segment changes and cardiac pain severity at the end of the second balloon inflation were similar to those at the end of the first inflation. Conversely, in placebo-treated patients, ST-segment changes and cardiac pain severity at the end of the second balloon inflation were significantly less than those at the end of the first inflation. (Courtesy of Tomai F, Crea F, Gaspardone A, et al: Phentolamine prevents adaptation to ischemia during coronary angioplasty: Role of α-adrenergic receptors in ischemic preconditioning. *Circulation* 96:2171–2177. Copyright 1997, American Heart Association. Reproduced with permission.)

Results.—Both groups of patients showed an increase in average peak velocity from baseline to the end of the first inflation, with no additional increase during the second inflation. For the phentolamine group, changes in the ST segment and in cardiac pain were similar during the first and second inflations. In contrast, the placebo group showed lesser changes during the second inflation (Fig 2).

Conclusions.—Human patients receiving phentolamine during coronary angioplasty do not show adaptation to ischemia after 2 sequential balloon inflations. This effect of phentolamine is independent of collateral recruitment, and thus is the result of ischemic preconditioning. α-Adrenergic

in the α-tocopherol–treated group. Mortality was highest in the β-carotene group and lowest in the placebo group (Fig 3).

Conclusions.—Both α-tocopherol and β-carotene increased the risk of a fatal coronary event in male smokers with a previous myocardial infarction.

► It has been speculated for years that LDL oxidation may be a key event in the initiation and progression of atherosclerosis. Similarly, there have been years of speculation that the antioxidants, including α-tocopherol (vitamin E), as well as β-carotene supplements may be clinically beneficial by protecting low density lipoprotein cholesterol from oxidation. The recently completed α-tocopherol/β-carotene cancer prevention study was conducted primarily to investigate the effects of α-tocopherol and β-carotene supplements on the incidence of lung cancer; however, a secondary end point was an investigation of these substances on cardiovascular disease. Unfortunately, the study was not only negative but, sadly, the risk of fatal coronary heart disease appeared to increase in the groups receiving either β-carotene or the combination of α-tocopherol and β-carotene. It is always sad when a well-conceived and entirely plausible hypothesis comes a cropper. To date the antioxidants have proved most disappointing. (See also Abstract 1–6.)

Follow-up Study of Patients Randomly Allocated Ramipril or Placebo for Heart Failure After Acute Myocardial Infarction: AIRE Extension (AIREX) Study

Hall AS, for the AIREX Study Investigators (Univ of Leeds, England)

Lancet 349:1493–1497, 1997 1–14

Objective.—Whether, when and for how long patients with acute myocardial infarction (AMI) should take angiotensin converting enzyme (ACE) inhibitors is controversial. Results of long-term survival of patients with AMI and clinical defined heart failure who took part in the Acute Infarction Ramipril Efficacy (AIRE) Study were reported.

Methods.—The 603 patients (average age, 65 years) in the independent, multinational, multicenter, double-blind, randomized, placebo-controlled, parallel-group study received placebo (n = 301, 71 women) or 1.25 or 2.5 mg ramipril twice daily (n = 302, 77 women), titrating to a maximum dose of 2.5 or 5 mg twice daily. Patients were followed for an average of 59 months after close of the study. Patients were treated with placebo for an average of 13.4 months and with ramipril for 12.4 months.

Results.—As of March 1996, 117 placebo patients (38.9%) and 83 ramipril patients (27.5%) had died (Fig 1). Treatment with ramipril reduced the relative risk of death by 36%. Survival rates were 11.4% higher in the ramipril group.

Conclusion.—Ramipril improved survival in patients after AMI. Patients with AMI who are treated with an ACE inhibitor should continue on the therapy unless intolerance develops.

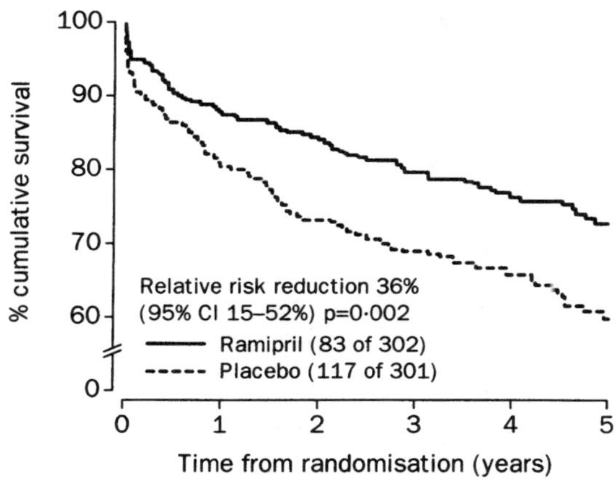

Numbers at risk						
Ramipril	302	263	253	239	202	93
Placebo	301	242	220	206	168	71

FIGURE 1.—Kaplan-Meier survival estimates for patients randomized to ramipril or placebo. Comparisons were made with the log-rank test (2-sided *P* value). (Courtesy of Hall AS, for the AIREX Study Investigators: Follow-up study of patients randomly allocated ramipril or placebo for heart failure after acute myocardial infarction: AIRE Extension (AIREX) Study. *Lancet* 349:1493–1497, copyright 1997 by The Lancet, Ltd.)

► The benefits of using ACE inhibitors in patients after myocardial infarction have been amply documented.[1] This important study examines the fate of patients with heart failure following myocardial infarction randomized to treatment with ACE inhibitors or placebo. A highly significant survival benefit was found in favor of the ACE inhibitor group after 3-year follow-up. Relative risk reduction was a very robust 36%, with an absolute mortality reduction of 11.4%. I believe the issue is settled that survivors of myocardial infarction should be on lifetime ACE inhibitor therapy. It appears that the absolute benefits will be even greater in patients with impaired ventricular function. Because so many of our vascular patients have suffered prior myocardial infarction, this is indeed important information for vascular surgeons.

Reference

1. 1998 YEAR BOOK OF VASCULAR SURGERY, p 190.

Body Iron Stores and the Risk of Carotid Atherosclerosis: Prospective Results From the Bruneck Study

Kiechl S, Willeit J, Egger G, et al (Innsbruck Univ, Austria)
Circulation 96:3300–3307, 1997 1–15

Background.—Body stores of ferritin may play a role in atherogenesis by accelerating lipid peroxidation. These authors examined the association

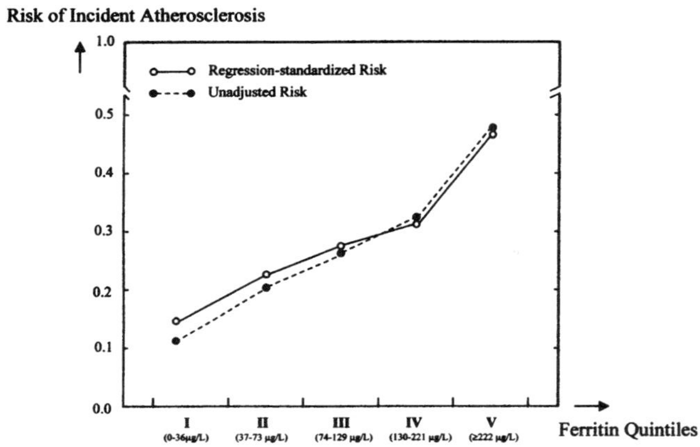

FIGURE 1.—Crude and regression-standardized risks of incident atherosclerosis (1990 to 1995) according to ferritin quintiles. Figure documents dose-response relation between ferritin measurements and risk of early atherogenesis. n = 476. (Courtesy of Kiechl S, Willeit J, Egger G, et al: Body iron stores and the risk of carotid atherosclerosis: prospective results from the Bruneck study. *Circulation* 96:3300–3397, 1997. Reproduced with permission, American Heart Association.)

between iron stores and carotid artery atherosclerosis over 5 years in normal subjects.

Methods.—Men (n = 414) and women (n = 412) between 40 and 79 years old underwent clinical and ultrasound examinations. Clinical evaluations included cardiologic, neurologic, and oral glucose tolerance tests. Levels of serum ferritin, apolipoproteins, HDL cholesterol, LDL cholesterol, antithrombin III, and fibrinogen were also measured. Ultrasound was used to scan the internal and common carotid arteries to determine any lesions. Differences between ultrasound scans at 1 year and at 5 years were used to determine the incidence and extension of atherosclerosis.

Findings.—The median ferritin concentration was 164 µg/L in men, 22 µg/L in premenopausal women, and 73 µg/L in postmenopausal women. Age-adjusted incidence rates controlling for sex and menopausal status were 4.4/100 person-years in men, 3.4 to 4.0 person-years in menopausal women, and 1.3/100 person-years in premenopausal women. When baseline atherosclerosis score, age, sex, risk attributes, and alcohol consumption were controlled for in analyses, the serum ferritin level was a significant and strong predictor of carotid atherosclerosis (odds ratio 1.50) (Fig 1). For each increase by 1 SD in the ferritin level, the higher the LDL level, and the greater the odds ratio for atherosclerotic disease; for example, a 1–SD increase in ferritin levels at LDL levels of 2.5, 3.6, and 4.9 mmol/L increased the odds ratios for atherosclerosis to 1.55, 1.77, and 2.05, respectively. In the 59 patients who developed cardiovascular disease, a synergistic association was found between ferritin levels and LDL cholesterol levels. Changes in iron levels between years 1 and 5 had an effect on atherosclerosis risk; lower ferritin levels were beneficial and higher levels had negative effects. The effects were similar both for the incidence of new plaques and the extension of disease in existing plaques.

Conclusions.—Iron stores are a major factor in atherosclerosis. These results indicate a pathologic role for lipid peroxidation in causing disease. Such a mechanism could help explain the sex differences in atherosclerotic vascular disease.

▶ The haunting question being asked by these investigators is whether elevated total body iron stores contribute to the development of atherosclerosis. For about the past 20 years, considerable evidence has been amassed that suggests iron has a role in the production of atherosclerosis, possibly participating in the oxidative modifications of lipoproteins. This 5-year clinical study supports the observation that increased iron stores are associated with atherosclerosis progression in a highly significant fashion. The authors have concluded that this study provides strong evidence for the role of iron stores in early atherogenesis, and suggests that lipid peroxidation may be a primary underlying pathogenetic mechanism. (See also Abstract 1–16.)

Association Between Body Iron Stores and the Risk of Acute Myocardial Infarction in Men

Tuomainen T-P, Punnonen K, Nyyssönen K, et al (Univ of Kuopio, Finland)
Circulation 97:1461–1466, 1998 1–16

Introduction.—Epidemiologic evidence is inconsistent regarding the role of iron, a lipid peroxidation catalyst, in coronary heart disease. The association between the concentration ratio of serum transferrin receptor to serum ferritin (TfR/ferritin) and risk of acute myocardial infarction (AMI) was evaluated in a prospective, nested case-control trial of men from eastern Finland.

Methods.—Transferrin receptors were measured by immunoenzymometric assay and ferritin concentration was calculated by radioimmunoassay from frozen baseline serum samples from 99 men who had an AMI and 98 controls nested from the Kuopio Ischemic Heart Disease Risk Factor Study. The AMIs were prospectively recorded.

Results.—The mean TfR/ferrin ratio was 15.1 among men who had AMI and 21.3 among controls, a significant difference. After adjusting for AMI risk factors and indicators of inflammation and alcohol intake, men in the lowest and second lowest thirds of the TfR/ferritin ratio, respectively, had a 2.9-fold and a 2.0-fold risk of AMI, compared with men in the highest third.

Conclusions.—There is a relationship between increased body stores of iron and excess risk of AMI. These data confirm earlier epidemiologic findings.

▶ These authors used the most sophisticated measure yet described to determine body iron stores, namely the TfR/ferritin ratio. These data showed a clear association between increased body iron stores and increased risk of AMI. This certainly complements the information presented in the preceding abstract. I know nothing about factors that control body iron stores, but I suspect it quite likely in the intermediate future that methods to reduce total body iron will become widespread. (See also Abstract 1–15.)

The Role of a Common Variant of the Cholesteryl Ester Transfer Protein Gene in the Progression of Coronary Atherosclerosis

Kuivenhoven JA, for the Regression Growth Evaluation Statin Study Group (Academic Med Ctr, Amsterdam; Leiden Univ, The Netherlands; Ottawa Heart Inst, Ont, Canada; et al)
N Engl J Med 338:86–93, 1998 1–17

Introduction.—There is an inverse relationship between high-density lipoprotein (HDL) cholesterol concentration and risk of coronary artery disease. The cholesteryl ester transfer protein (CETP) is key in the metabolism of this lipoprotein and may even alter susceptibility to atherosclerosis. The relationship between TaqIB, a polymorphism in the *CETP* gene associated with an effect on the lipid-transfer activity and HDL concentration, and the progression of coronary atherosclerosis was assessed in

TABLE 1.—Baseline Demographic and Coronary Artery Disease Characteristics, According to the *CETP* TaqIB Genotype*

Characteristic	*B1B1* (N=281)	*B1B2* (N=397)	*B2B2* (N=129)
Demographic			
Age—yr.	55±8	57±8	56±7
Body-mass index†	26±3	26±3	26±3
Systolic blood pressure—mm Hg	135±19	135±18	135±17
Diastolic blood pressure—mm Hg	82±10	82±10	81±9
Current or former smoker—no. (%)	246 (88)	346 (87)	118 (91)
Current smoker—no. (%)	76 (27)	113 (28)	30 (23)
Coronary artery disease			
History of myocardial infarction—no. (%)	129 (46)	183 (46)	68 (53)
Left ventricular ejection fraction—%	70±13	71±12	70±12
Mean luminal diameter—mm	2.80±0.45	2.81±0.49	2.81±0.45
Minimal luminal diameter—mm	1.90±0.53	1.92±0.55	1.86±0.56
Stenosis—%	35±13	35±12	37±15
Coronary artery disease—no. (%)‡			
1 vessel	115 (41)	165 (42)	54 (42)
2 vessels	103 (37)	128 (32)	45 (35)
3 vessels	62 (22)	101 (25)	30 (23)
Medications—no. (%)			
Pravastatin	136 (48)	212 (53)	63 (49)
Long-acting nitrates	149 (53)	229 (58)	70 (54)
β-Blocking agents	208 (74)	295 (74)	93 (72)
Calcium-blocking agents	163 (58)	252 (63)	73 (57)

*Plus-minus values are means ± SD. B1 denotes the presence of a restriction site for *TaqI* in intron 1 of the *CETP* gene, and B2 its absence. There were no significant differences between the subgroups.

†The body-mass index was calculated as the weight in kilograms divided by the square of the height in meters.

‡Data on 1 patient with the *B1B1* and 3 patients with the *B1B2* genotype were missing. Because of rounding, not all percentages total 100.

(Courtesy of Kuivenhoven JA, for the Regression Growth Evaluation Statin Study Group: The role of a common variant of the cholesteryl ester transfer protein gene in the progression of coronary atherosclerosis. *N Engl J Med* 338:86–93.)

TABLE 1.—Characteristics of Controls vs. Patients With Peripheral Arterial Disease (PAD)

	Control (n = 11)	PAD (n = 19)	p Value
Age	62 ± 6.9	66 ± 6.08	.66
Height (cm)	178.8 ± 5.19	173.5 ± 7.9	.54
Step length (cm)	73.4 ± 6.02	56.9 ± 7.9	<.001
Cadence (steps/min)	116.7 ± 7.57	107.2 ± 8.5	<.001
Speed (m/min)	84.2 ± 11.5	60.9 ± 9.6	<.001
Step length/height	.41 ± .03	.33 ± .04	<.001

*Values are mean ± SD; *P* values are given for differences between PAD and control group.

(Courtesy of Scherer SA, Bainbridge JS, Hiatt WR, et al: Gait characteristics of patients with claudication. *Arch Phys Med Rehabil* 79:529–531, 1998.)

Conclusions.—All patients with symptoms of claudication had abnormal gait patterns, compared with controls. Disease severity and pain symptoms did not affect the severity of gait abnormality.

► It had never really occurred to me that claudicants have a different walking pattern from nonclaudicants. We learn from this interesting study that claudicants walking at distances less than their claudication distance walk slower than normal, have decreased step length, and decreased cadence compared with nonclaudicants. It will be fascinating to learn whether these gait peculiarities are permanent or are returned to normal by successful treatment of claudication.

Chlamydia

Detection of *Chlamydia pneumoniae* in Atherosclerotic Plaques in the Walls of Arteries of Lower Extremities From Patients Undergoing Bypass Operation for Arterial Obstruction

Kuo C-c, Coulson AS, Campbell LA, et al (Univ of Washington, Seattle; Dameron Hosp Heart Inst, Stockton, Calif)

J Vasc Surg 26:29–31, 1997 1–23

Background.—*Chlamydia pneumoniae* has been detected in atherosclerotic lesions of the coronary and carotid arteries and aorta by various techniques. The studied specimens have been obtained from sources including autopsy, atherectomy, endarterectomy, vascular surgery, and heart transplantation. The finding of *C. pneumoniae* in atherosclerotic lesions from the lower extremities is reported.

Methods and Findings.—The study included femoral and popliteal artery biopsy specimens from 23 patients with claudication undergoing bypass surgery. The presence of *C. pneumoniae* was sought by immunocytochemical and polymerase chain reaction studies. In 48% of patients, atherosclerotic plaques from either artery showed *C. pneumoniae*. Thirty-eight percent of popliteal artery specimens and 17% of femoral artery specimens were positive for *C. pneumoniae* (Table 1).

TABLE 1.—*Chlamydia pneumoniae* Detected by ICC or PCR in Atherosclerotic Plaques of Arteries of Lower Extremities

Arteries	No. positive/No. tested *ICC*	*PCR*	*Either*
Popliteal	7/9	4/21	8/21
Femoral	2/11	1/18	3/18
Total	9/20	5/39	11/39

Abbreviations: ICC, immunocytochemical stain; *PCR*, polymerase chain reaction.
(Courtesy of Kuo C-c, Coulson AS, Campbell LA, et al: Detection of *Chlamydia pneumoniae* in atherosclerotic plaques in the walls of arteries of lower extremities from patients undergoing bypass operation for arterial obstruction. *J Vasc Surg* 26:29–31, 1997.)

Conclusions.—Extending the known association between *C. pneumoniae* and atherosclerosis, the organism is found in atherosclerotic plaques from lower extremity arteries. This suggests that *C. pneumoniae* is widespread in atherosclerosis of the vascular system, though any causal role remains to be determined.

▶ A number of infectious agents have been repeatedly noted in atherosclerotic deposits in arterial walls. In recent years, attention has focused primarily on *Chlamydia pneumoniae*, although other agents such as cytomegalovirus and herpes virus have also attracted attention. Using a complex immunocytochemical system including polymerase chain reaction, these investigators detected evidence of *C. pneumoniae* in 11 of 23 lower extremity atherosclerotic specimens. This and the information in the next article by Chiu et al. (Abstract 1–24) convincingly demonstrate that *C. pneumoniae* is widespread in atherosclerotic deposits. The question, of course, remains whether this is a fellow traveler or a potential cause of atherosclerosis. Would it not be wonderful if we determined that a significant percentage of atherosclerosis could be eliminated by use of antibiotics? (See also Abstracts 1–27 and 1–28.) Stay tuned. I am sure we shall hear a great deal more about this in time.

***Chlamydia pneumoniae*, Cytomegalovirus, and Herpes Simplex Virus in Atherosclerosis of the Carotid Artery**

Chiu B, Viira E, Tucker W, et al (Univ of Toronto)
Circulation 96:2144–2148, 1997 1–24

Background.—There is evidence that certain infectious agents are involved in the pathogenesis of atherosclerosis. Seroepidemiologic and histopathologic studies have shown that *Chlamydia pneumoniae*, cytomegalovirus, and herpes simplex virus type 1 are associated with atherosclerosis. The concurrent presence of *C. pneumoniae*, cytomegalovirus, and herpes simplex virus type 1 in patients having carotid endarterectomy was investigated.

TABLE 2.—Presence of *Chlamydia pneumoniae*, CMV, and HSV in Atherosclerotic vs. Control (Normal) Arteries

	Carotid Plaque (n=76)	Control (n=20)	*P*
C. pneumoniae	54 (71%)	0	<.0003
CMV	27 (35.5%)	0	.0004
HSV	8 (10.5%)	0	.09

Abbreviations: CMV, cytomegalovirus; *HSV*, herpes simplex virus type 1.

(Courtesy of Chiu B, Viira E, Tucker W, et al: *Chlamydia pneumoniae*, cytomegalovirus, and herpes simplex virus in atherosclerosis of the carotid artery. *Circulation* 96:2144–2148, 1997. Reproduced with permission *Circulation*. Copyright 1997 American Heart Association.)

Methods.—There were 76 patients with carotid artery stenosis undergoing carotid endarterectomy. The endarterectomy specimens were stained for *C. pneumoniae*, cytomegalovirus, and herpes simplex virus type 1 particles with IgG monoclonal antibodies using the avidin-biotin-peroxidase method. Serum IgG antibodies to *C. pneumoniae* and cytomegalovirus were also analyzed. Results were correlated to plaque morphologic characteristics and microorganisms in atherosclerotic plaques.

Results.—Among the 76 specimens, *C. pneumoniae* was detected in 54 specimens, cytomegalovirus was detected in 27 specimens, and herpes simplex virus type 1 was detected in 8 specimens (Table 2). *C. pneumoniae*, cytomegalovirus, and herpes simplex virus type 1 were not detected in 20 normal control carotid artery and aortic tissue autopsy specimens. In 59 of the 76 specimens, at least 1 microorganism was found; a single microorganism was present in 35 specimens, 2 microorganisms were present in 18 specimens, and all 3 microorganisms were present in 6 specimens. The incidence of *C. pneumoniae* or cytomegalovirus was higher in atherosclerotic plaques with thrombosis than those without thrombosis. No correlation was seen between the presence of *C. pneumoniae* and cytomegalovirus in atherosclerotic vessels and serum antibody titers.

Discussion.—These findings show that *C. pneumoniae* and cytomegalovirus are commonly present in atherosclerotic plaques of the carotid artery. Serum antibodies cannot predict the presence of these agents. Individuals with these microorganisms may have a higher risk of thrombosis in the plaques, but this needs to be confirmed in future studies.

► In this paper, which addresses a similar subject as Abstract 1–23, these investigators detected *Chlamydia pneumoniae* in 71% of carotid artery specimens, cytomegalovirus in 35%, and herpes simplex virus in 10.5%. Interestingly, they also examined normal control tissue and found no evidence of any infectious particle in normal carotid artery or aortic tissue obtained at autopsy. As these authors presciently note, further studies will be required to confirm the importance of this observation.

Distribution of *Chlamydia pneumoniae* Infection in the Atherosclerotic Carotid Artery

Yamashita K, Ouchi K, Shirai M, et al (Yamaguchi Univ, Japan)

Stroke 29:773–778, 1998 1–25

Background.—There is a positive correlation between *Chlamydia pneumoniae* infection and atherosclerosis. However, how this microorganism distributes in the carotid arterial wall and plaque is not known. The distribution of a *C. pneumoniae*–specific antigen in atheromatous lesions and carotid arterial walls was measured, and the relationship between immunohistochemical results and risk factors for atherosclerosis was determined.

Methods.—Carotid endarterectomy was performed in 19 patients (16 men and 3 women, aged 61–80 years) who had a transient ischemic attack (n = 8) or minor stroke (n = 11). Twenty carotid atherosclerotic lesions were stained with monoclonal antibodies for immunohistochemical examination. The monoclonal antibodies used were CF-2 (which identifies the lipopolysaccharide of *Chlamydia*), AY-6 (which recognizes an outer membrane protein of *C. pneumoniae*), Virostat 1641 (which recognizes an outer membrane protein of *C. trachomatis*), anti-human α-smooth muscle actin, and anti-human macrophage KP-1. Each patient's risk factors for atherosclerosis were determined and correlated with the severity of *C. pneumoniae* infection, as reflected by the intensity of immunoreactivity.

Findings.—All specimens had similar immunoreactivity to CF-2 and AY-6. More than half the specimens (11 of 20, or 55%) were positive for both of these antibodies, and 7 (35%) had intense immunoreactivity to AY-6. AY-6 immunoreactivity was present in endothelial cells of the intima near the plaque, in macrophages and smooth muscles within the plaque, and in the media, particularly in smooth muscle cells. Cells infected with *C. pneumoniae* formed clusters throughout the plaque and in the media, in a patchy pattern of distribution. Although many atherosclerotic risk factors were present, including hypertension (74%), smoking (32%), diabetes (32%), ischemic heart disease (16%), and hypercholesterolemia (11%), there was no significant relationship between risk factors and infection severity. Virostat 1641 immunoreactivity was not observed in any specimen.

Conclusions.—*Chlamydia pneumoniae* infection was found throughout the endothelial cells, macrophages, and smooth muscle cells of the carotid arteries and plaques from these patients with atherosclerosis. Although infection with *C. pneumoniae* may not be a cause of atherosclerosis, these results and other reports of clinical evidence warrant further examination of the role of *C. pneumoniae* in atherosclerotic disease.

► Immunoreactivity for the *C. pneumoniae*–specific antigen was present in endothelial cells, macrophages, and smooth muscle cells that had migrated into the atheromatous plaque, as well as in smooth muscle cells in small arteries in the media underlying the plaque from human specimens. Overall,

55% of human carotid atherosclerotic lesions revealed these findings. The widespread distribution of the *C. pneumoniae* antigen in multiple sites reported herein is new information.

Endovascular Presence of Viable *Chlamydia pneumoniae* is a Common Phenomenon in Coronary Artery Disease

Maass M, Bartels C, Engel PM, et al (Univ of Lübeck, Germany; Research Ctr Borstel, Germany)

J Am Coll Cardiol 31:827–832, 1998 1–26

Background.—Previous studies have shown that a seroresponse to *Chlamydia pneumoniae* may be a risk factor for cardiovascular disease. Furthermore, *C. pneumoniae* has been found in atheromatous plaques. If *C. pneumoniae* is a cause of coronary artery disease, then perhaps cardiac events could be prevented by antimicrobial treatment—if the pathogens in the plaque are viable. The viability of *C. pneumoniae* in atherosclerotic arteries and lesions was evaluated.

Methods.—Seventy patients (60 men and 10 women, mean age 63 years) underwent myocardial revascularization. Coronary samples during coronary endarterectomy were obtained from 53 patients, and atheromatous samples from restenotic bypass lesions were obtained from 17 patients. Samples were cultured and immunofluorescence was used to identify *C. pneumoniae* growth and the presence of antichlamydial IgG, IgA, and IgM. Polymerase chain reaction was used to measure *C. pneumoniae.*

Findings.—In 11 of the 70 samples (16%), viable *C. pneumoniae* were present. In 21 of the samples (30%), *C. pneumoniae* DNA was found. None of the control samples without atherosclerosis showed *C. pneumoniae* DNA. *Chlamydia pneumoniae* DNA was present in 15 of 53 endarterectomy samples (28%) and in 6 of 17 bypass samples (35%). Amplification of DNA could not distinguish vascular and respiratory strains of *C. pneumoniae*. Lesions with or without *C. pneumoniae* infection could not be identified by serology; for example, 33% of patients with infection had an elevated titer to IgA, but so did 51% of patients without infection. Cardiovascular risk factors did not differ between patients with and without *C. pneumoniae* coronary artery infection.

Conclusions.—Viable *C. pneumoniae* were found in about 1 of every 6 lesions, and almost 1 of every 3 lesions contained *C. pneumoniae* DNA. The strains found in the atheromata were the same as those commonly found in the respiratory tract. The role of *C. pneumoniae* in atherogenesis is not known, and more research is needed to identify whether infection with this microorganism plays a role in the etiology of coronary artery disease. Nonetheless, these results indicate that antibacterial treatment may help decrease the progression of coronary artery disease.

► The suggestion that infection by *Chlamydia pneumoniae* might be responsible for inflammatory changes in the atherosclerotic plaque has attracted

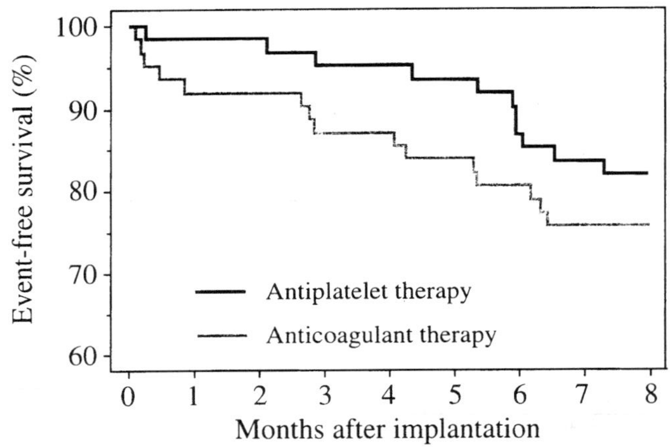

FIGURE 1.—Event-free survival curves for all cardiac events in both treatment groups. (Reprinted with permission from the American College of Cardiology from Schömig A, Neumann FJ, Walter H: Coronary stent placement in patients with acute myocardial infarction: Comparison of clinical and angiographic outcome after randomization to antiplatelet or anticoagulant therapy. *J Am Coll Cardiol* 29:28–34, 1997.)

late clinical and angiographic outcomes were compared in a subgroup of patients who underwent stent placement after acute myocardial infarction.

Methods.—Of 123 patients with successful stenting after acute myocardial infarction, 61 were randomized to receive aspirin plus ticlopidine and 62 were randomized to receive intense anticoagulant therapy. Of 101 eligible patients, 86.3% underwent 6-month repeat angiography.

Results.—Within the first 30 days after stenting, patients who underwent antiplatelet therapy had a significantly lower clinical event rate and stent vessel occlusion rate, and a trend toward fewer cardiac events, compared with the anticoagulation group (3.3%, 0%, and 1.6% vs. 21.0%, 9.7%, and 9.7%, respectively) Differences for clinical event rate and stent vessel occlusion rate were significant. At 6 month follow-up, the survival rate free of recurrent myocardial infarction was significantly higher in patients with antiplatelet therapy vs. antithrombotic therapy (100% vs. 90.3%) (Fig 1), and the rate of stent vessel occlusion was significantly lower (1.6% vs. 14.5%). Restenosis rates were comparable for both groups (26.5% vs. 26.9%).

Conclusion.—Combined antiplatelet therapy after stent placement in patients with acute myocardial infarction is related to better overall clinical and angiographic outcome than is anticoagulant therapy.

▶ A large number of studies involving coronary angioplasty have compared the efficacy of antiplatelet to anticoagulant therapy. In general, the antiplatelet therapy has proved superior. In this clinical study of coronary stent placement for acute myocardial infarction, 1 group was randomized to aspirin plus ticlopidine, and the other group received intense anticoagulant therapy. During the first 30 days, patients with antiplatelet therapy experienced a significantly lower clinical event rate and stent vessel occlusion rate than did the anticoagulated patients. The benefit persisted at 6 months. Although this study conclusively demonstrated that combined antiplatelet therapy was superior to anticoagulant therapy in this setting, we are unable to ascribe specific benefit to the aspirin component or to the ticlopidine component. With the recently released information on clopidogrel showing improved survival in vascular patients compared with aspirin, we are all going to have to consider the use of the more potent antiplatelet drugs in our patients. Although the newer types of antiplatelet drugs seem to have eliminated most of the former toxicity, expense remains a near prohibitive factor. One can only speculate on the cost of the oral GP IIb/IIIa inhibitors which may be available soon. (See also Abstract 1–29.)

Inhibition of Leucocyte and Platelet Adhesion Reduces Neointimal Hyperplasia After Arterial Injury

Golino P, Ambrosio G, Ragni M, et al (Univ of Naples, Italy; Boehringer-Ingelheim Pharmaceuticals, Ridgefield, Conn; Univ of Texas, Houston)
Thromb Haemost 77:783–788, 1997 1–32

Background.—The migration and proliferation of smooth muscle cells play an important role in restenosis after percutaneous transluminal coronary angioplasty (PTCA). Why this cell proliferation occurs is not known, but activated platelets and leukocytes release growth factors that may stimulate such proliferation. Whether platelets and leukocytes contribute to neointimal hyperplasia was examined in a rabbit model.

Methods.—Carotid arterial stenosis of about 75% was induced in New Zealand white rabbits. Then daily for 5 days after surgery, 8 animals each received either R15.7 (a monoclonal antibody against the leukocyte CD11/CD18 adhesion complex), aurintricarboxylic acid (ATA, which inhibits the interaction between platelet glycoprotein Ib and von Willebrand factor), both R15.7 and ATA, or no treatment. Animals were killed 21 days after surgery, and the carotid arteries were prepared for histologic examination. Planimetry was used to assess the extent of neointimal hyperplasia.

Findings.—Drug treatment significantly reduced the extent of the neointimal area. At 21 days, the neointimal area in controls averaged 0.51 mm^2, while the neointimal areas after either R15.7 or ATA alone were 0.12 and 0.20 mm^2, respectively ($P < 0.05$ compared with controls). Furthermore, the combination of R15.7 and ATA reduced neointimal area more than either treatment alone (to approximately 8 mm^2; $P < 0.05$ compared with ATA alone). Myeloperoxidase activity was significantly reduced by R15.7 administration, but neither R15.7 nor ATA caused any significant increases in circulating platelet and leukocyte counts.

Conclusions.—Two drugs that significantly reduced platelet and leukocyte adhesion at the site of vascular injury also significantly reduced the resultant neointimal hyperplasia. Thus, therapies to reduce or prevent platelet and leukocyte adhesion may help reduce the risk of restenosis after PTCA.

▶ It has been suspected for years that both activated platelets and leukocytes have an important role in the production of intimal hyperplasia. In this study, monoclonal antibodies against a leukocyte adhesion complex or an inhibitor of platelet glycoprotein Ib–von Willebrand factor interaction were given. Either of these alone and, more impressively in combination, greatly reduced neointimal hyperplasia occurring after a standard carotid arterial injury in the rabbit model. Thus, we have another entry on our growing list of substances shown to reduce intimal hyperplasia in certain settings. Won't it be wonderful if at least 1 of these 500 some odd compounds will prove transferable to the human model?

Endothelial Cell Adaptation to Chronic Thrombosis
Rose DA, Hertz SM, Eisenbud DE, et al (Newark Beth Israel Med Ctr, NJ)
Am J Surg 174:210–213, 1997 1–33

Background.—Autogenous vein is the longest lasting conduit for use in lower extremity vascular bypass grafting. Vein graft endothelial cells produce prostacyclin, which acts as a vasodilator and inhibitor of platelet aggregation. There is little information on how graft thrombosis affects the function and morphology of endothelial cells. In dog experiments, the investigators have showed that arterialized vein grafts recover function 5 days after exposure to thrombus. The endothelial cell response to longer periods of thrombosis was investigated.

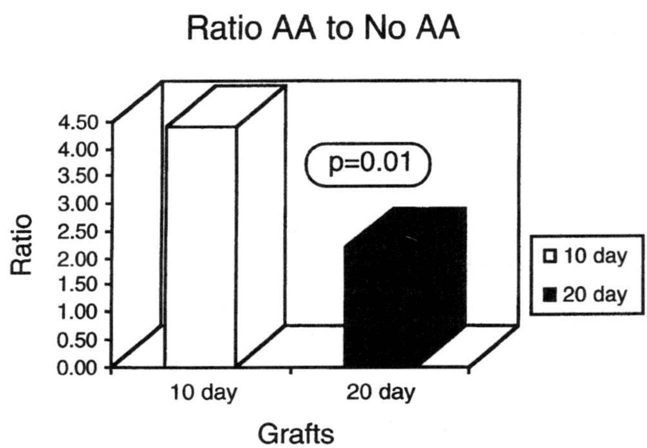

FIGURE 3.—Ratio of prostacyclin production with and without arachidonic acid comparing grafts thrombosed for 10 vs. 20 days. (Courtesy of Rose DA, Hertz SM, Eisenbud DE, et al: Endothelial cell adaptation to chronic thrombosis. *Am J Surg* 174:210–213. Copyright 1997. Reprinted with permission from Excerpta Medica Inc.)

Methods.—Experiments were carried out in a dog model of arterial vein grafts. One group of grafts was exposed to thrombus for 10 days and another for 20 days. After thrombectomy, the grafts were permitted to recover for 30 days. An ex vivo perfusion system was used to measure prostacyclin production in both groups, before and after addition of arachidonic acid. Scanning electron microscopic analysis of the grafts was performed.

Results.—Before the addition of arachidonic acid, prostacyclin perfusion at 5 minutes of perfusion was 4.31 pg/cm^2/min in the 20-day grafts vs. 2.42 pg/cm^2/min in the 10-day grafts. At 30 minutes, the difference was 1.86 vs. 0.95 pg/cm^2/min. After the addition of arachidonic acid, both groups showed increased prostacyclin production. The increase in response to arachidonic acid was 385% in the 10-day group vs. 229% in the 20-day group (Fig 3). Scanning electron microscopy showed the 2 groups were no different in endothelial coverage.

Conclusions.—In arterialized canine vein grafts, endothelial cells exposed to chronic thrombosis remain able to return to a baseline level of prostacyclin production. However, as the thrombus exposure time increases, the response to substrate stimulation decreases. This decreasing responsiveness could help to explain how vein grafts can survive after a period of thrombosis.

▶ My confidence in this experimental model is diminished by the use of mongrel dogs and by the simple assay techniques used. Nonetheless, the observation that vein grafts exposed to 20 days of intraluminal thrombus had important biochemical differences compared with vein grafts exposed to 10 days of intraluminal thrombus potential has profound importance. We have always had the clinical impression that thrombosed grafts never regain normal function no matter how meticulously thrombus was mechanically or enzymatically removed. Perhaps this study is beginning to give us a glimmer into the biochemical mechanisms underlying this clinical observation. We continue to believe that thrombosed vein grafts should be abandoned and replaced with new grafts. Thrombectomized leg vein grafts simply give lousy results.

Thrombin Binds to Soluble Fibrin Degradation Products Where It Is Protected From Inhibition by Heparin-Antithrombin but Susceptible to Inactivation by Antithrombin-Independent Inhibitors

Weitz JI, Leslie B, Hudoba M (McMaster Univ, Hamilton, Ont, Canada)

Circulation 97:544–552, 1998 1–34

Background.—A paradoxic effect of thrombolytic therapy is that it induces a procoagulant state of increased thrombin activity and higher levels of fibrinopeptide A (FPA). This increased activity may be responsible for reinfarction, although the mechanism for this effect remains unknown.

These authors offer a possible mechanism, via thrombin binding to soluble fibrin degradation products.

Methods.—Plasma clots were incubated in the presence or absence of tissue plasminogen activator (t-PA). Clot lysates were used to measure the extent to which soluble fibrin degradation products can generate FPA. Then various thrombin inhibitors were also studied to determine their effects on clot lysate–induced FPA generation.

Findings.—Significantly more clot-induced FPA was generated in the presence of t-PA than in its absence. FPA generation continued even after the clots were removed from plasma containing t-PA. In a lysing thrombus model, FPA generation in plasma containing t-PA continued after the clots were removed, whereas clot removal stopped the release of fibrin degradation products. Furthermore, as greater concentrations of clot lysate were added, FPA generation continued to increase, whereas FPA generation reached a plateau when free thrombin was incubated in plasma. These findings suggest that clot-bound, soluble thrombin is responsible for continued generation of FPA. The thrombin inhibitors hirugen and hirudin blocked FPA generation by both free thrombin and clot-bound thrombin. However, heparin had a significant effect on inhibition of FPA release by free fibrin but much less effect on inhibition of bound fibrin activity.

Conclusions.—When a clot undergoes t-PA–induced lysis, the increased FPA generation is caused by thrombin binding to soluble fibrin degradation products. Heparin is less effective in this situation, but other direct thrombin inhibitors are more successful in inactivating thrombin bound to fibrin degradation products. These findings help explain the greater success of thrombolytic therapies that include t-PA with a direct thrombin inhibitor.

▶ Thrombolytic therapy routinely induces a procoagulant state characterized by elevated plasma fibrinopeptide A, consistent with increased thrombin activity. This procoagulant state is believed to be potentially harmful and may partially explain arterial reocclusion, which occurs in 3% to 6% of patients despite successful initial thrombolysis. This study found that thrombin bound to soluble fibrin degradation products appeared to be responsible for the increase in fibrinopeptide A levels in this setting, and it further found that thrombin bound to fibrin derivatives was protected from inhibition by heparin. The fascinating observation is that such thrombin remains susceptible to inactivation by direct thrombin inhibitors. This may go a long way toward explaining the apparent superiority of hirudin over heparin when used in conjunction with t-PA. I have said before and I continue to believe that, as time passes, the use of unfractionated heparin will diminish and the use of specific thrombin inhibitors, as well as LMWH, will significantly increase.

► For years there has been a suspicion that hyperinsulinemia by itself conveys an unfavorable risk profile for atherosclerosis, including coronary heart disease. This interesting study examined the relationship between carotid atherosclerosis assessed in a large patient cohort over 5 years by duplex sonography, and compared this to their insulin status both at baseline and 2 hours after glucose loading (known diabetics were excluded). Interestingly, these investigators found a significant association between carotid atherosclerosis and both low and high insulin levels, leading them to conclude that both hypoinsulinemia and hyperinsulinemia are about equal independent risk factors for carotid atherosclerosis. Sounds a little fishy to me.

Improvement in Endothelial Function by Angiotensin Converting Enzyme Inhibition in Insulin-dependent Diabetes Mellitus

O'Driscoll G, Green D, Rankin J, et al (Royal Perth Hosp, Australia; Univ of Western Australia)

J Clin Invest 100:678–684, 1997 1–41

Introduction.—Endothelial dysfunction may be considered a manifestation of the genesis of the atherosclerotic process. Endothelial dysfunction has been detected in animal models of insulin-dependent (type 1) diabetes.

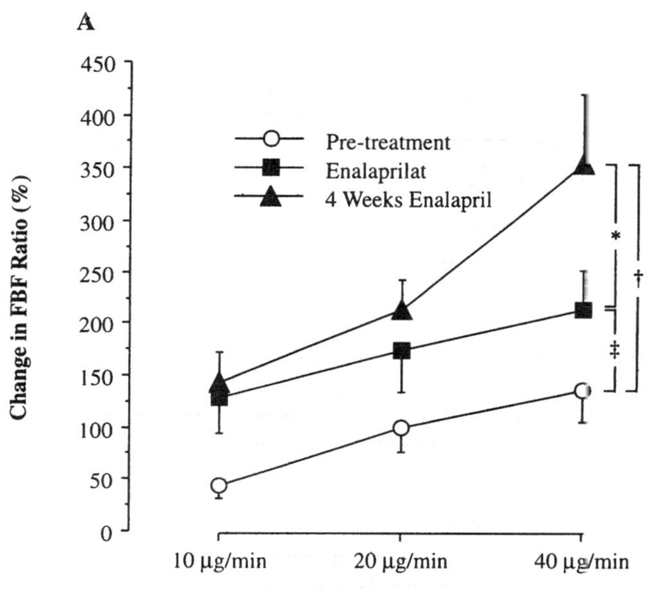

FIGURE 1.—The effects of enalaprilat and enalapril on forearm blood flow (FBF) ratios in diabetic patients, for 3 dose levels of ACh are illustrated. Results are expressed as mean ± SE. $^{*}P = 0.05$, ANOVA. $\dagger P < 0.005$, ANOVA. $\ddagger\ P < 0.001$, ANOVA. (Courtesy of O'Driscoll G, Green D, Rankin J: Improvement in endothelial function by angiotensin converting enzyme inhibition in insulin-dependent diabetes mellitus. *J Clin Invest* 100:678–684, 1997. Reproduced by copyright permission from Rockefeller University Press.)

It has been suggested that nitric oxide (NO)–mediated endothelial function might be improved by acute and short-term treatment with angiotensin converting enzyme (ACE) inhibitors in patients with type 1 diabetes mellitus. The effect of acute administration and short-term treatment with ACE inhibitors was evaluated in patients with type 1 diabetes mellitus.

Methods.—Nine male patients with type 1 diabetes and 8 healthy controls underwent forearm blood flow measurement using strain gauge plethysmography during intra-arterial infusion of incremental doses of endothelium-dependent (acetylcholine [ACh]) and endothelium-independent (sodium nitroprusside [SNP]) vasodilators.

Results.—Compared with controls, pretreatment ACh responses were depressed in patients with diabetes. There were no between-group differences in response to SNP. Acute ACE inhibition (with intrabrachial enalaprilat) significantly enhanced ACE responses in patients with diabetes. Further significant improvement was evident after 1 month of oral therapy with enalapril when ACh responses were normalized (Fig 1). The SNP responses were not affected by ACE inhibition.

Conclusion.—Acute administration of enalaprilat significantly enhances NO-mediated endothelial function in patients with type 1 diabetes mellitus, with further improvement observed after 4 weeks of enalapril therapy.

▶ Clearly, endothelial function is depressed in diabetics and appears improved by ACE. In the dramatic study in humans presented herein, enalapril normalized the abnormal vasodilatory responses to ACh in diabetics. We have learned in recent years that ACE inhibitors are dramatically effective in reducing the incidence of myocardial infarction, primarily, but not exclusively, in diabetics. ACE inhibition appears to improve endothelial NO-mediated dilator function, possibly through the suppression of angiotensin II production, possibly through inhibition of bradykinin breakdown, or through other unknown mechanisms. Whatever the mechanism, we must conclude that ACE inhibition clearly improves endothelial function in diabetics. I wonder if this may be related in some way to the dramatic effect of ACE inhibition in diminishing the incidence of myocardial infarction in this patient cohort.

Estrogen

A Comparison of Estrogen Replacement, Pravastatin, and Combined Treatment for the Management of Hypercholesterolemia in Postmenopausal Women

Davidson MH, Testolin LM, Maki KC, et al (Chicago Ctr for Clinical Research; Univ of North Dakota, Grand Forks)

Arch Intern Med 157:1186–1192, 1997 1–42

Objective.—Cholesterol levels increase in women after menopause. There is little information about the lipid-lowering effects and other health consequences of estrogen replacement therapy in postmenopausal women with hypercholesterolemia. The lipid-altering effects of conjugated estrogens, pravastatin, and their combination in postmenopausal women with hypercholesterolemia following a National Cholesterol Education Program (NCEP) Step 1 diet were compared in a double-blind, randomized, placebo-controlled clinical trial with 4 parallel groups.

Methods.—Of the 76 postmenopausal women with serum low-density lipoprotein cholesterol (LDL-C) concentrations greater than 3.88 mmol/L, 18 were in the placebo group, 19 in the conjugated estrogen (0.625 mg/day) group, 20 in the pravastatin (20 mg/day) group, and 19 in the combined treatment group. Dietary counseling was provided at week −6 and as necessary during study visits. Safety was assessed at baseline and at the end of the study (week 16). Dietary adherence was determined at weeks, −3, −1, 8, and 16.

Results.—Compared with the placebo group, non–high-density lipoprotein cholesterol (non–HDL-C) levels decreased significantly in the conjugated estrogen group (13.0%), the pravastatin group (23.7%), and the combined group (25.2%). The LDL-C decreased significantly by 13.5%, 25.4%, and 28.7%, respectively, compared with a gain of 1.1% in the placebo group. Compared with the placebo group, HDL-C increased significantly in the treatment groups by 22.5%, 3.7%, and 21.2%, respectively, Triglyceride concentrations increased by 11.3% in the placebo group and by 4.2% in the conjugated estrogen group, but decreased by 12.1% in the pravastatin group and by 0.9% in the combined treatment group. There were no significant changes in liver enzymes or creatine kinase concentration during treatment.

Conclusions.—Whereas both conjugated estrogens and pravastatin favorably altered the lipid profiles of postmenopausal women with hypercholesterolemia, results of the combined treatment were superior to either treatment alone.

▶ As everyone knows, premenopausal women are substantially protected from the ravages of atherosclerosis. At menopause a number of changes occur in the serum lipid profile, including an increase in LDL cholesterol and a decrease in HDL cholesterol. Without question, estrogen replacement therapy is effective in most women in reducing LDL cholesterol and increasing HDL cholesterol, and it has been noted in some studies that estrogen replacement therapy reduces the incidence of atherosclerotic cardiovascular disease by as much as 50%. To date, however, extremely little is known about the relative effects of estrogen replacement therapy vs. hypolipidemic medications in the treatment of the 30% to 35% of postmenopausal women who are clearly hyperlipidemic. In this 4 parallel group randomized trial of conjugated estrogens, pravastatin, estrogens plus pravastatin, or placebo, the favorable lipid changes, while slightly greater in the pravastatin group, were quite significant in the estrogen group, leading these authors to conclude that estrogen replacement should be given serious consideration as a therapeutic option for the management of hypercholesterolemia in postmenopausal women.

Contrasting Effects of Conjugated Estrogens and Tamoxifen on Dilator Responses of Atherosclerotic Epicardial Coronary Arteries in Nonhuman Primates

Williams JK, Honoré EK, Adams MR (Wake Forest Univ, Winston-Salem, NC)
Circulation 96:1970–1975, 1997 1–43

Objective.—Impaired normal vasodilation is one of the first signs of coronary artery disease. Whereas estrogen replacement improves arterial dilator response, the mechanism by which tamoxifen reduces progression of coronary artery atherosclerosis is not known. The vasodilator effects of tamoxifen in atherosclerotic coronary lesions was compared with the effects of conjugated equine estrogens (CEEs) in a nonhuman primate model.

Methods.—Fifty adult female cynomolgus monkeys were ovariectomized and fed an atherogenic diet for 34 months. Four months into the diet, 14 animals had CEEs (0.043 mg/kg/day) added to their diet, 21 animals had tamoxifen (1.3 mg/kg/day) added to their diet, and 15 control animals had no hormone replacement. Coronary artery vascular responses were measured angiographically during infusions of acetylcholine (10^{-8}, 10^{-7}, and 10^{-6} mol/L), nitroglycerin (15 μg/min), and 5% dextrose in water. Plaque size was measured at necropsy.

Results.—Animals treated with CEEs had plasma estradiol and estrone concentrations of 3.9 and 2.6 pmol/L, respectively, whereas control animals had concentrations of 0.3 and 0.6 pmol/L, respectively. Tamoxifen and CEEs significantly decreased low-density lipoprotein (LDL) molecular weight and increased triglyceride concentrations. Tamoxifen had no effect on total plasma cholesterol, high-density lipoprotein (HDL), intermediate-density lipoprotein plus very low density lipoprotein (IDL + VLDL), or LDL. Whereas arteries from control and tamoxifen-treated animals constricted when exposed to higher doses of acetylcholine, arteries of CEE-treated animals dilated at all concentrations of acetylcholine. Arteries of all animals dilated in response to nitroglycerin, although dilation in the CEE-treated group was significantly higher. Whereas plaque size was smaller in the treated animals, the differences were not clinically significant.

Conclusions.—Unlike CEEs, tamoxifen does not enhance arterial vasodilation in atherosclerotic monkeys.

▶ As with most basic science, it is frequently difficult to assess the ultimate importance of new information. Certainly tamoxifen has established itself as an extraordinarily important drug. This interesting study suggests that tamoxifen is a coronary vasoconstrictor, whereas conjugated estrogen appears to be a coronary vasodilator. This leads the authors to hypothesize that the estrogen receptor is a modulator of coronary artery dilator responses in ovariectomized atherosclerotic monkeys. If indeed these data are transportable to the human and tamoxifen is a coronary vasoconstrictor, this information may indeed be important.

Homocysteine

Plasma Homocysteine Levels and Mortality in Patients With Coronary Artery Disease

Nygård O, Nordrehaug JE, Refsum H, et al (Univ of Bergen, Norway; Haukeland Univ Hosp, Bergen, Norway)

N Engl J Med 337:230–236, 1997 1–44

Introduction.—Patients with elevated plasma homocysteine levels are at increased risk of coronary heart disease. For patients with established coronary artery disease, the prognostic significance of homocysteine levels is unknown. The relationship between plasma homocysteine levels and

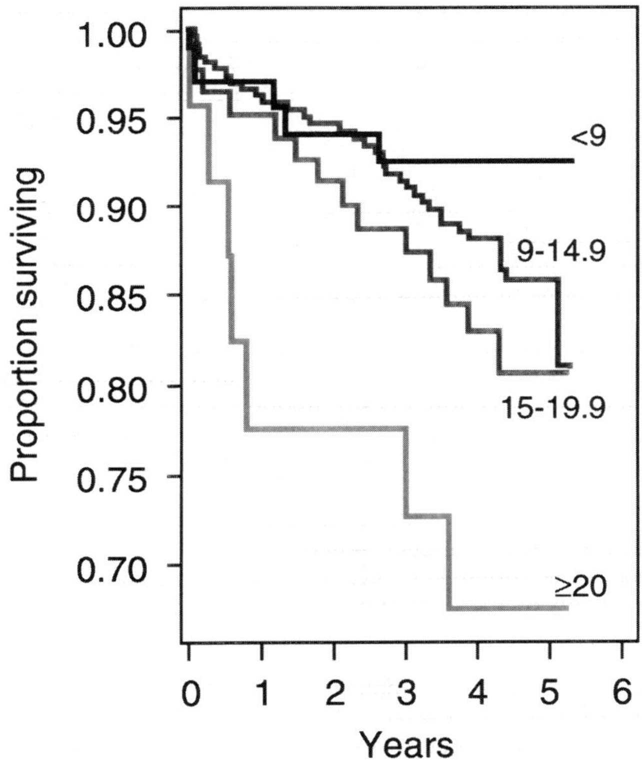

FIGURE 1.—Estimated survival among patients with coronary artery disease, according to plasma total homocysteine levels. The figure shows estimated survival for 55-year-old male former smokers with 3-vessel disease, a left ventricular ejection fraction of 55%, a creatinine level of 1.5 mg/dL (130 μmol/L), and a total cholesterol level of 241 mg/dL (6.24 mmol/L) at 4 different total homocysteine levels. Survival curves have been estimated in a stratified Cox regression analysis. (Courtesy of Nygård O, Nordrehaug JE, Refsum H, et al: Plasma homocysteine levels and mortality in patients with coronary artery disease. *N Engl J Med* 337:230–236. Copyright 1997, Massachusetts Medical Society. Reprinted by permission of *The New England Journal of Medicine*. All rights reserved.)

close correlation with the 1- and 5-hour apparent diffusion coefficient maps. Infarct size was 63% smaller in the CP101,606-treated animals.

Conclusion.—As in neurotrauma and hemorrhagic stroke, CP101,606 appears to have significant neuroprotective effects after occlusive stroke. Given its encouraging results in clinical trials and its excellent safety record, CP101,606 appears to be a promising agent for use in human occlusive stroke.

▶ One of the most exciting areas in neurologic research currently is exploration of methods to block the *N*-methyl-D-aspartate receptor ion channel complex at sites of neurologic injury. Stimulation of this receptor complex by glutamate appears to result in marked worsening of neurologic injury. Intensive research is currently under way to define agents that may be competitive antagonists at this binding site.

In the experimental model reported here regarding middle cerebral artery occlusion in adult cats, the control group showed a marked increase in brain lactate shortly after injury, compared with the drug-treated group. Interestingly, there was a significantly smaller lesion in the drug-treated group compared with the control group. On balance, this substance holds great promise as a significant neuroprotective agent. Time will tell whether it may have a role in neuroprotection during such vascular surgery as carotid endarterectomy and, possibly, thoracoabdominal aneurysm resection.

A Glycine Site Antagonist, ZD9379, Reduces Number of Spreading Depressions and Infarct Size in Rats With Permanent Middle Cerebral Artery Occlusion

Tatlisumak T, Takano K, Meiler MR, et al (Helsinki Univ; Univ of Massachusetts, Worcester; Worcester Polytechnic Inst, Mass)

Stroke 29:190–195, 1998 1–51

Background.—Experimental models of focal ischemia have demonstrated the presence of spreading depressions (SDs), which play a role in the evolution of ischemic injury. Spreading depressions are inhibited and infarct size limited by treatment with N-methyl-D-aspartate (NMDA) antagonists. The NMDA receptor includes a glycine site, which could be a useful therapeutic target for acute focal ischemia without the side effects noted with competitive and noncompetitive NMDA antagonists. The effects of the potent glycine antagonist ZD9379 on SDs and brain infarction were evaluated in rats.

Methods.—Middle cerebral artery occlusion (MCAO) was performed in male Sprague-Dawley rats. One group received a bolus of ZD9379 before MCAO, followed by an infusion afterward; another group received ZD9379 by both bolus and infusion after MCAO; and the third group received vehicle only, beginning before MCAO. For 4.5 hours after MCAO, continuous recording of cortical DC potentials and electrocorti-

TABLE 2.—Major Results of the Study

	Group 1 (Pre-MCAO Treatment)	Group 2 (Post-MCAO Treatment)	Group 3 (Controls)	P*
Infarct volume, mm^3				
All animals included	90.2±72.3	104.7±46.4	225.7±40.1	.00092
Premature deaths excluded	68.9±62.7	100.7±49.6	216.8±35.1	.0035
Number of SDs				
All animals included	8.2±5.8	8.1±2.5	16.0±5.1	.0084
Premature deaths excluded	6.0±3.5	7.3±1.5	15.3±3.5	.0011
Neurological score				
All animals included	2.6±1.3	1.9±1.5	3.7±1.1	.022
Premature deaths excluded	2.0±0.0	1.3±0.5	3.0±0.0	.0044

Note: Values are mean ± standard deviation. Values calculated by 1-factor ANOVA; values for neurologic scores calculated by Kruskal-Wallis *H* test.

(Courtesy of Tatlisumak T, Takano K, Meiler MR, et al: A glycine site antagonist, ZD9379, reduces number of spreading depressions and infarct size in rats with permanent middle cerebral artery occlusion. *Stroke* 29:190–195, 1998. Reproduced with permission of *Stroke*. Copyright 1998, American Heart Association.)

cography was performed to monitor the development of SDs. Infarct volume was measured at 24 hours.

Results.—Values for corrected infarct volume were 90 mm^3 in the group receiving ZD9379 before and after MCAO, 105 mm^3 in those receiving ZD9379 after MCAO, and 226 mm^3 in those receiving vehicle only. Both ZD9379–treated groups had about 8 SDs, compared with 16 in the vehicle group (Table 2). A significant correlation was noted between infarct volume and number of SDs across all groups.

Conclusion.—The glycine site antagonist ZD9379, given before and/or after MCAO in rats, significantly reduces both the number of SDs and the volume of ischemic infarct. ZD9379 appears to have neuroprotective effects, perhaps related to inhibition of ischemia-related SDs.

▶ Another manifestation of cortical neuronal damage which apparently contributes to lesion evolution is the phenomenon of SDs. Again, the occurrence of these SDs appears to be related to the NMDA receptor complex and the excitatory amino acid glutamate. The newly described glycine site antagonist described herein appears to be effective in limiting cerebral damage. See also Abstract 1–50 on the effect of CP101,606 at a similar site. I am certain that in the future, we shall hear a great deal more about the NMDA receptor complex and its relationship to progressive neurologic injury.

Enhancement of Heat Shock Protein Expression After Transient Ischemia in the Preconditioned Spinal Cord of Rabbits

Sakurai M, Hayashi T, Abe K, et al (Tohoku Univ, Sendai, Japan)

J Vasc Surg 27:720–725, 1998 1–52

Objective.—The exact mechanism of spinal cord injury in paraplegia is not completely known. Heat shock proteins (HSPs) may protect against neuronal injury and may also provide tolerance to future ischemic injury. Changes in HSP70 mRNA after transient ischemia in preconditioned rabbit spinal cords were evaluated using Northern blot and immunochemical analyses.

Methods.—White rabbits were sham operated (group 1) or subjected to 10 minutes of spinal cord ischemia (group 2), 15 minutes of spinal cord ischemia 2 days after sham operation (group 3), or 15 minutes of ischemic insult 2 days after previous exposure to 10 minutes of spinal cord ischemia (group 4). Neurologic assessments were performed at day 7 after operation, and HSP70 mRNA content in spinal cord was determined 7 days after operation or ischemic injury. The total number of intact motor neurons was determined in paraffin-embedded ventral gray matter.

Results.—There was a significant difference in Johnson's neurologic scores between groups 4 and 3 and between groups 3 and 2. Neuronal function was not affected by 15-minute ischemia in group 4, but was affected after 15-minute ischemia in group 3. HSP70 mRNA was induced in group 2 after 8 hours and 2 days of reperfusion; in group 3 after 8 hours of reperfusion (returning to sham level control by day 1); and in group 4 after 8 hours to 2 days of reperfusion. There was no HSP70 immunoreactivity in group 1 spinal cords, moderate immunoreactivity in group 2 spinal cords until 2 days of reperfusion, moderate immunoreactivity in group 3 at 8 hours of reperfusion, and strong immunoreactivity in group 4 at 8 hours of reperfusion that was sustained until 2 days of reperfusion.

Conclusions.—Expression of HSP70 was enhanced in the spinal cords of rabbits after 10-minute ischemic preconditioning, and motor neuron cells were preserved. These results suggest that HSP70 expression is involved in the acquisition of tolerance to spinal ischemia.

► Ischemic preconditioning, long popular among myocardial investigators, is finding its way now into spinal cord protective research. The fascinating results reported herein indicate that 10 minutes of ischemic preconditioning of the rabbit spinal cord significantly prevents motor cell death 2 days later after 15 minutes of ischemia, and that this protective effect is associated with the production of HSP, which appears to be a favorable event. Presently, it would appear that ischemic CNS preconditioning may be valuable in a few vascular procedures, perhaps most notably thoracoabdominal aneurysm resection. However, it is presently difficult to imagine ischemic preconditioning several days before the anticipated surgery. There clearly will be a great number of logistic considerations to be worked out. On balance, the information on the importance of blocking the effect of glutamate on the NMDA receptor complex, and this information concerning ischemic preconditioning may be pointing the way toward a future in which we may be able to actually modify ischemic neurologic damage. Maybe HSP itself will be of benefit.

Intracerebral Hemorrhage After Intravenous t-PA Therapy for Ischemic Stroke

Broderick JP, for the NINDS t-PA Stroke Study Group (Univ of Cincinnati, Ohio)
Stroke 28:2109–2118, 1997 1–53

Introduction.—Prompt treatment with tissue plasminogen activator (t-PA) increases the chances of normal functional outcome after stroke, even after adjustment for the increased risk of intracerebral hemorrhage (ICH). It remains to be determined whether some patient subgroups are at particularly increased risk of ICH after treatment with t-PA. Such risk factors were sought using data from a randomized, controlled trial of t-PA treatment for stroke.

Methods.—Subgroup analyses were performed using data from the NINDS t-PA stroke trial, in which patients received IV t-PA within 3 hours after stroke onset. The study included 312 patients treated with t-PA and 312 treated with placebo. Multivariate analyses were performed to examine the relationship of baseline and posttreatment variables to the occurrence of symptomatic and asymptomatic ICH within 36 hours after treatment.

Patients.—Patients receiving t-PA had a 6% increase in absolute risk of symptomatic ICH, with a 4% decrease in absolute mortality at 3 months. The only factors independently associated with increased risk of symptomatic ICH were severity of neurologic deficit as measured by the National Institutes of Health Stroke Scale score, odds ratio 1.8; and the CT finding of brain edema (that is, acute hypodensity) or mass effect before treatment, odds ratio 7.8. The final multivariate model was only 57% efficient in predicting which t-PA-treated patients would and would not have a symptomatic hemorrhage. Among patients with a severe neurologic deficit, those treated with t-PA were more likely to have a favorable outcome at 3 months. This was also so for patients with CT findings of edema or mass effect. Among patients with these characteristics, treatment with t-PA made no difference in the likelihood of severe disability or death.

Conclusions.—Patients with severe strokes or CT evidence of a mass effect have a higher risk of ICH after treatment with t-PA. However, as long as treatment is given within 3 hours of stroke onset, these patients are still reasonable candidates for t-PA. There is no evidence of a trade-off between an early excess in morbidity and mortality and an improvement in 3-month outcome.

► Few topics in recent years have more impressed the lay press than the use of thrombolytic therapy in the treatment of early thromboembolic stroke. In our city, we have had the usual number of unbelievable newspaper articles describing the dramatic recovery of "brain dead" patients after such therapy. The interest our patient population has in this matter is staggering. As covered, however, in previous editions of the YEAR BOOK OF VASCULAR SURGERY,[1] available supporting evidence is indeed scanty. This publication reports the results of a subgroup analysis of 600 patients with early stroke randomized to t-PA or placebo. The t-PA treated patients had an increase of 6% in the absolute risk of symptomatic intracerebral hemorrhage and a decrease of 4% in the absolute risk of 3-month mortality. Overall, the conclusion of the article is that patients with severe strokes, edema, or mass effect on the baseline CT have a higher rate of intracerebral hemorrhage than do other patients, but they are still reasonable candidates for t-PA if it is administered within 3 hours of the onset of symptoms. On balance, I continue to believe that intraarterial thrombolytic therapy for the treatment of early stroke is hazardous, associated with minimal benefits, and will require detailed additional evaluation. (See also Abstract, 1–54.)

Reference

1. 1997 YEAR BOOK OF VASCULAR SURGERY, p 360.

Systematic Review of Evidence on Thrombolytic Therapy for Acute Ischaemic Stroke

Wardlaw JM, Warlow CP, Counsell C (Univ of Edinburgh, Scotland)
Lancet 350:607–614, 1997 1–54

Background.—There are conflicting data on the effects of thrombolytic therapy in patients with acute ischemic stroke. Just 1 study concluded that thrombolysis was definitely beneficial in such patients. All randomized trials of thrombolytic therapy for acute ischemic stroke were reviewed.

Methods.—The review included 12 randomized trials of thrombolytic therapy vs. a control condition in patients with acute ischemic stroke. All trials included CT scanning before randomization. Data were collected on deaths during the first 2 weeks after treatment, deaths from all causes and functional outcome at the end of follow-up, and symptomatic and fatal intracranial hemorrhage.

Results.—Of 3,435 patients participating in the trials, 20% were dead and 39% were functionally dependent at a maximum follow-up of 5 months. Early symptomatic or fatal intracranial hemorrhage occurred in 6% of patients. Patients assigned to thrombolytic therapy had significant excesses of early deaths (91 per 1,000 patients treated) and total deaths (37 per 1,000). However, they had significantly fewer patients meeting the combined outcome of death or dependency (65 fewer per 1,000 patients treated). All recent studies showed that thrombolysis was associated with a significant excess of symptomatic and fatal intracranial hemorrhage. There were about 70 extra symptomatic intracranial hemorrhages per 1,000 patients treated, with 51 per 1,000 being fatal.

Among patients undergoing randomization within 3 hours after stroke, thrombolysis significantly reduced the number of patients dead or dependent at follow-up, by 141 per 1,000 patients treated. The number of patients who died increased insignificantly, by 9 per 1,000. The total

of activated complement C3a and tumor necrosis factor-α, but an increase was seen in levels of interleukin-6, interleukin-8 (IL-8), and elastase-α_1-antitrypsin. After surgery, slight neutrophilia was observed, and leukocyte counts were inversely related to levels of IL-8. Patients with the highest levels of IL-8 and the lowest leukocyte counts had the greatest increases in lung protein leak index but not in the leg protein leak index.

Discussion.—Protein permeability increases in the lung and leg early after aortic surgery. Leg injury from ischemia–reperfusion may cause activation of neutrophils and release of IL-8, which may then induce neutrophil sequestration and increased microvascular permeability in the lung. These results may help explain acute lung injuries seen after ischemia–reperfusion in humans.

► These investigators examined microvascular permeability in the lung and leg several hours after completion of lower extremity revascularization in patients. Using complex nuclear medicine techniques, they concluded that, after aortic surgery, microvascular protein permeability increased in the leg and the lung, with probable resultant neutrophil activation, including release of IL-8. Although the precise details of the conclusions reached by these authors differ moderately from those reached by the authors of the previous paper, the thrust of the observations is in the same direction. (See also Abstract 1–59.)

Direct In Vivo Measurement of Flow-dependent Nitric Oxide Production in Mesenteric Resistance Arteries

Hyre CE, Unthank JL, Dalsing MC (Indiana Univ, Indianapolis)

J Vasc Surg 27:726–732, 1998 1–61

Objective.—Whereas nitric oxide (NO) is thought to participate in flow-dependent or shear stress–dependent regulation of vascular diameter in large arteries to small arterioles, measuring its concentration is very difficult. Recently developed NO-specific electrodes were used to show that NO concentration at the arterial wall is increased with acute elevation of blood flow in small mesenteric arteries.

Methods.—The small bowel of 9 mongrel dogs was exteriorized, and a 2-mm ultrasonic flow probe connected to a flow meter was attached to a mesenteric artery close to the cecal end. The NO electrode was placed and calibrated. Nitric oxide concentration was increased slowly by adding 50-μm boluses of KNO_2 to a stirred solution of 100 mm of sulfuric acid. Adjacent mesenteric arteries were occluded to increase flow in the experimental artery. Increased flow was maintained for 2 hours in 4 dogs, and Nω-nitro-L-arginine-methyl ester (L-NAME), 10 mg/kg, was administered intravenously to inhibit NO production to check electrode response.

Results.—Eight dogs were evaluable. No ischemia or complications were observed. Nitric oxide current increased as arterial flow increased an average of 5.5 mL/min from a baseline value of 5.4 mL/min (Fig 3). The

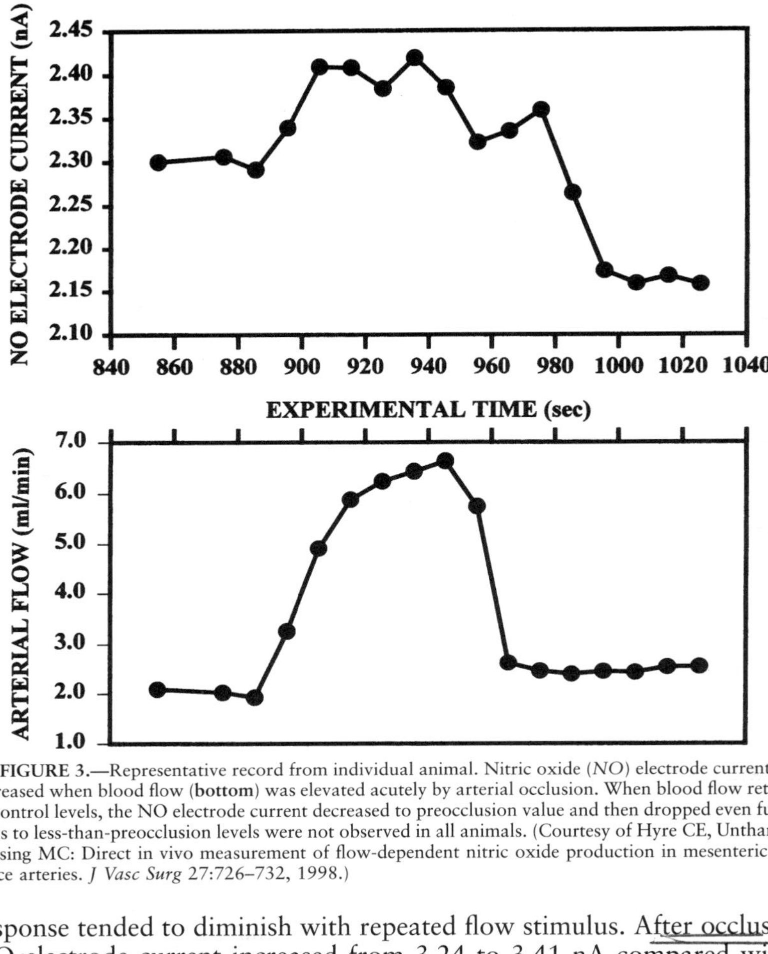

FIGURE 3.—Representative record from individual animal. Nitric oxide (*NO*) electrode current (**top**) increased when blood flow (**bottom**) was elevated acutely by arterial occlusion. When blood flow returned to control levels, the NO electrode current decreased to preocclusion value and then dropped even further. Falls to less-than-preocclusion levels were not observed in all animals. (Courtesy of Hyre CE, Unthank JL, Dalsing MC: Direct in vivo measurement of flow-dependent nitric oxide production in mesenteric resistance arteries. *J Vasc Surg* 27:726–732, 1998.)

response tended to diminish with repeated flow stimulus. After occlusion, NO electrode current increased from 3.24 to 3.41 nA compared with a baseline reading of 2.85 nA. After administration of L-NAME, mean arterial pressure increased 11 mm Hg, and current measured at the arterial wall decreased 0.24 nA.

Conclusions.—Increasing blood flow in canine mesenteric resistance arteries increases NO concentration at the outer arterial wall as measured with a NO-specific electrode.

► We are slowly beginning to appreciate the central role of NO in shear stress-related changes in arterial size. From the data contained in this paper it seems clear that NO plays an integral role in arterial enlargement accompanying the presence of an arteriovenous fistula. Furthermore, this effect appears to be independent of blood pressure. On balance, all available evidence suggests that endothelial NO is in fact the long sought shear stress effector in arteries.

Nitric Oxide Mediates Hyperglycemia-induced Defective Migration in Cultured Endothelial Cells

Gade PV, Andrades JA, Nimni ME, et al (Maimonides Med Ctr, Brooklyn, NY; Univ of Southern Calif, Los Angeles; Univ of Málaga, Spain)

J Vasc Surg 26:319–326, 1997 1–62

Background.—The integrity of the endothelial cell lining of the vasculature is essential for normal functioning. The ability of endothelial cells to migrate and proliferate is critical to the repair of endothelial lining defects. Exogenous nitric oxide (NO) has been shown to inhibit the proliferation of endothelial cells. Diabetics have an increased risk of atherosclerotic disease, which is linked in some way to their elevated levels of circulating glucose. To examine the relationship between these factors, the effect of glucose on levels of NO and the response of endothelial cells to wounding was examined.

Methods.—Bovine aortic endothelial cells were isolated and cultured. Migration was evaluated by scraping endothelial cell monolayers, and then measuring the distance, the number, and the area covered by migrating cells in the presence of physiological, elevated and non-metabolizable L-glucose (control). The effect of NO was evaluated by adding to these cultures the NO synthase inhibitor, NG-monomethyl arginine (NMMA), or S-nitrosylated penicillamine, which releases NO. Proliferation was evaluated in the presence of varying concentrations of serum, glucose, NMMA or S-nitrosylated penicillamine. Proliferation was quantified by estimating total cellular protein.

Results.—Glucose inhibited endothelial cell migration in a dose-dependent manner. Migration was also inhibited in the presence of S-nitrosylated penicillamine. Inhibition of NO synthase with NMMA prevented the glucose-mediated migration inhibition. Elevated glucose levels did not affect proliferation, except in the presence of 20% fetal bovine serum.

Conclusions.—Elevated glucose levels inhibited endothelial cell migration in an in vitro wound model. This inhibition appears to be mediated by increased NO levels.

► The protean manifestations of hyperglycemia on vascular wall function continue to attract the attention of many investigators. Clearly, endothelial injuries occur continuously and must be repaired. These authors present convincing evidence that hyperglycemia, interestingly, results in an elevation of nitric oxide, which, in turn, has a decidedly negative effect on endothelial cell migration and the ability of migrating endothelial cells to close an endothelial defect. This would appear to be one of the few harmful effects of nitric oxide yet described. (See also Abstract 1–59.)

Effect of Red Wine on Endothelium-dependent Relaxation in Rabbits

Cishek MB, Galloway MT, Karim M, et al (Univ of California, Davis)

Clin Sci (Colch) 93:507–511, 1997 1–63

Background.—Research has suggested that components of red wine protect against cardiovascular disease. The effects of red wine, ethanol, and flavonoids present in red wine on endothelium-dependent relaxation (EDR) of isolated rabbit aortic rings was investigated.

Methods.—Thoracic aortas were removed from rabbits, cut into rings, and suspended from force transducers in organ chambers. In some rings, the endothelium was first removed to serve as a control. All rings were contracted with noradrenaline before incubation with red wine, ethanol, catechin, epicatechin, quercetin, and polymeric phenols (PPs). In some experiments, the EDR response to cumulative doses of acetylcholine was determined before and after incubation with one of these compounds. The effects of sodium nitrate and noradrenaline on tissues incubated with these compounds were also examined. Cyclic guanosine monophosphate was extracted from aortic rings and measured by immunoassay.

Results.—Incubation of isolated aortic rings with red wine or PP caused dose-dependent ERD. These responses were inhibited by the nitric oxide (NO) synthase inhibitor, N^G-L-arginine methyl ester, and removal of endothelium. Incubation of aortic rings with either red wine, polymeric phenols, or sodium nitroprusside increased cGMP levels. When tissues were preincubated with red wine or PPs, the ERD response to acetylcholine was attenuated. This response was reconstituted by addition of arginine, a substrate for NO synthase.

Conclusions.—Exposure of isolated rabbit aortic rings to either red wine or PPs found in red wine evokes endothelium-dependent relaxation. Preincubation of these aortic rings with either red wine or PPs eliminated the EDR response to acetylcholine. This response could be restored by addition of arginine, indicating that preincubation with red wine or PPs depletes the supply of substrate for NO synthase. The endothelial response to flavonoids found in red wine may be a promising area for further clinical research.

▶ As faithful readers of the YEAR BOOK series have noted, I have a fascination with the effects of wine on vascular disease. I am delighted to learn here that exposure of arterial tissue to red wine results in an endothelium-dependent vasorelaxation, which appears mediated by nitric oxide. I shall, with pleasure, record this as another favorable effect of red wine on the vascular system, to be used ad libitum in justifying my continuing imbibition.

Spectroscopy

Dynamic Phosphorus-31 Magnetic Resonance Spectroscopy in Arterial Occlusive Disease: Correlation With Clinical and Angiographic Findings and Comparison With Healthy Volunteers

Schunk K, Romaneehsen B, Mildenberger P, et al (Univ Hosp Mainz, Germany)

Invest Radiol 32:651–659, 1997 1–64

Objective.—Individuals with arterial occlusive disease (AOD) are expected to have altered phosphate metabolism. The differences in muscular metabolism between patients with AOD and healthy age-matched volunteers were investigated by ^{31}P MR spectroscopy (MRS) during muscular exercise.

Methods.—Dynamic phosphorus MRS was performed in 56 patients (11 female), whose average age was 60 years, and 10 age-matched healthy volunteers, using a 60-mm single loop surface coil on the rectus femoral muscle to obtain transverse and sagittal spin echo images. Phosphorus-31 MRS was performed at rest, as participants lifted their weighted calf and maintained extension to fatigue, and after a few minutes rest, as participants lifted their weighted calf repeatedly at a rate of 1 per second to exhaustion. The intracellular pH was calculated from peak areas according to the following equation: $pH_i = 6.75 + \log_{10} [(\delta - 3.27)/(5.69 - \delta)]$, where δ is the frequency shift between P_i and PCr (Fig 2).

Results.—Cross-sectional area of quadriceps muscle was similar for both patients and controls. Inorganic phosphate (P_i/phosphocreatine (PCr) ratio continued to rise after the beginning of the exercise to the end of both exercises. P_i/PCr recovered 4 times faster than pH (Fig 3). Spectroscopic parameters at rest were similar for both groups except that diabetic pa-

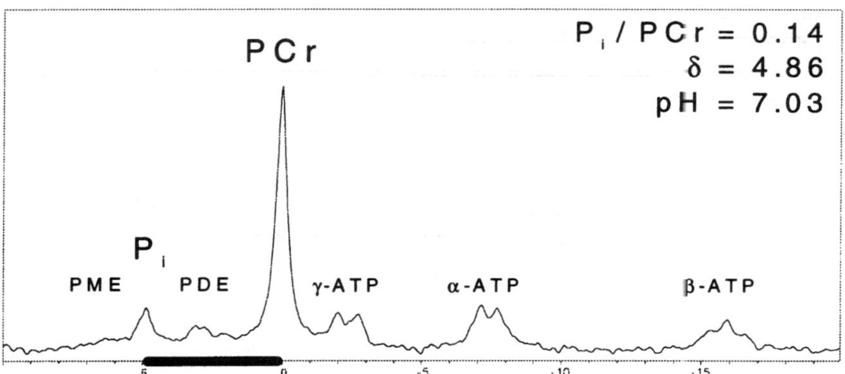

FIGURE 2.—Phosphorus-31 spectrum of the quadriceps muscle at rest. (Courtesy of Schunk K, Romaneehsen B, Mildenberger P, et al: Dynamic phosphorus-31 magnetic resonance spectroscopy in arterial occlusive disease: Correlation with clinical and angiographic findings and comparison with healthy volunteers. *Invest Radiol* 32:651–659, 1997.)

suggesed that IL-1β has a unique effect on human infragenicular VSMCs, as well as augmenting the production of fibronectin by these cells. I bet exactly the same effect would occur with VSMCs from any part of the body. The lack of the active control diminished the importance of this paper for me to near zero.

Protein Kinase C Isoforms in Human Aortic Smooth Muscle Cells

Grange JJ, Baca-Regen LM, Nollendorfs AJ, et al (Univ of Nebraska, Omaha)

J Vasc Surg 27:919–927, 1998 1–70

Objective.—Cytokines and growth factors promote the abnormal smooth muscle cell (SMC) proliferation that leads to atherosclerosis. Protein kinase C (PKC) isoforms are believed to regulate cellular processes including those involving human aortic SMCs. The specific PKC isoforms expressed in human arterial SMCs were identified, and their subcellular location and translocation with 12-O-tetradecanoylphorbol 13-acetate (TPA) activation were defined.

Methods.—Smooth muscle cells from human aortic tissue were cultured with and without TPA (100 nmol/L) and lysed. Protein kinase C isoforms were isolated from the soluble and particulate fractions and identified by immunoblot analysis as α, β_I, β_{II}, δ, ϵ, γ, and ζ. Bands were detected using enhanced chemiluminescence. Translocation was defined as a significant change in the proportion of isoform in the TPA-treated SMC fraction compared with results obtained in controls. Immunofluorescent microscopy was used to determine the location of each antibody-stained isoform before and after TPA stimulation.

Results.—Isoforms α and β_I were found mainly in the soluble fraction before TPA stimulation and primarily in the particulate fraction after TPA stimulation. Isoforms β_{II}, δ, and ϵ were found primarily in the particulate fraction before and after exposure to TPA. Immunofluorescent findings confirmed the locations. Isoforms γ and ζ were not detected.

Conclusions.—The subcellular location and response to TPA were defined in the 5 PKC isoforms identified in human aortic SMCs. These isoforms play a role in the pathogenic processes that are involved in vascular disease.

► Protein kinase C signal transduction pathway has a fundamental role in many vascular smooth muscle functions, serving as a signal transduction pathway. There are at least 11 distinct PKC isoforms that have subtle, but important differences in enzymatic properties and requirements for activation. Baxter and associates describe in this paper important preliminary studies attempting to characterize the role of specific PKC isoforms in human arterial smooth muscle cells. This is new information.

Plasma Concentration of C-Reactive Protein and Risk of Developing Peripheral Vascular Disease

Ridker PM, Cushman M, Stampfer MJ, et al (Harvard Med School, Boston; Harvard School of Public Health, Boston; Univ of Vermont, Burlington)

Circulation 97:425–428, 1998 1–71

Objective.—Elevated levels of C-reactive protein (CRP) are an indicator of systemic inflammation. Recent studies suggest that elevated CRP may also predict risk of myocardial infarction and thromboembolic stroke. The potential association between CRP levels and risk of symptomatic peripheral arterial disease (PAD) were assessed.

Methods.—The study used data on 144 men taking part in the Physicians' Health Study, apparently healthy at baseline, who went on to develop symptomatic PAD—intermittent claudication or need for revascularization. They were matched for age and smoking to control subjects who remained free of vascular disease. Mean follow-up was 60 months. Baseline levels of CRP were compared between groups.

Results.—Median CRP at baseline was 1.34 mg/L in the patients with PAD versus 0.99 mg/L in the controls (Figure). Relative risk of PAD was 1.3 for men in the second quartile of baseline CRP, 2.0 for those in the third quartile, and 2.1 for those in the fourth quartile. Median CRP level was higher, 1.75 mg/L, for patients with PAD who required revascularization. Again, risk of this outcome increased with each quartile of baseline CRP (1.8, 3.8, and 4.1). The risks were little changed by adjustment for

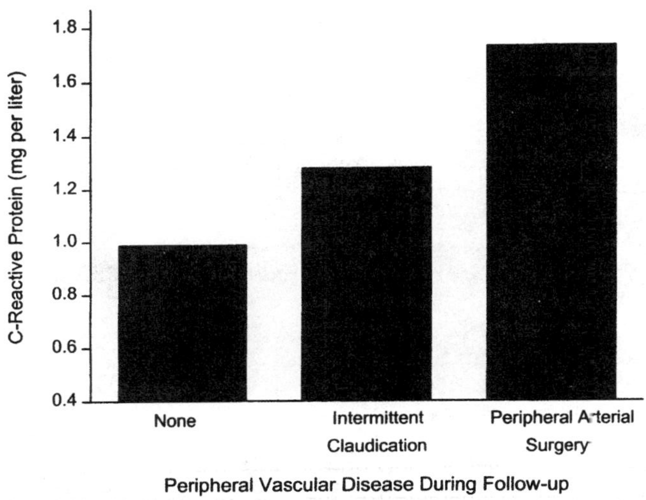

FIGURE.—Median levels of C-reactive protein at baseline among study participants who subsequently developed intermittent claudication or who required peripheral arterial revascularization (case subjects) and for those who remained free of vascular disease during follow-up (control subjects). (Courtesy of Ridker PM, Cushman M, Stampfer MJ, et al: Plasma concentration of C-reactive protein and risk of developing peripheral vascular disease. *Circulation* 97:425–428, 1998. Reproduced with permission, American Heart Association.)

body mass index, hypercholesterolemia, hypertension, diabetes, and family history of premature atherosclerosis.

Conclusions.—Baseline level of CRP significantly predicts future risk of symptomatic PAD, these results suggest. Patients with the highest CRP levels are also the most likely to require surgical revascularization. The findings are consistent with the hypothesis that chronic inflammation plays a pathogenetic role in atherothrombosis.

▶ The vascular community was recently stunned by an article in the *New England Journal of Medicine* showing that systemic inflammation, as manifest by the presence of CRP, had a high correlation with the risk of cardiovascular disease in apparently healthy men and that the benefits of aspirin on cardiovascular disease appeared significantly limited to just those patients who had elevated CRP.[1] The same authors herein extend these observations to the risk of developing PAD. Using the same Physicians Health Study they identified a cohort of 144 apparently healthy men who subsequently developed symptomatic PAD and an equal number of control subjects who remained free of vascular disease. The CRP level correlated closely with the development of peripheral arterial disease and, in fact, each increasing quartile of baseline CRP increased the relative risks significantly. They conclude that these prospective data indicate that baseline levels of CRP predict the future risk of developing symptomatic PAD and provide further support for the hypothesis that chronic inflammation is important in the pathogenesis of atherothrombosis. What fascinating information. Should we begin determining CRP in population screening studies with the specific intent of recommending aspirin in those patients who are positive? I wonder. (See also Abstract 1–20.)

Reference

1. Ridker, PM, Cushman, M, Stampfer, MJ, et al. Inflammation, aspirin, and risk of cardiovascular disease in apparently healthy men. *N Engl J Med* 336:973–979, 1997.

Vascular Endothelial Growth Factor Expression in Canine Peripheral Vein Bypass Grafts

Hamdan AD, Aiello LP, Misare BD, et al (Harvard Med School, Boston; Deaconess Hosp, Boston; Children's Hosp, Boston; et al)

J Vasc Surg 26:79–86, 1997 1–72

Background.—When placed as arterial bypass grafts, autologous veins initially lose their endothelial cell lining, after which reendothelialization occurs. The molecular and cellular mechanisms of this process remain unclear. Expression of vascular endothelial growth factor (VEGF), an endothelial cell–specific angiogenic mitogen, was studied in a dog vein grafting model.

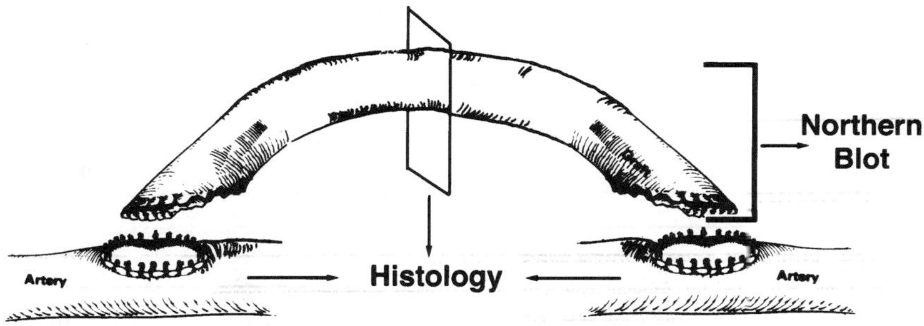

FIGURE 1.—Diagram depicts vein bypass graft in canine model. At time of harvesting, bypass grafts were disconnected from anastomotic sites to isolate specific areas for vascular endothelial growth factor (VEGF) mRNA expression determination. (Courtesy of Hamdan AD, Aiello LP, Misare BD, et al: Vascular endothelial growth factor expression in canine peripheral vein bypass grafts. *J Vasc Surg* 26:79–86, 1997.)

Methods.—Dog cephalic vein–femoral artery interposition grafts were harvested for study 48 hours or 4 weeks after bypass (Fig 1). After isolation of total RNA, Northern blotting was performed to determine VEGF mRNA expression. Immunohistochemical studies using anti-VEGF antibodies were performed as well.

Results.—At 48 hours, VEGF mRNA expression in vein grafts was elevated 2.5–fold over control veins. By 4 weeks, VEGF mRNA levels in grafts returned to control levels. Expression of VEGF in distal arterial segments—including the anastomotic site but not the attached vein graft—was increased by more than 21-fold at 48 hours and by nearly sevenfold at 4 weeks. Expression of VEGF was also increased in vessels subjected to arteriotomy or ischemia alone. Immunohistochemical studies showed VEGF protein in the endothelial cells and smooth muscle cells of the venous bypass graft, with peak levels seen in areas of intimal hyperplasia at the arterial anastomosis.

Conclusions.—High levels of VEGF were demonstrated in vein grafts and arterial anastomoses 48 hours after arterial reconstruction using venous conduits. Although VEGF expression in the vein graft normalizes within 4 weeks, it continues to be elevated in the adjacent arterial segment. The process of reendothelialization may be enhanced by increased VEGF production after arterial grafting, which could help to explain the optimal patency rates achieved with autologous vein grafts.

▶ This is an additional testimonial to the greatness of VEGF. My conclusion is that injured arteries and veins express increased levels of VEGF during the healing phase, which, at least in this experiment, appears to be more powerfully expressed in the artery than in the vein graft. In addition to facilitating endothelial repair, VEGF appears to have a desirable negative effect on smooth muscle migration and proliferation. Perhaps this substance will someday have an actual clinical role. We shall see.

Antisense Basic Fibroblast Growth Factor Gene Transfer Reduces Early Intimal Thickening in a Rabbit Femoral Artery Balloon Injury Model

Neschis DG, Safford SD, Hanna AK, et al (Univ of Pennsylvania, Philadelphia)

J Vasc Surg 27:126–134, 1998 1–73

Background.—There is evidence that basic fibroblast growth factor (bFGF) released by injured and dying cells is a major factor in the intimal hyperplastic response to injury. However, the importance of new bFGF production by arterial wall cells after injury is unclear. This issue was examined using a rabbit model of femoral artery balloon injury.

Methods.—After balloon injury of the superficial femoral artery, New Zealand White rabbits received intraluminal delivery of an adenoviral vector encoding a rat antisense bFGF (A*Sb*FGF) transcript at a concentration of 1×10^{10} plaque-forming units/mL. Control rabbits received either an adenovirus encoding the *lac Z* reporter gene (Ad.lacZ) or phosphate-buffered saline solution only. Two weeks later, the animals were killed for histomorphometric analysis of the femoral arteries. Measurements of in-

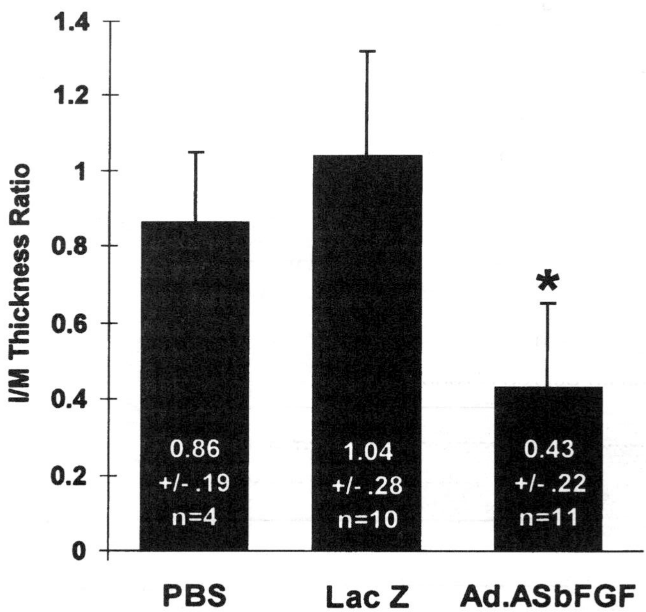

FIGURE 3.—Intimal-medial (*I/M*) thickness ratios 14 days after balloon injury immediately followed by a 20-minute local incubation of treatment solution. Treatment groups included phosphate-buffered saline (*PBS*) vehicle alone, an adenovirus encoding the *lacZ* reporter gene (*Ad.lacZ*) at 1×10^{10} plaque-forming units (pfm)/mL, and adenoviral gene transfer of antisense bFGF (*Ad.ASbFGF*) at 1×10^{10} pfu/mL. Graph demonstrates significant reduction in intimal thickening in Ad.ASbFGF group compared with phosphate-buffered saline and Ad.lacZ control groups ($P = 0.004$ and P less than 0.0001, respectively). There was no significant difference in intimal thickening between the phosphate-buffered saline and Ad.lacZ groups ($P = 0.27$). (Courtesy of Neschis DG, Safford SD, Hanna AK, et al: Antisense basic fibroblast growth factor gene transfer reduces early intimal thickening in a rabbit femoral artery balloon injury model. *J Vasc Surg* 27:126–134, 1998.)

TABLE 2.—Plasma ELAM-1, ICAM-1, VCAM-1, and vWf in Control Subjects and Patients With Chronic Venous Disease, Expressed as Median (Interquartile Range), Before and After Venous Hypertension Produced by Standing for 30 Minutes

Molecule/vWf	Controls	Patients LDS	VVs	Mann-Whitney U-test
ELAM				
Median (IQR) ng/mL				
Basal	41 (23–62)†,‡	57 (43–76)†	41 (34–59)‡	†=0.01, ‡=N.S.
Standing	52 (30–81)*,¶	61 (49–87)*	51 (39–66)¶	*=N.S., ¶=N.S.
Diff between median rise (95% CI, Wilcoxon)	11.5 (15–8)	3.5 (7–1)	6.75 (10–4)	
ICAM				
Median (IQR) ng/mL				
Basal	211 (196–229)†,‡	267 (230–341)†	251 (238–294)‡	†=0.002, ‡=0.001
Standing	272 (234–310)*,¶	312 (277–387)*	288 (253–363)¶	*=0.03, ¶=N.S.
Diff between median rise (95% CI, Wilcoxon)	60 (73.5–47)	34.8 (62–15)	34.8 (60–5.5)	
VCAM				
Median (IQR) ng/mL				
Basal	394 (333–445)†,‡	607 (552–776)†	513 (432–699)‡	†=0.003, ‡=0.01
Standing	559 (413–696)*,¶	899 (705–971)*	651 (505–907)¶	*<0.001, ¶=N.S.
Diff between median rise (95% CI, Wilcoxon)	144 (214–73.5)	202 (273.5–157)	103 (165–67.5)	
vWf iu/dL				
Median (IQR)				
Basal		138 (108–166)§	80 (61–105)§	§=0.002
Standing		141 (100–169)‡‡	92 (46–127)‡‡	‡‡=0.009
Diff between median rise (95% CI, Wilcoxon)		N.S.	N.S.	

P values: †, controls vs. LDS; ‡, controls vs. VVs; *, controls vs. LDS; ¶, controls vs. VVs; §, LDS vs. VVs; ‡‡, LDS vs. VVs.

Abbreviations: ELAM-1, endothelial leukocyte adhesion molecule-1; *ICAM-1,* intracellular adhesion molecule-1; *VCAM-1,* vascular cell adhesion molecule-1; *vWF,* von Willebrand factor; *LDS,* lipodermatosclerotic skin changes; *VVs,* skin change absent; *CI,* confidence interval, Wilcoxon; *N.S.,* not significant.

(Courtesy of Saharay M, Shields DA, Georgiannos SN, et al: Endothelial activation in patients with chronic venous disease. *Eur J Vasc Endovasc Surg* 15:342–349. Copyright 1998, by permission of WB Saunders Company Limited, London.)

that venous hypertension results in endothelial activation, which may aid endothelial leukocyte adhesion, and that patients with lipodermatosclerosis exhibit increased VCAM-1, a counterligand for receptors expressed by monocytes and lymphocytes, indicating these cells may be important in the development of skin changes. He has continued to elaborate upon his basic observation that some white blood cells may be trapped in areas of venous hypertension, and may undergo phenotypic modification. I would like to hear less about the method and more about the outcome at some point in the future.

Leukocyte Activity in the Microcirculation of the Leg in Patients With Chronic Venous Disease

Saharay M, Shields DA, Porter JB, et al (Univ College London)
J Vasc Surg 25:265–273, 1997 1–81

Background.—Although patients with chronic venous disease often develop skin damage, the mechanism is not well understood. Leukocyte trapping and activation in the microcirculation of the leg of these patients has been proposed to lead to ulceration. Patients with chronic venous disease were subjected to short-term venous hypertension to determine whether neutrophil and monocyte activation occurred.

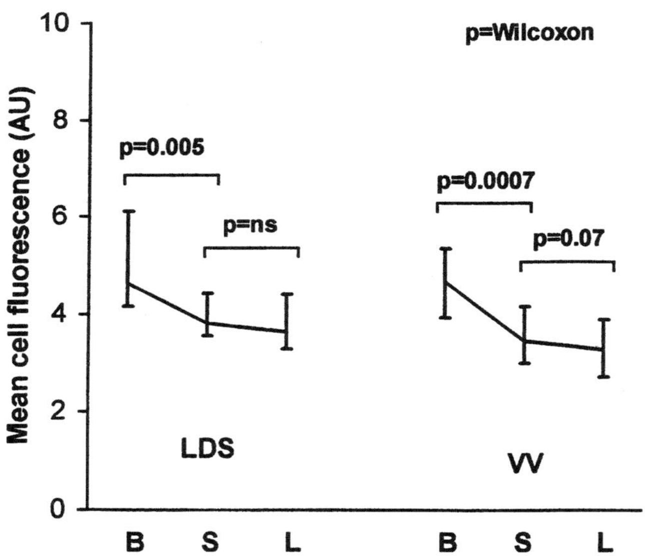

FIGURE 2.—Neutrophil surface CD11b expression expressed as a mean cell fluorescence in arbitrary units before, during, and after venous hypertension produced by standing for 30 minutes. Descriptors are medians and interquartile rages, statistics are Wilcoxon matched pairs signed rank test. *Abbreviations: B,* Basal; *S,* standing; *L,* lying; *NS,* not significant. (Courtesy of Saharay M, Shields DA, Porter JB, et al: Leukocyte activity in the microcirculation of the leg in patients with chronic venous disease. *J Vasc Surg* 25:265–273, 1997.)

Methods.—The study group included 15 patients with varicose veins and 15 patients with varicose veins and skin changes. Blood samples were obtained from a foot vein before and after 30 minutes of standing to raise venous pressure and again after lying supine for 10 minutes to relieve the pressure. These samples were examined for leukocyte surface CD11b and L-selectin (CD62L) expression by flow cytometry. An ELISA assay was also employed to detect plasma-soluble L-selectin.

Results.—In both groups of patients, median neutrophil CD11b levels decreased significantly after 30 minutes of venous hypertension induced by standing (Fig 2). Median monocyte CD11b levels also decreased after 30 minutes of venous hypertension and then decreased further after venous hypertension was removed. Neutrophil and monocyte L-selectin levels followed a similar pattern. After venous hypertension, there was an increase in soluble L-selectin in both groups of patients, which indicates leukocyte adhesion to the endothelium.

Conclusions.—In response to venous hypertension, both CD11b and L-selectin expression of circulating neutrophils and monocytes decreased in patients with chronic venous disease, because of the sequestration of the more activated population of neutrophils and monocytes through adherence to the endothelium. At the same time, a rise in soluble L-selectin levels was detected in the plasma, indicating L-selectin had been released preceding binding. These findings provide evidence of leukocyte activation and trapping in the microcirculation of the limb. These findings did not differ between patients with and without skin changes. Other aspects of the response to leukocyte adhesion may be involved in the development of the skin damage.

▶ Is leukocyte trapping in areas of venous hypertension a prime cause of lipodermatosclerosis and eventually venous ulceration? These investigators from the Middlesex Hospital in London are convinced this is the case. They, in fact, hypothesize two populations of leukocytes, one primed and the other unprimed. In the setting of acute venous hypertension, the primed leukocytes promptly bind to the endothelium and exit the circulation. Thus, they attribute the measured fall in the CD11B and L-selectin levels to the loss of the primed cells from the circulation. While this is an attractive explanation, I suspect that many other explanations are equally possible. While I accept this evidence as plausible, it is far from definitive. Cell trapping rears its ugly head again. (See also Abstract 1–80.)

The Fibrinolytic Effects of Intermittent Pneumatic Compression: Mechanism of Enhanced Fibrinolysis

Comerota AJ, Chouhan V, Harada RN, et al (Temple Univ, Philadelphia; Univ of North Carolina, Chapel Hill)

Ann Surg 226:306–314, 1997 1–82

Background.—For patients undergoing general surgery, intermittent pneumatic compression (IPC) can help to prevent deep vein thrombosis,

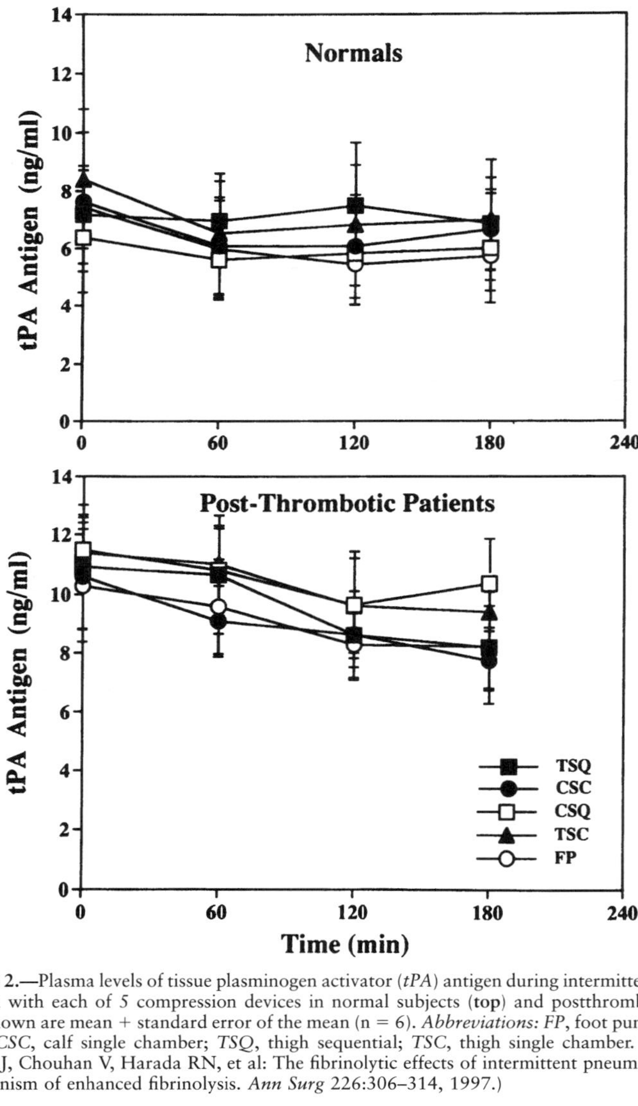

FIGURE 2.—Plasma levels of tissue plasminogen activator (*tPA*) antigen during intermittent pneumatic compression with each of 5 compression devices in normal subjects (**top**) and postthrombotic patients (**bottom**). Shown are mean + standard error of the mean (n = 6). *Abbreviations: FP*, foot pump; *CSQ*, calf sequential; *CSC*, calf single chamber; *TSQ*, thigh sequential; *TSC*, thigh single chamber. (Courtesy of Comerota AJ, Chouhan V, Harada RN, et al: The fibrinolytic effects of intermittent pneumatic compression: Mechanism of enhanced fibrinolysis. *Ann Surg* 226:306–314, 1997.)

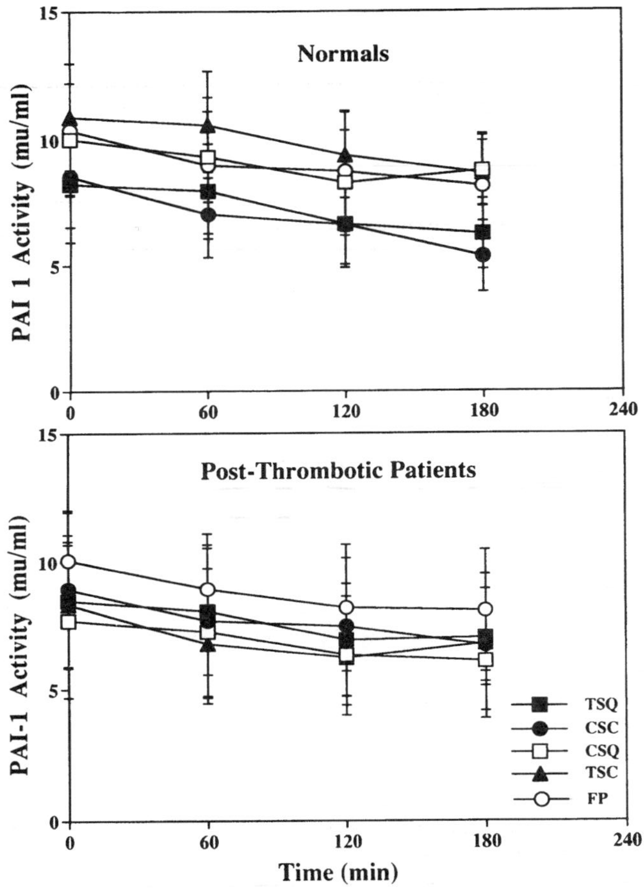

FIGURE 5.—Plasma levels of plasminogen activator inhibitor-1 (*PAI-1*) during intermittent pneumatic compression with each of 5 compression devices in normal subjects (**top**) and postthrombotic patients (**bottom**). Shown are mean + standard error of the mean (n = 6). *Abbreviations: FP*, foot pump; *CSQ*, calf sequential; *CSC*, calf single chamber; *TSQ*, thigh sequential; *TSC*, thigh single chamber. (Courtesy of Comerota AJ, Chouhan V, Harada RN, et al: The fibrinolytic effects of intermittent pneumatic compression: Mechanism of enhanced fibrinolysis. *Ann Surg* 226:306–314, 1997.)

presumably by increasing venous velocity and stimulating endogenous fibrinolysis. However, it remains unclear how fibrinolytic activity is increased and what the effects on normal and postthrombotic veins are. The effects of IPC on fibrinolytic activity were examined, including the mechanism of those effects. Differences in the responses of postthrombotic vs. normal individuals were studied as well.

Methods.—Participants were 12 volunteers, 6 with previous thrombosis and 6 without. In once-weekly sessions, the patients had 5 different IPC devices—including single-chamber, sequential, foot, calf, and long-leg

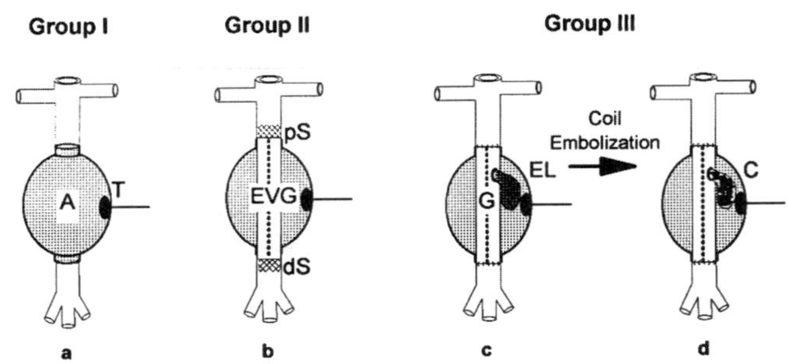

FIGURE 1.—Various types of models used in this study are shown. **A**, group I, untreated polytetrafluoroethylene aneurysms. **B**, group 2, aneurysms managed with endovascular graft (*EVG*) without endoleak. C, group 3, aneurysms managed with EVG with endoleak. These EVGs had a 4-mm–diameter hole in the graft to produce the endoleak. **D**, same model as in C after the endoleak was packed with coils. *Abbreviations: A*, Aneurysm; *T*, pressure transducer; *pS*, proximal stent; *dS*, distal stent; *G*, graft; *EL*, endoleak; *C*, coils. (Marty B, Sanchez LA, Ohki T, et al: Endoleak after endovascular graft repair of experimental aortic aneurysms: Does coil embolization with angiographic "seal" lower intraaneurysmal pressure? *J Vasc Surg* 27:454–462, 1998.)

(IAP) of large endoleaks from defects in the graft was assessed, together with the efficacy of coil embolization in the management of endoleaks.

Methods.—In 15 dogs, the infrarenal aorta was replaced by a polytetrafluoroethylene aneurysm containing a pressure transducer. Four dogs (group 1) had untreated aneurysms; 4 (group 2) had endovascularly excluded aneurysms without an endoleak; and 7 (group 3) had aneurysms excluded by grafts with a defect representing the source of an endoleak. Coil embolization was used after 4 weeks in group 3 dogs. Systolic IAP, measured daily, was expressed as a ratio of systolic blood pressure determined from a forelimb cuff. Endoleaks were assessed by arteriography, duplex US, and spiral contrast CT.

Findings.—The mean systolic IAP ratio in group 1 remained close to systolic blood pressure but declined to 0.34 in group 2. In group 3, the mean systolic IAP ratio initially decreased, then stabilized at 0.75. Aneurysms with an endoleak remained pulsatile, with a pulse pressure of 30 mm Hg, which was less than that of untreated aneurysms. Arteriography and CT showed "sealing" of endoleaks after coil embolization. However, the IAP ratio did not decline after coil embolization (Fig 1).

Conclusion.—Incomplete endovascular aneurysm exclusion resulting from an endoleak does not decrease the IAP ratio and may cause a continued risk for aneurysmal rupture. Although coil embolization produced angiographic and CT sealing in this study, it did not reduce the IAP ratio.

▶ This fascinating study indicates that in the experimental animal, coil embolization of an endoleak in an endovascularly repaired aneurysm initially lowers the pressure in the sac, but the pressure then rises to stabilize at about 75% of systemic pressure. In fact, in this setting, the aneurysm sac remained pulsatile and, as the authors presciently note, presented a continuing risk for rupture. It is fascinating to note that after coil embolization, all endoleaks were sealed angiographically, but this did not result in any permanent relief of the elevated pressure within the sac.

This study has profound implications for clinical management of patients with endoleaks. The only conclusion I can reach is that there must have been residual endoleaks after coil embolization that were too small to be angiographically visualized but, nonetheless, resulted in near systemic pressure within the aneurysm sac, including restoration of pulsatility. Perhaps this adverse outcome is specific for coil embolization. It appears that alternatives to coil embolization should be sought in this setting. On balance, this is most worrisome information.

Endovascular Grafts for Noninfected Aortoiliac Anastomotic Aneurysms

Yuan JG, Marin ML, Veith FJ, et al (Montefiore Med Ctr, New York)
J Vasc Surg 26:210–221, 1997 2–4

Background.—The reported incidence of anastomotic aneurysms of the aorta and iliac arteries ranges from 0.2% to 15%. Without treatment, these anastomotic aneurysms run the same risk of complications as true aneurysms. The use of endovascular grafts to treat anastomotic aneurysms was reported.

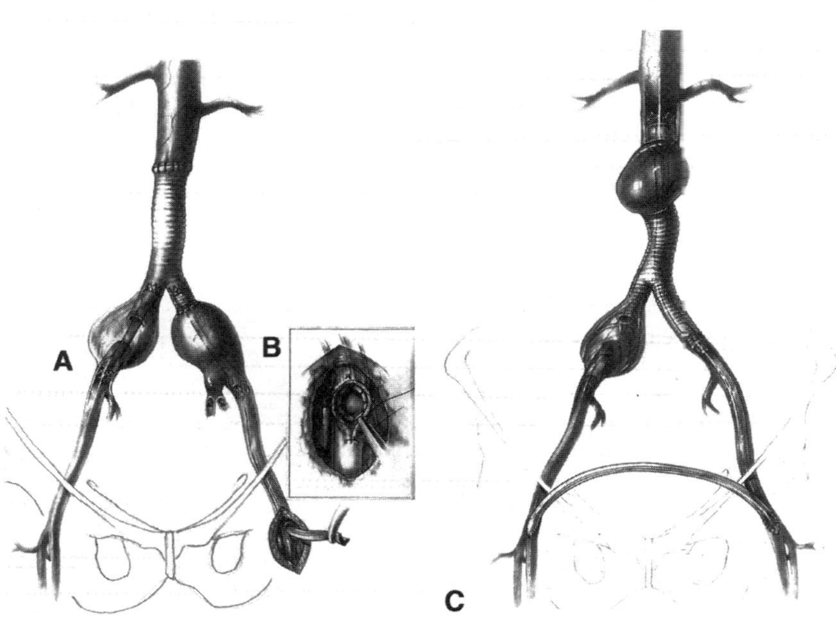

FIGURE 4.—Techniques **A, B,** and **C** used for endovascular repair of aortoiliac anastomotic aneurysms. *Inset* demonstrates endoluminal hand-sewn anastomosis through femoral arteriotomy. (Courtesy of Yuan JG, Marin ML, Veith FJ, et al: Endovascular grafts for noninfected aortoiliac anastomotic aneurysms. *J Vasc Surg* 26:210–221, 1997.)

Methods.—During a 21-month period, endovascular grafts were used to treat 12 aortic or iliac anastomotic aneurysms in 10 patients. The patients all had serious medical conditions that contraindicated surgical repair. There was no evidence of infection, such as fever, leukocytosis, or a periprosthetic fluid collection on CT. A femoral arteriotomy was used to place endovascular grafts composed of polytetrafluoroethylene and balloon-expandable stents. The grafts were placed under C-arm fluoroscopic guidance using over-the-wire techniques (Fig 4).

Results.—Endovascular graft placement was successful in every case. None of the patients died as a result of the procedure. One patient had a wound hematoma after graft placement, and another had perioperative myocardial infarction. The grafts maintained patency through a mean 16 months' follow-up. Computed tomography showed no evidence that the aneurysms were enlarging or that the grafts were leaking.

Conclusions.—Endovascular grafts were successfully used to manage aortoiliac anastomotic aneurysms in patients who were not good candidates for surgery. Graft placement may become an option for all patients with clinically significant lesions.

▶ Perhaps the endovascular graft may actually be a useful device for correction of certain types of pseudoaneurysms involving aortoiliac graft systems. For the life of me, however, I am unable to understand why these investigators choose to overdilate the proximal end of an 8-mm polytetrafluoroethylene graft. Does this not have the real potential to damage the polytetrafluoroethylene material to the point of loss of structural integrity?

Computed Tomographic Angiographic Imaging of Abdominal Aortic Aneurysms: Implications for Transfemoral Endovascular Aneurysm Management

Balm R, Stokking R, Kaatee R, et al (Univ Hosp Utrecht, The Netherlands)
J Vasc Surg 26:231–237, 1997 2–5

Introduction.—Having a proximal and distal segment of relatively nondiseased vessel wall is crucial to successful transfemoral endovascular aneurysm management (TEAM) of abdominal aortic aneurysms (AAAs). The anatomical features pertinent to patient selection and graft design for TEAM of the infrarenal aorta was evaluated using CT angiography.

Methods.—One hundred two spiral CT scans of the abdominal aorta of patients with AAAs were conducted during a prospective, noncomparative analysis. Slices were reconstructed perpendicular to the vessel axis (central lumen line) at a 10-mm interval from original CT data sets. Diameter measurements were taken in the reconstructed slices. Vessel length measurements were performed along the central lumen line. Patients were evaluated for suitability for TEAM. Suitability was defined as presence of a sufficient proximal aortic neck and either a sufficient distal aortic neck or 2 sufficient iliac necks.

Results.—Thirty-six scans had to be excluded for technical reasons. Of 66 patients remaining, only 18 were considered possible candidates for treatment with a bifurcated endovascular device. The infrarenal aortic diameter-to-iliac artery diameter ratio was less than 2 in most of this cohort. The vessel segments judged to be adequate for endovascular graft anchoring were noncylindrical in most patients.

Conclusions.—Very few patients with AAAs are able to be treated with an endovascular graft. Endovascular grafts should ideally be a combination of rigid and flexible components. The graft midsection can be relatively rigid, but both proximal and distal attachment systems should have some flexibility with an intrinsic maximum diameter.

► This detailed description of workstation reconstruction of CT angiograms of the infrarenal abdominal aorta describes how these authors approach the issue of imaging for endovascular aneurysm management. Interestingly, only 66 patient scans were adequate for analysis and less than one-fourth of these could be treated with a bifurcated endovascular device. There appeared to be not a single patient in whom a tube prosthesis would be possible. A primary reason for patient exclusion from the eligible group was absence of a sufficient proximal aortic neck. I note that others (see Abstract 2–1) are placing the proximal stent attachment directly across the renal orifices. There seems to be general agreement that successful deployment of endovascular aneurysm grafts will require detailed imaging studies and sophisticated imaging analysis. If such detailed analysis is mandatory, I wonder how well this device will travel to community hospitals? I continue to have the underlying suspicion that endovascular grafts are going to be ultimately applicable to far fewer patients than many enthusiasts currently suspect.

Conversion From Endoluminal to Open Repair of Abdominal Aortic Aneurysms: A Hazardous Procedure

May J, White GH, Yu W, et al (Univ of Sydney, Australia)

Eur J Vasc Endovasc Surg 14:4–11, 1997 2–6

Objective.—It has been suggested that if an attempted endoluminal repair of an abdominal aortic aneurysm (AAA) is unsuccessful, it can easily be converted to an open repair. Such conversions, however, may be more complicated than standard elective surgery. Technical problems in converting from endoluminal to open repair of AAAs were reviewed, including patient outcomes.

Patients.—The 4-year review included 113 patients in whom endoluminal repair of AAA was attempted. The series included 48 patients with comorbid conditions that caused them to be rejected for open AAA repair at other centers. Eighteen patients required conversion to open repair, including 13 at the initial operation and 5 at a later one. Serious comorbid

TABLE 2.—Causes of Failure Leading to Conversion

Primary conversion (13)	n
Access problems	2
Balloon-related problems	
Malfunction	1
Aortic rupture	1
Endograft migration	3
Graft thrombosis	1
Failed bifurcated graft deployment	5
Total	13
Secondary conversion (5)	
Renal arteries covered by endograft	2
Persistent endoleak	
AAA intact	2
AAA ruptured	1
Total	5

(Reprinted from *Eur J Vasc Endovasc Surg*, Vol. 14, July, May J, White GH, Yu W, et al, Conversion from endoluminal to open repair of abdominal aortic aneurysms: A hazardous procedure, 4–11, 1997, by permission of the publisher WB Saunders Company Limited, London.)

conditions were present in 7 of the 18 patients whose procedures were converted.

The choice of conversion technique depended on the cause of failure of endoluminal repair (Table 2). Three patients with access problems or balloon malfunction were treated with standard open AAA repair. Eleven patients with a correctly positioned endograft immediately below the renal arteries, part of the endograft within the common iliac arteries, or both were treated with a modification of the standard technique. The remaining 4 patients—with aortic rupture, renal arteries covered by the endograft, or trapping of the delivery catheter—required supraceliac control. Patients in the primary conversion group received a mean contrast volume of 225 mL and had a mean operative time of 5.25 hours.

Outcomes.—All procedures were successfully converted to open surgery. Three of 18 patients had renal impairment necessitating dialysis. Three patients died in the perioperative period, for a procedure-related mortality rate of 17%. There was 1 late death. All of the patients who died had preoperative comorbid conditions.

Conclusions.—Many patients undergoing conversion from an endoluminal to an open approach to AAA repair require modifications of the standard operative approach. This can lead to greatly elevated morbidity and mortality rates. The likelihood of conversion is no higher for patients with comorbid conditions, making them ineligible for open surgery. However, these patients have a greatly elevated risk of death.

▶ Dr. May and his associates from Sydney have one of the largest endovascular graft experiences in the world, and they have a well-deserved reputation for careful analysis. Thus, when they speak, the rest of us had best listen. During a recent experience with 113 endoluminal graft insertions, 18 patients required conversion to open repair, 13 initially and 5 at a later date. The conversion results were not good. Renal impairment neces-

Results.—Two-year outcomes were similar in terms of patient-reported maximum walking, treadmill distance to onset of claudication, treadmill maximum walking distance, and ankle-brachial pressure index. Number of occluded arteries and degree of stenosis of patent arteries were less in the PTA group. There were no significant differences in quality of life.

Conclusions.—Two years after treatment, patients with mild to moderate intermittent claudication treated with PTA had less extensive disease than did those treated by medical therapy only. However, the PTA-treated patients had no significant advantage in terms of walking or quality of life. These findings are relevant to patient management and clinical research.

▶ In this interesting study, 62 patients with claudication and short-segment femoral or iliac artery stenoses were randomly assigned to receive PTA plus medical treatment or medical treatment alone. Of considerable interest is the observation that at 2-year follow-up, the PTA group and the control group appeared identical in patient reported maximum walking distance, treadmill onset of claudication, treadmill maximum walking, and ankle-brachial index. The authors' statement that the PTA group had fewer occluded arteries and lesser stenoses, as measured by velocity ratios, appears a bit of a stretch to me. Quality of life did not differ between the 2 groups. My only conclusion is that in this carefully conducted randomized study, the 2 groups behaved identically. This is, of course, quite similar to the Creasy study[1] of a similar design reported from Oxford 7 years previously. Presently, I find little to objectively recommend femoral artery angioplasty at all, and certainly not for claudication. It appears neither durable nor particularly beneficial.

Reference

1. Creasy TS, McMillan PJ, Fletcher EWL, et al: Is percutaneous transluminal angioplasty better than exercise for claudication? Preliminary results from a prospective, randomised trial. *Eur J Vasc Surg* 4:135–140, 1990.

Subintimal Angioplasty of Infrapopliteal Occlusions in Critically Ischaemic Limbs

Nydahl S, Hartshorne T, Bell PRF, et al (Leicester Royal Infirmary, England)
Eur J Vasc Endovasc Surg 14:212–216, 1997 2–12

Background.—Most patients with critical limb ischemia have multilevel disease and have not been considered candidates for angioplasty. Distal angioplasty has been considered high risk because of the small caliber of the tibial arteries, the tendency for spasms to develop, and the difficulty of revascularization if angioplasty fails. Recent advances such as small strong low profile balloons, steerable hydrophilic guidewires, road-mapping capabilities, and the use of vasodilators have made infrapopliteal angioplasty feasible. The outcome of subintimal angioplasty of infrapopliteal occlusions in critically ischemic limbs was retrospectively reviewed.

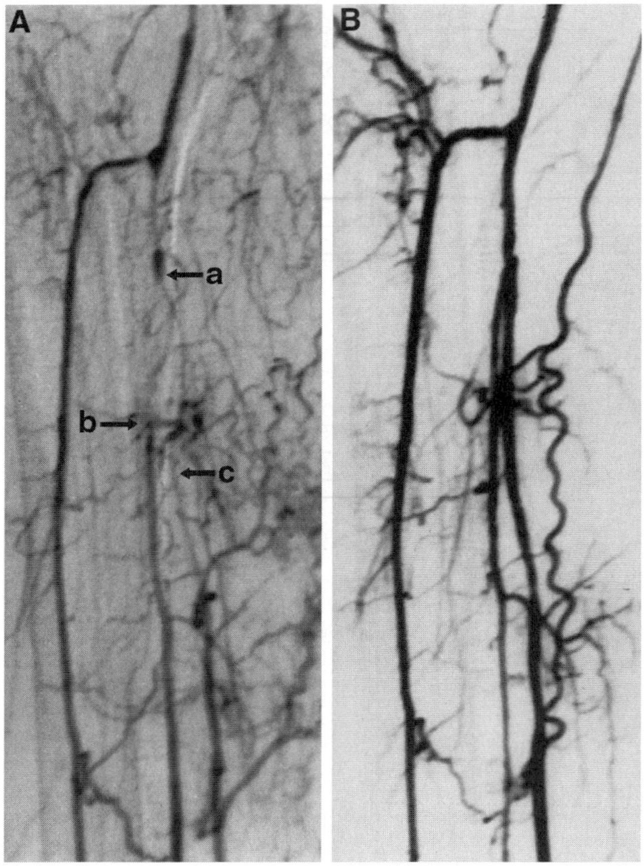

FIGURE 4.—A, tight stenosis of the tibioperoneal trunk leading into a 3-cm occlusion of the peroneal artery (*between arrows a and b*) and 4-cm occlusion of the posterior tibial artery (*between arrows a and c*). Before (**A**) and after (**B**) subintimal angioplasty. (Reprinted from Nydahl S, Hartshorne T, Bell PRF, et al: Subintimal angioplasty of infrapopliteal occlusions in critically ischaemic limbs. *Eur J Vasc Endovasc Surg* 14:212–216, copyright 1997 by permission of the publisher WB Saunders Company Limited, London.)

Methods.—The outcome of 28 consecutive limbs with critical ischemia in 27 patients who had subintimal angioplasty of infrapopliteal occlusions was examined. The median patient age was 81 years. Success, failure, complications, and long-term patency were defined according to the guidelines of the Society of Vascular Surgery and the International Society for Cardiovascular Surgery.

Results.—There were 32 infrapopliteal occlusions: 7 in the anterior tibial arteries, 7 in the peroneal arteries, and 6 in the posterior tibial arteries (Fig 4). Of the 28 limbs, 17 were ulcerated, 7 were gangrenous, and 4 had rest pain only. There were 25 procedures performed to a single calf vessel, and 3 procedures were performed to multiple calf vessels. The

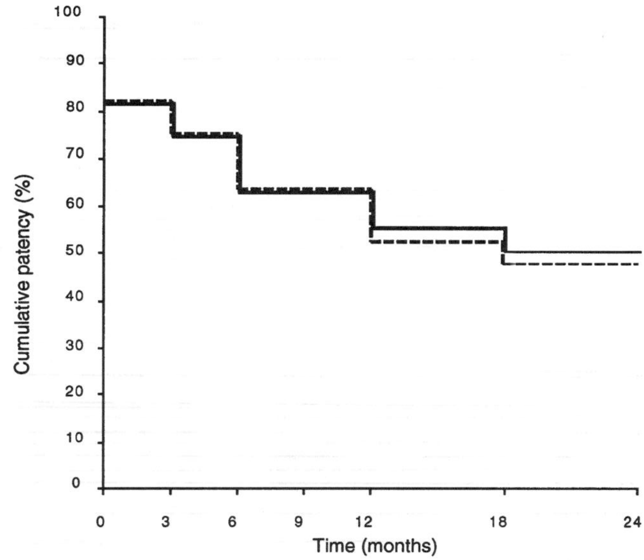

No. at risk	0	3	6	9	12	18	24
Haemodynamic	28	22	20	17	15	8	4
Symptomatic	28	22	20	17	15	9	4

FIGURE 5.—Cumulative hemodynamic (*dashed line*) and symptomatic (*solid line*) patency. The analysis includes initial technical failures, and the standard error of the mean is less than 10% up to 18 months. (Reprinted from Nydahl S, Hartshorne T, Bell PRF, et al: Subintimal angioplasty of infrapopliteal occlusions in critically ischaemic limbs. *Eur J Vasc Endovasc Surg* 14:212–216, copyright 1997 by permission of the publisher WB Saunders Company Limited, London.)

median occlusion length was 7 cm. The initial technical success rate was 84%. Three minor complications occurred: a groin hematoma, a vessel perforation, and a distal embolus. No limbs were lost as a result of the procedure. At 30 days, the mortality was 0. At 12 months, the hemodynamic patency was 53% and the symptomatic patency was 56%; both included initial failures (Fig 5). At 12 months, the limb salvage rate was 85%, and the patient survival rate was 81%.

Discussion.—These results show that subintimal angioplasty of infrapopliteal occlusions in patients with critically ischemic limbs is safe and effective. This approach is a low-risk alternative to distal reconstructive surgery. This technique should also be seen as a complement to surgery because it can be used to salvage limbs after failed femorodistal bypass and because surgery is technically feasible after failed angioplasty.

▶ Dr. Bell's group in England has told us for years that they have discovered a new way to perform angioplasty. Specifically, they deliberately direct the angioplasty catheter into the subintimal dissection plane and dilate this dissection plane. Although this sounds absolutely bizarre, they state that they have been able to successfully open long segments of completely occluded vessels. In fact, their initial success rate was 84%. To the best of my knowledge, they are currently a voice in the wilderness describing this technique. My friends in England tell me that they have not been able to duplicate this, and I am not aware of anyone in the United States trying this technique. Nonetheless, we shall record this as potentially another way to remove the integument from a feline (skin a cat).

A Combined Approach to the Treatment of Proximal Arterial Occlusions of the Upper Limb With Endovascular Stents

Whitbread T, Cleveland TJ, Beard JD, et al (Northern Gen Hosp, Sheffield, England)

Eur J Vasc Endovasc Surg 15:29–35, 1998 2–13

Background.—The traditional transfemoral approach to endovascular stenting is not ideal for the treatment of proximal arterial lesions of the upper limb. This is because the distance of the lesion from the femoral puncture site, flexibility and unsupported length of guidewires and delivery systems, and the often acutely angled origin of the great vessels make crossing the lesions and accurate deployment of the device difficult or impossible. Deploying the stent through a brachial arteriotomy should eliminate these problems. The treatment of proximal arterial occlusions of the upper limb by endoluminal stenting, using a combined surgical and radiologic approach, was reported.

Methods.—Eighteen proximal upper limb occlusions were treated. Eight were of brachiocephalic origin; 6 were of subclavian origin; 2 of the subclavian artery; and 2 of the axillary artery. When possible, primary stent deployment was used. The patients were given perioperative IV heparin followed by long-term aspirin treatment.

Findings.—Revascularization was successful in 15 of 18 proximal occlusions, completely alleviating symptoms. All stented vessels were patent up to 36 months after the procedure. No complications have arisen from the brachial arteriotomy sites.

Conclusion.—The treatment of choice for proximal occlusions of the upper limb vessels is primary stenting. A combined surgical and radiologic approach through a brachial arteriotomy can be used in such patients and is now the preferred treatment for such lesions at the authors' center.

▶ In Sheffield, England, a single regional vascular unit has been developed from a dispersed service previously delivered by competing hospitals. The mainspring was an equal partnership between surgeons and radiologists. This productive cooperation is not always achieved in the National Health Service, despite the absence of fee for service but it is particularly evident among younger consultants. The benefit of this cooperation—with radiologists expertly manipulating devices and surgeons expertly making and closing arteriotomies—is well illustrated here. We are reminded again that it is not always necessary to approach the thoracic or abdominal aorta from the groin, a route increasingly recognized as hazardous in patients with widespread atherosclerosis. A small operation in the arm certainly looks better than a big operation in the chest.

A.E.B. Giddings, M.D.

A Cost Comparison of Balloon Angioplasty and Stenting Versus Endarterectomy for the Treatment of Carotid Artery Stenosis

Jordan WD Jr, Roye GD, Fisher WS III, et al (Univ of Alabama, Birmingham)
J Vasc Surg 27:16–24, 1998 2–14

Introduction.—Percutaneous transluminal angioplasty with stenting (PTAS) is reported to offer reduced morbidity, a shorter recovery, and lower costs than carotid endarterectomy (CEA). To further define the role of PTAS as an alternative to CEA in the treatment of high-grade stenosis, a detailed cost analysis of the 2 procedures was performed

Methods.—All patients who underwent elective treatment of carotid artery stenosis at the study institution between August 1994 and October 1995 were retrospectively reviewed. During this period, 218 patients were admitted 229 times for the treatment of 239 carotid bifurcation stenoses. A total of 109 PTAS and 130 CEAs were performed. Hospital charges were reviewed and categorized for each procedure; professional fees were not included in calculations.

Results.—Although the PTAS and CEA groups were similar in patient characteristics and indications for treatment (Table 1), significantly more patients in the PTAS group had coronary artery disease and hypertension. One patient in the PTAS group and 2 in the CEA group died. Postprocedure strokes occurred at a rate of 7.7% in the PTAS group vs. 1.5% in the CEA group. Median postprocedure length of hospital stay was 2 days for PTAS patients vs. 3 days for CEA patients. Total hospital charges per admission were higher for PTAS ($30,140) than for CEA ($21,670), but the difference in average total charges was reduced when hospitalizations extended by complications were excluded ($24,848 and $19,247, respectively).

TABLE 1.—B, Indications for Treatment

	PTAS (*109 sides*)	*CEA* (*130 sides*)	*p*
Asymptomatic	44 (40%)	53 (41%)	0.917
Transient ischemic attack	37 (34%)	68 (52%)	0.015
Cerebrovascular accident	28 (26%)	9 (7%)	<0.001

Abbreviations: PTAS, percutaneous transluminal angioplasty with stenting; *CEA*, carotid endarterectomy.

(Courtesy of Jordan WD Jr, Roye GD, Fisher WS III, et al: A cost comparison of balloon angioplasty and stenting versus endarterectomy for the treatment of carotid artery stenosis. *J Vasc Surg* 27:16–24, 1998.)

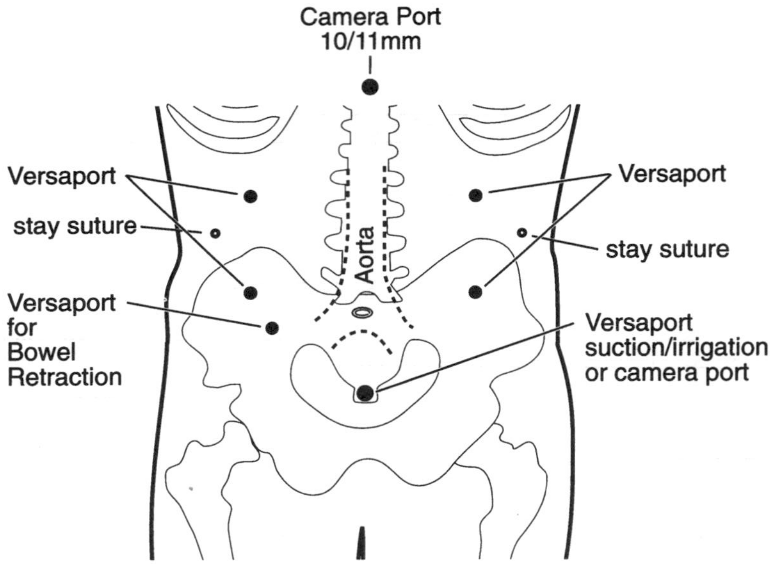

FIGURE 1.—Transperitoneal placement of 7 laparoscopic ports and trocars through stab incisions. Also note the lateral placement of 2 stay sutures. (Courtesy of Ahn SS, Hiyama DT, Rudkin GH, et al: Laparoscopic aortobifemoral bypass. *J Vasc Surg* 26:128–132, 1997.)

12 hours, with an aortic cross-clamp time of 3 hours and 30 minutes. Aortic graft anastomosis time was 2 hours and 15 minutes. Estimated blood loss was 1,800 mL. The patient stayed in the ICU overnight. He was ambulating and taking a regular diet by day 2. After the morning of the second day, the patient required no pain medication. He was discharged on day 2. The patient had no symptoms and a patent, intact graft and anastomosis at 18-month follow-up.

Discussion.—This study demonstrates the feasibility of laparoscopic aortobifemoral bypass grafting in humans. The laparoscopic approach can significantly reduce costs and rehabilitation time. Further studies of this less-invasive alternative to open surgery are required.

▶ In recent years, a few articles have appeared describing the somewhat painful procedure of laparoscopic aortobifemoral bypass. Herein, Dr. Ahn from UCLA throws his lobster pot into the ring. The procedure was justified by the patient being "reluctant" to undergo open abdominal surgery. Dr. Ahn honestly notes that the operative time for this procedure was 12 hours, with the aortic graft anastomosis taking 2 hours and 15 minutes and an estimated blood loss of 1,800 mL. The patient was discharged on the third postoperative day. I continue to be amazed at what is done from time to time in the name of progress. I somehow do not believe that a 12-hour aortobifemoral laparoscopic bypass in a slender man is going to be competitive with conventional surgery, despite the patient's preferences. (See also Abstract 7–9.)

Limitations of Intra-arterial Thrombolysis

Rickard MJFX, Fisher CM, Soong CV, et al (Royal North Shore Hosp, St Leonards, New South Wales, Australia)
Cardiovasc Surg 5:634–640, 1997 2–21

Introduction.—Although thrombolysis has long been used to treat patients with acute lower-limb ischemia caused by arterial occlusion, the indications for which the potential benefits of urokinase outweigh risks are unclear. A retrospective review assessed outcome, costs, and complications of initially treating acutely ischemic limbs with urokinase-induced thrombolysis.

Methods.—Data were reviewed from 37 patients undergoing 45 episodes of arterial thrombolysis in 37 limbs. The median age of the 21 men and 16 women was 72. Thrombolysis was performed to re-establish vascular patency or to convert an inoperable system to one with potential for limb salvage by surgical bypass. An initial bolus dose of urokinase was used in all limbs. Further boluses were given if thrombolysis was incomplete, and lacing with pulse spray was used in some cases. At any time during the procedure, percutaneous transluminal angioplasty or surgical intervention was undertaken if required.

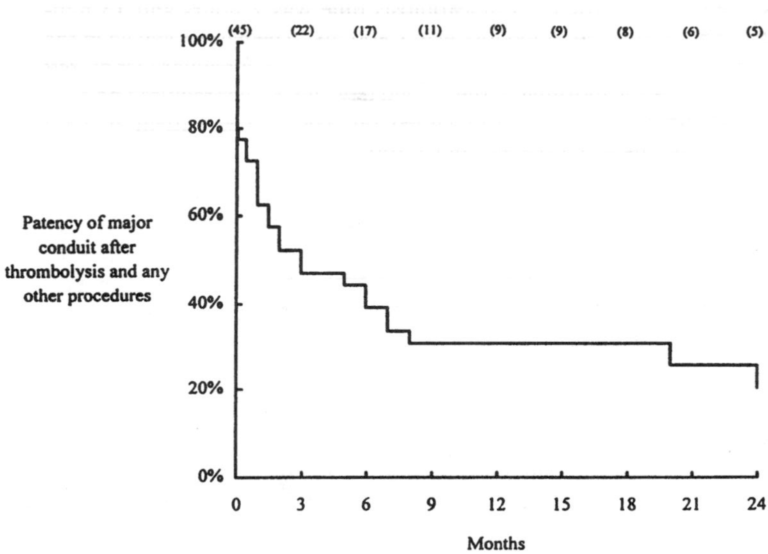

FIGURE 2.—Life-table patency of major vessels (including reconstructions when performed) for 45 episodes of thrombolysis. Numbers at risk shown in parentheses. Standard error of observed patency <0.10 for all data shown. (Courtesy of Rickard MJFX, Fisher CM, Soong CV, et al: Limitations of intra-arterial thrombolysis. *Cardiovasc Surg* 5:634–640, 1997. Reproduced with permission. Copyright 1997 American Heart Association.)

Results.—Occlusion occurred in 14 native arteries, 12 vein grafts, 16 prosthetic polytetrafluoroethylene grafts, and 3 composite grafts. Thrombolysis was initially successful in 73% of episodes (Fig 2). Percutaneous transluminal angioplasty was required in 23 of these, other surgery in 11, and bypass surgery in 7; only 3 required no additional procedure. Major surgery was performed in 8 of the 13 episodes with initial failure. Lysis-related complications were common (42% of episodes) and included distal embolization, major bleeding, minor bleeding, and arterial dissection. Both the 1 amputation and the 1 death that occurred within a month of treatment were directly attributable to thrombolysis. The mean 6-month patency rate of lysed vessels or replacement bypass grafts was 44%. Long-term patency was superior in cases involving a native artery or graft occlusion to the long-term patency in those cases with an occluded prosthetic graft. Costs of thrombolysis in excess of routine angiography were $2,440.

Conclusion.—Overall, thrombolysis in patients with acute lower-limb ischemia yielded a modest initial success rate and a poor early patency rate. Without better evidence of clinical evidence or cost advantage, thrombolysis should not be the routine first line management of lower-limb ischemia.

▶ We now know enough to predict with relative certainty the outcome of thrombolysis for lower extremity arterial or graft occlusion. If treatment is begun early, about two thirds of patients can be initially opened. A large majority of those opened, but not all, will require subsequent interventional procedures, using either an endovascular or an open surgical approach. There is always a small price to pay in terms of major bleeding and death—in this series, 16% major bleeding and 1 death among 45 patients. The real Achilles' heel, however, of this entire therapeutic exercise has been the 1-year patency following thrombolysis. The overall mean patency at 6 months in this series was only 44%. These results are simply abysmal. I do not believe one can justify the performance of a complex therapeutic treatment that has only a 44% likelihood of success at 6 months. I do believe we can regard these results as generally accurate, because they are quite similar to the randomized results in much larger patient groups reported in both the STILE and the TOPAS trials. As far as I am concerned, thrombolysis as primary treatment for lower extremity arterial or graft occlusion is a dead duck.

3 Vascular Laboratory and Imaging

Cerebrovascular

Transcranial Doppler Microembolus Detection in the Identification of Patients at High Risk of Perioperative Stroke

Levi CR, Roberts AK, Fell G, et al (Austin & Repatriation Med Centre, Melbourne, Victoria, Australia)

Eur J Vasc Endovasc Surg 14:170–176, 1997 3–1

Background.—In patients undergoing carotid endarterectomy (CEA), perioperative ischemic stroke is the major cause of morbidity and mortality. It has been suggested that transcranial Doppler US may be able to detect microembolic signals (MESs) in the intraoperative and postoperative periods, thus revealing patients at increased risk for perioperative stroke. This approach was tested in an open prospective study.

Methods.—The study included 81 consecutive patients undergoing CEA. All had preoperative, intraoperative, and interval postoperative monitoring of the middle cerebral artery ipsilateral to the operated side. Counts of MESs were made on-line in the preoperative and postoperative periods. After the operation, blinded analyses of MES counts were made off-line. The patients were followed up for 30 days after the operation for any focal neurologic deficit or death.

Results.—Ninety-four percent of patients had MESs detected in the intraoperative period, and 71% had them detected during the first hour after the operation (Fig 1). The rates of MES detection ranged from 0 to 25 MESs/hr during the operative phase and from 0 to 212 MESs/hr during the postoperative period. Ten percent of patients had postoperative MES counts greater than 50 MESs/hr. Frequent postoperative microemboli were strongly associated with the development of early cerebral ischemia, with 5 of 8 patients showing ischemic neurologic deficits in the territory of the monitored middle cerebral artery. Clinical outcome was unrelated to intraoperative MESs.

Conclusions.—In the early postoperative period after CEA, patients with MES counts greater than 50 MESs/hr are at significantly increased risk for ipsilateral focal cerebral ischemia. Thus, postoperative transcra-

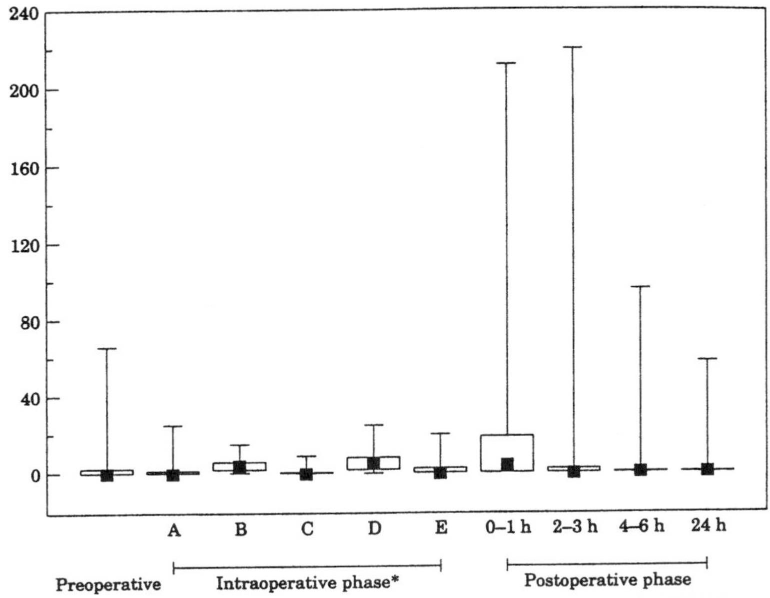

FIGURE 1.—Ranges with median values and 25th to 75th quartile ranges of MES counts detected preoperative, intraoperatively and postoperatively. (**Range bars,** minimum–maximum; **open square,** 25% to 75%; **filled square,** median value.) (Courtesy of Levi CR, Roberts AK, Hoare MC, et al: Transcranial Doppler microembolus detection in the identification of patients at high risk of perioperative stroke. *Eur J Vasc Endovasc Surg* 14:170–176. Copyright 1997. Reprinted by permission of WB Saunders Company Limited, London.)

nial Doppler US monitoring may have a role to play in revealing patients at high risk for embolic stroke. Further studies of this possibility, including preventive techniques and interventions, are needed.

▶ In this interesting study, 81 consecutive patients undergoing CEA were monitored with intraoperative and postoperative transcranial Doppler US. Embolic signals were detected in 94% of patients during intraoperation, and 71% of patients during the first postoperative hour, with the counts ranging widely from 0 to more than 200 MESs/hr. Eight patients had counts greater than 50 MESs/hr, and 5 of these 8 acquired ischemic neurologic deficits in the territory of the insonated middle cerebral artery. On balance, the 5% incidence of stroke after CEA is simply too high. The authors' observation that embolic counts in the middle cerebral artery greater than 50 MESs/hr in the early postoperative period are predictive of the development of ipsilateral focal cerebral ischemia is interesting and probably accurate, but I have no idea what to do with this information other than to conclude it appears to confirm the obvious. (See also Abstracts 2–15 and 3–2.)

protein levels could be used to predict the ultrasound echolucency—and thus the lipid content—of carotid plaque.

Methods.—The participants were 137 patients (96 men and 41 women, median age 64 years) who had carotid stenosis 50% or greater and symptoms of stroke, transient ischemic attack, or amaurosis fugax. The carotid artery on the symptomatic side was evaluated by high-resolution B-mode ultrasound. Images were processed by computer as gray-scale representations of the plaque (Figure). Plaques with a low gray-scale value were echolucent. After fasting overnight for 12 hours, patients ate a high-fat meal. Plasma lipid and lipoprotein levels were measured before and each hour after the meal for 4 hours. A subset of 58 patients underwent endarterectomy, and the plaque was examined histologically.

Findings.—Echolucent plaques were significantly associated with higher fasting and postprandial plasma triglyceride levels, IDL cholesterol levels, VLDL/chylomicron remnant cholesterol and triglyceride levels, the area under the plasma triglyceride curve up to 4 hours postprandial, and the body mass index. Analysis of covariance indicated that the body mass index, the fasting IDL cholesterol level, and the fasting plasma triglyceride level were independent predictors of plaque echolucency. Thus, plasma levels of triglyceride-rich lipoproteins were indeed predictive of echolucent plaques. Furthermore, the lower the plaque echolucency, the higher the plaque's lipid content, and thus the higher its vulnerability to rupture.

Conclusions.—Plasma levels of triglyceride-rich lipoproteins can predict the echolucency of carotid plaques. This echolucency is also significantly related to the plaque's lipid content. Thus, elevated plasma levels of triglyceride-rich lipoproteins should be measured as an indicator of carotid plaques that are especially vulnerable to rupture.

► In recent years, a number of investigators have found that increased echolucency of carotid atherosclerotic plaque on duplex is associated with a higher incidence of embolic symptoms, including brain infarcts and transient ischemic attacks.[1] These investigators have convincingly demonstrated that patients with increased echolucency of carotid plaques tend to have abnormally high serum lipids, and that the lucent plaques have an increased relative lipid content. While hardly surprising, this article does appear to be the first objective confirmation of this widely credited association.

Reference

1. 1997 Year Book of Vascular Surgery, p 152.

Oxygen Inhalation Can Differentiate Gaseous From Nongaseous Microemboli Detected by Transcranial Doppler Ultrasound

Droste DW, Hansberg T, Kemény V, et al (Univ of Münster, Germany; Univ of Lübeck, Germany)

Stroke 28:2453–2456, 1997 3–8

Introduction.—Transcranial Doppler ultrasound (TCD) can identify circulating, clinically silent, microemboli. There is uncertainty regarding the composition of these emboli under different clinical conditions. This study used oxygen inhalation to differentiate between gaseous and nongaseous microemboli detected by TCD.

Methods.—The study included 20 patients with mechanical prosthetic heart valves, 78 patients with an arterial embolic source, and 20 controls. Each subject underwent a 1-hr TCD recording from the middle cerebral artery or posterior cerebral artery. For half of this time, the subjects breathed room air only. For the other half, they breathed room air and oxygen, 6 L/min through a loose-fitting mask.

Results.—In patients with mechanical prosthetic heart valves, the number of embolic signals (ES) detected decreased from 144 with room air to 63 with oxygen. In patients with arterial embolic sources, the number of ES remained stable: 145 with room air and 135 with oxygen. No ES were detected in control patients.

Conclusions.—In patients with mechanical prosthetic heart valves, the ES detected by TCD reflect mainly gas bubbles. Bubbles are suppressed while the patient is breathing oxygen, either because oxygen inhibits the cavitation process or hastens the redissolution of bubbles produced by cavitation. Oxygen inhalation has no effect on solid microemboli. Thus having patients breathe oxygen during TCD should be useful in determining the nature of microemboli under various clinical and experimental conditions.

▶ I had no idea that the majority of clinically silent circulating microemboli in patients with mechanical cardiac valves were gaseous in origin. Apparently, these result from cavitation, which is the formation of bubbles from a gas dissolved in blood in patients with mechanical prosthetic cardiac valves. The inhalation of oxygen promptly decreases the number of gaseous embolic signals, probably by accelerated redissolution of gas bubbles generated by cavitation. This is indeed interesting information and suggests that if we are performing transcranial Doppler studies for detection of embolic signals in patients who have artificial heart valves, we should increase the FIO_2 to determine the percentage of the embolic signals caused by gaseous cavitation.

Valvular Strands and Cerebral Ischemia: Effect of Demographics and Strand Characteristics

Roberts JK, Omarali I, Di Tullio MR, et al (Columbia-Presbyterian Med Ctr, New York)

Stroke 28:2185–2188, 1997 3–9

Introduction.—Transesophageal echocardiography (TEE) has recently identified mobile, filamentous strands on the cardiac valves. These valvular strands appear to be associated with stroke and systemic embolization, but little is known about the association in different demographic subgroups. A case group and a control group were studied to identify the relationship between native valvular strands and cerebral ischemia, especially in different sex, age, and race-ethnic subgroups, and the effect of strand location.

Methods.—Study participants were drawn from a group of patients referred for TEE. Case patients had had a first ischemic stroke or transient ischemic attack (TIA) within 3 months before TEE. Age-matched control patients had no history of stroke or TIA. Stroke risk factor data were collected from patient histories. Images obtained at TEE were examined for the number and length of strands (Fig 1) by a single echocardiographer blinded to the case/control status of the patient.

Results.—The case group included 68 patients with ischemic stroke and 5 with TIA. Whites, blacks, and Hispanics were evenly represented among the case group, but the control group had a higher proportion of whites (53%) than of blacks (18%) and Hispanics (27%). Strands were seen in 47% of the case group vs. 16% of the control group. The association between valvular strands and cerebral ischemia was found for both men and women, and among all 3 race-ethnic groups. The odds ratio (OR) was

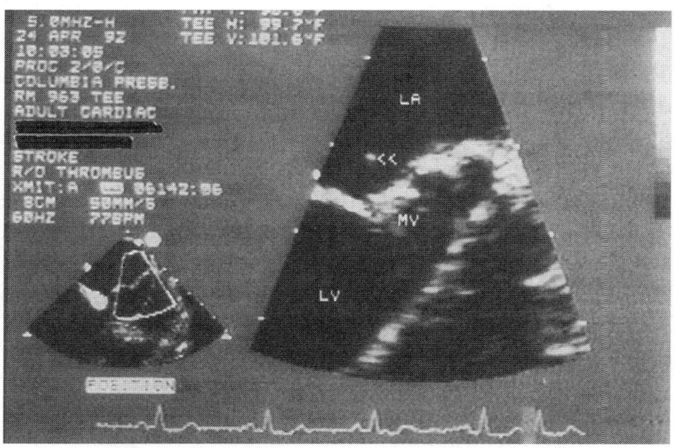

FIGURE 1.—Transesophageal echocardiographic view of a valvular strand (*double arrowhead*). *Abbreviations: LA*, left atrium; *LV*, left ventricle; *MV*, mitral valve. (Courtesy of Roberts JK, Omarali I, Di Tullio MR, et al: Valvular strands and cerebral ischemia: Effect of demographics and strand characteristics. *Stroke* 28:2185–2188, 1997.)

greater in younger (less than 60) patients (OR 12.5) than in older (70 or greater) patients (OR 1.8). Strands on both mitral and aortic valves were associated with cerebral ischemia, and the effect of strands was independent of valve thickness. The number and length of strands did not affect the association between strands and cerebral ischemia.

Conclusion.—Valvular strands were common, especially among younger patients with stroke. The association with cerebral ischemia was present for strands on both the mitral and aortic valves, and was seen in both men and women, and in all race-ethnic groups.

▶ With increasing experience in transesophageal echocardiography, investigators have begun noticing mobile filamentous strands attached to cardiac valves. The composition and pathogenesis of these strands are unknown, although the strands are believed to represent small endothelial-covered fibrinous protuberances, possibly resulting from mechanical trauma. Some researchers have termed these strands Lambl's excrescences. These filamentous strands have been suspected of having a causal role in thromboembolic stroke, but that role has previously not been convincingly demonstrated. In the careful study reported here, such strands were found in 47% of individuals with a recent stroke or TIA, and in 16% of control individuals, data clearly showing an association between cerebral ischemia and valvular strands, with an odds ratio of 4.4. I must confess that I was not familiar with valvular strands until recently. I am most impressed that almost 50% of patients with recent ischemic stroke or transient ischemic attack have such strands which can be detected by TEE. Presently, there is no consensus on optimal therapy after these strands are discovered. They have been variously treated with aspirin, ticlopidine, or warfarin. There are a few reports of strands resolving with warfarin therapy. Further information on this potentially important topic is needed.

Leg Arterial

Can Lower Limb Vascular Reconstruction Be Based on Colour Duplex Imaging Alone?

Pemberton M, Nydahl S, Hartshorne T, et al (Leicester Royal Infirmary, England)

Eur J Vasc Endovasc Surg 12:452–454, 1996 3–10

Background.—Color Doppler sonography is an accurate imaging technique in patients with lower limb arterial disease. However, preoperative arteriography is still considered essential before lower limb revascularization surgery is performed. The authors have been performing preoperative duplex assessment in this situation. The outcomes of lower limb revascularization after duplex scanning, without arteriography, were presented.

Methods.—The 2-year experience included 85 lower limbs in which vascular reconstruction was based on preoperative color duplex alone. Infragenicular reconstruction was done in 29 limbs; a wide range of other revascularization procedures were performed as well (Table 2). On-table

TABLE 2.—Type of Lower Limb Vascular Reconstruction Surgery Performed in 75 Patients on the Basis of Duplex Imaging Alone

Operation	Number performed
Aortobifemoral bypass graft	7 (9.3%)
Axillobifemoral bypass graft	3 (4.0%)
Ileofemoral bypass	5 (6.6%)
Ileofemoral crossover bypass	8 (10.6%)
Ileopopliteal bypass	4 (5.3%)
Femoral-above knee popliteal bypass	12 (16.0%)
Femoral-below knee popliteal bypass	9 (12.0%)
Femorodistal	14 (18.6%)
Amputation	2 (2.6%)
Combination of above	4 (5.3%)
Repeat femoral popliteal bypass (below knee)	4 (5.3%)
Distal extension from previous graft	3 (4.0%)

(Courtesy of Pemberton M, Nydahl S, Hartshorne T, et al: Can lower limb vascular reconstruction be based on colour duplex imaging alone? *Eur J Vasc Endovasc Surg* 12:452–454. Copyright 1996, by permission of WB Saunders Company Limited, London.)

preconstructive arteriography was performed in all limbs undergoing femoropopliteal or femorodistal procedures. Completion angiography was done in all cases.

Results.—There was a 14% rate of graft occlusion in the first month after infragenicular bypass surgery. However, no postoperative complications were thought to have resulted from failure of preoperative duplex imaging.

Conclusions.—For most patients undergoing lower limb revascularization surgery, the reconstruction can be safely done on the basis of duplex scanning alone. The need for trained and experienced vascular technologists to perform the duplex scans is emphasized.

► I suppose the simple answer to the haunting question posed in the title of this article is yes if you are determined to do so. I note, however, that the patients selected for fem-pop or fem-distal bypass had an on-the-table arteriogram performed at the beginning of the case, so I do believe this paper is just a bit deceptive. I further note that the 30-day graft failure rate was 14%, which is simply too high. Perhaps this center needs to consider improving the quality of their preoperative arteriography rather than performing surgery on the basis of duplex alone.

A Comparison Between Colour Duplex Ultrasonography and Arteriography for Imaging Infrapopliteal Arterial Lesions

Sensier Y, Fishwick G, Owen R, et al (Leicester Royal Infirmary, England)

Eur J Vasc Endovasc Surg 15:44–50, 1998 3–11

Background.—Although many researchers have studied the value of duplex US for imaging the lower limb arterial tree, few have assessed the

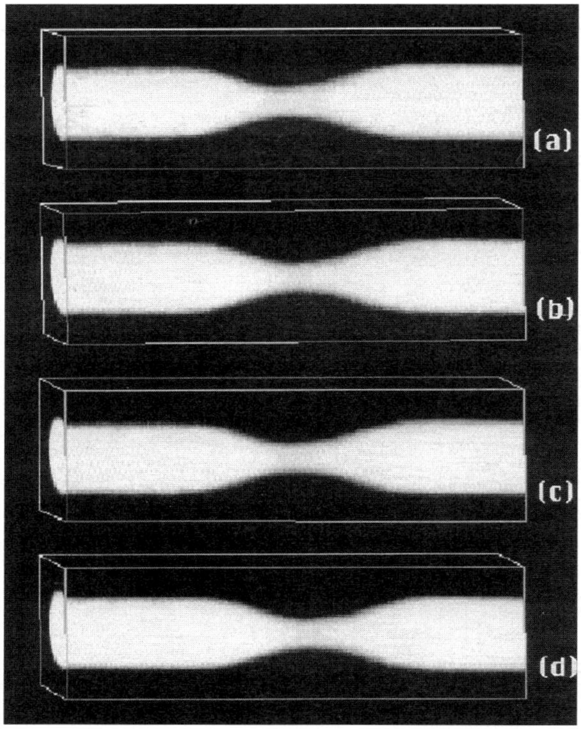

FIGURE 4.—Three-dimensional power Doppler angiograms of the central stenosis with an 80% area reduction generated with a steady flow of 10 mL/sec. **A**, without proximal and distal stenoses. **B**, with a 70% proximal stenosis. **C**, with a 70% distal stenosis. **D**, with proximal and distal stenoses of 70%. (Courtesy of Guo Z, Durand L-G, Allard L, et al: In vitro evaluation of multiple arterial stenoses using three-dimensional power Doppler angiography. *J Vasc Surg* 27:681–688, 1998.)

▶ This study provides more information about the potential of 3-dimensional power Doppler angiography. This may become a powerful tool in the future, allowing us to quantitatively grade multisegmental stenoses in an arterial system and possibly even permitting generation of a map for surgery planning. It appears that power Doppler has belatedly arrived. (See also Abstracts 3–5 and 3–14.)

Ability of Ankle-Brachial Index to Detect Lower-Extremity Atherosclerotic Disease Progression

McLafferty RB, Moneta GL, Taylor LM Jr, et al (Oregon Sciences Univ, Portland; Portland Veterans Affairs Hosp, Ore)
Arch Surg 132:836–841, 1997 3–16

Background.—Accurate information is needed on the progression of lower extremity arterial occlusive disease (LEAOD). It is unknown whether repeated measurements of ankle-brachial index (ABI) over time can detect the progression of LEAOD. The accuracy of serial ABI measurements to detect progression of LEAOD, compared with arteriography or duplex scanning, was assessed.

Methods.—A total of 193 extremities of 114 patients were studied. For those patients with a history of suprainguinal or infrainguinal lower extremity revascularization, preoperative arteriograms were compared with late follow-up arteriograms or duplex scans to determine the progression of LEAOD. These studies were used to grade the superficial femoral and popliteal arteries as being less than 50% stenosed, 50 % to 99% stenosed, or occluded, and to grade the tibial arteries as patent or occluded. Both revascularized and unaffected extremities were included. Measurements of ABI were made postoperatively and at each follow-up arteriogram or duplex scan. An ABI decrease of 0.15 or greater or an increase in 1 stenosis category on imaging studies was considered to represent progressive LEAOD. The patients were followed up for a mean of 3 years.

Results.—The follow-up arteriograms or duplex scans suggested progressive atherosclerosis in 37% of extremities. Compared with the findings of imaging studies, ABI had a sensitivity of 41% and a specificity of 84% in detecting progressive LEAOD. Positive and negative predictive value were 59% and 71%, respectively, with an accuracy of 68%.

Conclusions.—Progressive LEAOD, as determined by arteriography or duplex scanning, is not sensitively detected by changes in ABI over time. The results suggest that imaging studies are needed to accurately define the progression of LEAOD.

► I suppose it is not a revelation to learn that the ankle brachial index is relatively insensitive in identifying progression of lower extremity arterial occlusive disease. Clearly, it is not nearly as sensitive as imaging studies, including duplex and arteriography. I never thought this study was all that great, but Dr. Moneta seemed impressed by it.

Case Report: Delayed Superficial Femoral Artery Pseudoaneurysm Rupture Following Successful Compression Therapy

Birchall D, Fields JM, Chalmers N, et al (Univ of Manchester, England)

Clin Radiol 52:629–630, 1997 3–17

Introduction.—Ultrasound-guided mechanical compression is a safe and effective treatment for pseudoaneurysm formation complicating femoral artery catheterization. In the case presented here, however, the pseudoaneurysm ruptured after an apparently successful compression procedure.

Case Report.—Man, 66, was seen 10 days after cardiac catheterization with a 6F catheter via the right femoral artery. He reported pain and swelling, of 2 days' duration, in his right groin. Diffuse bruising was seen over the puncture site and a tender mass was palpable. Ultrasound revealed a 5 × 6 cm false aneurysm arising from the right superficial femoral artery. After 90 minutes of US-guided mechanical compression on the pseudoaneurysm neck, flow from the superficial femoral artery into the pseudoaneurysm was obliterated. The patient was discharged 4 hours after a 24-hour follow-up scan, but returned 2 hours later with a massive swelling in the right thigh. Blood transfusion was required when hemoglobin fell to 10.1 g/dL. A massive hematoma within the thigh was excavated and the defect in the superficial femoral arterial wall repaired. The patient made an uneventful recovery.

Conclusion.—This is the first report of late rupture of a femoral pseudoaneurysm after successful mechanical compression under US guidance. Immediate surgical repair is required for this life-threatening complication. A 48-hour period of gentle mobilization after compression therapy may help to detect late rupture.

▶ As careful readers of the YEAR BOOK OF VASCULAR SURGERY have recognized, I infrequently include case reports, but do make occasional exceptions. This article apparently represents the first documentation of a late rupture of a femoral pseudoaneurysm following successful mechanical compression under ultrasound guidance. I am not certain it is appropriate to take away any treatment recommendations based on a single case experience. These authors suggest a 48-hour period of gentle mobilization after compression therapy. However, if this is indeed the only case ever reported, such delayed discharge may be inappropriate. At any rate, we should be familiar with the possibility of this complication.

Treadmill Testing for Evaluation of Claudication: Comparison of Constant-load and Graded-exercise Tests

Cachovan M, Rogatti W, Creutzig A, et al (Herz-Kreislauf-Klinik Bevensen, Germany; Rogatti Consulting, Köln, Germany; Medizinische Hochschule Hannover, Germany; et al)

Eur J Vasc Endovasc Surg 14:238–243, 1997 3–18

Background.—The method of choice for assessment of the severity of intermittent claudication is measurement of treadmill walking distance, including initial claudication distance and absolute claudication distance (ACD). For comparability, 2 different treadmill protocols have been proposed: a constant-load test (C-test), in which speed is kept constant at 3 km/hr and the gradient is set at 12%, and a graded-exercise test (G-test), in which the subject walks at 3 km/hr for 3 minutes, with subsequent 3.5% increases in gradient every 3 minutes. These 2 tests were compared for correlation and practicability in the assessment of ACD.

Methods.—The randomized, open trial included 52 patients with peripheral arterial occlusive disease. Each patient performed the C-test and

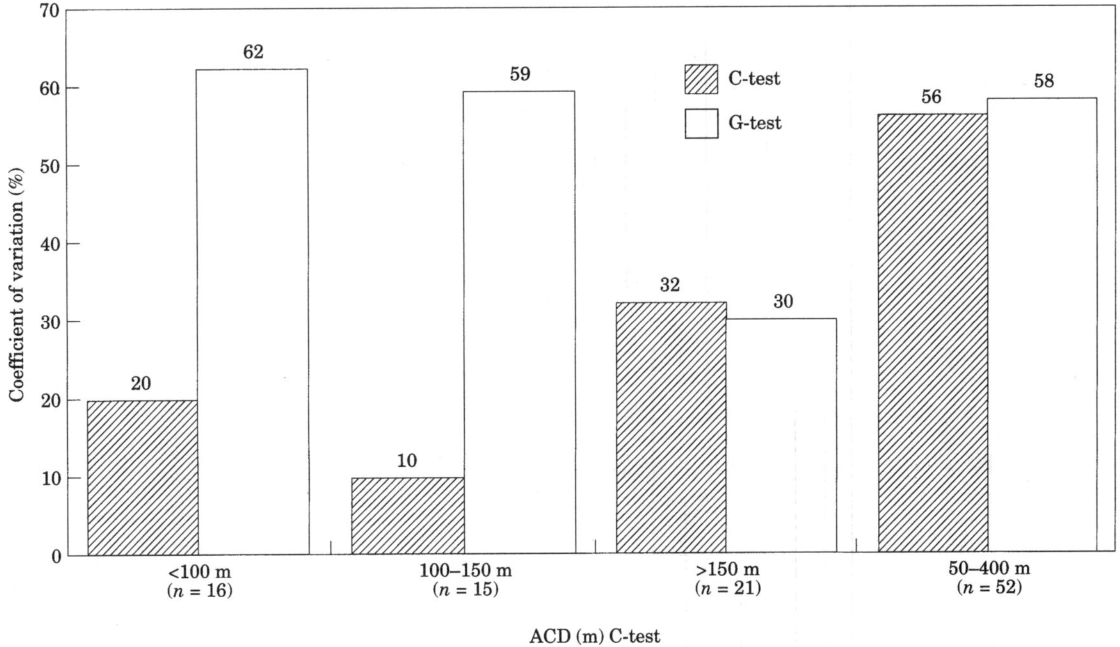

FIGURE 1.—Coefficients of variation of the C- and G-tests with respect to the ACD. *Shaded bars*, C-test; *open bars*, G-test. (Reprinted from *Eur J Vasc Endovasc Surg*, Vol 14, Oct, Cachovan M, Rogatti W, Creutzig A, et al: Treadmill testing for evaluation of claudication: Comparison of constant-load and graded-exercise tests, 238–243, 1997, by permission of the publisher, W B Saunders Company Limited, London.)

the G-test on the same day, in random order and under standardized conditions.

Results.—On the C-test, the patients' ACD values ranged from 50 to 400 m. Mean ACD was 360 m with the G-test versus 167 m on the C-test. However, the coefficients of variation were comparable at 58% and 56%, respectively. For patients with an ACD of 100 to 150 m, the difference in coefficient of variation was larger on the G-test (59%) than on the C-test (10%; Fig 1). The standard deviations were 340 and 122, respectively.

Conclusions.—The C-test seems a more appropriate measure of ACD than the G-test in patients with severe intermittent claudication. The overall level of agreement between the 2 tests is high.

▶ Those of us performing drug trials for claudication recognize that currently one of the hottest topics in the field is whether one should use a variable-load or a fixed-load treadmill for determining walking distance. A standard treadmill is 2½ miles/hr at a 12% grade, whereas the variable-load variety starts flat and increases the treadmill elevation at regular intervals during the test. Dr. Hiatt and his group from Colorado[1] have been sufficiently persuasive in recent years that most studies in America have converted to the variable-load treadmill on the presumption that it yields a more reproducible test with less internal variation. The carefully conducted randomized trial reported here examines the results of fixed-load (C-test) and variable-load (G-test) treadmill walking in a randomized fashion in the same group of patients. It concludes that, on balance, C-test appears to be superior to the G-test. Interestingly, at a recent claudication conference in Switzerland, the official position of the group was that either test was satisfactory and that neither one appeared superior to the other. For the present, variable lead does not appear superior.

Reference

1. Hiatt WR, Hirsch AT, Regensteiner JG, et al: Clinical trials for claudication. Assessment of exercise performance, functional status, and clinical end points. Vascular Clinical Trialists. *Circulation* 92:614–621, 1995.

Venous Imaging

Detection of Postoperative Deep-Venous Thrombosis Using Technetium-99m-labeled Tissue Plasminogen Activator

Butler SP, Rahman T, Boyd SJ, et al (St George Hosp, Sydney, Australia)
J Nucl Med 38:219–223, 1997 3–19

Introduction.—The formation of postoperative deep-venous thrombosis (DVT) and pulmonary embolism can be prevented in a significant proportion of patients by heparin prophylaxis, but the therapy is relatively ineffective in patients who have undergone total knee replacement. Current noninvasive methods of DVT detection in asymptomatic patients are too inaccurate to be used routinely. A group of asymptomatic postarthro-

TABLE 3.—Distribution of Acute Deep Vein Thrombosis (*DVT*)

	No. of patients	Percent of acute DVT	Percent of all patients
Symptomatic limb only	200	80.0	17.2
Bilateral	38	15.2	3.3
Asymptomatic limb only	12	4.8	1.0
Total	250	100.0	21.5

(Courtesy of Miller N, Obrand D, Tousignant L, et al: Venous duplex scanning for unilateral symptoms: When do we need a contralateral evaluation? *Eur J Vasc Endovasc Surg* 15:18–23. Copyright 1998, by permission of WB Saunders Company Limited, London.)

Results.—Acute DVT was diagnosed in 250 patients (22%). Of these, 80% had thrombus affecting the symptomatic limb only, 5% had thrombus in the asymptomatic limb, and 15% had bilateral DVT (Table 3). However, in no case did the finding of contralateral DVT alter the clinical management. Most cases of DVT diagnosed in the asymptomatic limb were localized to the infrapopliteal level. Nine of these 12 patients had advanced cancer, recent joint surgery, or a hypercoagulable state.

Conclusions.—Patients with unilateral symptoms of DVT should undergo Doppler scanning of the symptomatic extremity only. Bilateral duplex scanning should be performed only in patients with recent joint surgery who have normal duplex findings in the symptomatic limb, or in patients with advanced cancer or hypercoagulability. Such patients account for approximately 11% of those with unilateral DVT symptoms.

▶ This paper opines that the asymptomatic limb need not be studied. This is true if the only treatment to be offered is anticoagulation but not true if other treatments to remove thrombi or prevent embolism are to be used. Of their 250 patients, 50 (20%) had thrombus in the asymptomatic limb, a considerable potential source of embolism and late sequelae. *Message:* Know the devil you're dealing with, i.e., investigate both limbs so that you apply a logical treatment, rather than just hope things won't get any worse by giving heparin.

N. Browse, M.D.

▶ I agree! We always duplex both limbs to rule out DVT regardless of unilaterality of symptoms.

J.M. Porter, M.D.

Aortic

Abdominal Aortic Aneurysm: Rupture Associated With the High-attenuating Crescent Sign

Arita T, Matsunaga N, Takano K, et al (Yamaguchi Univ, Japan; Shimonoseki City Hosp, Japan; Tokuyama Central Hosp, Japan)
Radiology 204:765–768, 1997 3–25

Objective.—It has been suggested that a high-attenuating crescent sign on CT of an abdominal aortic aneurysm is an indicator of acute or impending rupture (Fig 1). Though this sign has been attributed to acute hemorrhage within the aneurysmal wall or adjacent mural thrombus, that hypothesis has had no histologic support. The histopathologic findings of ruptured abdominal aortic aneurysm associated with a high-attenuating crescent sign were investigated.

Methods.—The study included surgical specimens from 6 patients with ruptured abdominal aortic aneurysms who had exhibited a high-attenuating crescent sign. Specimens from 8 patients with nonruptured aneurysms and no such CT sign were studied for comparison.

Results.—All 6 specimens from patients with ruptured aneurysm showed acute hemorrhage in the mural thrombus or aneurysmal wall. Four of the specimens also showed clefts with seeping blood in the mural

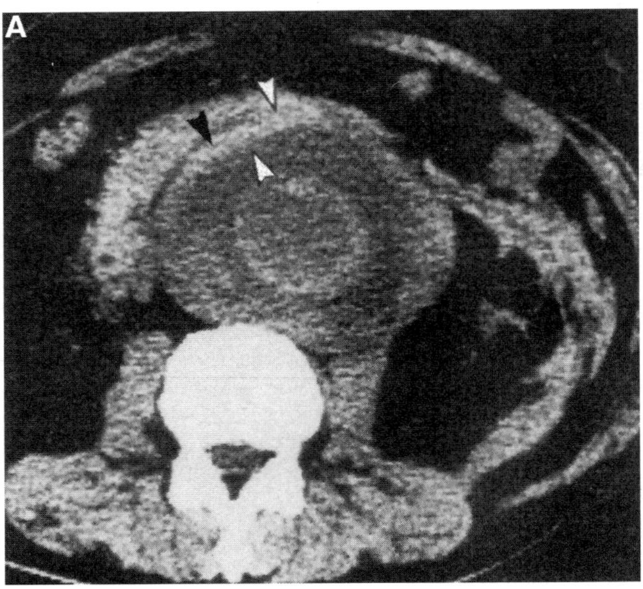

FIGURE 1.—Patient 1. Ruptured abdominal aortic aneurysm in a 64-year-old man. A, unenhanced CT scan shows the crescent-shaped area of high attenuation (*arrowheads*) in the aneurysmal wall and in the adjacent mural thrombus. (Courtesy of Arita T, Matsunaga N, Takano K, et al: Abdominal aortic aneurysm: Rupture associated with the high-attenuating crescent sign. *Radiology* 204:765–768, 1997. Radiological Society of North America.)

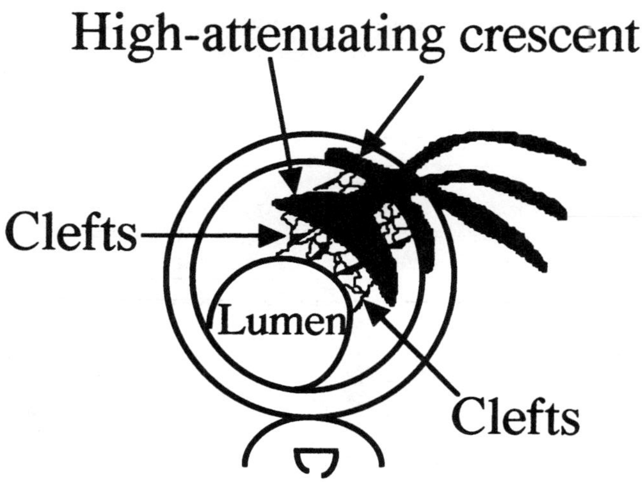

FIGURE 4.—Schema of the hypothesized mechanism of the rupture of an abdominal aortic aneurysm associated with the high-attenuating crescent sign. At the earliest stage, small clefts occur at a fragile site of the inner thrombus, and blood from the aortic lumen then penetrates into the clefts. Subsequently, clefts connected to each other expand to the other layer of the mural thrombus, with gradual seepage of flowing blood. At the last stage, large clefts with seeping blood penetrate through the fragile site of the aneurysmal wall and into the retroperitoneal space. (Courtesy of Arita T, Matsunaga N, Takano K, et al: Abdominal aortic aneurysm: Rupture associated with the high-attenuating crescent sign. *Radiology* 204:765–768, 1997. Radiological Society of North America.)

thrombus. No mural thrombus specimen was available for the other 2 patients. These clefts appeared from the inner to the outer layers of the thrombus. None of the patients with unruptured aneurysm had hemorrhage in the mural thrombus or aneurysmal wall, nor did any have clefts in the mural thrombus.

Conclusions.—The histopathologic findings of ruptured abdominal aortic aneurysm associated with a high-attenuating crescent sign indicate that high-attenuating crescents may reflect hemorrhage in the mural thrombus or aneurysmal wall. A possible mechanism for such ruptures (Fig 4) involves clefts at a fragile site of the inner thrombus.

► The high-attenuating crescent within the aorta has been noted sporadically for years on CT scan in certain patients with aneurysms. In this interesting study, such crescents were noted in 71% of 34 patients who proved to have a rupture or an impending rupture of an aortic aneurysm, and the finding was also present in 12% of 90 patients with a nonruptured aneurysm. Histopathologic examination confirmed hemorrhage within the aneurysmal wall in these patients, with hemorrhage absent in the patients who did not have this enhancing crescent sign. These authors present a persuasive case that dissection of blood into the aortic wall is an early event in aneurysm rupture that is detectable as an enhancing crescent. A number of publications in recent years suggest that the enhancing crescent is an important finding. The information provided by this careful histopathologic study appears both interesting and important.

CT Angiography Versus Intraarterial Digital Subtraction Angiography for Assessment of Aortoiliac Occlusive Disease

Rieker O, Düber C, Neufang A, et al (Johannes Gutenberg-Universität Mainz, Germany; Univ of Mainz, Germany)

AJR 169:1133–1138, 1997 3–26

Introduction.—Helical CT angiography (CTA) is now routinely performed before abdominal aneurysm repair, and other applications of this technique are under evaluation. This study examined the accuracy of CTA with a single helical acquisition for assessment of stenoses and occlusions of the iliac artery.

Methods.—Intra-arterial digital subtraction angiography and IV CTA were compared in 30 patients with peripheral arterial occlusive disease. The 2 techniques were performed within 1–4 days of each other. With CTA, a single helical acquisition, covering the volume from the upper pole of the kidneys to a level below the groin, was obtained. Left and right anterior oblique series of the pelvis and leg arteries were always performed with digital subtraction angiography. Two observers independently interpreted the studies. Occlusive disease was graded on a scale from 0 (no stenosis) to 4 (occlusion).

Results.—Observers were in complete agreement differing only about degree of stenosis, for all normal and occluded segments. Iliac artery occlusions were identified by CTA with a sensitivity and specificity of

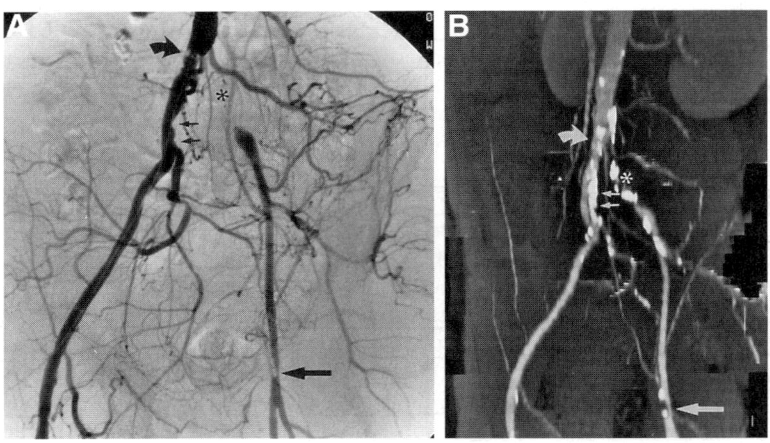

FIGURE 3.—Example of limited z-axis resolution of CT angiography in 58-year-old man with claudication of both legs. **A**, digital subtraction angiogram (left anterior oblique view) shows short high-grade stenosis (*curved arrow*) and low-grade stenosis (*small straight arrows*) of right common iliac artery, occlusion of left common iliac artery (*asterisk*), and high-grade stenosis of left common femoral artery (*large straight arrow*). **B**, maximum intensity projection of CT angiography shows low-grade stenosis of right common iliac artery caused by calcified plaques (*small straight arrows*). Short stenosis of right common iliac artery (*curved arrow*) is not seen because of partial-volume averaging. High-grade stenosis of left common femoral artery (*large straight arrow*) correlates with findings of catheter angiography (A). Calcified plaques (*asterisk*) indicate position of occluded left common iliac artery. (Courtesy of Rieker O, Düber C, Neufang A, et al: CT angiography versus intraarterial digital subtraction angiography for assessment of aortoiliac occlusive disease. *AJR* 169:1133–1138, 1997.)

100%. Fourteen of 15 high-grade (greater than 75%) stenoses were recognized when axial scans were interpreted. Because calcified plaques obscured 6 stenoses, sensitivity for the diagnosis of 15 high-grade stenoses was only 53% when maximum intensity projections alone were analyzed. One stenosis was overlooked (Fig 3) because of partial volume averaging.

Conclusion.—The accuracy of CTA for iliac artery occlusions was quite high, and the length of occlusions was always confidently described. Occlusion length is important because surgery is usually the preferred treatment for long occlusions. In rare instances, observers of CT angiograms may overlook short stenoses. Results support the consideration of CTA for the preinterventional assessment of aortoiliac occlusive disease.

► CTA is a newly described imaging technique which, at some institutions, is beginning to compete with both catheter angiography and MR angiography (MRA). In this comparative study, CTA was generally as accurate as IV digital subtraction angiography in detecting aortoiliac lesions, although the presence of heavy calcification did diminish the accuracy of CTA in certain circumstances. Unfortunately, CTA requires at least as much iodinated contrast material as conventional arteriography. Recently, however, MRA has improved with the application of breath hold 3-dimensional protocols and the bolus administration of gadolinium. It appears that in the near future imaging services in major hospitals are going to have many techniques, including conventional arteriography, MRA, and CTA, with which to image arteries. I suspect with time each of these will be superior in specific applications. It does appear essential that 1 imaging service have familiarity with all available techniques. To me, this suggests that if vascular surgeons are determined to retake angiography, they will also have to become equally facile with CTA and MRA. It seems inescapable that if one is going to acquire competitive familiarity with all these techniques, one must, in effect, become a radiologist. Why in the world would a vascular surgeon want to do that?

Visceral–Renal

Hemodynamically Significant Atherosclerotic Renal Artery Stenosis: MR Angiographic Features

Prince MR, Schoenberg SO, Ward JS, et al (Univ of Michigan Med Ctr, Ann Arbor)

Radiology 205:128–136, 1997 3–27

Introduction.—Several MR and MR angiographic techniques have been developed for imaging the kidneys and renal arteries. An outcomes study was conducted to identify MR angiographic features of hemodynamically significant renal artery stenosis.

Methods.—Over a 2-year period, 413 consecutive patients underwent renal artery MR angiography at the study institution. Severe renal artery stenoses were found in 60 patients, renal artery occlusion in 23, and both in 9. Excluded were 2 patients whose severe stenoses were the result of

images per segment and segment lengths between 9.6 and 40.0 mm. Automated contour detection took 34.3 plus or minus 7.3 minutes per segment, and the resultant 3D reconstruction was remarkably clear of "saw-shaped" artifacts due to cyclic movements (Fig 2). To determine intra-observer variability, 2 independent observers analyzed the images off-line via a computerized algorithm; furthermore, 200 planar images were examined manually by a third investigator.

Findings.—Area and volume measurements of the lumen, the external elastic membrane, the cross-sectional areas of plaques and media, and the cross-sectional area of the plaque plus media burden were basically the same regardless of whether they were measured manually or via an automated algorithm (correlation coefficients between manual measurements and those calculated automatically were r equal to or greater than 0.98). Furthermore, correlation coefficients for interobserver and intra-observer measurements of these parameters were also high (all r equal to or greater than 0.97).

Conclusions.—The ECG-gated stepwise acquisition of 3D IVUS images was accurate and relatively quick. The resultant contour tracings were clear, with little cyclic artifact. Both lumen and plaque cross-sectional areas and volumes could be measured reproducibly. This method can substantially reduce the time needed to evaluate atherosclerotic segments.

► Volumetric analysis of conventionally obtained IVUS images is possible and does yield additional information, although the technique is quite time consuming. Automated 3-D image reconstruction systems have been developed to reduce the time required for volumetric analysis. These systems have significant limitations, including an inconsistent ability to detect the external arterial boundary and imaging artifacts produced by cyclic movements in vascular dimensions, as well as by actual movements of the IVUS catheter itself relative to the vessel. These authors have developed an analysis system that uses a 3-D IVUS image acquired with an ECG-gated image acquisition work station and a pull back device to limit cyclic artifacts. Their improved system detects both the luminal and external vascular boundaries of atherosclerotic coronary arteries, permitting much improved plaque volume measurements. The usefulness of this technique appears significant as related to coronary artery disease detection and quantitation. So far the device has only been used in the coronary arteries. I suspect, however, it will have application to other arteries.

Perflenapent Emulsion: A US Contrast Agent for Diagnostic Radiology—Multicenter, Double-blind Comparison With a Placebo

Robbin ML, for the EchoGen Contrast Ultrasound Study Group (Univ of Alabama, Birmingham; Sonus Pharmaceuticals, Bothell, Wash; Massachusetts Gen Hosp, Boston; et al)

Radiology 207:717–722, 1998 3–32

Background.—There is a need for new ultrasound contrast agents, especially for use in abdominal imaging. Perflenapent is a phase-shift emulsion that has given promising results in ultrasound studies of the liver, kidneys, spleen, prostate, testes, and peripheral vessels in animals. Perflenapent was evaluated as an ultrasound contrast agent for examination of the liver, kidneys, and vasculature.

Methods.—The phase III randomized, controlled trial included 151 patients referred for diagnostic ultrasound examination. They received both perflenapent emulsion, 0.05 mL/kg IV, and placebo in randomized order for sonographic investigation. The scans were interpreted in blinded fashion.

Results.—The rate of contrast enhancement was 94% after perflenapent administration vs. 8% after placebo. The duration of enhancement was 5–15 minutes with perflenapent vs. 0–2 minutes with placebo. In 94% of patients, perflenapent aided visualization of blood flow, structural abnormalities, masses, or lesions, compared with just 8% with placebo. This improvement contributed to the diagnosis in 73% vs. 3% of patients, respectively. The diagnostic information provided by perflenapent affected patient management in 48% of patients, compared with 6% with placebo. Perflenapent had few significant adverse effects. Most such effects took place within the first 30 minutes and resolved without treatment.

Conclusions.—This trial demonstrates the safety and effectiveness of perflenapent emulsion as an ultrasound contrast agent for examination of the liver, kidneys, and blood vessels. It provides extended contrast enhancement that improves visualization and aids patient management with few adverse effects. Perflenapent could become an important new tool in diagnostic ultrasound examination.

► This ultrasound contrast agent is a phase-shift liquid-in-liquid emulsion that converts to a dispersion of microbubbles as a result of ex vivo activation. When injected after activation, microbubbles circulate within the intravascular space and provide strong back scatter during ultrasound. These microbubbles are small enough to cross the lung capillary bed, persist in solution longer than microbubbles of carbon dioxide or other gases, and are eliminated without metabolism by means of expiration, with an elimination half-life from blood of 1.8–6.0 minutes. This material appears to provide prolonged Doppler and gray-scale enhancement of the liver, kidney, spleen, prostate, testes, and peripheral vessels. The images accompanying the article are dramatic but, unfortunately, cannot be shown here because they are in color. It does appear that perflenapent emulsion is a safe and effective contrast agent for ultrasound of the liver, kidneys, and vasculature, and may well become an important aid in diagnostic imaging.

Utility of Magnetic Resonance Arteriography for Distal Lower Extremity Revascularization

Huber TS, Back MR, Ballinger J, et al (Univ of Florida, Gainesville; Gainesville VA Med Ctr, Fla)

J Vasc Surg 26:415–424, 1997 3–33

Background.—The role of MR arteriography (MRA) in the evaluation of patients undergoing lower extremity arterial revascularization remains unclear. It offers several potential advantages over conventional contrast arteriography (CA). The accuracy of MRA of the infrageniculate vessels was compared with that of preoperative CA in evaluating a series of patients undergoing surgical revascularization for limb-threatening ischemia.

Methods.—Fifty-three extremities in 49 patients were evaluated prospectively. Before surgery, all patients underwent both infrageniculate time-of-flight MRA and standard CA of the aortoiliac and runoff vessels. The costs of these studies were $170 and $1,310, respectively. An operative plan was made according to the results of these studies. During surgery but before bypass, arteriography was performed (cost $46) to confirm the presence of adequate distal runoff. The preoperative bypass plan, based on MRA and CA, was compared with the actual bypass performed, based on intraoperative arteriography (IOA). The results were assessed in terms of number of patent vessel segments and number of segments with less than 50% stenosis.

Results.—Seventeen percent of extremities were amputated because of lack of a suitable bypass target. The remaining limbs were successfully revascularized. Effectiveness in predicting the optimal operative plan was 77% for CA and 75% for MRA. Conventional arteriography showed more patent vessels than MRA. However, the difference was reduced on analysis excluding the vessels of the foot. Compared with IOA, CA offered better accuracy and sensitivity than MRA, although there was no difference in specificity. In 96% of cases, the combination of MRA and IOA would have successfully identified the optimal operative plan. Using MRA plus IOA rather than CA plus IOA would have produced a cost savings of more than $60,000.

Conclusions.—In patients undergoing revascularization of the lower extremity, the combination of MRA and IOA is an accurate, cost-efficient strategy for visualization of the infrageniculate vessels. More research is needed to determine whether MRA can accurately replace CA at more proximal levels.

► I have a different opinion of this material. These authors used an intraoperative arteriogram as the definitive test upon which to base their operative bypass decision. They found that preoperative contrast arteriogram was 77% accurate and MRA was 75% accurate in predicting the optimal operative plans. I am of the firm opinion that if an intraoperative arteriogram is required to define the outflow tract, then preoperative arteriography is inadequate. I also note parenthetically that these authors found 17% of ischemic limbs they undertook for treatment required amputation because of inadequate arteries available for bypass. Our need for initial amputation because of inadequate bypass vessels is approximately 2%. This information suggests to me that these authors desperately need improved preoperative arteriography.

Livedo Reticularis, Rhabdomyolysis, Massive Intestinal Infarction, and Death After Carbon Dioxide Arteriography

Rundback JH, Shah PM, Wong J, et al (Weschester County Med Ctr, Valhalla, NY)

J Vasc Surg 26:337–340, 1997 3–34

Background.—Iodinated contrast material cannot be used in patients with a history of hypersensitivity reactions or renal insufficiency. For such patients, carbon dioxide gas (CO_2) is regarded as a safe alternative for vascular imaging, with very few major complications. A patient who died of systemic complications of CO_2 angiography was described.

Case.—Man, 67, was undergoing predialysis evaluation to determine the cause of his renal insufficiency. He also had hypertension and congestive heart failure. The patient underwent transfemoral digital subtraction abdominal aortography using 250 mL of CO_2 and 10 mL of nonionic contrast medium. The images showed extensive atherosclerosis of the abdominal aorta with single patent renal arteries on both sides. Forty-eight hours after angiography, the patient reported severe muscular pain in the buttocks, thighs, and legs, which had a mottled appearance suggestive of livedo reticularis. The patient received IV mannitol, hydration, and analgesics for suspected angiography-related peripheral atheroemboli and rhabdomyolysis. Skin necrosis and sloughing developed over the next several days, and peritonitis developed after 10 days. At surgery, the small bowel showed ischemic areas with multiple gray lesions over the antimesenteric border (Fig 2). The patient underwent segmental jejunal resection, followed 48 hours later by complete resection of the small intestine. On histopathologic examination, there was full-thickness necrosis of the antimesenteric wall, with no evidence of thrombosis or atheroemboli. The patient's condition continued to worsen, and he died 1 month after angiography of multiorgan failure.

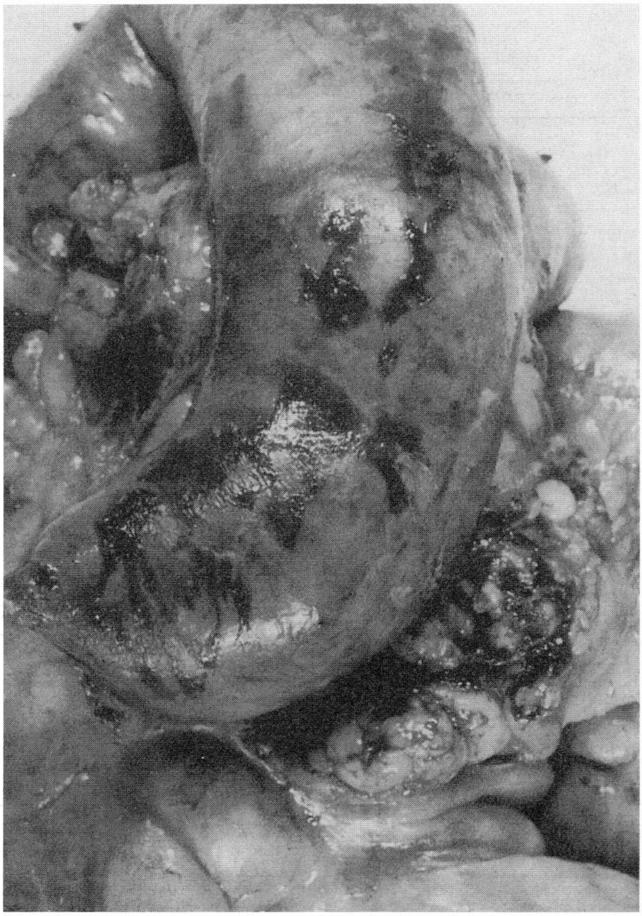

FIGURE 2.—Small intestine shows raised necrotic grey area over the antimesenteric border. (Courtesy of Rundback JH, Shah PM, Wong J, et al: Livedo reticularis, rhabdomyolysis, massive intestinal infarction, and death after carbon dioxide arteriography. *J Vasc Surg* 26:337–340, 1997.)

Discussion.—This patient with acute renal dysfunction and congestive heart failure died of complications related to CO_2 angiography. In conditions of reduced arterial inflow or excessive partial pressure of intravascular CO_2—both of which may have been present in this patient—CO_2 may remain undissolved for a long time. The pathogenic mechanism of this complication may involve delayed clearing of CO_2 from the mesenteric and peripheral circulation, as well as reduced microvascular blood flow. Previous studies have shown that intra-arterial CO_2 injections may reduce intrarenal blood flow. Prolonged intra-arterial stasis of CO_2 may cause vasoconstriction, thus producing tissue ischemia.

5 Perioperative Conditions

Coronary Disease

Perioperative Ischemia and Cardiac Complications in Major Vascular Surgery: Importance of the Preoperative Twelve-lead Electrocardiogram

Landesberg G, Einav S, Christopherson R, et al (Hadassah Hosp, Jerusalem; Johns Hopkins Hosp, Baltimore, Md)

J Vasc Surg 26:570–578, 1997 5–1

Purpose.—The value of preoperative ECG in predicting postoperative cardiac complications in patients with known or suspected coronary artery disease has not been thoroughly examined. Data from 2 unrelated prospective studies of patients who underwent major vascular surgery were analyzed to determine the associations among specific preoperative 12-lead ECG abnormalities, perioperative ischemia, and postoperative myocardial infarction or cardiac death.

Methods.—The 2 studies were analyzed both separately and with all patients combined. Enrolled in the first study were 115 patients who underwent elective carotid endarterectomy, 68 with abdominal artery repair, and 122 with lower extremity revascularization. Patients were assessed for signs or symptoms of cardiac complications before and after surgery. In the second study, data from 100 patients who had been enrolled in the Perioperative Ischemia–Randomized Anesthesia Trial were analyzed. All preoperative ECGs were analyzed at each center by 2 investigators blinded to the patients' clinical courses and outcomes.

Results.—There were 19 postoperative cardiac complications in the 2 patient groups (2 cardiac deaths and 17 myocardial infarctions). A significant association was found between these 2 events and preoperative ECG findings of voltage criteria for left ventricular hypertrophy and S-T segment depression greater than 0.5 mm. These ECG findings were also significantly associated with longer intraoperative and postoperative myocardial ischemia. And in both study groups, a preoperative ECG abnormality involving voltage criteria and/or S-T segment depression was more predictive of postoperative cardiac complications than was any other preoperative clinical value.

Conclusion.—Data from 2 independent prospective studies of vascular surgery patients with different preoperative and clinical features show that in those patients with known or suspected coronary artery disease, voltage criteria for left ventricular hypertrophy and S-T segment depression greater than 0.5 mm are markers of an increased risk of postoperative myocardial infarction or death.

▶ On balance, there appears to be less here than meets the eye. Nineteen of 405 patients undergoing vascular surgery in 2 hospitals suffered either fatal or nonfatal myocardial infarction following surgery. Preoperative ECGs and Holter monitoring had been obtained on these patients, and 15 of the 19 patients who had cardiac events had voltage criteria for left ventricular hypertrophy or S-T depression. Interestingly, pathologic Q waves and T-wave inversion were not associated with postoperative cardiac events. Unfortunately, the positive predictive value of these findings was a dismal 14%. While 33% of vascular patients presented these findings, cardiac events occurred in only 5%. Keep in mind, even if the positive predictive value of these tests had been considerably higher, there is not one shred of evidence that coronary artery intervention would have altered the outcome. It seems that our vascular surgery literature frequently proceeds in concentric circles of ever-diminishing diameters.

Coronary Bypass in Vascular Patients: A Relatively High-risk Procedure

Mesh CL, Cmolik BL, Van Heekeren DW, et al (Case Western Reserve Univ, Cleveland, Ohio; Jewish Hosp of Cincinnati, Ohio)

Ann Vasc Surg 11:612–619, 1997 5–2

Introduction.—Successful coronary artery bypass grafting (CABG) is reported to reduce mortality for subsequent major vascular reconstruction (VR) among patients with peripheral vascular disease (PVD). A retrospective review of patients who had undergone isolated, nonemergent CABG was conducted to determine the risk of CABG in the PVD patient.

Methods.—The study cohort included 680 CABG patients who underwent the procedure in 1993 or 1994. Mean age of the group was 64.7; 75.1% were men and 63 had diabetes mellitus. Data were collected on patient characteristics, operative variables, and outcome. Only patients with a history of VR or those with standard indications for VR were defined as having severe PVD.

Results.—Fifty-eight patients (8.5%) had severe PVD. In 30 cases, VR antedated CABG; the procedure was performed in 18 cases in preparation for subsequent vascular surgery. Thirty-day mortality for CABG for the entire cohort was 2.5%. Compared with patients who survived, those who died were older, required longer cardiopulmonary bypass time, and were less likely to have diabetes mellitus. Major postoperative morbidity oc-

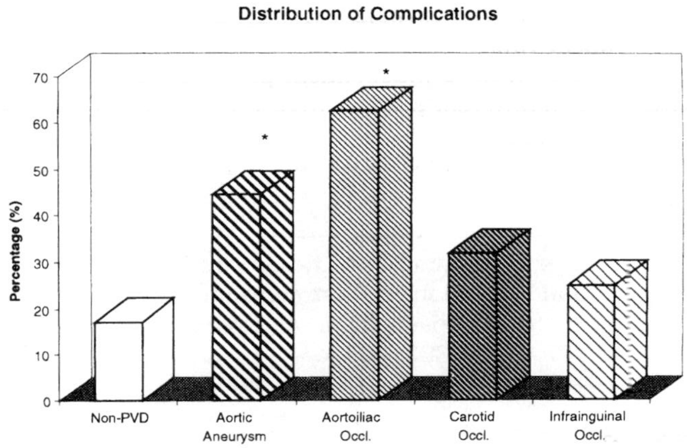

FIGURE 2.—Likelihood of complications among PVD types. The frequency of complications in patients with aortoiliac occlusive disease and aortic aneurysm was significantly higher than that for disease-free patients. (*, p less than 0.05). *Abbreviation: PVD*, peripheral vascular disease. (Courtesy of Mesh CL, Cmolik BL, Van Heekeren DW, et al: Coronary bypass in vascular patients: A relatively high-risk procedure. *Ann Vasc Surg* 11:612–619, 1997.)

curred in 129 (18%) patients; these patients were older and had more PVD than the complication-free survivors. Although operative mortality was higher in patients with PVD than in those without (5.2% vs. 2.3%), this difference was not statistically significant. Major morbidity, however, was significantly higher for surviving patients with PVD (41%) than for disease-free survivors (17%). This increase in morbidity occurred in all subtypes (Fig 2) of PVD.

Conclusion.—Patients with PVD who undergo CABG have an increased risk of major morbidity, and PVD was found to be the strongest predictor of morbidity. Findings indicate a need to define the appropriate timing of peripheral and coronary revascularization.

► It has been increasingly apparent for years that the morbidity and mortality of coronary artery bypass in elderly arteriopaths was quite different from that routinely reported in younger patients. These differences may become quite important when we consider recommending prophylactic coronary intervention for elderly arteriopaths in preparation for vascular surgery. In this interesting study of a small group of vascular patients undergoing coronary bypass, relatively higher rates of mortality were encountered, but the major difference noted was that major morbidity occurred 3.6 times more frequently in the peripheral vascular disease patients. Coronary bypass morbidity was most likely in patients with underlying aortoiliac disease or aortic aneurysmal disease. The authors appropriately concluded that the major morbidity occurring with coronary bypass in peripheral vascular disease patients may preclude or alter the timing of subsequent vascular reconstruction. I am willing to take the matter a bit further. It is obvious that morbidity and mortality of coronary artery bypass grafting is considerably increased in arteriopaths, especially the elderly. This, combined with a remarkable absence of convincing data that coronary bypass in elderly arteriopaths prolongs life, leads me to conclude that vascular patients should have coronary disease evaluated only on its own merits and certainly with no consideration of prophylactic intervention in preparation for subsequent arterial vascular surgery. It is always gratifying to find additional scientific support for my carefully thought-out positions.

Drug Therapy

Duration of Estrogen Replacement Therapy in Relation to the Risk of Incident Myocardial Infarction in Postmenopausal Women

Heckbert SR, Weiss NS, Koepsell TD, et al (Univ of Washington, Seattle)

Arch Intern Med 157:1330–1336, 1997 5–3

Introduction.—A decreased risk for first coronary heart disease events is said to be associated with estrogen replacement therapy in women after menopause. Little is known about whether the risk declines with increased duration of therapy. Estrogen is known to have procoagulant activity, to affect the endothelium and vascular smooth muscle, to favorably affect the lipid profile, decrease formation of new plaques, and stabilize existing plaques. Hormone replacement therapy in relation to a risk of cardiovascular disease in women was examined in a population-based case-control study.

Methods.—Telephone interviews with consenting survivors of 850 postmenopausal women aged 30–79 years who had an incident fatal or nonfatal myocardial infarction during a 7-year period were conducted. They were compared with control postmenopausal women who did not have myocardial infarction. An assessment was made of the use of estrogen or estrogen and progestin.

Results.—After adjustment for age, year of identification, diabetes mellitus, angina, and smoking, a longer duration of use of estrogen was inversely associated with a risk for myocardial infarction among women who were currently using estrogen. There were 27% of women with myocardial infarction who used estrogen replacement therapy at any time, and there were 33% of women without myocardial infarction who used estrogen replacement therapy at any time. There was a 28% decrease in the risk of myocardial infarction with the use of estrogens at any time. The odds ratio for myocardial infarction was 1.00 for estrogen use of 0 years; 0.91 for estrogen use of less than 1.8 years; 0.70 for estrogen use of 1.8–4.2 years; 0.65 for estrogen use of 4.2–8.2 years; and 0.55 for estrogen use of 8.2 years or more. There was no evidence of decreasing risk with increasing duration of estrogen use among women who had used estrogen in the past.

Conclusions.—A reduced risk for first myocardial infarction was associated with a long duration of hormone replacement therapy among women currently using estrogen. Those who had used estrogen for 8.2 years or more had a 45% reduction in risk for myocardial infarction compared to those who had never used estrogen replacement therapy.

▶ This very large case-control study among women participants in the Group Health Cooperative of Seattle clearly established that a long duration of hormone replacement therapy with estrogen, with or without associated progesterone, is associated with a significant reduction in the risk for first myocardial infarction. This and abundant other information has shown that estrogen replacement therapy should be considered routinely in postmenopausal women. Vascular surgeons need information in this area.

Warfarin Use Among Patients With Atrial Fibrillation

Brass LM, Krumholz HM, Scinto JM, et al (Yale–New Haven Hosp, Conn; VA Connecticut Healthcare System, West Haven; Yale Univ, New Haven, Conn; et al)

Stroke 28:2382–2389, 1997 5–4

Introduction.—Anticoagulation therapy offers a potent means of stroke prevention in patients with atrial fibrillation, a group at high risk for stroke. Randomized trials have shown warfarin to be safe, effective, and with cost benefits, especially for those at moderate to high risk. Current patterns of warfarin use were examined in a study of Medicare patients.

Methods.—Study participants were discharged from Connecticut hospitals from January–June of 1994. All were Medicare patients aged 65 or older and had a history of atrial fibrillation before hospitalization. Excluded were patients with a principal diagnosis of myocardial infarction. The retrospective study was conducted by the Connecticut Peer Review Organization. Variables examined in the chart review included age, sex, race, stroke risk factors, classes of medication, and potential contraindications to anticoagulants. Differences were sought between patients who used warfarin and those who did not.

Results.—The patient group was predominantly female and white (308 and 457, respectively, of a total of 488); 173 were aged 85 or older and 184 (38%) had a relative contraindication to anticoagulation. Only 38% of the 304 patients with atrial fibrillation and no contraindication to anticoagulation had been prescribed warfarin, and of those not prescribed warfarin, 63% were not taking aspirin. In multiple logistic regression analysis, patients more likely to receive warfarin were younger, had a previous stroke or transient ischemic attack, and used diuretics, β-blockers, or angiotensin-converting enzyme inhibitors. Less likely to receive warfarin were patients who were older, had possible contraindications, and were limited in activities before admission.

Conclusion.—Among patients with atrial fibrillation, warfarin appears to be vastly underused for stroke prevention. Even ideal candidates may not receive the anticoagulant, and those who do are often undertreated.

▶ It is sobering to consider that atrial fibrillation has a prevalence of over 6% among patients older than 65 years, and accounts for approximately 10% to 15% of all ischemic strokes in this age group and for nearly 25% of strokes

The Utility of Hemodynamic Measurements Acquired by Pulmonary Artery Catheterization

Mostafa G, Kumar M, Schlotthauer J, et al (Mayo Clinic and Found, Rochester, Minn)

Am J Surg 175:293–296, 1998 5–10

Introduction.—There is considerable debate regarding the risks and benefits of the pulmonary artery catheter (PAC). In addition, the information obtained by the PAC may not be fully understood or uniformly applied. A prospective observational study was designed to assess the impact of 1 of the parameters measured by the PAC—the pulmonary capillary wedge pressure (PCWP)—on clinical practice.

Methods.—Study participants were postoperative patients in a thoracic and vascular ICU. Over a 6-month period, all those admitted with a PAC in place after abdominal aortic reconstructive surgery were studied. The primary surgeons, intensivists, ICU nurses, and respiratory therapists were not aware of the study. Recordings of PCWP were obtained at 4- to 6-hour intervals on 50 patients for the first 48 hours after surgery. Researchers then reviewed patients records for evidence that PCWP measurements were used to guide therapy.

Results.—Patients were 38 men and 12 women with a mean age of 71.7 years. There were 243 hemodynamic observations adequate for analysis, and these observations were divided into 2 subgroups: PCWP readings of 18 mm Hg or greater and PCWP readings of 8 mm Hg or less. Patients with PCWPs of less than 8 mm Hg were more likely to be treated with volume resuscitation, but no other correlation was found between PCWP measurements and fluid or pharmacologic management.

Conclusion.—The clinical benefit of the PAC has not been scientifically established despite is widespread use in cardiac surgical patients and noncardiac vascular surgical patients. In this series of patients undergoing abdominal aortic reconstructive surgery, there was a correlation between a low PCWP and use of volume resuscitation. But because data derived from PAC are generally not applied to therapy, routine placement of the PAC is not indicated.

▶ These authors conclude, remarkably, that data from PACs are infrequently used to guide therapy in patients undergoing abdominal aortic reconstructive surgery. They found that patients with low PCWPs were more likely to receive volume resuscitation, but there was no other correlation between the PCWP and patient management. The preceding abstract concluded that routine pulmonary artery catheterization does not reduce morbidity or mortality during elective vascular surgery, and this conclusion appears to be slightly amplified by the data contained in this abstract.

Isn't it interesting that the more experience we acquire, the less use we have for certain of the more detailed invasive monitoring parameters that have been proposed for use during vascular surgery? We gave up use of transesophageal cardiac wall monitoring long ago, and it now looks as though we may well be able to give up the PAC. Time passes, things change, but, unfortunately, all change is definitely not for the better. (See also Abstract 5–9.)

Walking

Effects of Walking on Mortality Among Nonsmoking Retired Men
Hakim AA, Petrovitch H, Burchfiel CM, et al (Univ of Virginia Charlottesville; Univ of Hawaii, Honolulu; Kuakini Med Ctr, Honolulu, Hawaii, et al)
N Engl J Med 338:94–99, 1998 5–11

Introduction.—Low-intensity activities are thought to reduce the risk of cardiovascular disease and increase longevity, but the benefits of such regimens for older men have not been documented. A cohort of nonsmoking retired men was studied to determine the association between walking and mortality.

Methods.—The study subjects were 707 men who were participants in the Honolulu Heart Program. Those eligible for the study of walking and mortality were considered physically capable. At the time of the evalua-

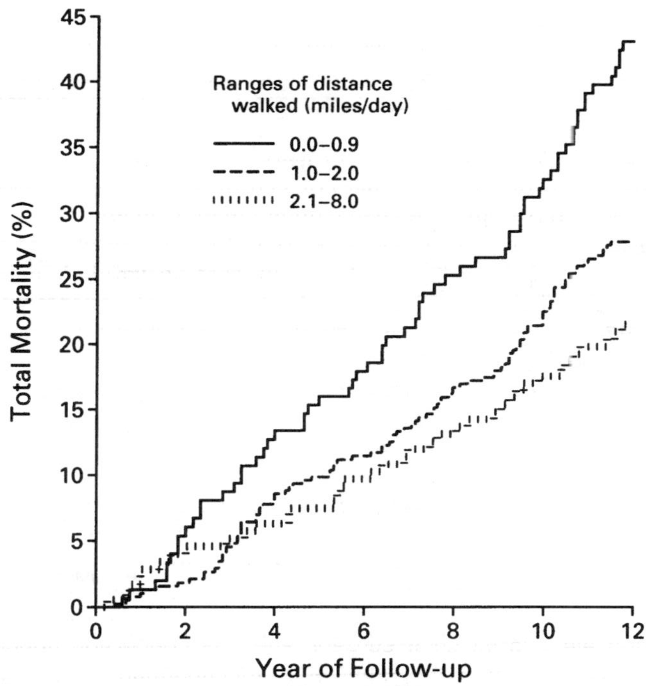

FIGURE 1.—Cumulative mortality according to year of follow-up and distance walked per day. To convert distance to kilometers, multiply by 1.609. (Reprinted by permission of *The New England Journal of Medicine* courtesy of Hakim AA, Petrovitch H, Burchfiel CM, et al: Effects of walking on mortality among nonsmoking retired men. *N Engl J Med* 338:94–99, copyright 1998, Massachusetts Medical Society. All rights reserved.)

tion, the men ranged in age from 61 to 81 years (average age, 68.9 years). The distance they walked in miles per day was recorded at a baseline examination between 1980 and 1982. Over a 12-year period, the men were followed for overall mortality from any cause.

Results.—The average distance the men walked was 1.8 miles per day. All participated in at least 1 hour of slight activity on a daily basis and most (589) spent at least 1 hour in moderate daily activity. Only 45 men reported heavy activity on a daily basis. Of the 208 deaths during the 12 years of follow-up, 68 were attributable to cancer, 33 to coronary heart disease, and 19 to stroke. Unadjusted mortality was more than halved among men who walked more than 2 miles per day compared with those who walked less than 1 mile per day (21.5 vs. 42.1 deaths per 100 men) (Fig 1). Walking appeared to protect against deaths from coronary heart disease and stroke, although findings were not statistically significant. In the case of cancer deaths, the risk was statistically significantly lower for men who walked more than 2 miles per day.

Conclusion.—Older, physically capable nonsmoking men who walked more than 2 miles on a daily basis had a lower overall mortality rate than similar men who were less active. The distance walked remained inversely related to mortality after adjustment for overall measurements of activity and other risk factors.

▶ It is always risky to attempt to ascribe an inherently multivariate outcome to a single variable. Although this study purports to show that walking more than 1 mile per day by reasonably healthy elderly men reduces mortality, one must face the obvious question of why the 1 group chose to walk less. Perhaps there were many less conspicuous medical reasons leading to the decision to restrict walking. I subscribe to the notion that walking is excellent exercise and makes sense for the population at large. However, I am not willing to accept the suggestion that walking more than 1 mile per day prolongs life.

Exercise Therapy for Intermittent Claudication: A Review of the Quality of Randomised Clinical Trials and Evaluation of Predictive Factors

Robeer GG, Brandsma JW, van den Heuvel SP, et al (Cardiac and Pulmonary Rehabilitation Centre "Rijnlands Zeehospitium," Katwijk aan Zee, The Netherlands; Dutch Natl Inst of Allied Health Professions, Amersfoort, The Netherlands; St Franciscus Hosp, Rotterdam, The Netherlands)

Eur J Vasc Endovasc Surg 15:36–43, 1998 5–12

Introduction.—Few patients with claudication progress to rest pain or critical ischemia, and most are advised to undertake exercise therapy. A methodologic study of randomized clinical trials was conducted to establish the effect of exercise therapy in patients with intermittent claudication and to identify outcome predictors for exercise training.

Methods.—Relevant studies were identified through MEDLINE, the database of the Dutch National Institute of Allied Health Professions, and other sources. Included studies were randomized clinical trials published in English, German, French, and Dutch and had as their outcome walking capacity as assessed on a treadmill. Eligible studies were examined for quality by 2 independent investigators.

Results.—Ten studies, most with a small sample size, were included in the analysis. Seven randomized clinical trials were considered to be of good quality, with a methodologic score of 60 or greater on a scale of 0 to 100. The mean of the methodologic score was 62.5. Most of the studies included men aged 60 to 76 years. Only 1 study added a smoking cessation program to the exercise training. All studies reported beneficial effects of exercise therapy on walking capacity. Improvement in walking distance/time ranged from 28% to 210%. There was no correlation between increases in walking distance and age, sex, history of myocardial ischemic disease, diabetes, or level of stenosis.

Discussion.—As reported in other review articles, exercise therapy improves walking performance in patients with intermittent claudication. Yet to be determined are the optimal exercise therapy and the factors predictive of the outcome of therapy.

► Although this paper had many goals—including a general assessment of the methodologic quality of randomized clinical trials of exercise for claudication and an attempt to evaluate the general effects of exercise therapy in claudicating patients—a specific objective was to identify predictors of outcome of exercise therapy in individual patients. This, the investigators accurately note, could help in the selection of patients for structured exercise therapy. The remarkable conclusion of this extensive review is that we know almost nothing about exercise therapy, including the optimal frequency, type, mode, intensity, and duration, or the value of supervision. The dramatic variation in the details of exercise programs is sobering and indicates that we have a great deal of work left to do in this area. At present, there is absolutely no consensus on the optimal components of a therapeutic exercise program for claudication. I always suspected that this was true and now I have confirmation.

Miscellaneous

Duration of Antimicrobial Prophylaxis in Vascular Surgery

Hall JC, Christiansen KJ, Goodman M, et al (Royal Perth Hosp, Australia)
Am J Surg 175:87–90, 1998 5–13

Introduction.—Short-term antimicrobial prophylaxis is considered adequate in many types of surgery, but vascular surgeons often prefer extended regimens. A randomized clinical trial was conducted to compare the incidence of wound infection in patients undergoing vascular surgery who received either a single-dose or a multiple-dose regimen of antimicrobial prophylaxis.

Methods.—The patients were operated on at the study institution between January 1993 and October 1995. Each of the 302 enrolled patients received ticarcillin 3.0 g/clavulanate 0.1 g by slow IV infusion immediately after the induction of anesthesia. An additional dose was administered if the duration of the procedure was prolonged beyond 3 hours. Patients in the multiple-dose group received ticarcillin 3.0 g/clavulanate 0.1 g IV at 6 hourly intervals after the initial dose (maximal total of 20 doses). Outcome was compared for the 153 single-dose and the 149 multiple-dose patients.

Results.—Most patients were elderly, debilitated men; nearly half had undergone previous cardiovascular surgery. The 2 groups were comparable in risk factors for wound infection at baseline and during the perioperative period. The overall incidence of wound infection was 14.2%. Patients receiving single-dose prophylaxis were twice as likely as those given the multiple-dose regimen to have a wound infection and were also at higher risk for wound morbidity. Both groups had similar patterns of postoperative adverse events. No major side effects were associated with the parenteral administration of ticarcillin.

Conclusion.—The multiple-dose antibiotic regimen used in this trial provided optimal prophylaxis against wound infection for patients undergoing vascular surgery. The authors conclude that single-dose antibiotic prophylaxis is inappropriate in this setting.

▶ The conclusion drawn by the authors that "it is inappropriate to use single-dose antibiotic prophylaxis for patients undergoing vascular surgery" has wide consequences for daily practice, mainly of an economic nature. Instead of using, on average, 2 doses, we presumably have to administer, on average, 14 doses, which—with the use of Zinaceff, which is our preferred antibiotic—would incur an additional cost of approximately $8,000 per 100 vascular surgical cases, not to mention the cost of administering the drug, the ecological consequences, etc. Therefore, the basis for this firm statement must be scrutinized.

First, the study did not involve the use of placebo agents, which potentially induces a bias, because the decision as to whether or not an infection was present relied on partially soft criteria ("the discharge of pus or a serous discharge that contains pathologic organisms" and only 25 of the 43 wound infections had positive wound cultures). Secondly, the overall rate of infections was high (14%), and I wonder to what extent the long-term use of IV lines may have contributed to this.

Thirdly, infections appeared relatively late (a median of 13 days postoperatively, 4 days after discharge). The authors state that "the follow-up schedule was maintained until 42 days after the date of surgery," but the paper contains no information on the completeness of follow-up and, clearly, it was less than 100%. Finally, the attained level of significance was modest and carried no consequences for treatment, i.e., the number of reoperations or deaths or the length of the postoperative stay. My conclusion is that this study has generated an hypothesis that should be further addressed in a double-blinded (single dose vs. multiple dose) study in which tubes and lines are left in situ for as short a time as possible

T.V. Schroeder, M.D., D.M.Sc.

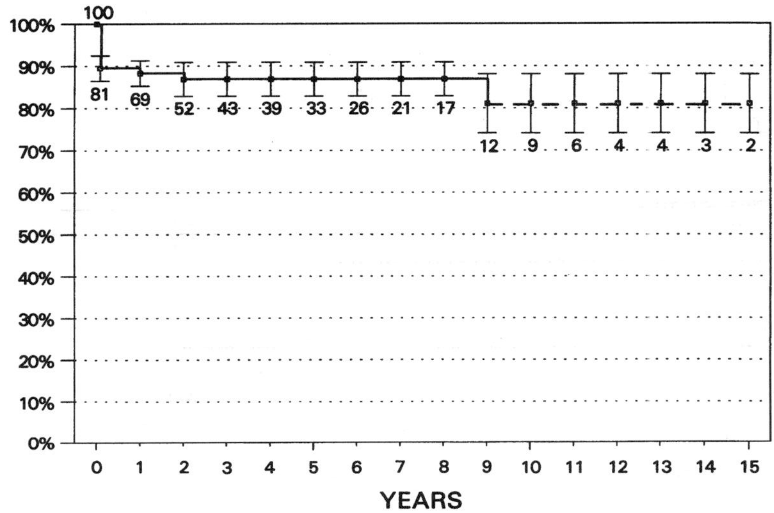

FIGURE 3.—Supra-aortic trunk reconstruction protection from stroke. (Courtesy of Berguer R, Morasch MD, Kline RA: Transthoracic repair of innominate and common carotid artery disease: Immediate and long-term outcome for 100 consecutive surgical reconstructions. *J Vasc Surg* 27:34–42, 1998.)

among the perioperative complications. There were 21 late deaths. Late revision was performed in 2 supra-aortic trunk reconstructions. At 5 years, the cumulative primary patency rate was 94% ± 3%, and at 10 years, it was 88% ± 6%. At 5 years, the stroke-free survival rate was 87% ± 4%, and at 10 years, it was 81% ± 7%. A median stroke-free life expectancy of 10 years, 7 months occurred for patients who survived beyond 30 days (Fig 3).

Conclusion.—Acceptable death/stroke rates, with long-term patient benefit, can be achieved with direct reconstruction of complex symptomatic supra-aortic trunk lesions. A less morbid cervical or endovascular approach should be used for asymptomatic lesions in patients who have significant concomitant conditions, even if long-term outcome of the concomitant condition is inferior.

▶ Multiple procedures, generally based on inflow using the ascending aorta or the proximal innominate artery were used by these authors to revascularize the supra-aortic trunks. Clinical outcome and freedom from subsequent neurologic events were commendable. Although not supported by any data that I can detect, the authors have concluded that direct transthoracic repair of lesions of the supra-aortic trunk should be limited to patients with neurologic symptoms. The authors further recommend that asymptomatic stenoses be reconstructed using a cervical surgical repair, or even endovascular techniques. I would have been more impressed with their recommendation had they provided at least a little supporting data.

Innominate Artery Occlusive Disease: Management With Central Reconstructive Techniques

Ligush J Jr, Criado E, Keagy BA (Bowman Gray School of Medicine, Winston-Salem, NC; Univ of North Carolina, Chapel Hill)

Surgery 121:556–562, 1997 6–5

Background.—Innominate artery (IA) occlusive disease is a rare vascular condition. However, stenoses and occlusions of the IA can cause serious problems with cerebral and arm circulation. An experience with IA occlusive disease and its treatment by central vascular reconstruction was reviewed.

Patients.—The 8-year experience included 18 patients: 12 women and 6 men (mean age, 59 years). All patients had symptoms, including amaurosis fugax in 55%, transient ischemic attacks in 44%, vertebrobasilar insufficiency in 44%, and arm claudication in 33%. Three patients had complete occlusion of the IA, whereas 15 had stenosis. Three patients had undergone previous, unsuccessful extrathoracic bypass procedures for IA lesions.

Techniques.—Seventeen patients were managed via a median sternotomy, including aortocarotid bypass with reimplantation of the subclavian in 10 patients and aortoinnominate bypass in 7. One patient underwent ligation of the IA; the rest had transection and oversewing of the IA. Retrograde-transluminal IA angioplasty, with endovascular stenting, was performed via the carotid artery in a patient with severe chronic obstructive pulmonary disease and a history of coronary artery bypass grafting. Carotid endarterectomy was performed at the same surgery in 4 patients, and coronary artery bypass grafting was performed in 2 patients.

Outcomes.—One patient died of myocardial infarction in the operative period. In the perioperative period, there were 3 cases of dysrhythmia, 3 of respiratory insufficiency, 2 of subendocardial myocardial infarction, 2 of cerebrovascular accident with complete recovery, 1 of hemorrhage, and 1 of acute graft occlusion. The mean follow-up was 21 months, with all grafts remaining patent. At 4 months after carotid bypass, the patient who underwent IA ligation had an embolic event requiring conversion to IA transection and oversewing. The patient managed by angioplasty remained symptom free with a patent IA at 12 months. Patients undergoing transthoracic repair had an average hospital stay of 14 days.

Conclusion.—For patients with symptomatic stenosis or occlusion of the IA, innominate artery bypass using the ascending aorta provides effective symptom relief and a high patency rate. Because innominate artery reconstruction carries a high morbidity rate, it should be used only in patients with symptoms. Transection and oversewing of the IA is necessary to prevent recurrent embolism. Stenoses of the IA or proximal common carotid artery can also be managed by transcarotid, retrograde angioplasty. Proper patient treatment requires an aggressive approach to defining the extent of coronary artery disease.

▶ These authors describe a modest and generally successful experience with IA bypass in 18 patients over 8 years. Their operative preference was median sternotomy with transection and oversewing of the IA and bypass from the ascending aorta to either the carotid with subclavian reimplantation, or the IA. I totally agree with their conclusion that IA bypass based on the ascending aorta is effective and has a high patency rate. I do note the relatively high complication rate in these patients. In recent years, we have begun to use a variety of extrathoracic revascularizations to accomplish IA. We agree with these authors that embolic events require direct IA surgery, but I am not certain that any other types of pathology require it. I am inclined to use extrathoracic bypass techniques whenever possible.

Intramural Hematoma

Fate of Intramural Hematoma of the Aorta: CT Evaluation

Sueyoshi E, Matsuoka Y, Sakamoto I, et al (Nagasaki Univ, Japan; Natl Nagasaki-chuo Hosp, Omura, Japan)

J Comput Assist Tomogr 21:931–938, 1997 6–6

Introduction.—The availability of CT has made it easy to identify the false lumen—sometimes unappreciated by angiography—in patients with aortic dissection. The mechanism of aortic dissection remains unclear; the initial event may be either an intimal tear or intramural hemorrhage from the vasa vasorum. The ultimate fate of intramural hematoma was evaluated.

Methods.—The study included 32 patients with intramural hematoma of the aorta seen between 1984 and 1995. All patients had CT scans available for review, and 22 had MRI scans. The diagnosis was made and followed up by CT in each case. The CT and MRI findings and sequential changes of each patient were reviewed.

Results.—In each case, the intramural hematoma decreased in size. (See Fig 1 for an example). Six patients showed ulcer-like projections (ULPs) when first studied, and 14 on later follow-up. In 12 patients, these ULPs progressed to saccular aneurysms within a mean of 47 days. Another 6 patients without ULPs went on to develop fusiform aneurysms within a mean of 348 days. Two patients showed progression to overt aortic dissection.

Conclusions.—Most intramural hematomas decrease in size over time. However, the aorta can still show progression to aneurysm or overt aortic dissection. In aortas with ULPs, saccular aneurysms can develop as an early complication. In other cases, the late complication of fusiform aneurysm can occur. The initial imaging findings cannot predict the final

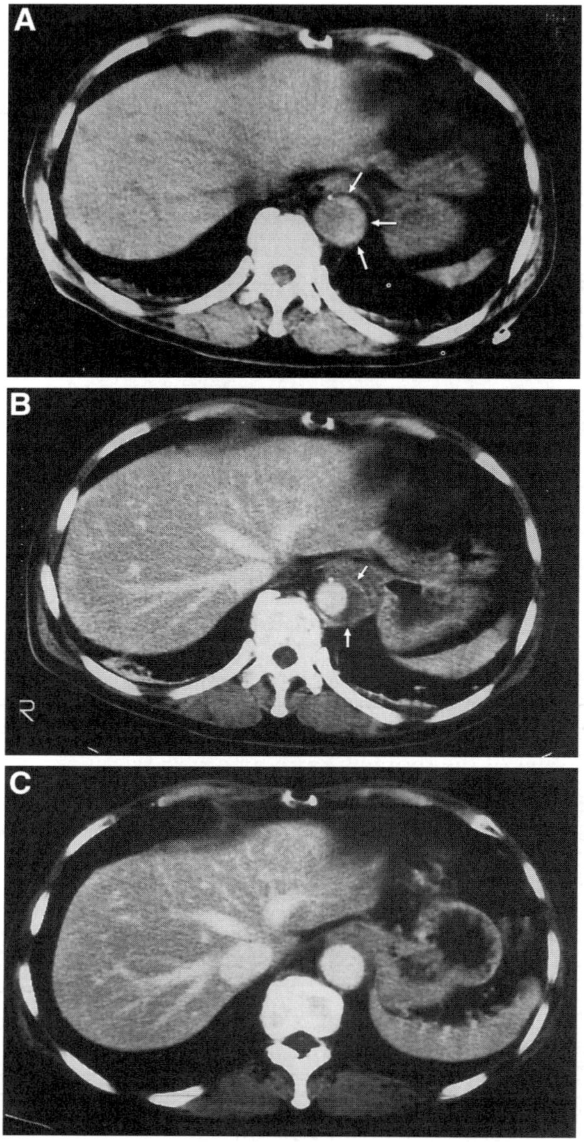

FIGURE 1.—Case 3. **A,** nonenhanced CT immediately after the onset shows high density crescent-shaped area (*arrows*) in the descending thoracic aorta. **B,** contrast-enhanced CT shows same crescent-shaped area (*arrows*), which is not enhanced. **C,** contrast-enhanced CT 16 months after onset shows almost complete resolution of intramural hematoma. (Courtesy of Sueyoshi E, Matsuoka Y, Sakamoto I, et al: Fate of intramural hematoma of the aorta: CT evaluation. *J Comput Assist Tomogr* 21:931–938, 1997.)

outcome of intramural hematomas; thus, all patients need long-term imaging follow-up.

▶ Intramural hematoma of the thoracic aorta has attracted increasing attention in recent years. We really do not know if this is a unique disease entity or an early form of aortic dissection. The remarkable study reported herein followed 32 patients with intramural hematoma with serial CT scans, the majority of whom had a penetrating aortic ulcer at the site of the intramural hematoma. Intramural hematomas progressed to saccular aneurysm in 12 patients and fusiform aneurysm in 6 patients. In 2 patients, the affected aorta progressed to overt aortic dissection. The recommendation of these authors that intramural hematoma should be followed carefully by CT scan appears prudent, as 20 of 32 intramural hematoma patients developed aneurysm or dissection over time.

Intramural Hematoma of the Thoracic Aorta: MR Image Findings and Their Prognostic Implications

Murray JG, Manisali M, Flamm SD, et al (Cleveland Clinic Found, Ohio)

Radiology 204:349–355, 1997 6–7

Introduction.—Magnetic resonance imaging findings of intramural hematoma of the thoracic aorta were first described in 1988 and has since been described only in small series of patients. Only preliminary data are available regarding the changes over time in MRI findings and how those changes relate to clinical outcome. Characteristic MRI findings of intramural hematoma of the thoracic aorta and their relationship to prognosis were assessed.

Methods.—The MR images of 22 patients with intramural hematoma of the thoracic aorta were retrospectively reviewed to ascertain site, thickness, degree of mural involvement, and signal intensity on spin-echo (SE) and cine gradient-echo (GRE) images of the hematoma. A comparison was made between patients who did and did not have complications develop.

Results.—The only finding that correlated significantly with patient outcome was hematoma site. Complication frequencies were significantly higher for patients with hematoma of the ascending aorta, compared with patients who had hematoma of the descending aorta (80% [4 of 5] vs. 12% [2 of 17]). The correlation between days after symptom onset and signal intensity of the hematoma on SE and GRE images was moderately strong. Two of 3 patients with early subacute complications had signal intensity changes of the hematoma that were consistent with recurrent bleeding (Fig 6).

Conclusions.—Patients with MRI findings consistent with hematoma of the ascending aorta should undergo surgery. Patients with hematoma of

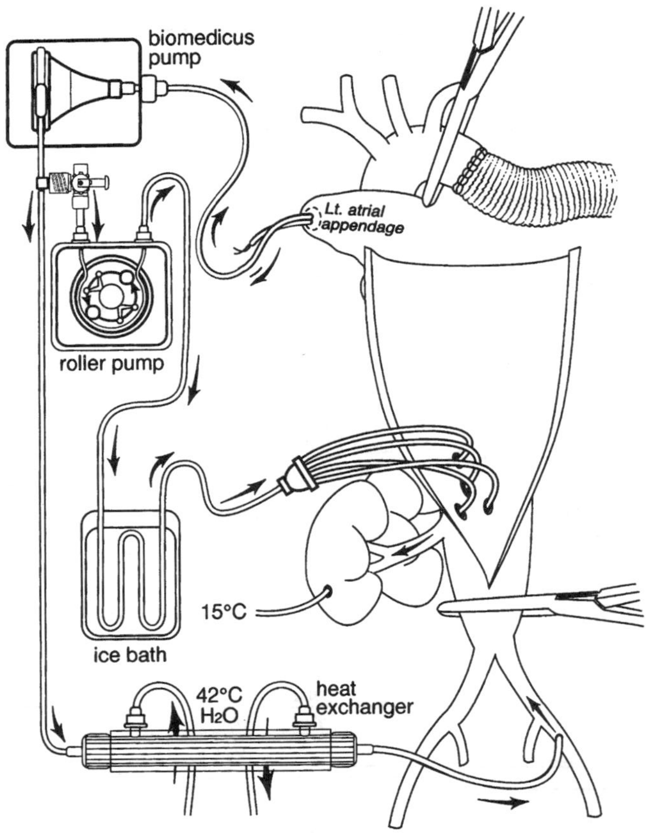

FIGURE 1.—Visceral perfusion of celiac axis, superior mesenteric artery, and renal arteries. (Courtesy of Safi HJ, Miller CC III, Yawn DH, et al: Impact of distal aortic and visceral perfusion on liver function during thoracoabdominal and descending thoracic aortic repair. *J Vasc Surg* 27:145–153, 1998.)

visceral perfusion on liver function was examined. A comparison of baseline to postoperative enzymes was made to determine the impact of visceral and sital perfusion on liver function, after thoracoabdominal and descending thoracic aortic repair.

Methods.—Thoracoabdominal and descending thoracic aortic repair was performed on 367 patients in a 5-year period. For 286 patients, baseline and postoperative total bilirubin, alanine aminotransferase, alkaline phosphatase, aspartate aminotransferase, fibrinogen, lactate dehydrogenase, partial thromboplastin time, and prothrombin time were measured. The impact of distal aortic and direct visceral perfusion on liver function-related clinical laboratory values was examined.

Results.—A statistically significant multivariate association with abnormal laboratory values was found with type II thoracoabdominal aortic aneurysm, history of hepatitis, and emergency presentation. Statistically significant predictors of postoperative alkaline phosphatase, prothrombin time, and partial thromboplastin time were type II thoracoabdominal aortic aneurysm and visceral perfusion. Postoperative liver function-related laboratory values were significantly increased by type II aneurysms, more than by other types. A concomitant decrease was associated with visceral perfusion.

Conclusion.—The rise in postoperative liver function-related clinical laboratory values, which is associated with type II thoracoabdominal aortic aneurysm repair, is negated by visceral perfusion (Fig 1).

► As one might predict, the type II thoracoabdominal aortic aneurysm had the greatest association with abnormal liver function in the immediate postoperative period. Other associated factors, in addition to type II aneurysm, included a history of hepatitis and emergency presentation. Interestingly, visceral perfusion appeared to mitigate the rise in postoperative liver function-related abnormal laboratory values associated with type II thoracoabdominal aortic aneurysm repair. On our service we have not yet come to use routine visceral perfusion. However, we do perform a preliminary right-sided axillary-femoral bypass, which appears to provide adequate retrograde perfusion during performance of the proximal anastomosis. The only visceral ischemia time is that required for the performance of the single anastomosis to the multiple visceral orifices, a matter of minutes. I do, however, acknowledge the remarkable experience of Dr. Safi and his associates, and we shall give careful consideration to this technique in the future.

Staged Repair of Extensive Aortic Aneurysm: Improved Neurologic Outcome

Safi HJ, Miller CC III, Iliopoulos DC, et al (Methodist Hosp, Houston)
Ann Surg 226:599–605, 1997 6–13

Purpose.—Surgical repair of massive aortic aneurysms must consider not only the diseased part of the aorta but also the necessity of protecting the brain and spinal cord. The 2-staged "elephant trunk" technique has effectively accomplished surgical repair, but with a high morbidity rate. The authors report their results with staged repair of extensive aortic aneurysms, including technical modifications and adjuncts for brain and spinal cord protection.

Methods.—Over a 5-year period, the investigators performed surgical repair in 512 patients with thoracic aortic aneurysm. Sixty-three of these patients underwent a staged elephant trunk procedure (Figs 4 and 7). Preoperative, intraoperative, and postoperative factors associated with morbidity were evaluated.

Results.—None of 53 patients undergoing retrograde cerebral perfusion had a stroke after the first stage of the procedure. In contrast, 2 of 10 patients who did not undergo retrograde cerebral perfusion had strokes. Four patients died, for an early mortality rate of 6%. During follow-up, mortality rate among patients who survived the initial operation was 10%.

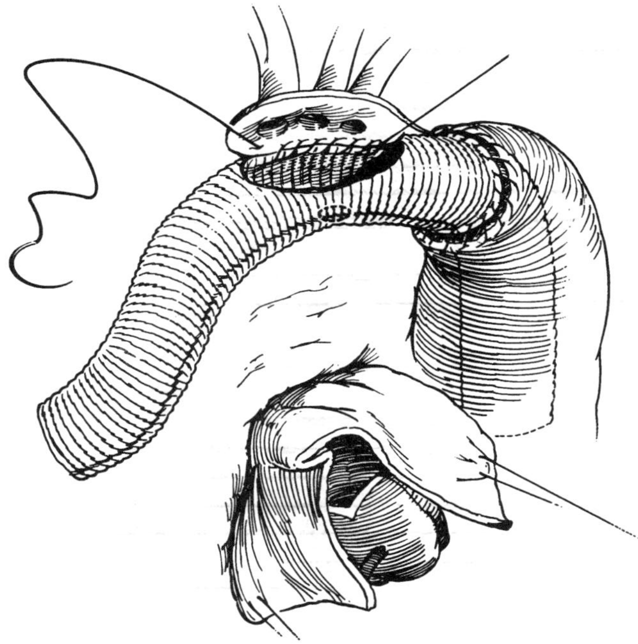

FIGURE 4.—The brachiocephalic arteries are sewn to the graft. (Courtesy of Safi HJ, Miller CC III, Iliopoulos DC, et al: Staged Repair of Extensive Aortic Aneurysm: Improved Neurologic Outcome. *Ann Surg* 226:599–605, 1997.)

Three of the 6 late deaths resulted from distal rupture of the aortic aneurysm. The second stage of the repair was completed in 28 patients. None of these patients was left with a neurologic deficit; 1 died, for an early mortality rate of 3%.

Conclusions.—The effective use of the elephant trunk technique to treat extensive aortic aneurysms is reported. The risk of neurologic complications can be avoided through the use of retrograde cerebral perfusion. Timely completion of the second stage of the procedure is necessary to avoid death from distal aneurysmal rupture.

► As the authors note, extensive aneurysms of the transverse aortic arch are seldom limited to just this area. They usually involve the ascending aorta, the arch, and the descending thoracic aorta. These authors have had a remarkable experience in dealing with this extraordinarily complex arterial problem. They perform the elephant trunk anastomosis in stage I, taking care to provide retrograde cerebral perfusion with the patient in the head down position by pumping oxygenated blood through the superior vena cava into the internal jugular vein and then to the brain. The second stage repair adds the adjuncts of distal aortic perfusion, cerebrospinal fluid drainage, and moderate hypothermia. The overall results were absolutely superb. Interest-

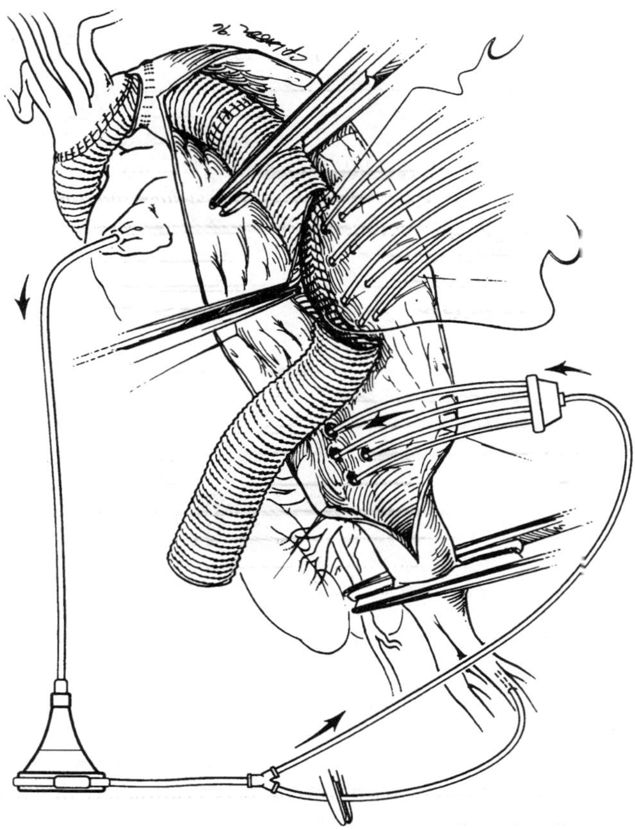

FIGURE 7.—Proximal clamping after anastomosis of elephant trunk to thoracoabdominal aortic graft, perfusion of visceral vessels, and reimplantation of intercostal arteries. (Courtesy of Safi HJ, Miller CC III, Iliopoulos DC, et al: Staged Repair of Extensive Aortic Aneurysm: Improved Neurologic Outcome. *Ann Surg* 226:599–605, 1997.)

ingly, one of the primary causes of mortality was distal aneurysm rupture during the interval between stage I and stage II surgery. These authors are commended for their outstanding results.

Thoracoabdominal Aneurysm Repair: Perspectives Over a Decade With the Clamp-and-Sew Technique

Cambria RP, Davison JK, Zannetti S, et al (Massachusetts Gen Hosp, Boston; Harvard Med School, Boston)

Ann Surg 226:294–305, 1997 6–14

Background.—There is ongoing debate over the best surgical technique for repair of thoracoabdominal aneurysm (TAA). Advocates of bypass-distal perfusion techniques suggest that these approaches are associated with reduced rates of operative mortality, postoperative renal failure, and lower extremity neurologic deficit. The authors review their 10-year experience with the clamp-sew technique for TAA repair.

Patients.—The experience included 160 TAA repairs in 157 patients. There were equal numbers of men and women, mean age 70. Thirty-two percent of TAAs were type I, 15% type II, 34% type III, and 19% type IV. Ten percent of repairs were done for ruptured TAAs. Twenty-three percent of cases were urgent, and 18% involved aortic dissections. The surgeons followed a clamp-sew technique, including regional hypothermia to protect the spinal cord and kidneys. In the latter years of the experience, epidural cooling was used. Factors associated with operative mortality, spinal cord injury, and other forms of morbidity were analyzed. Late survival was assessed as well.

Outcomes.—In-hospital mortality during the experience was 9%. Death was more likely for patients with ruptured TAA and other acute presentations. Postoperative renal failure and spinal cord injury were independently associated with operative mortality, with relative risks of 6.5 and 16.5, respectively. The rate of paraparesis/paraplegia was 7%, significantly lower than the 19% rate predicted using previously published models. On univariate analysis, paraparesis/paraplegia was associated with ruptured TAA, dissection and other acute presentations, operative time longer than 6 hours, and more than 3 L of blood transfusion. Factors independently associated with this complication on multivariate analysis were acute presentation or dissection and prolonged surgery, with relative risks of 7.9 and 7.5, respectively. Postoperatively, 2.5% of patients required dialysis. One-year survival, as estimated using the Kaplan-Meier method, was 86% at 1 year and 62% at 5 years.

Conclusions.—An extensive experience with the clamp-sew technique for TAA repair is reported. The results are as good or better than reported with other techniques. The experience suggests that bypass-distal perfusion—increasingly emphasized in recent reports—is not necessarily the preferred technique for repair of TAAs.

▶ Dr. Cambria, from Massachusetts General Hospital, is one of the most vocal advocates of the clamp-and-sew technique. Herein he reports his 9-year experience with 160 aneurysms, with an in-hospital mortality of 9% and spinal cord injury in 7%. These authors conclude their data compare favorably with those from other centers using different operative strategies, and the authors do not support the adoption of routine distal perfusion. I agree that their results are excellent, and I am presently uncertain as to which technique is superior. We have made the decision to use the right ax-fem bypass without selective visceral perfusion for now. (See also Abstract 6–18.)

Patients.—The experience included 75 patients with acute aortic transection following blunt trauma. Seventy-one patients were treated surgically, all with the clamp-sew method. Average aortic cross-clamp time was 24 minutes—just 4 patients had a cross-clamp time of longer than 30 minutes. Sixty-eight percent of the operated patients had significant associated injuries, including intrathoracic injuries in 49%, orthopedic injuries in 39%, intra-abdominal injuries in 34%, and CNS damage in 24%.

Outcomes.—Paraplegia developed in 1 patient with a cross-clamp time of 28 min. There were no deaths in the first 24 hr after surgery. Mortality within the first 30 days was 12%, with 7 of 9 deaths occurring in patients with multiple associated injuries and 5 in patients with CNS damage. The other 2 deaths were associated with low hemoglobin in a Jehovah's Witness who declined operative intervention with sepsis, respectively.

Conclusions.—In the authors' experience, the "clamp-sew" technique is a simple, safe, and effective approach to the treatment of traumatic aortic transection. The results provide no evidence that this technique is superior to the others that may be used, however.

▶ This article presents a nice overview of a large series of traumatic transections of the thoracic aorta operated upon by highly experienced surgeons using the clamp-and-sew technique. Only 12.6% of the patients survived to get to the operating room, indeed a remarkable achievement. Most of the patients who died did so from associated injury for which no effective treatment was available. New postoperative paraplegia was observed in only one patient. Remarkably, aortic cross-clamp time averaged only 24 minutes. There is a general belief that aortic cross-clamp time of less than 30 minutes is highly important in dealing with traumatic aortic transections. Paraplegia is distinctly uncommon with a short clamp time and becomes much more frequent with clamp times exceeding 30 minutes. An unresolved controversial question is whether these patients should be treated with the clamp-and-sew technique attempting short clamp time, or whether they should be treated with heparinization and a bypass technique, which is strongly recommended by some. This article does not resolve the controversy, but if results this good can be obtained with clamp-and-sew, it appears that the bypass technique may be unnecessary for a majority of patients. These indeed represent excellent results from a very difficult patient group.

Successful Repair of Mega Aorta Using Reversed Elephant Trunk Procedure

Coselli JS, Oberwalder P (Baylor College of Medicine, Houston)
J Vasc Surg 27:183–188, 1998 6–22

Introduction.—In more than 65% of untreated patients with aortic aneurysms, the life expectancy is less than 5 years. Patients with multiple or extensive aneurysms benefit from graft replacement, the standard form of treatment which prevents rupture and prolongs life. The preferred technique for treating patients with multifocal aneurysmal disease of the entire thoracic aorta is the "elephant trunk" procedure, which remains the gold standard for the staged repair of aneurysms involving the entire thoracic aorta. Patients with fusiform aneurysmal disease or aortic dissection benefit from this method, which allows replacement of the ascending aorta and transverse aortic arch. A patient with mega aorta who was treated with the "elephant trunk" procedure was reviewed.

Case Report.—Man, 70, had chronic fusiform medial degenerative disease and chronic type III aortic dissection. He had a symptomatic thoracoabdominal portion of the aneurysm, which necessitated replacement of the distal aorta at the initial operation. His aortic aneurysm extended from the subclavian artery to the renal arteries. After excision of the septum from the origin of the left subclavian artery to the renal arteries, a 28-mm woven Dacron tube graft was inverted, with the proximal part invaginated into the tubular graft. Within 5 months, he had the second stage of his procedure. Total cardiopulmonary bypass was established. A left ventricular sump was inserted. He was systematically cooled and circulatory arrest was initiated. The graft segment left invaginated was withdrawn and brought to its full length, and the left common carotid and left subclavian arteries were reattached. Just above the coronary artery ostia, the aortic graft was sutured end-to-end to the native aorta.

Results.—The patient had successful replacement, in 2 stages, of the entire thoracic aorta down to the suprarenal abdominal aorta. He had a total pump time of 94 minutes and a circulatory arrest time of 48 minutes. When he awoke, he had no neurologic deficit, and was extubated 18 hours after operation. Satisfactory repair was confirmed with postoperative aortography.

Conclusion.—The second stage of treatment in the "reversed elephant trunk" technique is facilitated by eliminating the need for distal anastomosis upon replacement of the transverse aortic arch, and by reducing the time of circulatory arrest and potential for hemorrhage. The technique of "reversed elephant trunk" is an alternative approach to the staged treatment of patients with mega aorta, in whom replacement of the descending thoracic or thoracoabdominal aorta is required as the initial procedure.

▶ An innovative "reversed elephant trunk procedure" was used to treat this patient with a chronic type III aortic dissection involving the ascending, transverse, and descending aorta as far as the renals. The typically excellent Baylor illustrations accompany this article. Retrograde cerebral perfusion during the repair of the ascending component of the aneurysm was accomplished by inflow through the superior vena cava at 300–600 mL/min.

7 Aortic Aneurysm

Epidemiology

Relationship of Age, Gender, Race, and Body Size to Infrarenal Aortic Diameter

Lederle FA, and the Aneurysm Detection and Management (ADAM) Veterans Affairs Cooperative Study Investigators (Veterans Affairs Med Ctr, Minneapolis)

J Vasc Surg 26:595–601, 1997 7–1

Introduction.—Abdominal aortic aneurysm (AAA) has been defined as at least a 50% increase in the infrarenal aortic diameter (IAD), compared with the expected value. However, there are few data on the expected IAD. This study examined the influence of age, sex, race, and body size on IAD, and calculated the expected values for IAD based on these variables.

Methods.—The study included 50- to 79-year-old subjects recruited at 15 Department of Veterans Affairs medical centers. After completing a questionnaire, the subjects underwent ultrasound measurement of IAD. Data on 69,905 subjects with no history or ultrasound evidence of AAA—defined as an IAD measuring 3.0 cm or greater—were analyzed.

Results.—Multivariate linear regression showed that age, sex, African-American race, height, weight, body mass index, and body surface area all had small but significant effects on IAD. Being females was linked to a 0.14-cm reduction in IAD and being African-American to a 0.01cm increase. Large changes in the independent variables—including 29 years of age, 19 or 40 cm in height, 35 kg in weight, 11 kg/m^2 in body mass index, and 0.35 m^2 in body surface area—were associated with a 0.1 cm change in IAD. For almost all height-weight groups, IAD was within 0.1 cm of the mean for sex (Fig 1). Before adjustment, the mean values for sex differed by only 0.23 cm. There was greater variation in IAD by medical center than by age, gender, race, and body size combined.

Conclusion.—Factors such as age, sex, race, and body size have significant effects on IAD. However, these effects are so small that using them to define AAA may offer no important advantages over simpler definitions, i.e., an IAD of 3.0 cm or greater.

▶ The slices are beginning to role off the salami cutter at the headquarters of the Aneurysm Detection and Management study. In this very thin slice,

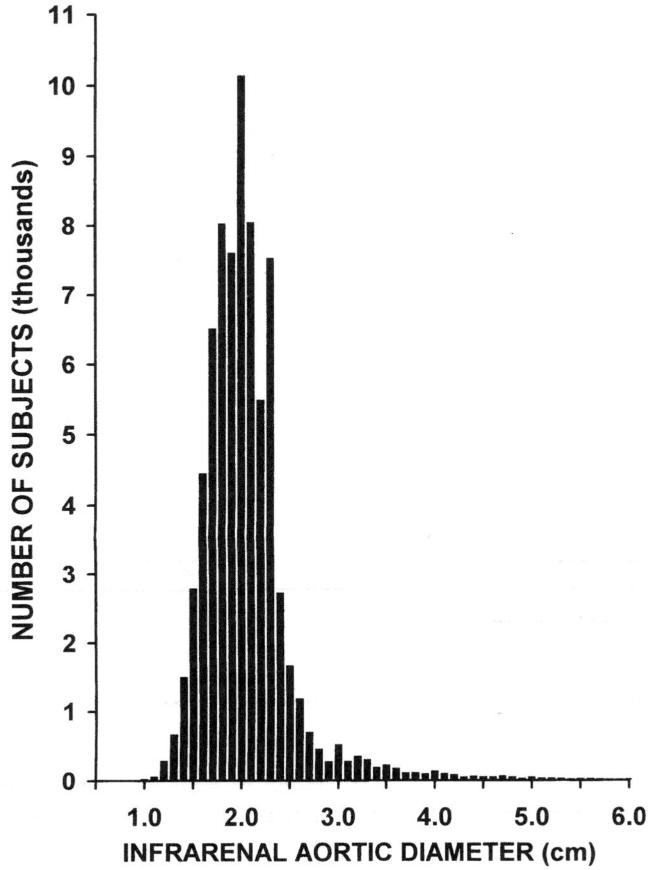

FIGURE 1.—Distribution of infrarenal aortic diameter measurements in 73,271 veterans aged 50 to 79 years. (Courtesy of Lederle FA, and the Aneurysm Detection and Management (ADAM) Veterans Affairs Cooperative Study Investigators. *J Vasc Surg* 26:595–601, 1997.)

the authors have assessed the effects of age, gender, race, and body size on IAD. Although they found a statistically significant relationship between each of these variables and IAD, the effects were very small, generally a fraction of a centimeter. They concluded, and I believe appropriately, that use of these complex relationships does not offer any significant advantage over a simpler definition of aneurysm, such as an IAD of greater than 3 cm. This information is hardly surprising.

Prevalence of Abdominal Aortic Aneurysms in Men With Diabetes

Mattes E, Davis TME, Yang D, et al (Univ of Western Australia, Fremantle, Australia)
Med J Aust 166:630–633, 1997 7–2

Objective.—Patients with diabetes have elevated rates of arterial disease, and can benefit from early detection and treatment of vascular complications. The prevalence of abdominal aortic aneurysms (AAAs) among patients with diabetes is unknown. Community-based data on the prevalence of AAAs in elderly men with diabetes were reported.

Methods.—The study used data from a large, community-based study of diabetes in an urban area of Australia. Three hundred three men with diabetes, aged 60 years or older, were invited to participate. The study definition of AAA was an aortic diameter of 30 mm or greater on ultrasonography or a history of surgery for AAA.

Results.—Of the 303 men studied, 3 had an ultrasound diagnosis of AAA and 4 had undergone surgery for AAA. In 3 obese subjects, it was not possible to visualize the aorta. Surgery was required for 1 AAA. The study found a 2.3% prevalence of AAA, lower than reported for the general population. Factors significantly associated with AAA on multivariate logistic regression analysis were fasting triglyceride levels and a history of intermittent claudication.

Conclusion.—Screening ultrasonography identifies AAA in a small percentage of older men with diabetes. However, the prevalence of AAA in this population does not seem high enough to warrant targeted screening programs.

▶ These authors note that the prevalence of AAA in a well-characterized diabetic population had never been reported. They set out to address this omission with a large community-based study of diabetics in an urban Australian setting, using abdominal ultrasonography. They found only 1 aneurysm requiring surgery in 303 study patients, with an overall aneurysm prevalence of 2.3%; this is actually lower than that previously reported in the general population. The authors have concluded there is presently no indication for extending detailed ultrasonographic screening to diabetics to detect aneurysms. At last, a genuinely negative study.

Prevalence of Abdominal Aortic Aneurysms in Patients Undergoing Coronary Artery Bypass

Bergersen L, Kiernan S, McFarlane G, et al (Univ of Vermont, Burlington)
Ann Vasc Surg 12:101–105, 1998 7–3

Introduction.—Only a single study has examined the prevalence of abdominal aortic aneurysm (AAA) in patients who have previously undergone coronary artery bypass grafting (CABG). Researchers hypothesized

relative, and medicolegal considerations were factors that influenced few surgeons.

Conclusion.—Few surgeons were influenced by patients' social circumstance. For patients with ruptured abdominal aortic aneurysm, almost all vascular surgeons practiced some selection of patients.

▶ As the population continues to age and as the percentage of GDP society is willing to spend on health care continues to diminish, we are inevitably going to be forced to make decisions about which patients should not be treated. This interesting study begins to brush the surface of this difficult question concerning ruptured aortic aneurysms by contacting physicians in Great Britain. Unfortunately, the study suffers from all the defects of a postal survey. Nonetheless, some interesting trends were noted. The most impressive is that 97% of physicians surveyed thought the proper decision was not to operate on at least certain selected patients with ruptured aneurysm. Interestingly, age over 80 years and severe neurologic deficit seemed to be the most important correlates with the hypothetical decision not to operate. I do believe that in the near future we are going to have to carefully examine the role of advancing age on many of our vascular operations. After all, if a patient is going to die 1 or 2 years after a most successful vascular operation, will the duration of survival benefit be sufficient to justify the expense of the procedure? Ultimately, of course, there are no right or wrong answers, only choices. I am certain that we are facing a painful period of difficult choices.

Natural History of the Residual Infrarenal Aorta After Infrarenal Abdominal Aortic Aneurysm Repair

Lipski DA, Ernst CB (Henry Ford Hosp, Detroit)

J Vasc Surg 27:805–812, 1998 7–8

Introduction.—Before the development of endovascular technology, the success and acceptance of conventional abdominal aortic aneurysm repair remained unchallenged. The natural history of the native aortic segment proximal to a graft placed for aneurysmal disease is not known because postoperative imaging is not routinely performed after conventional infrarenal aneurysm repair. For patients who returned for follow-up examinations, aortic reconstruction was followed by surveillance translumbar aortograms, which provided a unique opportunity to observe the natural history of the residual infrarenal aortic segment after conventional repair of an abdominal aortic aneurysm.

Methods.—Eight hundred translumbar aortograms were obtained for 272 patients before and after conventional abdominal aortic aneurysm repair in this retrospective arteriographic case series. Changes in the aortographic diameter and the length of the infrarenal aortic segment, corrected and uncorrected for magnification by normalization to the first lumbar vertebral body height, were the main outcome measures.

Results.—There was a mean follow-up time of 42 months from the preoperative translumbar aortogram to the most recent postoperative translumbar aortogram. There was no change in vertebral body height. The length of the native infrarenal aorta cephalad to the proximal anastomosis increased a mean of 3 mm from 23 to 26 mm. This aortic segment elongated more than 5 mm in 1,125 patients (43%) and more than 10 mm in 63 patients (24%). There was a mean dilation of 1 mm of the native residual infrarenal aorta above the proximal anastomosis, from 23 to 24 mm. It dilated more than 5 mm in 21 patients (8%). There was a weak positive correlation between the increase in residual native aortic diameter and duration of follow-up. There was a negative correlation between this increase and the initial size. There was no change in the diameters of the proximal anastomosis and the proximal graft. There was marked variability in the changes in aortic dimensions.

Conclusion.—The native infrarenal aortic segment elongates and dilates at a mean period of 42 months after conventional abdominal aortic aneurysm repair. The average increase appears to be small, although such enlargement is statistically significant. In a significant number of patients, residual aortic cuff diameter increased more than 5 mm and neck length increased more than 10 mm, with potentially serious implications for endovascular treatment of abdominal aortic aneurysm.

► The Henry Ford Hospital has had a long-standing policy whereby patients undergo routine aortography at various times after infrarenal aortic aneurysm resection. Sequential films of 272 patients were available over the past 30 years. These were reviewed with special attention to changes in the diameter and the length of the infrarenal aortic segment. It is hardly surprising to note that after a period of months, the native infrarenal aortic segment both elongates and dilates more than 5 mm in a number of patients. The authors present this as interesting information against which to balance the potential disadvantages of endovascular aortic aneurysm repair, in which the quality of the proximal stent seal is always suspect. If the native infrarenal aortic cuff dilates significantly, I wonder if we are going to find a number of patients with endoleak first developing years after apparently successful endovascular grafting? At the very least, patients with endovascular aneurysms are going to require careful imaging studies for the rest of their lives.

Laparoscopically Assisted Abdominal Aortic Aneurysm Repair: First 20 Cases

Kline RG, D'Angelo AJ, Chen MHM, et al (Long Island Jewish Med Ctr, New Hyde Park, NY)

J Vasc Surg 27:81–88, 1998 7–9

Introduction.—Over the past 50 years, abdominal aortic surgery has advanced dramatically. Open abdominal aortic aneurysms require exposure of the abdominal aorta, with a long midline or flank incision and

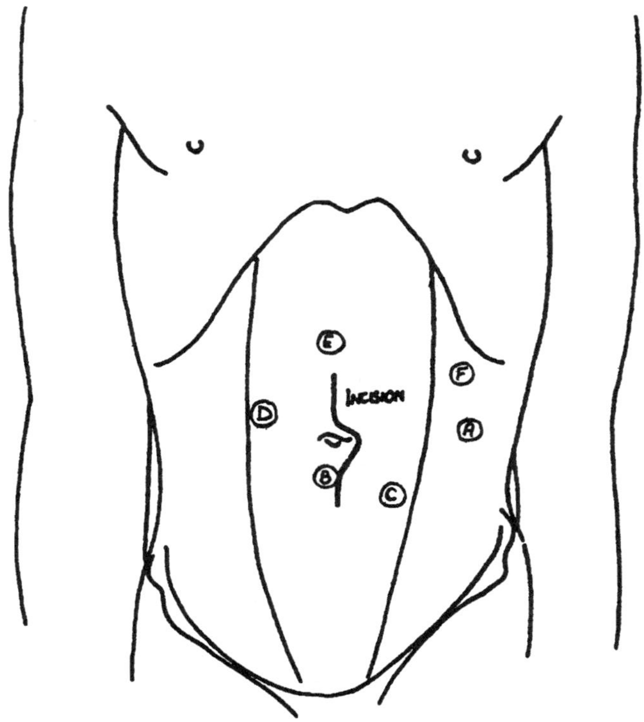

FIGURE 1.—Placement of trocars for aortic dissection and location of minilaparotomy. **A**, camera; **B**, dissector; **C**, dissector; **D**, bowel retractor; **E**, bowel retractor; **F**, suction. (Courtesy of Kline RG, D'Angelo AJ, Chen MHM, et al: Laparoscopically assisted abdominal aortic aneurysm repair: First 20 cases. *J Vasc Surg* 27:81–88, 1998.)

extensive retroperitoneal dissection, and cause significant postoperative pain. The technical feasibility of laparoscopic vascular surgery for occlusive and aneurysmal disease has been demonstrated in several animal studies and small series. The feasibility of laparoscopically assisted abdominal aorta aneurysm repair was established. Laparoscopic techniques for application to abdominal aortic aneurysm repair were evaluated.

Methods.—Laparoscopically assisted abdominal aortic aneurysm repair was performed on 20 patients who had abdominal aortic aneurysms that required a tube graft. Transperitoneal laparoscopic dissection of the aneurysm neck and iliac vessels was performed. A standard endoaneurysmorrhaphy was then performed through a minilaparotomy using the port sites for the aortic and iliac clamps (Fig 1). Operative times, duration of nasogastric suction, intensive care unit days, and postoperative hospital days were recorded. Seven patients had pulmonary artery catheters and transesophageal echocardiography. Heart rate, pulmonary artery systolic and diastolic pressures, mean arterial pressure, central venous pressure, pulmonary capillary wedge pressure, cardiac index, and end diastolic area were recorded for these patients. Before induction, during and after insufflation, during aortic cross-clamp, and at the end of the procedure, data were obtained.

Results.—In 18 of 20 patients, laparoscopically assisted abdominal aortic aneurysm repair was completed. Laparoscopic time was 1.44±0.44 hours, and total operative time was 4.1±0.92 hours. Nasogastric suction time was 1.3±0.7 days. The time for intensive care unit stay was 2.2±0.9 days. Excluding 3 patients who had other procedures, the mean length of hospital stay was 5.8 days. There were 2 minor complications, a colectomy after colon ischemia, and no deaths. No changes were noted in heart rate, pulmonary artery systolic pressure, pulmonary capillary wedge pressure, or cardiac index for the 8 patients who had intraoperative transesophageal echocardiographic monitoring. During insufflation, pulmonary artery diastolic pressure and central venous pressure were greatest, without changes in end-diastolic area. There was no change in volume status, as reflected by end-diastolic area and pulmonary capillary wedge pressure.

Conclusion.—Performing laparoscopically assisted abdominal aortic aneurysm repair is technically challenging but feasible. Early removal of nasogastric suction, shorter intensive care unit and hospital stays, and prompt return to full functional status are the potential advantages. Transesophageal echocardiography may be sufficient for evaluating volume status, and gives the added benefit of detecting regional wall motion abnormalities and aortic insufficiency, according to the hemodynamic data obtained from the pulmonary artery catheter and transesophageal echocardiogram during pneumoperitoneum. With further refinement in technique and instrumentation, total laparoscopic abdominal aortic aneurysm repair will become a reality.

▶ I do not know what to make of the current status of laparoscopically assisted abdominal aneurysm repair. In this series, 1 of the largest to date, patients with small infrarenal aortic aneurysms requiring tube grafts were selected for surgery. Surgery required an average of 4 hours, 6 trochar punctures, and a minilaparotomy 8–11 cm in length. There appeared to be no particular reduction in length of intensive care, or length of hospital stay, or in rate of complications. The authors accurately note that this procedure is technically challenging, although feasible. Frequently, we get caught up in surgical research in the performance of what is possible, rather than the performance of what makes sense. This procedure will make sense only if it can be shown to be broadly applicable and associated with some objectively verified benefit, which may or may not be related to diminished length of hospital stay, diminished operative time, diminished complication rate, or diminished charges. I have no interest in the performance of a procedure simply because it is possible. (See also Abstract 2–20.)

Complementary Surgical/Interventional Techniques for Nonresective Management of "Inoperable" Aneurysms: A Second Look

Todd GJ, DeRose JJ, Martin EC (Columbia Univ, New York)

Ann Vasc Surg 12:248–254, 1998 7–10

Introduction.—Elective repair of aortoiliac aneurysms involves an operative risk of about 3%. Even the most difficult types of aneurysm can be repaired with a very acceptable operative risk. For some patients, however, conventional surgical techniques or endovascular repair are not appropriate. Results from a group of patients who had nonresective aneurysm repair by a combined surgical/interventional radiologic approach during the 1990s was reviewed.

Methods.—Two hundred thirty-one patients had standard aortic aneurysm repair with 99.1% survival, 6 patients had endovascular aortic aneurysm repair with 83.3% survival, and 10 patients had combined surgical/interventional "nonresective" repair of a variety of aneurysms with 100% survival. The group had a mean age of 67.9 years. There were 4 aortoiliac aneurysms, 3 common iliac aneurysms, 2 internal iliac aneurysms, and 1 large proximal subclavian artery pseudoaneurysm.

Results.—No patient had aneurysm rupture, but one patient with presumed thrombosed subclavian pseudoaneurysm had postcoil-induced thrombosis with progressive aneurysm enlargement caused by incomplete aneurysm thrombosis at 26 months. The patient required repair with circulatory arrest. At a mean follow-up of 40.3 months, 8 patients remain alive (80%). By 30 months 1 patient had died of cancer, and by 15 months 1 patient had died of cardiac disease.

Conclusion.—In the rare instances in which conventional or endovascular aneurysm repair is not advisable but complete aneurysm thrombosis is essential and occasionally difficult to achieve, combined surgical/interventional techniques can be lifesaving. Contrast angiographic documentation of complete aneurysm thrombosis is essential before hospital discharge because small proximal portions of the aneurysm may remain patent and not be visualized on MRI or CT. To ascertain long-term adequacy of the repair, close follow-up is necessary. In earlier reports of aneurysm rupture after seemingly successful nonresective therapy, incomplete thrombosis is suspected.

▶ I am surprised by this revisitation of aneurysm thrombosis with extra-anatomic bypass as definitive therapy. The group at Columbia Presbyterian has treated 10 patients in the past 8 years in this fashion, and apparently no delayed aneurysm rupture has been recognized. The authors believe that therapeutic failure in past patients was due to incomplete thrombosis of the aneurysms. I disagree. It is my opinion that the proximal portion of an aneurysm is prone to rupture, even if completely thrombosed, and I am uncomfortable with the technique described herein. In fact, I thought it was a surgical principle that aneurysm thrombosis was nondefinitive and inher-

8 Aortoiliac Disease

Experience With the Use of Polytetrafluoroethylene Pericardial Membrane (Preclude Pericardial Membrane) for Retroperitoneal Closure After Abdominal Aortic Surgery

Abad C (Hosp Ntra Sra del Pino, Las Palmas de Gran Canaria, Spain)

J Cardiovasc Surg 38:283–286, 1997 8–1

Background.—Experimental and clinical studies have shown good results with the Preclude Pericardial Membrane (PPM), an artificial mesh of expanded polytetrafluoroethylene, as a pericardial substitute for cardiac operations. An experience with PPM patching for closure of the retroperitoneum after abdominal aortic surgery is reported.

Patients.—The investigators review 7 consecutive patients who had a PPM patch placed for retroperitoneal closure after surgery on the infrarenal abdominal aorta. The patients were all men, mean age 62. Six of the patients had a small infrarenal abdominal aortic aneurysm, diameter 4 to 5 cm. These patients were managed with aneurysmal resection, followed by interposition of a straight vascular graft in 2 cases, a bifurcated aortobifemoral graft in 2, and a straight vascular graft with extension to the femoral artery in 1. The remaining patient had Leriche syndrome, with total obliteration of the distal abdominal aorta. He was managed with an end-to-end aortobifemoral bypass graft. The patients' clinical outcomes and complications were evaluated.

Outcomes.—At a mean follow-up of 25 months, all patients were alive. Two required early reoperation, in 1 case involving limited jejunal resection. However, there were no complications related to PPM closure of the retroperitoneum.

Conclusions.—The use of a PPM patch for closure of the retroperitoneum after surgery for abdominal aortic aneurysm is reported. This technique can separate the arterial graft from the gastrointestinal system when it is not possible to obtain complete coverage and isolation of an artificial vascular graft in the abdominal aorta. Preclude Pericardial Membrane patching appears to be a useful technique for prevention of secondary aortointestinal fistulae.

▶ This article must be regarded only as a feasibility study, because the follow-up is short and the numbers are low. The author does not tell us why it was impossible to obtain autogenous coverage in these patients. We have all encountered the occasional patient in whom it seems impossible to achieve a complete coverage of an abdominal aortic graft, usually in reoperative patients. In certain of these patients, we have considered moving down the omentum, but this has always introduced the possibility of intestinal obstruction if a loop of bowel should torque around the omental pedicle. The author suggests that simple suturing of a pericardial PTFE membrane to the wall of the aneurysm around the graft will ensure adequate separation of the graft from the viscera and, hopefully, preclude the future development of aortoenteric or periprosthetic fistulae. Clearly, the short follow-up and small number of patients in this series do not prove this technique successful. However, it does indicate that this method of closure is feasible and causes no particular complications up to 25 months. I shall await further information.

Clostridium difficile Colitis After Aortic Surgery

Bulstrode NW, Bradbury AW, Barrett S, et al (Imperial College School of Medicine, London)

Eur J Vasc Endovasc Surg 14:217–220, 1997 8–2

Background.—*Clostridium difficile* infection is becoming an increasingly common problem in surgical patients. In elderly patients undergoing aortic surgery for peripheral vascular disease, the risk of *Clostridium difficile* colitis (CDC) is elevated. This retrospective study looked at the incidence and outcome of CDC in patients having aortic surgery for aneurysmal or occlusive disease.

Methods.—One hundred eighty such patients were treated over a 2-year period. Fifteen had CDC, for an incidence of approximately 8%. The patients were 12 men and 3 women with a median age of 65 years. The patients' records were reviewed to analyze the diagnosis, treatment, and clinical significance of CDC.

Findings.—There were 2 deaths from multiple organ failure. In 1 of these patients, the possibility of CDC was not suspected, and repeat laparotomy results were negative for suspected bowel ischemia. Most patients had several known risk factors for CDC, including high dependency unit care in 14 patients, H_2 antagonist therapy in 13, intensive therapy unit care in 9, age older than 65 years in 8, chronic obstructive airways disease in 7, renal impairment in 4, admission from another hospital in 4, and concomitant malignancy in 3. Diarrhea began after a median of 9 days postoperatively, and CDC was diagnosed at a median of 14 days. The patients received IV cefuroxime, initially used as a prophylactic agent, for a median of 6 days before the start of CDC. Before CDC onset, 2 patients received 1 additional antibiotic, 1 received 2 antibiotics, 2 received 3 antibiotics, and 1 received 4 antibiotics.

Conclusion.—Patients undergoing vascular surgery particularly aortic surgery—are at high risk of the serious complication of CDC. These patients usually have several known risk factors for CDC. However, the condition often occurs after prolonged "prophylactic" treatment with cephalosporin, suggesting that such treatment should be avoided.

► I am amazed that in 8.4% of 180 patients undergoing aortic surgery over 2 years, *Clostridium difficile* colitis developed. Two patients died of the CDC. Among several important points in this paper included diagnosis of CDC a median of 14 days after operation with the onset of diarrhea diagnosed a median of 9 days after operation. The authors point out that this is the first documentation of the frequency of CDC in vascular patients. I suppose they are right, but their experience is certainly different from ours. Although we recognize the occasional patient with CDC, it certainly is not 8.4% of our aortic cases.

Rupture of a Nonaneurysmal Atherosclerotic Infrarenal Aorta

Goldstein DJ, Flores RM, Todd GJ (Columbia Presbyterian Med Ctr, New York)

J Vasc Surg 26:700–703, 1997 8–3

Background.—There have been very few reports of spontaneous rupture of a nonaneurysmal aorta through an atheromatous plaque. A patient with such a ruptured aorta is reported.

Case.—Man, age 67, was seen in the emergency department for back pain and weight loss. He had undergone endoaneurysmorraphy for an 8 cm left internal iliac artery aneurysm 8 years previously and coronary artery bypass surgery for triple-vessel coronary disease 4 years earlier. Computed tomography (CT) showed concentric calcification and atherosclerosis of the aorta with no sign of aneurysm, dissection, or leakage. There was no flow in the left hypogastric artery aneurysm; the hematocrit was 40%. The pain was thought to be musculoskeletal in origin, and the patient was given anti-inflammatory drugs. However, he returned to the emergency department 4 weeks later with another episode of back pain with syncope.

On this occasion, the patient reported midepigastic and left groin pain. The abdomen was soft and nondistended with a pulsatile mass in the left upper quadrant. Stool was positive for occult blood; hematocrit was 29% with a mean corpuscular volume of 85 fL. Repeated abdominal CT scan showed a large left retroperitoneal collection adjacent to the aorta, extending from the renal arteries to the aortic bifurcation (Fig 2). This finding was located at the L3 level, the site of a previously documented area of atheromatous thinning. Enhancement of the collection was noted after IV contrast injection. Emergency surgery was performed and showed a 3.5 cm hole in the infrarenal aorta. The aorta was not ectatic nor aneurysmal and showed no signs of dissection, infection, or inflammation. The aorta had ruptured through the atheromatous plaque, followed by bleeding into the left retroperitoneum. The old left internal iliac aneurysm showed no flow or leakage. The patient

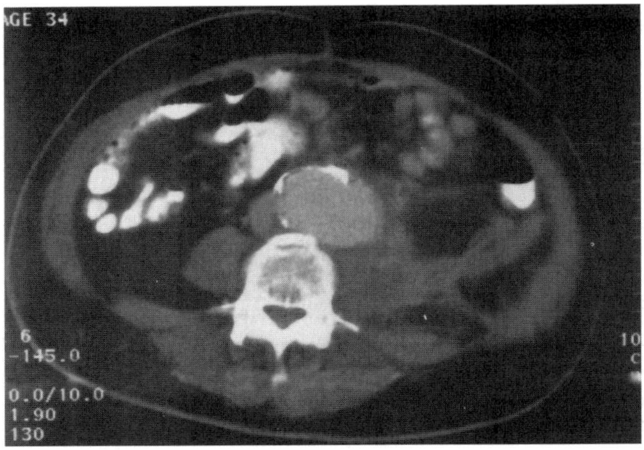

FIGURE 2.—Contained retroperitoneal rupture of the abdominal aorta at the level of L3 is noted. No flow through the iliac aneurysm is documented (not shown). (Courtesy of Goldstein DJ, Flores RM, Todd GJ: Rupture of a nonaneurysmal atherosclerotic infrarenal aorta. *J Vasc Surg* 26:700–703, 1997.)

underwent extensive iliac endarterectomies and placement of an 18 × 9 mm bifurcated Dacron prosthesis to restore vascular continuity. He recovered without complications.

Conclusions.—This patient had spontaneous rupture of a normal-caliber abdominal aorta through an atheromatous plaque. The finding of an aortic ulceration in an asymptomatic patient warrants close follow-up, aggressive antihypertensive therapy, and serial imaging studies. If symptoms develop, surgery should be done so as to avoid transmural aortic rupture.

▶ This single case report is included because of its rarity. This 67-year-old patient clinically suffered a ruptured aneurysm and the preop CT scan showed a contained rupture, although no aneurysm was noted. At surgery, a large hole was found in the left posterolateral aspect of the infrarenal aorta where spontaneous aortic rupture had apparently occurred through an area of atheromatous plaque. Inclusion of this interesting case report is simply to remind everyone that occasionally atherosclerotic infrarenal aortas rupture in the absence of aneurysm. (See also Abstract 8–4.)

Spontaneous Rupture of the Abdominal Aorta Without Pre-existing Aneurysm—Two Case Reports

Does RTC, Brouwer KJ (Zuiderziekenhuis, Rotterdam, The Netherlands)

Eur J Vasc Endovasc Surg 14:408–409, 1997 8–4

Introduction.—Rupture of an abdominal aortic aneurysm is a catastrophic event that can occur in a nonaneurysmal aorta, generally as a result of abdominal trauma, abdominal surgery, interventional radiology, or infection. Two patients had a rupture of a nonaneurysmal aorta. The first patient was seen with a false aneurysm, and the second with a frank and severe retroperitoneal hemorrhage. Neither patient had a rupture of a nonaneurysmal aorta for any of the common reasons above.

Case 1.—Man, 56, had mild abdominal discomfort and swelling. He had had myocardial infarction and hairy cell leukemia previously and was on anticoagulants and heart medication. A slightly tender pulsatile mass to the right of the umbilicus, with maximum diameter of 4 cm, was revealed with abdominal examination. An aneurysm of the distal aorta was confirmed by ultrasound. A Dacron tube graft was interposed and the postoperative course was uneventful. He had a false aneurysm without signs of infection.

Case 2.—Woman, 69, had excruciating pain in the abdomen and back. Previously, she had had a right-sided nephrectomy. A large, ill-defined pulsatile mass was found on examination of the abdomen. A large retroperitoneal hematoma was found at immediate laparotomy. The patient had a Dacron tube graft interposed. Cardiac arrhythmia and hypotension developed on the seventh day after surgery, with unsuccessful resuscitation. Multiple system organ failure was the cause of death.

Conclusion.—Although rupture of the abdominal aorta rarely occurs spontaneously, it can occur without the precipitating factors known to be causative for pseudo-aneurysm formation. These spontaneous ruptures were probably caused by degenerative changes, such as atherosclerotic changes in 1 patient and cystic medical degeneration in the other. Both of these causes are known to be underlying factors for aneurysmal dilation.

► Spontaneous rupture of a nonaneurysmal infrarenal aorta appears to result from transmural wall penetration of an atherosclerotic ulcer. In a few patients this rupture may occur without the formation of an intervening false aneurysm. Spontaneous rupture is an extraordinarily uncommon clinical entity, but one with which vascular surgeons must be familiar. The similarity of these patients to the patients reported in Abstract 8–3, is apparent. I wonder if we will begin to see more of these patients in our aging population?

Axillobifemoral Bypass: Elective Versus Emergent Operation

Jain KM, O'Brien SP, Munn JS, et al (Michigan State Univ, Kalamazoo)

Ann Vasc Surg 12:265–269, 1998 8–5

Introduction.—The mainstay of treatment for aortoiliac occlusive disease is direct aortic revascularization; however, this approach is not used

Conclusion.—The development of arteriolar nephrosclerosis in the contralateral kidney is associated with a unilateral hemodynamically significant atherosclerotic renal artery stenosis. These results have important implications for blood pressure control, renal function, and response to renal revascularization in this patient population.

► I have been confused for decades about the relationship between unilateral renal artery stenosis and contralateral renal disease, and the 1- and 2-clip model of renal hypertension described by Goldblatt. It does seem clear that virulent hypertension resulting from unilateral renal artery hypertension may cause considerable disease in the contralateral kidney. This study presents convincing evidence of the widespread incidence of significant contralateral disease as measured by the end-diastolic ratio in the contralateral renal artery. The authors make the cogent point that the functional status of the contralateral kidney must be considered when planning renal artery intervention. I do wish, however, the actual differences in the end-diastolic ratio had been a little greater (0.27 ± 0.08 vs. 0.30 ± 0.08; $P = 0.001$—but does it mean anything?).

Carotid and Lower Extremity Arterial Disease in Patients With Renal Artery Atherosclerosis

Zierler RE, Bergelin RO, Polissar NL, et al (Univ of Washington, Seattle; Mountain-Whisper-Light Statistical Consulting, Seattle)

Arch Intern Med 158:761–767, 1998 9–4

Introduction.—Information on atherosclerotic involvement in carotid and lower extremity arteries may be meaningful in the clinical management of patients with renal artery disease. The prevalence and severity of extracranial carotid and lower extremity occlusive disease in patients with varying degrees of artery atherosclerosis was prospectively assessed in 149 patients with renal artery stenosis.

Methods.—All patients had at least 1 abnormal renal artery as determined by duplex scanning. Ankle/brachial indices were used to evaluate lower extremity arteries. Duplex scanning was used to assess carotid artery disease. Involvement at renal artery, carotid artery, and extremity artery sites were classified as mild, moderate, or severe, based on the extent of disease on both sides. Blood was obtained for determination of serum urea nitrogen, creatinine, and lipid levels.

Results.—Severe renal, carotid, and lower extremity arterial disease was observed in 44%, 19%, and 21% of patients, respectively. There was a tendency for patients with increasing degrees of renal artery disease to have increasing degrees of carotid and lower extremity arterial disease. The rate of severe carotid artery disease rose from 7% in patients with mild renal artery disease to 28% in patients with severe renal artery disease. Clinical factors associated with severe renal artery, carotid artery, and lower extremity artery disease were elevated apolipoprotein B levels, high serum urea nitrogen or creatinine levels, and smoking, respectively.

Conclusion.—There was a highly significant correlation between severe renal artery atherosclerosis and severe carotid artery disease.

► I don't know whether to give Dr. Zierler credit for rediscovering or minimally extending our knowledge of the wheel. Is there any vascular surgeon in the world sufficiently stuporous to not realize that atherosclerosis is a systemic disease, and people who have symptomatic manifestations in 1 place will invariably have significant disease in other places? We learn in this monumental paper that patients who have atherosclerotic lesions in the renal arteries have a significant prevalence of atherosclerotic lesions in the carotid arteries and the lower extremity arteries. The incremental information we get from this publication is the percentage of patients with mild, moderate, and severe disease in the other locations. Although I have absolutely no idea what I will do with this information, I am reminded of the famous statement ascribed to the founder of Faber College in the movie "Animal House": "Knowledge is Good."

Renal Artery Repair: Consequence of Operative Failures

Hansen KJ, Deitch JS, Oskin TC, et al (Wake Forest Univ, Winston-Salem, NC)

Ann Surg 227:678–690, 1998 9–5

Introduction.—Most reports characterizing operative failure of renal artery (RA) repair focus on the technical aspects of repeat RA reconstruction and the immediate blood pressure response to secondary surgery. Eventual renal function and estimated survival in 20 patients who underwent repeat RA reconstruction were described.

Methods.—Of 534 patients undergoing operative repair of renovascular disease, 20 (12 with recurrent hypertension and 8 with recurrent hypertension with worsening excretory renal function) had a failed RA repair at a mean of 27 months. Primary methods of RA reconstruction, primary blood pressure and renal function responses, and causes of failed RA repair were examined and compared with secondary procedures. Eventual blood pressure, renal function responses, and estimated survival were compared in the 20 patients who underwent repeat procedures and 514 patients managed by primary renal revascularization during the same period.

Results.—There was a significant correlation between failure of primary RA repair and complex fibromuscular dysplasia requiring branch ex vivo reconstruction. Nephrectomy was required in 83% of patients with RA thrombosis. Renal artery stenosis was successfully repaired in 91% of patients. Blood pressure responses were similar for patients in the primary and secondary repair groups (94% and 95%, respectively). There was a significant between-group difference in renal function responses; 7 patients in the secondary group required dialysis. Eventual dialysis dependence was significantly correlated with preoperative azotemia, bilateral failure of primary RA repair, and increased risk of follow-up death. With regard to all 534 patients evaluated, failed RA repair showed a significant and independent correlation with eventual dialysis dependence and diminished dialysis-free survival.

Conclusion.—A high rate of blood pressure and renal function benefit and a low rate of reoperation after surgical RA repair were observed in this series of 534 patients. The risk of eventual dialysis in patients who required repeat RA procedures is significantly high.

▶ This abstract presents fascinating information concerning the outcome of patients requiring secondary renal revascularization after a failed primary operative repair. From their extremely large experience, these authors could identify only 20 reoperative patients. It is sobering to note that 9 of these patients required nephrectomy and that during follow-up, 7 of the patients either died or required dialysis. Even though some of the patients enjoyed a favorable blood pressure response, the overall outcome was, indeed, poor. Hopefully, we will all encounter few patients with failed primary RA revascularization requiring repeat surgery.

Visceral Ischemia

Current Results of Surgical Therapy for Chronic Mesenteric Ischemia
Moawad J, McKinsey JF, Wyble CW, et al (Univ of Chicago)
Arch Surg 132:613–619, 1997 9–6

Background.—The prevalence of chronic mesenteric ischemia (CMI) appears to have increased in recent years. However, it continues to be a difficult condition to diagnose and treat. The authors reviewed their experience with the surgical treatment of CMI.

Patients.—The 10-year review included 24 patients (19 women and 5 men; mean age, 58 years) undergoing surgery for CMI. Seventy-five percent of patients complained of postprandial abdominal pain and 58% had weight loss. Other, less common symptoms included nausea and vomiting, diarrhea, and constipation. Many patients had risk factors for atherosclerosis—83% were tobacco users, 42% had coronary artery disease, and 42% had hypertension. Atherosclerosis was the cause of CMI in 21 patients; a pair of monozygotic twins had median arcuate ligament compression, and 1 patient had Takayasu's arteritis. Eight patients had lesions localized to all 3 major visceral vessels; 13 had lesions localized to the celiac artery and superior mesenteric artery (SMA), 2 to the SMA alone, and 2 to the SMA and inferior mesenteric artery. Antegrade reconstruction from the supraceliac aorta to the SMA and/or the celiac artery was performed in 17 patients. In 7 patients, a retrograde bypass from the infrarenal aorta or a prosthetic graft was used.

Outcomes.—None of the patients died during the operative period, although 1 patient died of early graft failure and sepsis at 6 weeks. Thus, the in-hospital mortality rate was 4%. The patients were followed up for a median of 2.4 years. According to contrast angiography or duplex scanning, the mean 5-year primary graft patency rate was 78%. Three patients had primary failure, occurring between 3 weeks and 7 months postoperatively. Thrombectomy was required in 2 patients, 1 of whom died of an intestinal infarction. According to life-table analysis, the mean 5-year survival rate was 71%. As long as the grafts remained patent, there were no symptomatic recurrences.

Conclusion.—Atherosclerosis is the most frequent cause of CMI, with symptoms resulting from midgut ischemia in the distribution of the SMA. Antegrade bypass from the supraceliac aorta is a relatively safe reconstructive technique and is the current procedure of choice. For most patients, surgical therapy for CMI permits long-term, symptom-free survival.

▶ I disagree with these authors on several important points. They dismiss a graft originating from the infrarenal aorta or iliac arteries as "anatomically unfavorable." They also favor multiple visceral artery revascularization, including the celiac artery and the SMA. Our experience is quite different. We prefer to originate grafts from the iliac artery as our first choice and the infrarenal aorta as our second choice. We prefer prosthetics, which are then routed toward the left shoulder and make a 180-degree U-turn under the lower edge of the pancreas, coming back to the SMA in an antegrade direction. Our patient survival and clinical success rates have been every bit as good as the authors report for their techniques described herein. Furthermore, I am convinced that revascularization of the SMA alone is adequate in a large majority, if not all patients. I identify no persuasive benefit in revascularizing the hepatic or celiac artery and frankly think it is a waste of time. Otherwise, I find myself in full agreement with the authors.

ascribed to the use of thrombolytics. As I have repeatedly stated, as time passes I find fewer and fewer indications for the clinical use of thrombolytic agents in the peripheral circulation. This may be an explanation for the results presented in Abstract 10–1.

Effect of Ticlopidine on the Long-term Patency of Saphenous-Vein Bypass Grafts in the Legs

Becquemin J-P, for the Etude de la Ticlopidine Après Portage Fémoro-Poplité and the Association Universitaire de Recherche en Chirurgie (Centre Hospitalier Universitaire Henri Mondor, Créteil, France)

N Engl J Med 337:1726–1731, 1997 10–6

Introduction.—Late graft failure after infrainguinal arterial bypass surgery is often caused by progressive stenosis of the arteries on either side of the bypass. Platelet-inhibiting drugs have been evaluated as a way of improving the patency of saphenous-vein grafts, but the optimal treatment to prevent late occlusions has not been determined. A double-blind trial assessed the efficacy of ticlopidine, an inhibitor of platelet aggregation, on the long-term patency of below-the-knee saphenous-vein grafts.

Methods.—The multicenter study enrolled 243 patients with femoropopliteal or femorotibial saphenous-vein bypass grafts. Randomization was to ticlopidine (250-mg tablets) or matching placebo. Patients were instructed to take 1 tablet twice daily for 24 months. They were also given

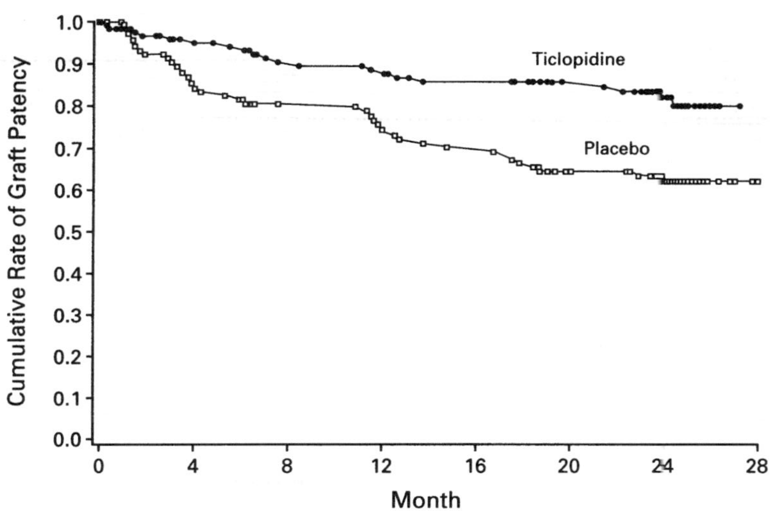

FIGURE 1.—Cumulative rates of graft patency according to the intention-to-treat analysis. There was a significant difference between groups ($P = 0.002$ by the log-rank test). (Courtesy of Becquemin J-P, for the Etude de la Ticlopidine Après Pontage Fémoro-Poplité and the Association Universitaire de Recherche en Chirurgie: Effect of ticlopidine on the long-term patency of saphenous-vein bypass grafts in the legs. *N Engl J Med* 337:1726–1731, 1997. Reprinted by permission of *The New England Journal of Medicine*.

a list of anticoagulants and antiplatelet drugs to avoid during the study period. Graft patency was evaluated at 1, 3, 6, 12, 18, and 24 months.

Results.—Study participants had a mean age of 67.4; 77.4% were men. Treatment and placebo groups did not differ significantly in sex, age, preoperative risk factors, site of proximal anastomosis, runoff, immediate graft patency, or mean duration of therapy. Bypass patency was assessed in 192 patients at 24 months by either duplex US (171) or angiography (21); 12 patients were assessed on the basis of clinical evaluation. The percentage of patients alive with a patent graft was greater in the ticlopidine group (66.4%) than in the placebo group (51.2%) at 2 years. The ticlopidine group also had a 2-year cumulative patency rate (Fig 1) superior to that of the placebo group (82% vs. 63%). Overall mortality (18 patients in each group) and the rate of major ischemic events did not differ significantly between the 2 groups. Nonischemic adverse events were more common in the ticlopidine group, a difference almost entirely accounted for by gastrointestinal disorders.

Conclusion.—Treatment with ticlopidine significantly improved the long-term patency of below-the-knee saphenous-vein grafts and reduced the need for major amputations. The drug's efficacy and lack of serious adverse effects recommend its use after femoropopliteal or femorotibial saphenous-vein bypass grafting.

▶ This prospective, randomized study compared 2 groups of patients undergoing leg vein bypass to the popliteal or tibial arteries, with 1 group receiving ticlopidine and the other group matching placebo, for 2 years. The 2-year patency rate was 82% in the ticlopidine group and 63% in the placebo group, with a highly significant $P = 0.002$. This is clearly impressive work, but I would have personally found the results much more convincing had the placebo patients received active control with aspirin. Certainly, in today's world we attempt to place all bypass patients on aspirin, and we rarely have patients on no treatment at all. Nonetheless, we have to note that there is a very large difference between the active and the placebo patients in this study, although I am not sure whether this should be regarded more as a testimonial for antiplatelet drugs in general, or ticlopidine in particular. Based on this study, I am not prepared to use ticlopidine routinely, but I shall pay close attention to further information. I do note this article is from France.

Should Vein Be Saved for Future Operations? A 15-Year Review of Infrainguinal Bypasses and the Subsequent Need for Autogenous Vein

Poletti LF, Matsuura JH, Dattilo JB, et al (HH McGuire and Syracuse Veterans Affairs Med Ctr, NY; Virginia Commonwealth Univ, Richmond)

Ann Vasc Surg 12:143–147, 1998 10–7

Background.—Infrainguinal bypass using autogenous saphenous vein is standard procedure for revascularization of lower extremities. Some have advocated the initial use of prosthetic material to spare vein for the

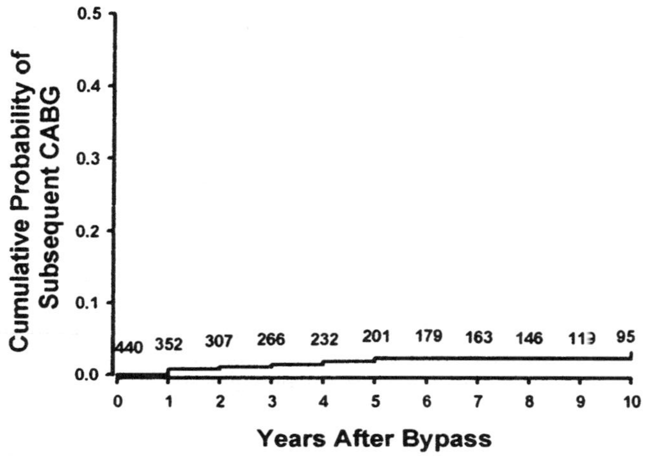

FIGURE 3.—Life-table curve of cumulative probability of having a coronary artery bypass (*CABG*) subsequent to an infrainguinal bypass. (Courtesy of Poletti LF, Matsuura JH, Dattilo JB, et al: Should vein be saved for future operations? A 15-year review of infrainguinal bypasses and the subsequent need for autogenous vein. *Ann Vasc Surg* 12:143–147, 1998.)

subsequent potential use in other leg and heart bypasses. To determine whether vein should be spared, a large series of infrainguinal bypasses were retrospectively analyzed with respect to the need for subsequent bypasses and the availability of autogenous vein.

Study Design.—The operating room database of the H.H. McGuire Veterans Affairs Medical Center was retrospectively searched for infrainguinal bypasses, coronary artery bypasses (CABG), and lower extremity amputations from 1980 to 1995. During this period, 572 infrainguinal bypasses, 2,592 CABGs, and 622 lower extremity amputations were performed. Subsequent operations were noted. Life-table analysis estimated the probability of subsequent bypasses per year. Prosthetic vs. autogenous vein use was determined.

Findings.—Autogenous vein was used in 84% of first operations in this series. In these patients, the use of prosthetic material increased to 27% in second operations. The rate of subsequent CABG was only 3% at 10 years (Fig 3). The cumulative probability of subsequent infrainguinal bypass was 27% at 5 years and 32% at 10 years. Considering only tibial bypasses, the cumulative 5-year rate of subsequent leg bypass was only 13%. Most subsequent bypasses occurred within 3 years of the initial surgery.

Conclusions.—After primary infrainguinal bypass with autogenous vein, most patients do not require an additional bypass. When one is required, adequate vein is usually still available. The probability of requiring a subsequent CABG is quite low. Therefore, most patients would benefit from the use of autogenous vein in their first operation.

▶ The issue of saving the vein for future use has been used repeatedly by scoundrels to justify the use of a prosthetic material for the initial lower-extremity bypass. I have always considered this to be the product of distorted thinking. My overall summary, and one substantially supported by the data presented herein, is that although about 15% of patients requiring lower extremity bypass have already undergone coronary bypass at the time of presentation with leg symptoms, only about 5% will subsequently require coronary bypass. Thus, saving the vein in most patients to benefit a maximum of 5% for subsequent CABG makes no sense at all. It is also clear that a certain number of patients will require subsequent leg bypasses, for which the vein may be used. Fortunately, we are able to piece together autogenous venous conduits in 96% of all patients undergoing leg bypass at the present time, using both arms and both legs as vein sources. I firmly believe that one should not perform a second-class operation because of some concocted potential future benefit requiring saving the vein. My philosophy is simple: do the best operation first. I hope I make myself clear.

Optimal Methods for Autogenous Bypass to the Anterior Tibial Artery

Eslami MH, Belkin M, Mannick JA, et al (Brigham and Women's Hosp, Boston; Harvard Med School, Boston)

Am J Surg 174:198–201, 1997 10–8

Background.—From 10% to 20% of infrainguinal bypass procedures use the anterior tibial artery (AT) for distal anastomosis. Surgical bypass to the AT requires routing of the conduit through the interosseous membrane, a pretibial tunnel, or through a lateral thigh and calf tunnel. A retrospective study of 130 consecutive vein grafts to the AT evaluated the potential advantages and disadvantages of the 3 routing options.

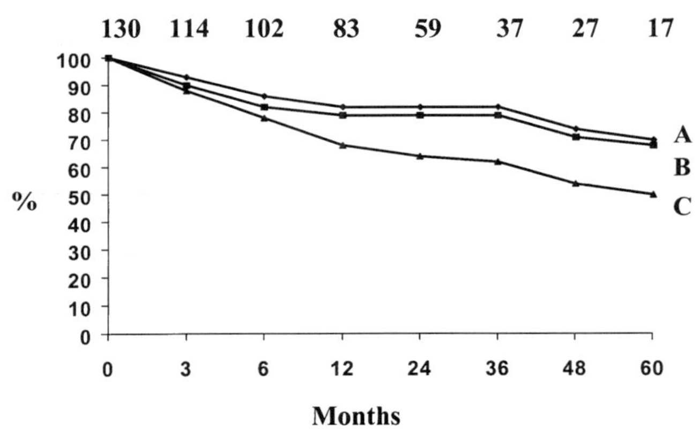

FIGURE.—Five-year cumulative patency rates of 130 consecutive autogenous anterior tibial artery grafts. **Curve A,** secondary patency. **Curve B,** primary revised patency. **Curve C,** primary patency. Number of grafts entering each time interval is noted at the top of figure. Standard error less than 6.8. (Reprinted by permission of the publisher from Eslami MH, Belkin M, Mannick JA, et al: Optimal methods for autogenous bypass to the anterior tibial artery. *Am J Surg* 174:198–201. Copyright 1997, by Excerpta Medica Inc.)

Methods.—The routing technique was chosen by the vascular surgeon in each case. During the study period (January 1985 through June 1995), the interosseous route was used in 50 procedures, the pretibial route in 51, and the lateral route in 29. Patients were followed up postoperatively at 1 month, every 3 months for a year, and every 6 months thereafter. Outcomes analyzed were cumulative graft patency, limb salvage, and patient survival rates.

Results.—One hundred thirty vein grafts to the AT were performed in 121 patients; indications were critical ischemia in 114 and claudication in 16. The 3 graft-routing subgroups were generally comparable in preoperative risk factors, except for a smaller prevalence of coronary artery disease in the pretibial route group. All conduits were of autogenous vein, with the greater saphenous vein used in 78% of cases. Seven procedures (5.3%) involved major postoperative morbidity within 30 days of surgery. Early graft failure occurred in 7.7% of procedures overall, with no difference among the 3 routing subgroups. There was a significantly higher rate of postoperative wound complications in the interosseous group (20%) than in the pretibial group (8%) or the lateral group (7%), but only 1 of 9 infections in the interosseous group occurred in the distal tunnel portion of the wound. Overall 5-year primary, primary revised, and secondary graft patency rates were 50.0%, 67.8%, and 70.4%, respectively (Figure).

Conclusion.—Autogenous bypass grafts to the AT yielded excellent results, as measured by wound morbidity and graft patency, regardless of the routing method used. Factors to be considered when selecting the optimal method for AT bypass include the location of suitable AT, the length of adequate vein conduit, and surgeon preference.

▶ It is obvious that the way one routes a graft from the femoral artery to the AT makes little difference. As long as one is using a reversed vein, one has the choice of routing through the lateral subcutaneous, the interosseous membrane using a medial approach, or a medial approach using a pretibial tunnel. In this study, during a mean follow-up of 2 years, the overall secondary patency rate was 70%, with no difference among routing techniques. We, too, have used all of these routing techniques, but in recent years we have come to prefer the lateral subcutaneous route for passing a vein graft from the femoral artery to the AT. This has seemed easier to us and has given quite satisfactory results. I am especially wary of passage through the interosseous membrane, as I seem to have a unique ability to routinely harpoon some enormous vein while attempting to blindly perforate this membrane. I will stick with the lateral subcutaneous, thank you.

procedures. The mortality rate (2%) and the nonfatal myocardial infarction rate (2%) were comparable with other reports of patients who underwent regional or general anesthesia. Cooperation between surgeon and anesthesiologist is required so that additional sedation can be administered if required.

► Although one can obviously do lower extremity vascular reconstruction in high-risk patients under local anesthesia, why would one want to? I would only be interested in so doing if there were persuasive evidence of cardiac benefit resulting from local anesthesia. In fact, at least one influential report of a large retrospective anesthesia review found an increased 30-day mortality rate with local anesthesia.[1] I am of the opinion that frequent episodes of leg pain associated with inadequate local anesthesia can lead to a detrimentally heightened state of catecholamine release and other noxious substances in these high-risk cardiac patients. I hereby present these authors the Honorable Mention Camel Dung Award in recognition of their undertaking a radical form of therapy in high-risk patients in the total absence of proof of efficacy. (See also Abstract 10–14.)

Reference

1. Cohen MN, Duncan PG, Tate RB: Does anesthesia contribute to operative mortality? *JAMA* 260:2859–2863, 1988.

Local Anaesthetic for Lower-Limb Revascularization in High-risk Patients

Mackay CA, Razik W, Simms MH (Selly Oak Hosp, Birmingham, England)
Br J Surg 84:1096–1098, 1997 10–14

Background.—In some medically compromised patients with critical limb ischemia, the decision to perform primary amputation may be based on unfitness for prolonged anesthesia. The outcome of a group of high-risk patients undergoing lower-limb revascularization using local anesthetic techniques was analyzed.

Patients.—Forty-six patients with critical limb ischemia who received local and regional anesthesia for revascularization procedures were studied. The patients were 28 men and 18 women, with a mean age of 76 years. Most patients were in American Society of Anesthesiologists grade 4. The most frequent indications for local anesthesia were impaired cardiac function and chronic obstructive pulmonary disease. A wide range of arterial reconstructive procedures were performed, most commonly femorodistal bypass (Table 2).

Outcomes.—Ten of 46 patients died within 30 days, and another 4 died before discharge, at 31–78 days. Cumulative survival was 67% at 6 months, 57% at 1 year, and 51% at 2 years. Primary patency rates were 77%, 67%, and 53%, respectively. The limb salvage rate was 87% at 6 months and 1 year, and 79% at 2 years.

TABLE 2.—Arterial Reconstructions Under Local Anesthetic Included in the Study

Procedure	No. of procedures
Axillofemoral graft	2
Femoral crossover graft	2
Sequential jump graft	4
Femorodistal bypass	27
Femoropopliteal bypass	6
Popliteal–pedal bypass	5

(Courtesy of Mackay CA, Razik W, Simms MH: Local anaesthetic for lower-limb revascularization in high-risk patients. *Br J Surg* 84:1096–1098. Copyright 1997, Blackwell Science Ltd.)

Conclusions.—For selected high-risk patients with critical limb ischemia, lower-limb revascularization can be carried out using local anesthesia. This approach offers the benefits of limb salvage to patients who are medically unfit for conventional anesthesia.

► I am absolutely amazed at this study. I cannot believe these authors undertook 46 lower extremity revascularization procedures for the treatment of critical limb ischemia using local anesthesia only. I fail to find any convincing evidence that local anesthesia for extensive surgery is the least bit better tolerated than carefully administered general or spinal anesthesia. The fact that these authors had an operative mortality rate of 22% with local anesthesia would appear to support my position. At the very least, they should give us a randomized comparison of local anesthesia to alternate anesthetic techniques. It seems to me that a critically ill patient having at least intermittent pain under local anesthesia will experience far more significant systemic stress than a patient under well-conducted general anesthesia. For their naive assumption that local anesthesia is safer in this patient cohort, I am pleased to present these authors the coveted Camel Dung Award (CDA). I urge them to return with a properly randomized study to lend credence, if possible, to their peculiar position. (See also Abstract 10–13.) Perhaps I am being too generous in awarding both these papers the coveted CDA. I am just an old softie.

Skin Perfusion Pressure Measurement Is Valuable in the Diagnosis of Critical Limb Ischemia

Castronuovo JJ Jr, Adera HM, Smiell JM, et al (Morristown Mem Hosp, NJ)
J Vasc Surg 26:629–637, 1997 10–15

Objective.—An accurate, noninvasive test for critical limb ischemia (CLI) would be beneficial in selecting patients in need of arterial reconstruction and increasing the odds of limb salvage. Whether skin perfusion pressure (SPP) measurements could be used to identify patients with CLI who need major amputation or vascular reconstruction and distinguish

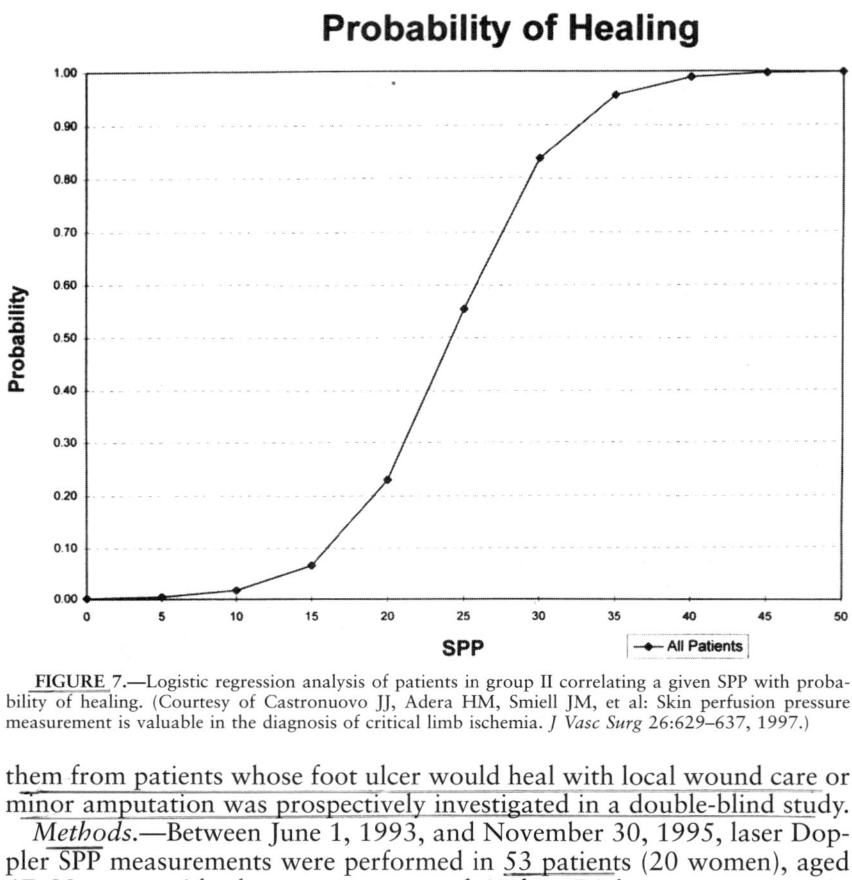

FIGURE 7.—Logistic regression analysis of patients in group II correlating a given SPP with probability of healing. (Courtesy of Castronuovo JJ, Adera HM, Smiell JM, et al: Skin perfusion pressure measurement is valuable in the diagnosis of critical limb ischemia. *J Vasc Surg* 26:629–637, 1997.)

them from patients whose foot ulcer would heal with local wound care or minor amputation was prospectively investigated in a double-blind study.

Methods.—Between June 1, 1993, and November 30, 1995, laser Doppler SPP measurements were performed in 53 patients (20 women), aged 47–88 years, with ulcers or gangrene of 61 feet. Diabetes was present in 75%. The size and site of ulcers and gangrene were recorded. Group I patients (n = 32) required vascular reconstruction or major amputation, in the opinion of the surgeon; and group II patients (n = 29) were thought to require local débridement, minor amputation, or both. Treatment decisions were based on clinical judgment alone. SPP results, measured at the proximal margin, and clinical judgment were compared with outcome (healed or not healed) for group II patients.

Results.—Three patients, all in group II, had palpable foot pulses. An ankle-brachial systolic pressure index (ABI) could not be obtained in 17 feet. In group II, 15 limbs healed and 14 did not. The SPP test was negative in 13 ulcers, 11 of which healed, for an SPP-negative predictive value of 85%, a specificity of 73%, a sensitivity of 85%, and a diagnostic accuracy of 79.3% as compared with a clinical judgment accuracy of slightly more than 50%. Twelve of 16 limbs with SPP of less than 30 mm Hg failed to heal, for a positive predictive value of 75%. Whereas ABI was not predictive of the need for reconstruction or major amputation, SPP measurements correctly identified 31 of 32 limbs with CLI. When logical regression analysis was used to correlate SPP with the probability of healing, there was no significant difference between diabetic and nondiabetic patients (Fig 7).

Conclusion.—SPP measurements are an accurate, noninvasive method for identifying patients with CLI who need vascular reconstruction or major amputation.

▶ I have always been impressed by the determination of skin perfusion pressure by using a combination of cuff compression associated with some sort of flow detection, such as the laser Doppler. Although the determination of skin perfusion pressure does correlate with the healing of ischemic ulcers in about 80% of patients, there is clearly too big an overlap to use this as a definitive basis for clinical decision making. For now, I will take this as one more interesting method for the assessment of limb ischemia but certainly not as a definitive method for assessment of ulcer-healing potential.

Implications for the Vascular Surgeon With Prolonged (3 to 89 Days) Intraaortic Balloon Pump Counterpulsation

Manord JD, Garrard CL, Mehra MR, et al (Ochsner Clinic and Alton Ochsner Med Found, New Orleans, La)

J Vasc Surg 26:511–516, 1997 10–16

Objective.—Whereas the intra-aortic balloon pump (IABP) has long been used for acute short-term treatment of failing hearts, prolonged therapy is sometimes required in patients who are awaiting cardiac transplantation. The outcome and vascular implications of long-term IABP therapy and the factors contributing to complications in these patients were retrospectively assessed.

Methods.—Between January 1993 and March 1995, 50 patients (10 women), aged 32–77 years, awaiting cardiac transplantation, underwent placement of an IABP for more than 72 hours. Patients received heparin anticoagulation therapy. Incidences of ischemia, hemorrhage, local infection, and general sepsis were recorded, and 31 variables possibly predictive of these complications were evaluated.

Results.—Twelve patients required insulin for diabetes, 28 had hypertension, 1 had peripheral vascular disease, and 37 had mild renal insufficiency. The average duration of IABP support was 23.2 days, and the average duration of any single IABP was 13 days. Sixteen patients (32%) had 21 complications, including 16 ischemic episodes in 12 patients (24%), sepsis in 3, and hemorrhage in 2. Five complications occurred during insertion, and 4 during removal. All ischemic complications occurring during maintenance were thrombolic or embolic, and all but 1 were treated surgically (Table 2). The complication rate was 0.13 per patient-week of therapy. Significant predictors of complications included total days on IABP support, use of more than 1 IABP, and unsuccessful percu-

TABLE 2.—Surgical Procedures Resulting From Vascular Complications

Surgical procedures	*No.*
Thrombectomy and patch angioplasties	5
Major amputations	2
Ileofemoral bypass	1
Axillofemoral bypass	1
Femorofemoral bypass	1
Femoropopliteal bypass	1
Fasciotomy	1
Groin exploration for hemorrhage	1
Removal infected Dacron patch	1

(Courtesy of Manord JD, Garrard CL, Mehra MR, et al: Implications for the vascular surgeon with prolonged (3 to 89 days) intraaortic ballon pump counterpulsation. *J Vasc Surg* 26:511–516, 1997.)

taneous insertions. Patients having percutaneous removal were significantly more likely to experience an ischemic complication.

Conclusion.—Use of IABP for long-term cardiac support is feasible but is accompanied by complications, many of which occur during insertion and removal of the IABP. Significant predictors of complications included total days on IABP support, use of more than 1 IABP, and unsuccessful percutaneous insertions. Patients having percutaneous removal have a 14% complication rate compared with patients having operative removal.

▶ The intra-aortic balloon pump has obviously been a great boon to cardiac support in selected patients, but its use has been associated with a disturbing number of vascular complications. In the main, these have been lower extremity ischemic complications, although occasionally infectious. This article nicely documents the large number of complications one can expect from the use of the intra-aortic balloon. It is again noted that percutaneous removal of these devices carries a 14% complication rate compared with none after operative removal. Clearly, operative removal should be considered when feasible. On balance, this is a nice review of an important clinical topic.

Effects of Vascular Surgery on Amputation Rates and Mortality

Karlström L, Bergqvist D (Älvsborgs Länssjukhus, Trollhättan, Sweden; Akademiska Sjukhuset, Uppsala, Sweden)

Eur J Vasc Endovasc Surg 14:273–283, 1997 10–17

Introduction.—The increasing number of vascular surgical procedures—many of them performed to avoid amputation—has not been shown to reduce the need for amputation. Some studies show increasing rates of both vascular reconstruction and amputation. This retrospective study examined the effect of vascular surgery rate on amputation rate and mortality in a well-defined population.

Methods.—Data were drawn from a Swedish district hospital covering a defined population. Patients from 2 consecutive 4-year periods—with

sumed mode of action of vein cuffs at the distal end of crural prosthetic grafts.

T.V. Schroeder, M.D., D.M.Sc.

Vein Transposition in the Forearm for Autogenous Hemodialysis Access

Silva MB Jr, Hobson RW II, Pappas PJ, et al (Univ of Medicine and Dentistry of New Jersey, Newark)

J Vasc Surg 26:981–988, 1997 11–3

Objective.—Primary arteriovenous fistulas (AFs) in the forearm of patients undergoing chronic hemodialysis have several advantages over synthetic bridging grafts. To increase options for formation of AFs, a technique of superficial venous transposition in the forearm using veins and arteries not in immediate proximity was designed.

Methods.—Over a period of 3 years, a primary AF was placed in 89 patients (36 women), aged 25 to 82. Ultrasound scans were used to map veins and arteries and assess compressibility and diameters. When the most suitable site for cannulation was identified, the selected vein was dissected and prepared for transposition (Fig 2). A subcutaneous tunnel was constructed, and the vein was passed through (Fig 3). The vein was heparinized, an arteriotomy was performed, and an end-to-end anastomosis was created (Fig 5).

Results.—There were 13 type A transpositions (15%) performed in immediate proximity to the radial artery using a single incision. Veins on the dorsal aspect were transposed to the volar aspect and anastomosed to the appropriate artery in 30 type B transpositions (33%). Volar-to-volar

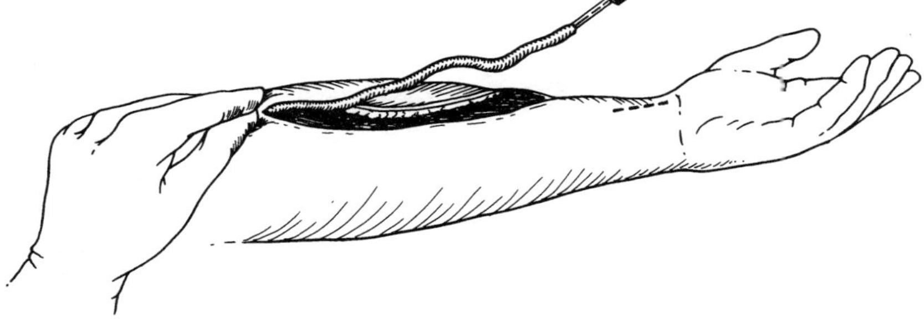

FIGURE 2.—Complete dissection of vein and dilation with heparinized saline solution; separate radial artery incision marked. (Courtesy of Silva MB Jr, Hobson RW II, Pappas PJ, et al: Vein transposition in the forearm for autogenous hemodialysis access. *J Vasc Surg* 26:981–988, 1997).

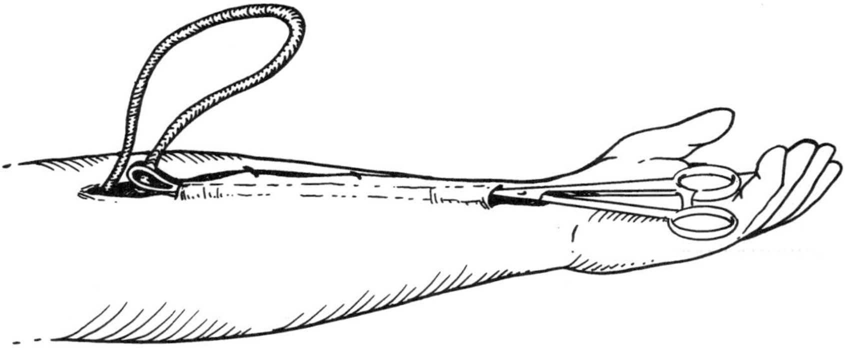

FIGURE 3.—Construction of subcutaneous tunnel. (Courtesy of Silva MB Jr, Hobson RW II, Pappas PJ, et al: Vein transposition in the forearm for autogenous hemodialysis access. *J Vasc Surg* 26:981–988, 1997).

type C transpositions were performed in 46 veins (52%). Cannulation and hemodialysis was successful in 81 patients (91%). Of the 8 initial failures, 4 became occluded, 2 had stenosis and underwent revision, and 2 had insufficient flows. Ten fistulas failed during follow-up. Of the total 18 fistulas that failed, 4 were salvaged by revision, 3 were converted to contralateral forearm AFs, 6 were converted to ipsilateral bridging grafts, 2 were converted to contralateral forearm bridging grafts, 2 patients received permanent central venous catheters, and 1 patient died. Patency rates at 1 and 2 years were 84% and 69%, respectively. Patients were followed up on average for 14.3 months.

Conclusion.—Vein transposition in the forearm for formation of autogenous hemodialysis access yields a high hemodialysis success rate, and primary patency rates at 1 and 2 years of 84% and 69%.

▶ This is a rather complex procedure that does require considerable dissection. However, this extra effort appears to be abundantly rewarded with a primary patency of 84% at 1 year and 69% at 2 years. This is the best patency I have ever seen with hemodialysis access. I am impressed with this procedure, and we are beginning to use it in a few selected cases.

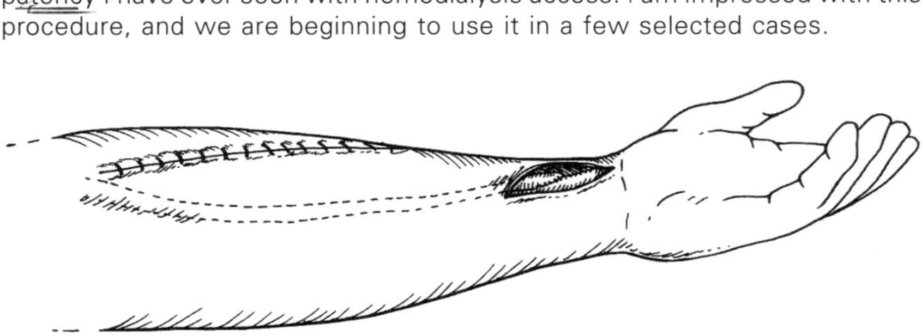

FIGURE 5.—Completed fistula. Mid-forearm volar location facilitates cannulation and comfortable arm positioning during dialysis. (Courtesy of Silva MB Jr, Hobson RW II, Pappas PJ, et al: Vein transposition in the forearm for autogenous hemodialysis access. *J Vasc Surg* 26:981–988, 1997).

A Prospective Comparison of Two Expanded Polytetrafluoroethylene Grafts for Linear Forearm Hemodialysis Access: Does the Manufacturer Matter?

Kaufman JL, Garb JL, Berman JA, et al (Baystate Med Ctr, Springfield, Mass)

J Am Coll Surg 185:74–79, 1997 11–4

Background.—Two manufacturers, W.L. Gore and Associates (Goretex) and Impra, Inc. (Impra), dominate the market for the expanded polytetrafluoroethylene (PTFE) grafts used in hemodialysis access sites. The grafts differ in gross appearance and handling characteristics, but it is not known whether these differences affect outcomes and long-term patency. This question was examined in a randomized clinical trial.

Methods.—Patients were drawn from 2 community dialysis centers and 1 hospital-based center. Those eligible for linear forearm access had palpable radial pulses with a normal Allen test and normal digital Doppler flow in the hand. Graft type, Goretex or Impra, was determined by randomization. Linear grafts were placed using end-to-side anastomoses to the artery and vein. All grafts were followed for at least 2 years. Primary patency was defined as function to the first thrombosis episode and secondary patency as function thereafter to the time when the graft is no longer clinically usable.

Results.—Linear forearm grafts were placed in 117 patients (131 grafts). The Impra and Goretex groups were similar in gender distribution and major risk factors, except that the Goretex group had more smokers. Differences in primary patencies between the groups were not statistically significant: 43% for Impra and 47% for Goretex at 1 year and 30% and

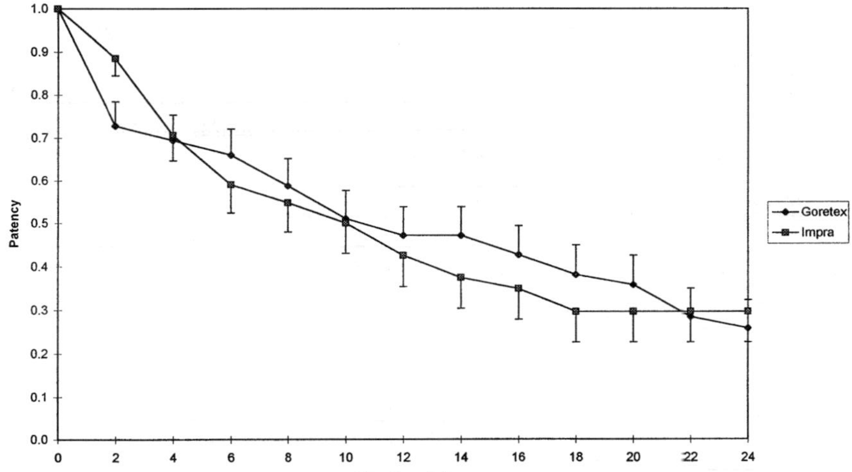

FIGURE 1.—Life-table curves for primary patency of grafts. *Bars* indicate standard error. (Courtesy of Kaufman JL, Garb JL, Berman JA, et al: A prospective comparison of two expanded polytetrafluoroethylene grafts for linear forearm hemodialysis access: Does the manufacturer matter? *J Am Coll Surg* 185:74–79, 1997. By permission of the Journal of the American College of Surgeons.)

26%, respectively, at 2 years (Fig 1). The 2 groups were also similar in discontinuation of use of a patent graft, complications, episodes of thrombosis, and need to replace the original graft.

Conclusion.—Prosthetic grafts are commonly required for hemodialysis in the forearm, and PTFE is the most widely used material. In this study—the first randomized clinical trial to compare Goretex and Impra grafts and to control for potential confounding factors—the 2 products showed no difference in primary or secondary patency. Selection of a PTFE graft on the basis of the surgeon's preference or cost of the product should not affect overall long-term function of the access site.

► I am relieved to note that the Goretex and Impra grafts yielded identical outcomes when used as a linear forearm fistula from the radial artery to an antecubital vein. In fact, the overall patency rates of these grafts appeared superior, with secondary patency at 1 year of about 50% to 69%. I am glad I am not going to have to worry about which brand of graft to use.

Distal Revascularization-Interval Ligation for Limb Salvage and Maintenance of Dialysis Access in Ischemic Steal Syndrome

Berman SS, Gentile AT, Glickman MH, et al (Univ of Arizona, Tucson; Carondelet St Mary's Hosp, Tucson, Ariz; Virginia Vascular Associates, Norfolk)

J Vasc Surg 26:393–404, 1997 11–5

Background.—About 150,000 patients in the United States are currently treated by renal replacement and hemodialysis. Maintenance of vascular access grafts and fistulas and resulting complications in this population are very costly. Ischemic steal syndrome, related to a functioning dialysis access graft or fistula, is traditionally treated by banding or ligation, although these methods often result in inconsistent limb salvage, loss of a functional access, or both. The authors describe their experience with the distal revascularization-interval ligation (DRIL) procedure as an alternate method of limb revascularization that eliminates steal while maintaining continuous dialysis access (Fig 1).

Methods.—The medical records of 21 patients who underwent the DRIL procedure for severe limb ischemia related to a functioning arteriovenous access site were reviewed. Patients underwent color-flow duplex scanning, digital photoplethysmography, and arteriography. Arterial ligation distal to the arteriovenous fistula origin eliminated the steal physiologic mechanism, and arterial bypass grafting from above to below the arteriovenous fistulae revascularized the extremity.

Results.—Of the 21 patients, 11 had chronic ischemia with rest pain, paresthesia, or ulcerations related to 9 native fistulae and 2 prosthetic bridge grafts. Acute ischemia related to 3 native fistulae and 7 prosthetic bridge grafts was seen in 10 patients. The DRIL procedure was used in all 21 patients. Three patients were treated for ischemia at the time of arteriovenous fistulae construction. Of the 21 bypass procedures, 19 were

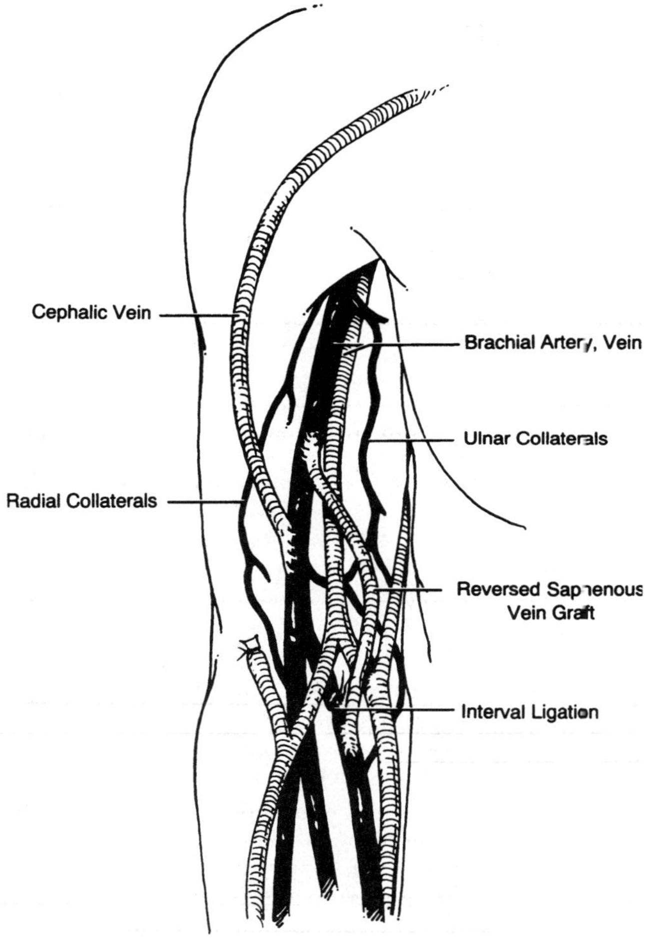

FIGURE 1.—DRIL procedure. (Courtesy of Berman SS, Gentile AT, Glickman MH, et al: Distal revascularization-interval ligation for limb salvage and maintenance of dialysis access in ischemic steal syndrome. *J Vasc Surg* 26:393–404, 1997.)

performed with autogenous vein; there were 9 brachial-brachial, 3 brachial-radial, 2 radial-radial, 2 brachial-ulnar, 1 popliteal-popliteal, 1 femoral-popliteal, and 1 femoral-peroneal. Polytetrafluoroethylene grafts were used in 1 external iliac-popliteal and 1 axillary-brachial bypass graft. At 18 months, life-table analysis showed a patency rate/limb salvage rate of 100% and an access site patency rate of 94% for the DRIL procedures.

Discussion.—The results in these patients show that the DRIL procedure can restore antegrade flow to an ischemic limb, eliminate the potential pathway for the steal physiologic mechanism, and maintain continuous dialysis access. Although the DRIL procedure is given little attention in most vascular textbooks that discuss complications of arteriovenous

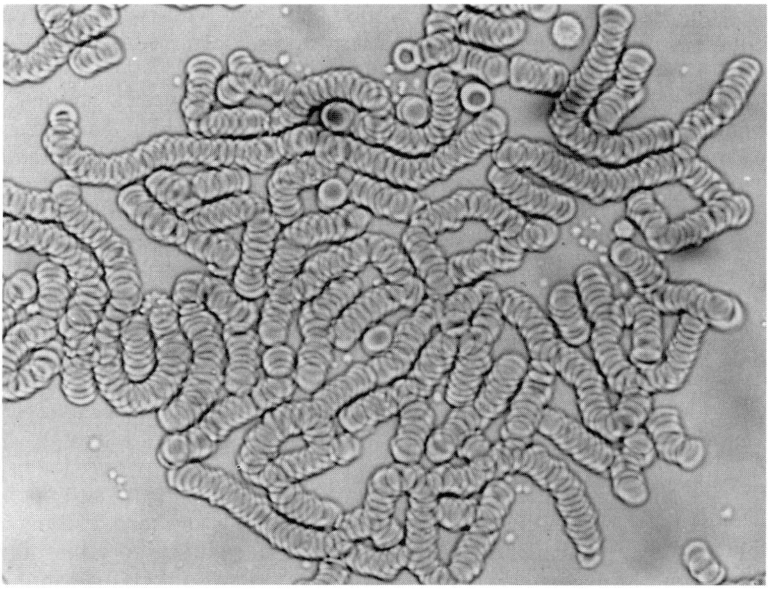

FIGURE 3.—Cover-slip preparation of patient's blood shows rouleaux formation in long chains. (Courtesy of Kwaan HC, Levin M, Sakurai S, et al: Digital ischemia and gangrene due to red blood cell aggregation induced by acquired dysfibrinogenemia. *J Vasc Surg* 26:1061–1068, 1997.)

sodilators brought no relief. Over the following 3 weeks, gangrene continued in the 2 fingers and amputation was needed. The patient's blood showed a marked RBC aggregation with rouleaux formation in long chains (Fig 3), and the presence of an abnormal fibrinogen capable of aggregating normal RBC. Raman spectroscopy showed this fibrinogen to have an increased α-helical content and a decreased β-sheet content. The patient's symptoms were dramatically reduced within 6 hours after defibrinogenation therapy with ancrod was initiated. The therapy continued for 2 weeks. Aggregation of RBCs disappeared after 2 months and no further symptoms appeared.

Conclusion.—Because the rouleaux formation was concentration-dependent, symptomatic relief in this case appears to have resulted from the decreased plasma fibrinogen level. The disappearance of abnormal fibrinogen and an absence of family history indicate an acquired dysfibrinogenemia.

► I chose this article because of my impression that this disease may be considerably more prevalent than suggested by a single case report. This patient clearly had an abnormal fibrinogen, producing rouleaux formation of red cells with arterial occlusion. Defibrinogenation with ancrod resulted in dramatic clinical improvement. Interestingly, a test 6 months later showed that the abnormal fibrinogen had disappeared, revealing this to be an acquired dysfibrinogenemia. I wonder how many patients presenting with digital gangrene in our clinical practice have this condition, which we are missing simply because of lack of familiarity?

12 Carotid and Cerebrovascular Disease

Clinical Series

Early Outcome Assessment for 2228 Consecutive Carotid Endarterectomy Procedures: The Cleveland Clinic Experience From 1989 to 1995

Hertzer NR, O'Hara PJ, Mascha EJ, et al (Cleveland Clinic Found, Ohio)

J Vasc Surg 26:1–10, 1997 12–1

Objective.—Whereas a number of prospective randomized trials have shown the benefits of carotid endarterectomy (CEA) vs. nonoperative management for stroke prevention in patients with severe carotid stenosis, the safety of CEA relies on a number of factors including patient selection. The cumulative experience with CEA at the Cleveland Clinic from 1989 through 1995 was reviewed to study the feasibility of a prospective early outcome assessment.

Methods.—During the study period, 2,228 CEAs, including 153 reoperations for recurrent stenosis, were performed in 2,046 patients (Table 1).

Results.—The early mortality rate was 0.5% for isolated operation and significantly higher (5.3%) for combined CEA and coronary artery bypass grafting (CABG) surgeries. Mortality tended to be higher in women (8.9%) and in patients who had had a prior stroke (12%). The perioperative stroke rate was 1.8% for isolated operations and significantly higher (4.3%) for combined CEA-CABG surgeries. The stroke rate for isolated procedures was 2.8% in women and 1.3% in men. The stroke rate for CEA-CABG procedures was 3.1% in asymptomatic patients and 5.7% in patients with a history of stroke. Patients with vein patches had a significantly lower stroke rate than patients with synthetic patches (1.3% vs. 3.3%). In reoperated patients, the mortality rate was 1.5% for isolated surgeries. The perioperative stroke rates were 4.4% for isolated procedures, 2.1% for patients with a history of transient ischemic attacks (TIAs), 4.0% for patients with asymptomatic recurrence, and 15% for patients with prior strokes. Multivariate analysis showed that the material

TABLE 1.—Basic Demographic Data

	Isolated CEA		Combined CEA-CABG		Total	
	No.	%	No.	%	No.	%
Procedures	1924	86	304	14	2228	100
Men	1272	66	213	70	1486	67
Women	652	34	90	30	742	33
Age (yr)						
Range	35 to 92		45 to 87		35 to 92	
Mean	69		69		69	
Indications						
Asymptomatic Stenosis	1174	61	227	75	1401	63
TIA or amaurosis	514	27	53	17	566	25
Prior stroke	236	12	24	8	261	12

Abbrevations: CEA, carotid endarterectomy; *CABG*, coronary artery bypass grafting; *TIA*, transient ischemic attack.
(Courtesy of Hertzer NR, O'Hara PJ, Mascha EJ, et al: Early outcome assessment for 2228 consecutive carotid endarterectomy procedures: The Cleveland Clinic experience from 1989 to 1995. *J Vasc Surg* 26:1–10, 1997.)

used to patch the arteriotomy was significantly related to stroke and mortality rates.

Conclusions.—In this study, women had significantly higher risks than men for stroke and for death. Although patients with synthetic patches had a higher incidence of perioperative stroke, there were too few patients to validate this observation. The value of this prospective outcome assessment is its ability to reconcile indications for CEA with results.

▶ Isn't it interesting to note that the authors of this large carotid series from the Cleveland Clinic report that 61% of all CEAs were performed prophylactically on asymptomatic patients? Considering the minimal patient benefit described in the Asymptomatic Carotid Atherosclerosis Study,[1] I wonder whether we may have gone a bit overboard in our performance of prophylactic carotid surgery. I am especially concerned when such prophylactic surgery is extended to the extremes of age, especially those older than 80 years. If the bean counters forced a significant reduction in prophylactic CEA, I suspect a number of our patients may actually be better off.

Reference

1. Young B, Moore WS, Robertson JT, et al: An analysis of perioperative surgical mortality and morbidity in the asymptomatic carotid atherosclerosis study. ACAS Investigators. Asymptomatic Carotid Atherosclerosis Study. *Stroke* 27:2216–2224, 1996.

Completion Angiography, Is It Really Necessary?

Ricotta JJ, O'Brien-Irr MS (State Univ of New York at Buffalo)
Am J Surg 174:181–184, 1997 12–2

Background.—Many investigators recommend routine completion imaging after carotid endarterectomy to detect unsuspected defects and to

Methods.—Data from 999 patients who were treated with best medical care and CEA and from 997 patients who had best medical care alone were analyzed. All patients were recruited by the North American Symptomatic Carotid Endarterectomy Trial (NASCET). Patients made regular clinic visits. About 69% of the patients were men, and the mean age was about 65 years.

Results.—At baseline, mean blood pressure was 146.2/81.9 mm Hg for patients who had surgery and 145.2/81.2 mm Hg for patients who had medical treatment only. In the first month after randomization, mean systolic and diastolic pressure increased by about 2.5%, then decreased during the next year, and remained relatively stable thereafter. During follow-up, patients who underwent surgery had slightly higher blood pressure than patients who had medical treatment only. At 2 years, mean systolic pressure in the two patient groups converged at 147.6 mm Hg. Mean diastolic pressure in patients who had medical treatment alone returned to baseline values, but blood pressure in patients who had surgery was slightly elevated by 0.5 mm Hg. The percentage of patients taking antihypertensive medication reflected the rise and fall seen in patients' blood pressure. The use of antihypertensive medication declined sharply at 1 month in both treatment groups but then increased. At the end of 2 years, about 63% of the patients were taking antihypertensive medication.

Discussion.—These findings indicate that CEA does not affect long-term blood pressure. The use of antihypertensive medication seems to be the key element in the treatment of blood pressure. Strict regulation of blood pressure is vitally important in patients with cerebrovascular disease because hypertension is related to neurologic morbidity and mortality.

► Another thin slice rolls off the giant salami roll at the headquarters of the NASCET study. The authors accurately observe that a number of studies have found an increase in blood pressure, both intraoperatively and postoperatively after CEA, generally attributed to accidental operative damage to the carotid sinus baroreceptor and carotid sinus nerve. These authors also accurately observe that heretofore it has been unclear whether blood pressure elevation persists in the long-term, as few studies have followed patients beyond the postoperative period. The present study examined the long-term pattern of blood pressure in patients after CEA in comparison with patients undergoing medical treatment only. In a total of almost 2,000 patients, half of whom received medical therapy and half of whom had CEA, and a mean follow-up in excess of 2 years, they concluded that CEA did not affect long-term blood pressure. What a relief!

Carotid Resection and Replacement With Autogenous Arterial Graft During Operation for Neck Malignancy

Sessa CN, Morasch MD, Berguer R, et al (Wayne State Univ, Detroit, Mich)

Ann Vasc Surg 12:229–235, 1998 12–9

Background.—The use of carotid artery resection as part of the treatment of advanced head and neck cancer is controversial. Since 1991, the authors have performed resection of the carotid artery with immediate reconstruction using superficial femoral artery as the replacement conduit in 30 patients.

Methods.—Thirty patients with primary, metastatic, or recurrent squamous cell cancer involving the carotid artery in the neck had carotid replacement with autogenous superficial femoral artery during radical resection of the tumor. The 30 patients consisted of 22 men and 8 women with a mean age of 60 years. A history of tobacco use was reported by 97% of the patients, and a history of alcohol use was reported by 80%. The mean follow-up was 20 months (range, 3 to 76 months).

Results.—Among the 30 patients, there was 1 stroke-related death. Neck wound problems developed in 43% of the patients, but no grafts failed or hemorrhaged. From the time of operation, the mean life expectancy was 16 months. At the time of death, 58% patients had no local recurrence. At 2 years, the disease-free survival rate was 35% (Fig 1).

Discussion.—These results compare favorably with results of alternative treatments, including carotid ligation and shaving of tumor from the carotid artery. Because cerebral perfusion and local tumor control are so important, the authors suggest the use of superficial femoral artery as a durable conduit for immediate extracranial carotid reconstruction. Size, mechanical strength, and resistance to infection and thrombosis make this

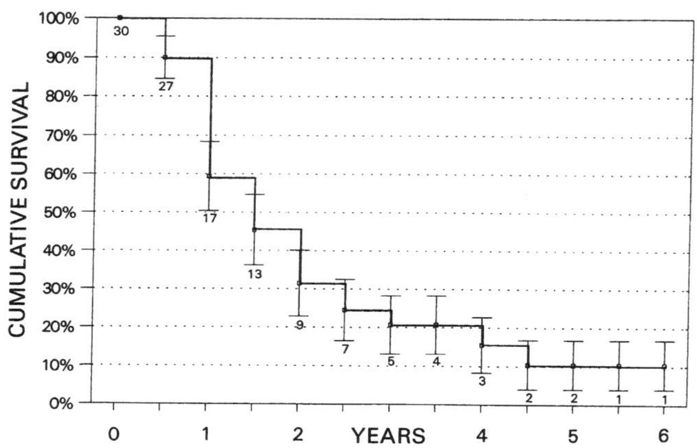

FIGURE 1.—Overall cumulative patient survival curves (numbers indicate patients at risk). (Courtesy of Sessa CN, Morasch MD, Berguer R, et al: Carotid resection and replacement with autogenous arterial graft during operation for neck malignancy. *Ann Vasc Surg* 12:229–235, 1998.)

artery a good alternative conduit in the often hostile environment associated with resection of extensive cancer of the neck.

▶ Many of us are called upon with some frequency to assist head and neck cancer surgeons when they find malignant tumors involving the carotid artery. We have routinely replaced the carotid artery, when necessary, with saphenous vein and have recognized no difficulty with this conduit. These authors believe that the use of a vein graft in potentially contaminated, frequently irradiated fields may be attended by an occasional blowout. I am sure this is true, but we have not seen it to date. They have made the peculiar decision to use the superficial femoral artery (SFA) as a carotid replacement, followed by prosthetic replacement of the femoral artery. I reiterate that I have absolutely no use for prosthetic graft replacement below the inguinal ligament. I believe the authors' selection of the SFA makes no sense unless they have a peculiarly bad local problem with carotid replacement vein blowout, which, as stated above, we have never seen. At the very least, I have to state that I respectfully disagree with the authors' choice of replacement conduit.

Prophylactic Carotid Endarterectomy

Natural History and Management of the Asymptomatic, Moderately Stenotic Internal Carotid Artery

Rockman CB, Riles TS, Lamparello PJ, et al (New York Univ)
J Vasc Surg 25:423–431, 1997 12–10

Objective.—Indications for prophylactic carotid endarterectomy in patients with asymptomatic severe stenosis published in the Asymptomatic Carotid Atherosclerosis Study (ACAS) are controversial. Results of a retrospective review of the natural history of 496 arteries in 425 patients with

TABLE 1.—Neurologic Events and Progression of Stenosis Occurring in Follow-up

	Clinical only (%)	Duplex and clinical (%) Stable (50–79%)	Duplex and clinical (%) Progressive (>80%)	Totals (%)
ASX	208 (97.2)	217 (92.7)*	30 (62.5)*	455 (91.7)
TIA	0 (0)	12 (5.1)†	13 (27.1)†	25 (5.0)
CVA	6 (2.8)	5 (2.1)‡	5 (10.4)‡	16 (3.2)
Total	214	234	48	496

*(92.7% vs. 62.5%) $P < 0.001$.
†(5.1% vs. 27.1%) $P = 0.001$.
‡(2.1% vs. 10.4%) $P < 0.02$.
Abbreviations: ASX, asymptomatic; *CVA*, cerebrovascular accident.
(Courtesy of Rockman CB, Riles TS, Lamperello PJ, et al: Natural history and management of the asymptomatic, moderately stenotic internal carotid artery. *J Vasc Surg* 25:423–431, 1997.)

TABLE 2.—Life Table Analysis for Stroke, TIA, and Progression of Stenosis

Year	*Stroke (N = 496) (%)*	*TIA (N = 496) (%)*	*Stenosis progression (N = 282) (%)*
1	0.85 (±0.4)	1.9 (±0.6)	4.9 (±1.3)
2	1.6 (±0.6)	3.6 (±0.9)	11.8 (±2.1)
3	3.6 (±0.9)	5.5 (±1.1)	16.7 (±2.5)
4	3.6 (±0.9)	6.3 (±1.3)	22.6 (±3.2)
5	5.4 (±1.6)	6.3 (±1.3)	26.5 (±4.0)
6	5.4 (±1.6)	6.3 (±1.3)	33.9 (±7.9)

Note: Results expressed as cumulative percentage by year (±standard error of cumulative percentage).

(Courtesy of Rockman CB, Riles TS, Lamperello PJ, et al: Natural history and management of the asymptomatic, moderately stenotic internal carotid artery. *J Vasc Surg* 25:423–431, 1997).

asymptomatic moderate carotid artery stenosis (50% to 79%) are presented.

Methods.—Patients (48.5% female), average age 74.5, were followed up on average for 38 months, during which time 51 died. Degree of stenosis was determined with pulsed-wave duplex Doppler scans. Data were analyzed statistically.

Results.—Significant events occurring during the follow-up period were documented (Table 1). New ipsilateral strokes occurred in 1 artery in each of 16 patients (3.8%), new transient ischemic attacks (TIAs) in 25 patients (5.9%), and progression of stenosis in 48 of 282 arteries (17%) that underwent follow-up Doppler scanning. Patients with documented progression had significantly more new ipsilateral strokes and significantly more TIAs than did patients with stable stenosis (10.4% vs. 2.1% and 27.1% vs. 5.1%, respectively). Patients with diabetes were significantly more likely to have a TIA than patients without diabetes (9.8% vs. 3.3%). Arteries without progression of stenosis were significantly more likely to remain asymptomatic than arteries with stenotic progression (92.1% vs. 62.5%). Life table analysis of stroke, TIA, and progression of stenosis for years 1 to 6 were calculated (Table 2). Overall survival at 1, 3, and 5 years was 98%, 92.2%, and 77%. The cumulative stroke rate was significantly higher in patients with arteries with progression of stenosis than in patients with arteries that remained stable.

Conclusion.—Based on the low incidence of neurologic events at 5 years, prophylactic endarterectomy is not recommended for patients with moderate carotid artery stenosis. Prophylactic endarterectomy is recommended for patients with greater than 80% carotid artery stenosis.

► It appears that these authors have attempted to duplicate the ACAS in their own department. They found a large number of patients with moderate (50% to 79%) carotid stenosis defined by the University of Washington criteria, and followed these for a number of years and found that very few had trouble. The 5-year stroke rate in these patients was only 5.4%. However, of course, some arteries did progress, and those that showed progressive stenosis were much more likely to cause mischief than those that did not. I suppose I will take this study as a vindication of the ACAS study, although I am not quite sure why the authors went to so much trouble.

Prophylactic Carotid Endarterectomy in Patients With High-Grade Carotid Stenosis Undergoing Coronary Bypass: Does It Decrease the Incidence of Perioperative Stroke?

Hines GL, Scott WC, Schubach SL, et al (Winthrop-Univ Hosp, Mineola, NY)

Ann Vasc Surg 12:23–27, 1998 12–11

Background.—Many factors are involved in the etiology of perioperative stroke in patients who have isolated coronary artery bypass grafting (CABG), although high-grade internal carotid artery stenosis is believed to be a significant cause.

Methods.—Between April 1992 and June 1995, isolated CABG was performed in 2,188 patients. Results of preoperative carotid duplex scanning were available for 1,686 of those patients. There was 80% to 99% stenosis of at least one carotid artery in 4% of the patients. Group 1 consisted of 15 patients who had coronary bypass without carotid intervention, and group 2 consisted of 53 patients who had carotid endarterectomy (CEA) either before coronary bypass or simultaneously with coronary bypass. The age, sex, history of neurologic events, ejection fraction, number of distal bypasses, total pump time, and aortic cross clamp times were similar in both groups.

Results.—In group 1, a permanent postoperative neurologic defect ipsilateral to the high-grade stenosis developed in 3 patients, and a transient defect ipsilateral to the appropriate carotid lesion developed in 1 patient. No transient or permanent neurologic deficits were seen in group 2. In group 1, one patient with a global neurologic deficit died. In group 2, one patient who had prophylactic CEA before coronary bypass died 2 weeks after coronary bypass.

Discussion.—Statistical analysis of these results showed a significant decrease in total neurologic events and permanent neurologic deficits in patients who had prophylactic CEA. Patients with 80% to 99% carotid stenosis who have CEA before or at the same time as isolated CABG have a lower risk of postoperative neurologic events.

► We have all been swamped in recent years by the controversy surrounding the patient who has an urgent need for CABG and is also found to have high-grade carotid stenosis, be it symptomatic or asymptomatic. In an attempt to shed at least a thin ray of light on this controversial topic, these authors screened a large number of patients undergoing CABG and discovered 68 patients from a cohort of 1,686 who had 80% to 99% carotid stenosis. We are not told whether these patients had symptoms from a carotid standpoint. Fifteen of these patients proceeded directly to CABG

ties in our area. I commend these authors for their excellent results, and I hope that one day soon we will find a patient on whom to perform the operation.

Randomised Trial of Endarterectomy for Recently Symptomatic Carotid Stenosis: Final Results of the MRC European Carotid Surgery Trial (ECST)

Warlow C, for the European Carotid Surgery Trialists' Collaborative Group (Western Gen Hosp, Edinburgh, Scotland)

Lancet 351:1379–1381, 1998 12–18

Objective.—Results of a multicenter, randomized controlled trial designed to test the risk and benefit of carotid endarterectomy in patients with symptomatic internal carotid artery (ICA) are presented.

Methods.—Between 1981 and 1994, 3,024 patients with at least 1 transient or mild symptomatic ischemic vascular event in the carotid artery were randomly assigned to surgery (n = 1,811) or to avoidance of surgery as long as possible (n = 1,213). Patients were followed up for an average of 6.1 years. Stroke, surgical events, nonstroke vascular death, and nonvascular death were the outcomes measured.

Results.—There were 3,018 patients in the trial analysis. The surgery group had 669 events, and the nonsurgery group had 442 (Fig 1). Whereas the risk of major stroke or death associated with surgery was 7% regardless of the degree of stenosis, the risk of same-side major ischemic stroke increased with the degree of carotid artery stenosis during the first 2 to 3 years of the trial. After that there was no relation between stroke risk and degree of stenosis. There was an advantage to surgery when stenosis

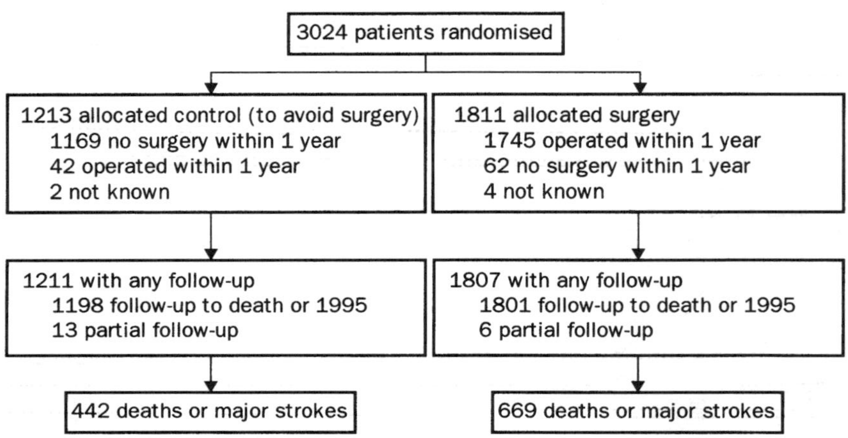

FIGURE 1.—Trial profile. (Courtesy of Warlow C, for the European Carotid Surgery Trialists' Collaborative Group: Randomised trial of endarterectomy for recently symptomatic carotid stenosis: Final results of the MRC European carotid surgery trial (ECST). *Lancet* 351:1379–1381, 1998. Copyright by The Lancet Ltd.)

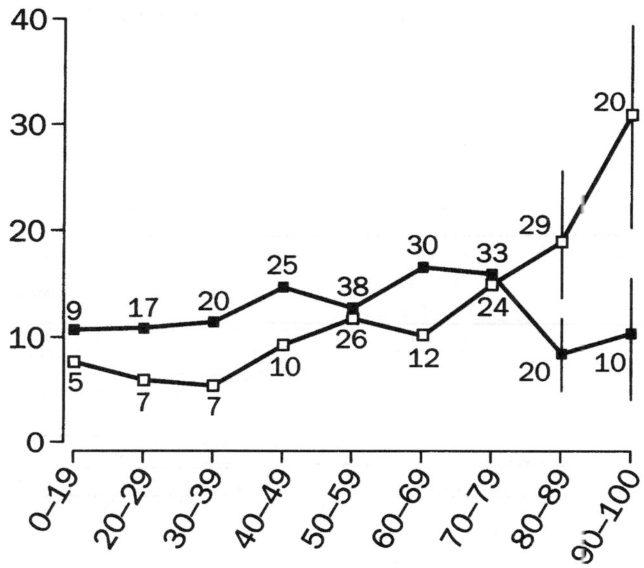

FIGURE 2.—Predicted risk of any major stroke at 3 years and actual risk of a surgical event. For surgical events, the actual risk is plotted. For ipsilateral major ischemic stroke and other major strokes, the predicted risk at 3 years is plotted. The combined outcome is predicted risk of any major stroke at 3 years and actual risk of a surgical event. *Numbers above curves*-numbers of patients with event. *Vertical bars*-95% CI. (Courtesy of Warlow C, for the European Carotid Surgery Trialists' Collaborative Group: Randomised trial of endarterectomy for recently symptomatic carotid stenosis: Final results of the MRC European carotid surgery trial (ECST). *Lancet* 351:1379–1381, 1998. Copyright by The Lancet Ltd.)

exceeded 80% (Fig 2). At 3 years the absolute benefit of surgery was 11.6%, although the effects of age and sex were significant mitigating factors. A model for estimating change in total life expectancy free of major stroke for men and women depends on age and severity of stenosis.

Conclusion.—Carotid endarterectomy is recommended for patients with a recent ischemic event and symptomatic stenosis greater than 80%. Risk of major stroke is significantly associated with age and sex.

▶ The ECST has always stood as the continental equivalent of NASCET, although clear differences were apparent in the recruitment requirements for the two groups. The ECST randomized 1,811 patients to surgery and 1,213 to control, and the mean follow-up is now in excess of 6 years. Overall, the 3-year risk of major stroke or death was 26.5% for the control group and 14.9% for the surgery group, with the greatest benefit occurring in patients with severe stenosis above 70% to 80% when first seen. A rather complex algorithm for patient selection is presented in this article, including the adverse effects of female gender and age in estimating risk. On balance, this article is complex and, in my opinion, adds little substantive information to that already published.

Natural History of Stenosis From Intracranial Atherosclerosis by Serial Angiography

Akins PT, Pilgram TK, Cross DT III, et al (Washington Univ, St Louis; Mercy Healthcare Sacramento, Calif)
Stroke 29:433–438, 1998 12–19

Introduction.—Patients with intracranial atherosclerosis are at increased risk for stroke, heart disease, and death. Management of such patients has included both aspirin and warfarin, but no prospective studies have compared these 2 treatments. The value of cerebral percutaneous transluminal angioplasty in patients refractory to medical treatment is also uncertain. A retrospective review sought to determine the natural history of stenoses caused by intracranial atherosclerosis.

Methods.—A review of files at the study institution identified 28 patients with moderate or severe atherosclerosis in an intracranial vessel. Angiograms from 5 patients were incomplete or missing, and 2 additional patients did not fulfill study criteria, leaving 21 patients with a total of 45 stenoses suitable for serial measurement. Quantitative measurements were made in a blinded manner and clinical outcomes reviewed.

Results.—The average age of the patient group was 62; 62% were men and 81% were white. Carotid bifurcation disease was present in 86%, hypertension in 76%, and ischemic stroke in 48%; 71% were smokers. Patients had undergone repeat angiography at an average interval of 26.7 months. The average stenosis for all intracranial lesions was 43.9% at initial evaluation vs. 51.8% at follow-up. Progression occurred in the average stenosis in anterior cerebral (ACA), middle cerebral (MCA), and posterior cerebral (PCA) arteries (range 32.4% to 49.7%), whereas the average stenosis in the intracranial internal carotid artery (ICA) was stable (51.2% vs. 52.6%). Progression of at least 10% was seen in 20% of intracranial ICA lesions, and in 61% of ACA, MCA, and PCA lesions. Regression was also seen in 14% of intracranial ICA lesions, and in 28% of ACA, MCA, and PCA lesions. Four transient ischemic attacks and 1 intracerebral hemorrhage occurred during follow-up.

Conclusion.—Among stenoses associated with intracranial atherosclerosis, lesion progression occurs frequently. Medium-sized vessels are most likely to show progression, and intracranial ICA lesions are more stable than ACA, MCA, and PCA lesions. However, regression can also occur during follow-up.

▶ It is surprising how limited our database is concerning progression of intracranial atherosclerotic stenoses. Clearly, a significant number of atherothrombotic clinical events result from this source. This interesting study from Washington University provides considerable important information. Far more intracranial lesions progressed than extracranial lesions. Regression was infrequent. This focused article is recommended as a source of information concerning the progression of intracranial atherosclerotic lesions.

Lipid-Rich Carotid Artery Plaques Appear Echolucent on Ultrasound B-Mode Images and May Be Associated With Intraplaque Haemorrhage

Grønholdt M-LM, Wiebe BM, Laursen H, et al (Univ Hosp of Copenhagen)

Eur J Vasc Endovasc Surg 14:439–445, 1997 12–20

Objective.—One recent study found that echolucent and heterogeneous carotid artery plaques are associated with a higher risk of neurologic

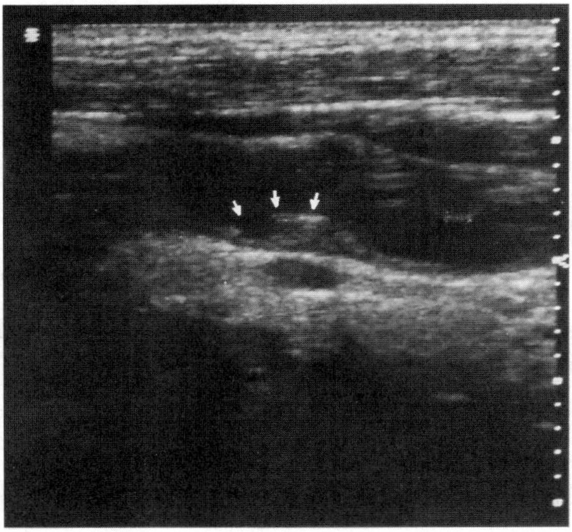

(a)

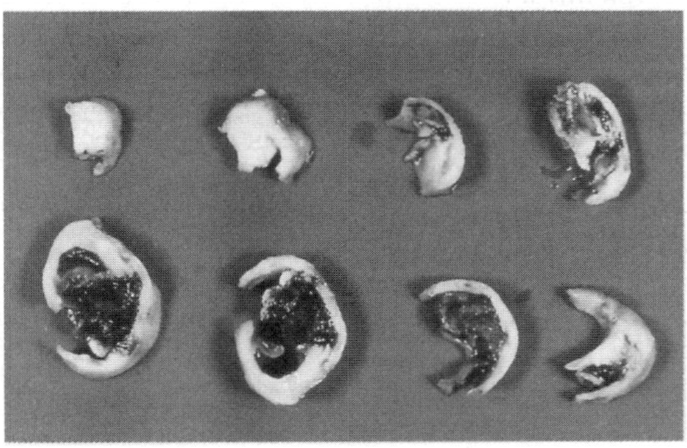

(b)

FIGURE 1.—An echolucent plaque: **a**, Ultrasound B-mode image of the plaque, indicated by arrows. Distance between dots on right-hand scale is 2 mm. *Abbreviations: CCA*, common carotid artery. *ICA*, internal carotid artery. **b**, Photograph of the sliced plaque after removal by endarterectomy. The atheromatous regions indicated by *arrows* are associated with a high lipid/hemorrhage content. (Courtesy of Grønholdt M-LM, Wiebe BM, Laursen H, et al: Lipid-rich carotid artery plaques appear echolucent on ultrasound B-mode images and may be associated with intraplaque haemorrhage. *Eur J Vasc Endovasc Surg* 14:439–445, 1997. Reprinted by permission of the WB Saunders Company Limited, London.)

symptoms than are echo-rich and homogeneous plaques. Ultrasonic plaque morphology, risk factors, and plasma lipids were prospectively compared to detailed histomorphometric analysis of removed carotid specimens in a consecutive, single-center trial.

Methods.—Plaque morphology of 78 patients (22 women), aged 44 to 79, undergoing carotid endarterectomy, was evaluated preoperatively with the use of ultrasound Duplex scanning. Echogenicity was classified as echo rich, intermediate, or echolucent (Fig 1). Endarterectomy specimens were analyzed morphometrically to determine lipid content and degree of hemorrhage, calcification, and fibrous tissue. Ultrasonic features, histomorphometric results, and risk factors for atherosclerosis were correlated by means of nonparametric analysis.

Results.—Degree of stenosis ranged from 50% to 79% in 26 (33%) patients and from 80% to 99% in 53 (67%) patients. Age, sex, clinical history, and lifestyle were not significantly related to plaque echogenicity or histomorphometric results. Plaque echogenicity was significantly related to calcification and fibrous tissue and inversely related to lipid content. There was significantly more calcification in heterogeneous and irregular plaques than in homogeneous and regular-surface plaques. The amount of intraplaque hemorrhage was significantly correlated with lipid content and inversely correlated with fibrous tissue content. Patients whose neurologic symptoms had been present for more than 3 months had significantly higher amounts of calcification than patients with more recent neurologic symptoms.

Conclusion.—With B-mode ultrasonography, echolucent carotid artery plaques show a higher lipid and a lower fibrous tissue content than echo-rich plaques.

► See also Abstract 12C-17. If the risks of hemorrhage, plaque rupture, and brain infarcts were all related to echolucent lipid-rich plaques, we should have an important window through which to study some big killers, especially stroke and probably myocardial infarction. Both of these catastrophes may be initiated by plaque causing hemodynamically unimportant stenosis. Plaque morphology may prove to be as important in the selection of patients for operation as the degree of stenosis. At present, we have only histologic snapshots but the prospect of plaque surveillance and risk modification is now in view.

A.E.B. Giddings, M.D.

► Two of the obvious problems with this study are the very low number of autogenous grafts, only 25, and the inclusion of 21 prosthetic grafts. Numerous publications call into question the value of duplex surveillance of prosthetic grafts, and their inclusion in this article, in my opinion, severely weakens the results. The authors conclude that a significant number of grafts predicted to fail by duplex actually remained patent during their mean follow-up of 10 months. I am not at all sure what this means. Abundant literature attests to the benefit of graft surveillance, and a randomized, prospective study confirmed enhanced patency results owing to preemptive revision of failing grafts.[1] I regard the conclusions of the authors herein as only interesting, certainly not definitive.

Reference

1. Lundell A, Lindblad B, Bergqvist D, et al: Femoropopliteal-crural graft patency is improved by an intensive surveillance program: A prospective randomized study. *J Vasc Surg* 21:26–34, 1995.

Percutaneous Angioplasty for Infrainguinal Graft-related Stenoses

Houghton AD, Todd C, Pardy B, et al (Guys Hosp, London)

Eur J Vasc Endovasc Surg 14:380–385, 1997 13–7

Background.—Stenoses can occur after both venous and polytetrafluoroethylene (PTFE) grafts. These authors report their experience with percutaneous transluminal angioplasty (PTA) in treating infrainguinal graft-related stenoses.

Methods.—Forty-two patients had a total of 56 dilated stenoses in 42 infrainguinal grafts. The site of the stenosis, its length, and its type were recorded for both venous (34) and PTFE (8) grafts. Follow-up continued until the patient was discharged, the graft was irretrievably occluded, or the patient died (median follow-up 13 months).

Findings.—Each of the 56 stenoses was treated by PTA; 4 were lost to follow-up. Of the remaining 52 stenoses, PTA was successful in treating the occlusion in 48 stenoses. In the 48 successful cases of PTA, 36 stenoses were patent, 8 were occluded, and 4 were lost to follow-up. In the 36 patent stenoses, 14 required further intervention (repeat PTA, jump grafts, or vein patch). Causes of the 8 occluded stenoses were occluded veins, multiple stenoses, and a PTFE graft that occluded soon after PTA. Overall graft patency at 1 year was 84% (27 of 32 grafts). Short localized stenoses responded better to PTA (9 of 11 venous grafts) than did long stenoses (5 of 5 long venous grafts required re-operation or occluded). Also, grafts with 2 or fewer stenoses fared better than those with 3 or more stenoses.

Conclusions.—PTA was successful in treating localized stenosis in 84% (48 of 57) cases. It was most successful when the stenosis was less than 2 cm long and when 2 or fewer stenoses were present. Also, mid-graft stenoses in PTFE grafts responded less well to PTA. Thus PTA should be considered for treating graft-related stenoses in vein grafts and anastomotic stenoses in PTFE grafts.

▶ Transluminal angioplasty for correction of stenoses occurring in infrainguinal vein grafts makes no sense to me. The very poor results reported here appear to support my opinion. Forced dilatation of collagenous stenosis can only result in tearing of the collagen and the real possibility of graft disruption. Even if this does not occur, the torn collagen would appear to be a very poor substrate for wound healing, and I am sure significantly explains the poor results experienced by most who have tried this procedure. (See also Abstract 2–19.)

Allografts

Immunosuppression for Human Saphenous Vein Allograft Bypass Surgery: A Prospective Randomized Trial

Carpenter JP, Tomaszewski JE (Univ of Pennsylvania, Philadelphia)

J Vasc Surg 26:32–42, 1997 13–8

Introduction.—Autogenous saphenous vein is the graft material of choice in patients undergoing lower extremity peripheral bypass surgery. Vein allografts are an alternative bypass conduit for patients with inadequate autogenous vein, but transplant rejection remains a problem. Animal trials have shown that vein patency can be augmented by low-dose immunosuppression using azathioprine. The effects of low-dose immunosuppression with azathioprine were assessed in human saphenous vein allograft recipients in a prospective, randomized, controlled, parallel group trial.

Methods.—Forty patients (20 men, 20 women) with pain or tissue loss requiring bypass grafting to pedal or crural outflow and inadequate autogenous saphenous vein were randomized to receive (n = 17) or not receive (n = 23) azathioprine 1 mg/kg/day after undergoing cryopreserved vein allograft bypass grafting. Anti-HLA antibody screens were conducted before and after surgery. Biopsies were taken of allografts at implantation and at all subsequent opportunities. Patients underwent postoperative physical and vascular laboratory assessments every 3 months.

Results.—Ten patients died during a 31-month follow-up interval, of causes unrelated to immunosuppression. Rates of primary graft patency and limb salvage were 13% and 42%, respectively, at 12 months. Positive preoperative anti-HLA antibody screen in 8 patients approached significance ($P = 0.09$) as a predictor of graft failure. Thirteen of 22 (59%) explanted grafts had histologic evidence of rejection (6 immunosuppressed, 7 control). In 7 patients with negative preoperative anti-HLA antibody screens, results were positive after surgery. In 6 patients with positive preoperative anti-HLA screens, results became more strongly positive after surgery.

Conclusion.—Vein graft failure is partly mediated by rejection that includes both humoral (antibody) and cellular reactions to vein allografts.

This response is not halted by low-dose azathioprine. It is possible that patency rates of vein allograft bypass grafts may be enhanced by more potent immunosuppression and improvement in allograft procurement, preservation, and matching.

▶ Forty patients receiving cryopreserved venous allografts as lower extremity bypass grafts for limb salvage, accompanied by randomized administration of azathioprine, experienced a primary graft patency rate at 12 months of 13%, and limb salvage rate of 42%, with no difference between immunosuppressed and control grafts, as measured by mortality, primary graft patency, or limb salvage. Clearly, azathioprine, as used in this study, was of no demonstrable benefit. I continue to find no indication for the clinical use of the cryopreserved venous allograft with or without immunosuppression. In my opinion, a polytetrafluoroethylene prosthesis, especially with the Miller cuff, is a distinctly superior conduit for the occasional patient who simply has no vein available.

In Situ Arterial Allografts: A New Treatment for Aortic Prosthetic Infection

Ruotolo C, Plissonnier D, Bahnini A, et al (Pitié-Salpêtrière Univ Hosp, Paris)
Eur J Vasc Endovasc Surg 14 (suppl A):102–107, 1997 13–9

Background.—Total graft removal, aortic stump closure, and extra-anatomic grafting through uninfected tissues has been the accepted approach to management of aortic graft infection. However, the results can be disappointing in terms of thrombosis and recurrent infection. The risk of aortic stump blowout is unclear. To avoid these problems, various autogenous reconstructions have been proposed. The authors report an in situ arterial allograft technique for treatment of aortic prosthetic infection.

Methods.—The experience included 100 consecutive patients with infected infrarenal aortic prosthetic grafts who were treated by in situ replacement with preserved allografts. The allografts were obtained from cadavers in a multi-organ transplant tissue retrieval program. All were implanted after being preserved for 48 hours, to decrease antigenicity, to 21 days, to avoid late degeneration. Blood and tissue compatibility matching were not performed. Before implantation, bacteriologic culture was performed on the periprosthetic fluid and part of the infected prosthetic graft. The allograft was implanted in situ; the infected prosthetic material was usually removed at the same operation.

Results.—Overall mortality was 24%, with most deaths resulting from septic complications. Mortality was 38% in patients with aorto-enteric fistulas and 19% in those with isolated prosthetic infections. Mortality was 46% for patients undergoing emergency operations vs. 16% for those undergoing planned operations. Of the 13 late deaths, 2 were caused by aortic rupture. Twenty occlusive lesions were detected during follow-up, with successful reoperation in 15 of these. Five patients showed aortic dilation and mural thrombosis on ultrasound and CT scans, although none had to be operated on during follow-up. Three major amputations were performed because of preexisting, irreversible ischemia, but no secondary amputations were required.

Conclusions.—An experience with arterial allografting for the treatment of aortic prosthetic infections is reported. Although not ideal, this technique warrants further investigation. The authors continue to use in situ allograft replacement in patients with infected abdominal aortic grafts.

▶ As I have repeatedly stated, I continue to believe that the optimal treatment for graft infection is the established surgical principle of remote bypass grafting through a clean field followed by excision of the infected graft. This has worked well. Three new methods of dealing with abdominal prosthetic graft infection include in situ prosthetic grafting with rifampicin bonding to Dacron, femoral vein graft in situ replacement, and cryopreserved aortic allograft in situ replacement. Convincing experimental data supporting the use of cryopreserved arterial allograft in this setting are skimpy. I am aware of no persuasive evidence suggesting that the cryopreserved allograft should be uniquely favored when used in an infected field. Kieffer, reporting here, has one of the largest experiences to date with the use of cryopreserved allografts for infection. Unfortunately, the results reported in the present series of 100 patients operated upon for graft infection are not particularly impressive, with an overall mortality of 24%. For the present, I continue to regard graft excision and remote bypass as choice number one, gelatin-Dacron graft impregnated with rifampicin as choice number two, and cryopreserved aortic allograft as last choice. (See also Abstract 13–10.)

Treatment of Vascular Graft Infection by In Situ Replacement With Cryopreserved Aortic Allografts: An Experimental Study

Knosalla C, Goëau-Brissonnière O, Leflon V, et al (Pitié-Salpêtrière Univ Hosp, Paris; Ambroise-Paré Univ Hosp, Boulogne-Billancourt, France; Broussais Univ Hosp, Paris; et al)

J Vasc Surg 27:689–698, 1998 13–10

Objective.—Infection of prosthetic grafts, particularly of aortic grafts, is a serious complication. In an effort to avoid extra-anatomic repair techniques, in situ replacement methods have been investigated. The efficacy of cryopreserved aortic allografts to treat established vascular graft infection by in situ replacement was tested in an animal model, and the role of antibiotics normally used for decontamination of the allograft during the cryopreservation process was evaluated.

Methods.—The infrarenal aortas in 23 dogs were replaced with gelatin-sealed knitted polyester grafts contaminated with *Staphylococcus epidermidis* RP-62. A week later, grafts were removed from 18 surviving animals and replaced with untreated gelatin-sealed knitted polyester vascular prostheses (control group I) (n = 6), untreated cryopreserved allografts (group

TABLE 4.—Bacteriologic Evaluation of Graft Infection With *S. epidermidis* RP-62

	No. with positive culture/total examined		
	Grafts	*Fragments*	*Viable counts (CFU/cm^2): median (range)*
Group I			
Initial grafts	6/6	12/12	7.9×10^4 (6×10^3 to 1×10^6)
Control grafts	6/6	12/12	9.8×10^4 (1.6×10^4 to 1.1×10^6)
Group II			
Initial grafts	6/6	12/12	2.03×10^4 (1.94×10^3 to 4.61×10^5)
Untreated allografts	1/6*	2/12†	5.54×10^4
Group III			
Initial grafts	6/6	12/12	3.32×10^3 (1.03×10^3 to 2.95×10^4)
AB-treated allografts	0/6*	0/12‡	0

Initial grafts, colonized gelatin-sealed knitted polyester implanted for 7 days; *control grafts*, in situ replacement with gelatin-sealed knitted polyester grafts; *untreated allografts*, cryopreserved aortic allografts prepared without antibiotics; *AB-treated allografts*, cryopreserved aortic allografts prepared with antibiotics.

*P <0.01 when compared with control grafts and initial grafts.

†P <0.001 when compared with control grafts and initial grafts.

‡P <0.0001 when compared with control grafts and initial grafts. (Courtesy of Knosalla C, Goëau-Brissonnière O, Leflon V: Treatment of vascular graft infection by in situ replacement with cryopreserved aortic allografts: An experimental study. *J Vasc Surg* 27:689–698, 1998.)

II) (n = 6), or antibiotic-treated allografts (group III) (n = 6). Four weeks later, the grafts were harvested for bacteriologic and histologic analysis.

Results.—All initial grafts removed were infected. At 4 weeks, all 6 control replacement grafts were infected, 3 group II grafts were incompletely incorporated, and all group III grafts were completely incorporated (Table 4). The 3 incompletely incorporated grafts in group II showed signs of perigraft inflammation. Whereas 3 group II allografts grew bacteria, all of the antibiotic-treated group III allografts were sterile.

Conclusion.—In this study, cryopreserved, antibiotic-treated allograft replacements for infected vascular grafts were more resistant to reinfection than were untreated gelatin-sealed knitted polyester grafts.

▶ Results from this animal model suggested that antibiotic-soaked allografts produced superior results in the treatment of infected infrarenal aortas. I wish they had used an active control of a rifampicin-bonded sealed Dacron graft. Unfortunately, such was not the case. Thus, I conclude that it is virtually impossible to interpret this article. As stated in Abstract 13–9, I do not accept aortic allografts as superior for treatment of arterial infection.

In Situ Repair of Aortobronchial, Aortoesophageal, and Aortoenteric Fistulae With Cryopreserved Aortic Homografts

Vogt PR, Pfammatter T, Schlumpf R, et al (Univ Hosp Zurich, Switzerland)
J Vasc Surg 26:11–17, 1997 13–11

Objective.—Because of the lack of a consistently effective surgical treatment, fistulas that originate from aortic aneurysms or prosthetic aortic grafts are associated with high mortality rates of 30% to 80%. The

14 Vascular Trauma

Arterial

Popliteal Artery Trauma: Systemic Anticoagulation and Intraoperative Thrombolysis Improves Limb Salvage

Melton SM, Croce MA, Patton JH Jr, et al (Univ of Tennessee, Memphis)
Ann Surg 225:518–529, 1997 14–1

Background.—In both wartime and civilian settings, advances in vascular surgery techniques have continued to lower amputation rates after popliteal artery injuries. Nevertheless, these injuries remain associated with a fairly high rate of amputation and disability. A review of patients treated from April 1985 through November 1995 sought to identify factors related to popliteal artery injury that influence amputation.

TABLE 1.—Mangled Extremity Severity Score (MESS) Variables

A. Skeletal/soft-tissue injury	
Low energy (stab; simple fracture; "civilian" GSW)	1
Medium energy (open or multiple fractures; dislocation)	2
High energy (close-range shotgun or "military" GSW, crush injury)	3
Very high energy (above + gross contamination, soft-tissue avulsion)	4
B. Limb ischemia*	
Pulse reduced or absent but perfusion normal	1
Pulseless: parasthesias, diminished capillary refill	2
Cool, paralyzed, insensate, numb	3
C. Shock	
Systolic BP always >90 mmHg	0
Hypotensive transiently	1
Persistent hypotension	2
D. Age (yr)	
<30	0
30–50	1
>50	2

*Score doubled for ischemia >6 hr.
GSW, gunshot wound; *BP*, blood pressure.
(From Johansen K, Daines M, Howey T, et al: Objective criteria accurately predict amputation following lower extremity trauma. *J Trauma* 30:568–573, 1990. Courtesy of Melton SM, Croce MA, Patton JH Jr, et al: Popliteal artery trauma: Systemic anticoagulation and intraoperative thrombolysis improves limb salvage. *Ann Surg* 225:518–529, 1997.)

TABLE 2.—Ischemia and Ischemia Times (Hours)

Interval	Ischemic (50) AMP (7)	Ischemic (50) No AMP (43)	Nonischemic (38) AMP (5)	Nonischemic (38) No AMP (33)
Inj to TC	1.9	1.9	2.2	2.2
TC to OR	1.8	2.2	3.2	6.0
OR to repair	6.4	5.0	6.3	4.3
Inj to repair	10.1	8.9	11.7	12.0

AMP, amputation; *Inj*, injury; *TC*, trauma center; *OR*, operating room.
(Courtesy of Melton SM, Croce MA, Patton JH Jr, et al: Popliteal artery trauma: Systemic anticoagulation and intraoperative thrombolysis improves limb salvage. *Ann Surg* 225:518–529, 1997.)

Methods.—Patients were identified through the trauma registry of a regional center. Their charts were reviewed for demographics, severity of injury, details of the vascular examination, ischemic times, methods of repair, and the use of heparin and urokinase. The Mangled Extremity Severity Score (MESS) was calculated to quantitate severity of lower limb injury (Table 1). Patients with a MESS of 7 or higher have usually required amputation. Amputations were classified as primary (no attempt at vascular repair) or secondary (after vascular repair).

Results.—Over the 10-year study period, 88 men and 14 women were treated for popliteal artery trauma. Penetrating trauma was the cause of 62 injuries, and blunt trauma was the cause of 40. There were 25 amputations in the patient group; 11 were primary, and 14 were performed after attempts at vascular repair. Blunt trauma was associated with an overall amputation rate of 36% and a secondary amputation rate of 24%. These rates were lower for penetrating injuries (18% and 10%, respectively). Patients with totally ischemic extremities also were more likely to undergo amputation (31% vs. 13%). Although ischemic times did not differ significantly in the salvaged limb and amputated limb groups, the time from operation to repair was longer in the amputated limb group (Table 2). The average MESS in the primary amputation group was 7.6, and all these patients had severe soft tissue injury. Independent factors associated with secondary amputation were blunt injury, vein injury, MESS, and heparin–urokinase therapy.

Conclusion.—The correlation between degree of ischemia and limb salvage in patients with popliteal artery trauma confirms the importance of minimizing ischemia. Morbidity can be reduced by the use of anticoagulation and intraoperative thrombolysis and optimal organization of trauma care.

▶ Isn't it sobering to note that a major trauma center in the modern world still experiences a 25% incidence of lower extremity amputation associated with popliteal artery injury? Only a few of these had nerve transection. I still believe in the old, established principles in the treatment of these patients. They should be revascularized as rapidly as possible, without the delay required for detailed preoperative arteriography. An intraoperative arteriogram can be obtained if absolutely mandatory, although I find in most cases an equally satisfactory repair can be achieved without any arteriography, based entirely on clinical examination.

Traumatic Internal Carotid Artery Dissections Caused by Blunt Softball Injuries

Schievink WI, Atkinson JLD, Bartleson JD, et al (Mayo Clinic, Rochester, Minn)

Am J Emerg Med 16:179–182, 1998 14–2

Background.—Injuries while playing softball or baseball are the leading cause of sports-related emergency department visits in the United States. Most injuries are musculoskeletal, although a few vascular injuries do occur. A patient with an internal carotid artery dissection resulting from blunt trauma from a softball injury was treated by the authors, which prompted them to examine the incidence of this type of injury in their county.

Case Report.—Man, 39, was playing first base and was hit on the right side of his neck when the softball was deflected off his

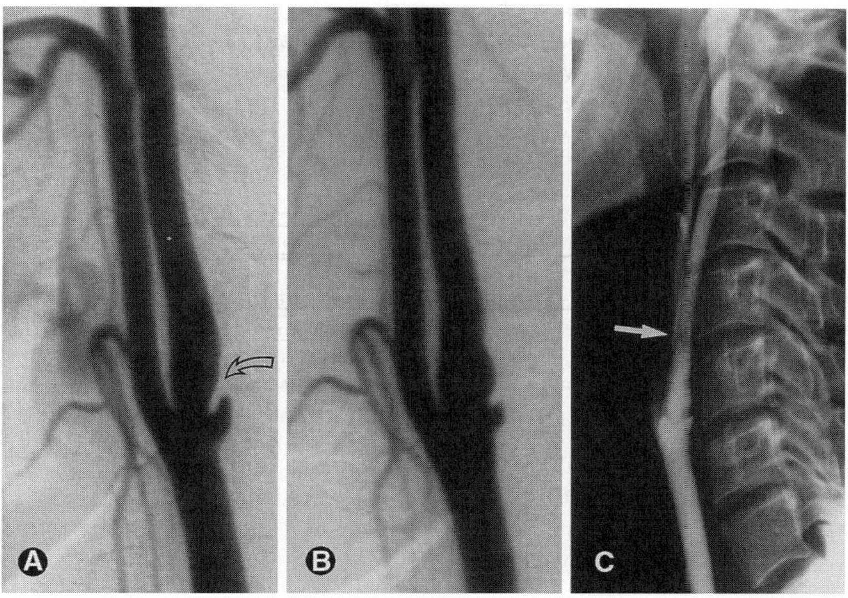

FIGURE 2.—A, right carotid angiogram shows an intimal flap (*curved arrow*) of the proximal internal carotid artery with associated aneurysmal dilatation, consistent with dissection. B, three months later, a repeat angiogram shows improvement in this area of dissection. C, an area of lumina irregularity several centimeters distal to the bifurcation (*arrow*), consistent with thrombosis or intimal flap, has not changed since the previous examination. Note the long neck and low carotid bifurcation. (Courtesy of Schievink WI, Atkinson JLD, Bartleson JD, et al. Traumatic internal carotid artery dissections caused by blunt softball injuries. *Am J Emerg Med* 16:179–182, 1998.)

glove. Soon thereafter he dropped the ball from his glove, presumably because of transient hand weakness. When he was seen in the emergency department 2 hours later, results of clinical examination and CT were normal except for an area of erythema on the right anterolateral neck. Angiography showed an acute dissection of the right extracranial internal carotid artery (Fig 2), with an intimal flap, aneurysmal dilatation, and suspected thrombosis. The carotid artery was bifurcated at the C6 level. After intravenous heparin and a 3-month course of oral anticoagulants, repeat angiography showed improvement (Fig 2). The patient had no evidence of cerebral infarction, and he has had no further neurologic events in the 4 years since the injury.

Findings.—Analysis of medical records covering all of Olmsted County, Minnesota (which includes the Mayo Clinic) identified 4 cases of traumatic carotid artery dissection from 1987 through 1994. Two patients (the man described above and a 35-year-old woman) had carotid artery dissection caused by a blunt softball injury, 1 patient had carotid artery dissection caused by an all-terrain vehicle accident, and 1 patient, by an automobile accident. During this same period, there were 16 cases of spontaneous carotid artery dissection in the county.

Conclusions.—Half of the 4 cases of traumatic carotid artery dissection that occurred in the authors' county were the result of blunt trauma with a softball. All patients who are hit in the anterolateral neck by a softball or baseball and who complain of unusual ipsilateral neck pain or headache should be evaluated for possible carotid artery dissection, even when cerebral ischemic symptoms are absent or mild.

► I include this article because of the thin ray of light it sheds on the contentious issue of carotid dissection caused by blunt trauma. Anyone who consults regularly with the State Industrial Accident Board recognizes that this issue comes up with some modest degree of frequency. Many of the contentious cases that I have seen have first had symptoms days after the apparent traumatic event. I am fascinated to learn that in both of these cases of presumed blunt softball injury, symptoms were immediate. While this adds nothing but a thin shred of anecdotal evidence, I suppose that is marginally better than nothing. I have generally taken the position that if a blunt injury is not followed by symptoms very shortly after the injury, but rather by delay of many days, there is no clear cause and effect relationship apparent. Based on this information, I believe I will stick with this position.

an arm amputated because of extensive soft tissue and bony injury. None of the 20 patients without associated neurologic injury had functional defects at discharge or at follow-up. However, of the 15 patients who did have associated brachial nerve injury, 8 had very severe functional deficits. Functional impairment was still evident at follow-up in these patients, although the disability had improved slightly.

Conclusions.—Patients with thoracic outlet vascular injuries can be successfully treated with an aggressive surgical approach that includes arteriography. Arteriography helps in localizing the injury and planning the surgical approach. Functional results should be good, unless there is associated injury to the brachial nerve. In these latter cases, short- and long-term functional deficits are likely.

▶ In this series of 35 patients with vascular injury of the thoracic outlet, 15 had associated nerve injury, about average. The authors' observation that no functional deficits occurred in patients with an isolated vascular injury is about what we have come to expect. Severe disability occurs in patients with associated brachial plexus injury, exactly as described in this series. I believe we will all have to accept the authors' conclusion that arteriography and enlightened vascular repair is generally quite successful in detecting and repairing major vascular injuries of the "thoracic inlet." (Note: this is the correct term. It is *not* the "thoracic outlet.") As repeatedly stated, however, this is really not the problem. The problem is the functional disability resulting from associated nerve injuries which, as far as I know, lends itself to no solution, save consideration of early amputation. (See also Abstract 14–7.)

Venous

Long-term Results of Lower-Extremity Venous Injuries

Bermudez KM, Knudson MM, Nelken NA, et al (Univ of California, San Francisco)

Arch Surg 132:963–968, 1997 14–9

Introduction.—Venous injuries have been simply ligated during military conflicts, whereas venous repairs with complex interposition grafts are successfully performed in the civilian setting. Little is known, however, about the long-term function of a repaired or ligated venous system. A cohort study of patients with lower extremity injuries was conducted to compare long-term venous function of ligated, simple, and complex repairs and to evaluate long-term patency in repaired veins.

Methods.—The study group included 21 patients with 41 involved extremities. Twenty patients were men, and the mean age of the group was 32.7 years. All had sustained iliac, femoral, or popliteal venous injuries. The patients underwent a thorough history and a physical examination, followed by color flow duplex (CFD) US imaging. They also were studied with air plethysmography (APG), concentrating on the injured extremity and using the contralateral limb as a control. The time from the date of injury ranged from 6 weeks to 336 weeks.

Results.—Six patients underwent venous ligation, 11 had simple repairs, and 4 had complex repairs of venous injuries with interposition grafts. Penetrating trauma was the most common cause of injury (85.7%). All repairs were patent, and CFD venous imaging showed no evidence of deep vein thrombosis. When APG data from all 3 levels of venous injuries were combined, there were significant differences between injured extremities and control extremities in outflow fraction, outflow fraction with compression, venous filling index, and residual volume fraction. In 17 patients, CFD venous imaging findings and APG data were consistent with chronic venous insufficiency. Changes were greatest in those who underwent complex repairs together with perioperative fasciotomies.

Conclusion.—A study published in 1980 challenged the aggressive approach in the treatment of civilian venous injuries when the authors reported that primary venous interruption was a quick, safe, and effective means of managing venous injuries. In this small series, no long-term advantage of either ligation or repair could be detected. Although long-term patency is excellent, most patients exhibit evidence of chronic venous insufficiency after ligation or repair. The most severe functional changes were found after complex venous repairs and fasciotomy.

▶ Abundant data indicate that simple ligation of complex venous injuries seems to produce about the same clinical results as the much more complicated venous repair. This article from the San Francisco Trauma Center concludes that although complex venous repair following trauma had a patency of 100%, a majority of patients had clinical symptoms and lab findings of chronic venous insufficiency. These authors conclude, and I believe appropriately, that most patients show evidence of chronic venous insufficiency after either venous repair or venous ligation following trauma. I continue to find little persuasive evidence in favor of detailed venous repair. If the 2 ends of a transected vein are in your face, then repair, I suppose, is appropriate. However, I am not going to make any substantial effort to accomplish a venous repair when simple ligation is equally plausible.

15 Venous Thrombosis and Pulmonary Embolism

Deep Venous Thrombosis

The Origin of Lower Extremity Deep Vein Thrombi in Acute Venous Thrombosis

Hill SL, Holtzman GI, Martin D, et al (Community Hosp of Roanoke Valley, Va)
Am J Surg 173:485–490, 1997 15–1

Introduction.—The origin of a lower extremity deep venous thrombosis (DVT) is difficult to pinpoint, but the common view is that most begin in the calf veins and propagate proximally. Yet newer and more accurate noninvasive techniques, including the duplex scan, have revealed that many thrombi do not have their origin in the calf. Duplex scans have also showed several types of thrombi. A retrospective review of duplex scans examined the pattern, distribution, and types of acute DVT.

Methods.—Over a 5-year period, 3,585 duplex scans were performed on 2,654 patients at a 200-bed acute care hospital. Data recorded for each patient included demographic information, associated diseases, and the location and type of thromboses. All vascular studies were recorded on a video cassette for review and evaluation.

Results.—Venous thromboses were detected in 461 patients (17.4%), 189 men and 272 women with a mean age of 63.4. The mean age of the women was significantly greater than that of the men (65.5 versus 60.3). Thromboses were present in 854 locations and were equally divided between the right leg (51%) and left leg (49%). Locations of thromboses were the iliofemoral segment (16%), the common femoral vein (13%), the superficial femoral vein (19%), the popliteal vein (18%), the veins of the calf (24%), and the superficial veins (11%). Of the 4 types of venous thrombosis identified, approximately one-half (52%) extended over 2 or more contiguous segments and one-third (34%) were isolated in 1 venous segment. Less common were multiple thromboses in noncontiguous segments (8%) and bilateral thrombi in different locations (6%). Overall, most patients (57%) had DVT without calf involvement. Age and past or coexistent disease were associated with the presence and type of thromboses.

Discussion.—In contrast to the previous view that most DVT begin in the deep veins of the calf, calf vein thrombi represented only 24% of DVT in this series. A thrombus can occur at any location in the lower extremity, and the most significant DVT arise in the proximal thigh or groin.

▶ Again the haunting question is asked: Just where do lower extremity deep vein thrombi start? Heretofore, it has been widely believed that some started below the knee, some started above the knee, and some started in both places simultaneously. These authors conclude about the same, pointing out that somewhat more DVT appeared to originate proximal to the calf than at the calf. While I suppose they may be correct, I am hard pressed to understand the importance of this finding.

Occult Cancer in Patients With Venous Thromboembolism: Which Patients, Which Cancers

Monreal M, Fernandez-Llamazares J, Perandreu J, et al (Hosp Universitari Germans Trias i Pujol, Badalona, Spain)

Thromb Haemost 78:1316–1318, 1997 15–2

Objective.—The association between venous thromboembolism (VTE) and visceral cancer is unclear. Results of a 5-year retrospective study focused on identifying patients who can potentially benefit from screening procedures and the sensitivity of the diagnostic workup and possible survival advantages for patients with identified and treated cancers are discussed.

Methods.—Between January 1990 and October 1996, 832 patients were admitted for treatment of VTE of the lower limbs. Predisposing risk factors were found for all except 112 patients, who were assumed to have idiopathic VTE. Patients were screened for malignancies and were followed up at 4-month intervals for 1 year after discharge; patients with idiopathic VTE were followed up for 3 years. The incidence of occult cancer was compared in patients with idiopathic vs. secondary VTE. Clinical characteristics of these patients were compared with those of 147 patients diagnosed with cancer prior to VTE.

Results.—Cancer was diagnosed in 15 patients with VTE during hospitalization and in an additional 8 after discharge. The frequency of occult cancer was significantly higher in patients with idiopathic VTE (13/105, 12.4%) than in patients with risk factors for VTE (10/569, 1.8%) (Table 2). Venous thromboembolism was the first sign of malignancy in most patients with prostate and pancreatic cancer; and developed months or years later in patients with breast, brain, uterus, or unknown origin cancer. In most patients with VTE whose cancers were detected during admission, the cancer was at an early stage.

TABLE 2.—Frequency of Occult Cancer According to Risk Factors for Venous Thromboembolism

	Specific tests*	Follow-up	Total
Secondary DVT			
Surgery	2	3	5/220
Bedrest	0	0	0/165
Previous VTE	3	1	4/107
Leg varicosities	1	0	1/43
Miscellanea	0	0	0/34
Total	6	4	10/569
Idiopathic DVT	9	4	13/105
Total	15	8	23/674

(Courtesy of Monreal M, Fernandez-Llamazares J, Perandreu J, et al: Occult cancer in patients with venous thromboembolism: Which patients, which cancers. *Thromb Haemost* 78:1316–1318, 1997).

Conclusion.—Cancer was detected significantly more frequently in patients with idiopathic VTE than in patients with risk factors for VTE. Additional studies need to be conducted to determine if routine screening for cancer is cost-effective for patients with idiopathic VTE.

► The relationship between idiopathic VTE and occult cancer is unclear, although potentially extraordinarily important. These investigators found that 12% of patients with idiopathic VTE proved to have cancer. The tests most useful in the diagnosis of cancer were CT scan, CEA, and PSA. Interestingly, VTE was the first sign of malignancy in most patients with prostatic and pancreatic cancer, but not other cell types. The relationship of idiopathic VTE to occult cancer has been previously described in the YEAR BOOK.[1] The real question is: With what degree of enthusiasm should we pursue screening for occult cancer in patients who present with idiopathic venous thrombosis? At the present time, I am recommending to the patient's internist that basic screening for cancer be carried out. I believe this is the prudent course. (See also Abstracts 15–3 and 15–4.)

Reference

1. 1997 YEAR BOOK OF VASCULAR SURGERY, p 426.

Venous Thromboembolism and Cancer

Baron JA, Gridley G, Weiderpass E, et al (Dartmouth Med School, Hanover, NH; Karolinska Inst, Stockholm; Natl Cancer Inst, Bethesda, Md)
Lancet 351:1077–1080, 1998 15–3

Background.—Some studies suggest that venous thromboembolism (VTE) may be a presenting marker of cancer. In particular reports suggest that cancer risk is increased in the first few years after VTE. The long-term risk of cancer for patients with VTE was determined, as well as whether

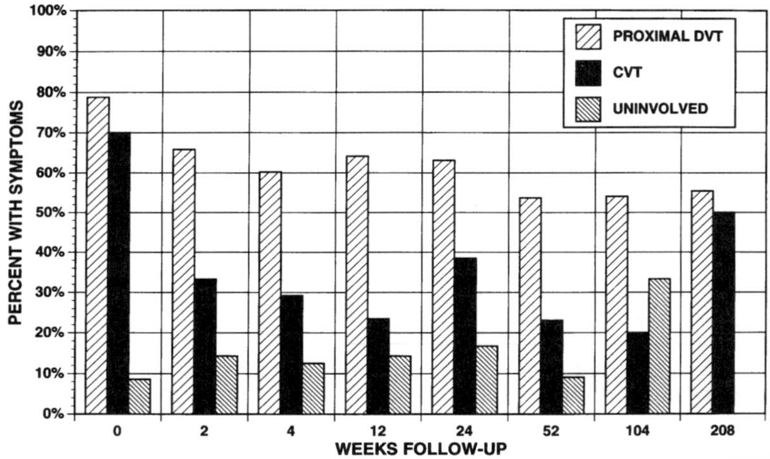

# LIMBS	0	2	4	12	24	52	104	208
PROXIMAL DVT	368	179	128	123	111	95	61	56
CVT	50	27	24	17	13	13	5	2
UNINVOLVED	35	21	16	14	12	11	3	1

FIGURE 2.—Prevalence of symptoms (edema, pain, hyperpigmentation, or ulceration) during follow-up among extremities with proximal deep venous thrombosis (*DVT*), calf vein thrombosis (*CVT*), and in uninvolved limbs contralateral to a CVT. Differences among the 3 groups are statistically significant at 12 months ($P = 0.004$). Table shows total number of extremities within each group evaluated at each follow-up interval. (Courtesy of Meissner MH, Caps MT, Bergelin RO, et al: Early outcome after isolated calf vein thrombosis. *J Vasc Surg* 26:749–756, 1997.)

Results.—At referral, 70% of extremities in the CVT group were symptomatic. Clinical signs and symptoms were present in only 29% of patients by 1 month. However, at 1 year, 23% of patients had pain and/or edema. At the same time, 9% of unaffected contralateral extremities and 54% of those with proximal DVT were symptomatic (Fig 2). The affected veins quickly recanalized—mean thrombus load decreased to 50% by 1 month and to zero by 1 year. Valvular incompetence became progressively more prevalent, found in 24% of extremities by 1 year. Pulmonary embolism was found at referral in 11% of patients and developed during follow-up in 3%.

Conclusions.—About one fourth of patients with CVT have persistent symptoms with valvular incompetence. The risk of persistent lower extremity symptoms can make isolated DVT of the calf vein a clinically relevant problem.

► A number of fascinating conclusions concerning isolated CVT are apparent from this article. About one fourth of patients had symptoms at presentation, the mean thrombus load was reduced to 0 at 1 year, valvular incompetency progressively increased such that reflux was present in 24% of extremities at 1 year, and remarkably, pulmonary embolism occurred in association with isolated CVT in 14% of patients. I believe the only logical conclusion is that we should not regard venous thrombosis as a one-hit event. I strongly suspect that patients who have venous thrombosis have recurrent venous thrombosis in both legs repeatedly over time, with many episodes going unrecognized. How else could we explain the consistently noted high prevalence of venous insufficiency in the opposite leg? It also seems well established that isolated CVT presents a real risk of pulmonary embolism. I consider one of the most pressing questions presently to be whether patients with CVT should receive systemic anticoagulation therapy just as if they had proximal DVT. As years pass, we are inclined to treat CVT vigorously. Presently, I believe this is the decision best supported by available evidence. Our choice of therapy will probably be outpatient low–molecular weight heparin.

Incidence of Deep Venous Thrombosis Associated With Femoral Venous Catheterization

Mian NZ, Bayly R, Schreck DM, et al (Muhlenberg Regional Med Ctr, Plainfield, NJ)
Acad Emerg Med 4:1118–1121, 1997 15–10

Introduction.—Femoral vein catheterization (FVC) is an alternative method of obtaining central venous access, which is particularly useful in unstable patients. Although FVC has been successfully employed in critically ill adults and children, a recent study reported that large-bore femoral vein catheters were associated with an increased incidence of deep vein thrombosis (DVT). A prospective study sought to determine the incidence of DVT in adult medical patients who underwent FVC.

Methods.—The study involved patients treated at a 420-bed community hospital from August 1993 through October 1994. Eligible patients were older than 18 and had received triple-lumen femoral venous catheters in the Emergency Department, medical inpatient floors, or critical care units. Excluded were patients with trauma. Heparin-coated 7 Fr 20-cm femoral vein catheters were inserted unilaterally into a femoral vein. Data recorded for each patient included age, gender, number of FVC days, DVT risk factors, DVT prophylaxis, and DVT formation and site. Each patient underwent bilateral venous duplex sonography within 7 days of femoral vein catheter removal.

Results.—Forty-two patients had femoral vein catheters inserted. With the contralateral leg serving as the control vein, a total of 84 femoral veins were studied. Eleven of 42 FVC sites (26%), but no control leg, had a femoral DVT. One patient with no evidence of femoral DVT had popliteal and posterior tibial DVT in both legs. There was a highly significant association between DVT formation and FVC insertion but no statistically significant associations between DVT and age, gender, number of DVT risk factors, number of FVC days, use of DVT prophylaxis, or site (right vs. left lower extremity) of insertion.

Discussion.—Despite the use of heparin-coated catheters, the placement of femoral catheters was associated with a significant incidence of femoral

DVT at the site of catheter insertion. Physicians managing critically ill patients should be aware of the DVT risk associated with the femoral venous access route.

▶ The high incidence of femoral vein thrombosis associated with FVC has been noted repeatedly. A 26% incidence was found in these patients despite the fact that everyone received seemingly adequate DVT prophylaxis. Despite the small size of this study, the results continue to demonstrate that FVC is associated with an extraordinary incidence of femoral DVT in the catheterized limb of critically ill adults. Individuals managing these patients must be familiar with this information. The femoral vein access route should be chosen only when all else has failed.

Saphenous Vein Thrombophlebitis (SVT): A Deceptively Benign Disease
Hanson JN, Ascher E, DePippo P, et al (Maimonides Med Ctr, Brooklyn, NY)
J Vasc Surg 27:677–680, 1998 15–11

Background.—Although acute thrombosis of the branches of the saphenous vein is generally self-limiting, the clinical effects of acute thrombosis of the main trunk of this vein may not be so benign. There is a well-known association between deep venous thrombosis (DVT) and hypercoagulability. Whether a relationship exists between saphenous vein thrombophlebitis (SVT) and abnormal coagulation profiles was examined.

Methods.—A total of 17 patients (6 men and 11 women, mean age 60.8 years) with isolated SVT (no DVT and no underlying malignancies) were studied. One patient had been taking Coumadin because of DVT 4.5 months earlier, but no patient was taking heparin or had liver disease, diffuse intravascular coagulation, or a history of lower extremity trauma. Superficial and deep venous systems were examined bilaterally with duplex scans. The coagulation profile determined for all patients included antithrombin III antigen and activity levels, protein C antigen and activity levels, activated protein C resistance, protein S antigen and activity levels, factor V DNA mutations, and coagulation factors II and X levels. Coagulation profiles were repeated at least once up to 5 months after the initial examination to examine how coagulation profiles changed over time.

Findings.—Ten of the 17 patients (59%) had an abnormal coagulation profile when first investigated. At repeat testing, 6 of these 17 (35%) remained hypercoagulable. Four of these 6 patients had antithrombin III deficiency, either alone or in combination with another coagulation abnormality. Of the 7 patients whose initial coagulation profile was normal, repeat tests were also normal. Fourteen patients had great saphenous vein thrombophlebitis (GSVT) and 3 had saphenofemoral junction thrombophlebitis (SFJT). Repeat coagulation profiles were abnormal in 5 of the 14 patients with GSVT (36%) and in 1 of the 3 patients with SFJT (33%). All but 4 of the patients also underwent repeat duplex examination; in 6 patients duplex results were unchanged, in 1 they were improved, but in 6 results were worse. Three of the patients with unchanged duplex results and 3 of the 6 patients with worse results were hypercoagulable.

Conclusions.—About one third of these patients with isolated GSVT or SFJT had consistently abnormal coagulation profiles up to 5 months after the initial examination. Thus, patients with isolated SVT may be prone to develop DVT, and their coagulation profiles should be closely monitored. All 7 patients whose coagulation profile was normal at the initial evaluation also had a normal profile at follow-up, which suggests that coagulation tests in these patients need not be repeated if the initial coagulation profile is normal.

▶ It seems well established that some version of hypercoagulability appears as a cause of DVT in 5% to 10% of afflicted patients. To date, we have had little information concerning the relationship of hypercoagulability to superficial vein thrombosis of the saphenous vein system.

In this article, the group from Maimonides found remarkably that 59% of patients with saphenous vein thrombosis had abnormal coagulation profiles, and 35% remained abnormal when repeated months later. I have no idea whether this finding will prove to be real or is an aberrancy based on the small number of patients studied (only 17). I also wonder what we should do with this information. If we have a patient who has superficial vein thrombosis and we test for and discover a hypercoagulable state such as factor V Leiden, should this patient receive long-term anticoagulation? Certainly we would routinely give a patient who had had DVT with a hypercoagulable state long-term warfarin, but I have no idea whether we should extend the same risky therapy to a patient who has only had a single episode of superficial vein thrombosis.

This paper raises a number of questions with few answers in sight. The primary take-home message is that I shall begin to screen for hypercoagulability in patients who have superficial vein thrombosis. As noted above, however, I really do not know what to do with the information. I suppose over time we shall sort this out.

Incidence of Idiopathic Deep Venous Thrombosis and Secondary Thromboembolism Among Ethnic Groups in California

White RH, Zhou H, Romano PS (Univ of California, Davis, Sacramento)

Ann Intern Med 128:737–740, 1998 15–12

Background.—Studies in various ethnic groups suggest differences in the incidence of deep venous thrombosis (DVT) and secondary venous thromboembolism. The incidence of these events was examined among the 4 major ethnic groups in California.

Methods.—The California Patient Discharge Data Set was used to determine the incidence of idiopathic and secondary DVT in adults (18 years or older) of 4 ethnic groups: white individuals, African Americans, Hispanic individuals, and Asians and Pacific Islanders. Secondary thrombo-

TABLE.—Standardized Incidence of Idiopathic Deep Venous Thrombosis, Incidence Risk Ratio, and Relative Risk for Acute Recurrent Thromboembolism Within 3 Months of the Index Event in Ethnic Groups in California

Ethnic Group	Directly Standardized Incidence of Idiopathic DVT per 1 000 000 Persons Older Than Age 18 Years*	Incidence Risk Ratio for Idiopathic DVT (95% Cl)†	Relative Risk for Recurrence of DVT (95% Cl)†‡
White	230	1.0	1.0
African American	293	1.27 (1.07–1.51)	1.03 (0.91–1.15)
Hispanic	139	0.60 (0.54–0.67)	0.95 (0.84–1.06)
Asian or Pacific Islander	60	0.26 (0.22–0.30)	0.65 (0.49–0.85)

*Age- and sex-standardized incidence calculated by using the 1990 California census.
†White persons used as the reference group.
‡Age- and sex-adjusted relative risk for recurrent thromboembolism within 91 days of hospitalization for venous thrombosis.
Abbreviations: DVT, deep venous thrombosis; *CI*, confidence interval.
(Courtesy of White RH, Zhou H, Romano PS: Incidence of idiopathic deep venous thrombosis and secondary thromboembolism among ethnic groups in California. *Am Intern Med* 128:737–740, 1998.)

embolism was defined as venous thrombosis or pulmonary embolism that occurred during hospitalization for the index event or within 91 days of that admission. The incidence of secondary thromboembolism was determined by counting such events after myocardial infarction (without bypass surgery or revascularization), partial or total colectomy with or without cancer, hip fracture requiring internal fixation or hip replacement, stroke with paralysis but without carotid endarterectomy, and childbirth. The 1990 U.S. Census figures were used to determine age- and sex-adjusted standardized annual incidences of DVT.

Findings.—Idiopathic DVT was identified in 17,991 patients, and secondary thromboembolism occurred in 5,573 patients. The age- and sex-standardized risks for DVT and secondary thromboembolism differed according to ethnicity (Table). The annual incidence for DVT (per 1,000,000 adults) was 230 for white individuals, 293 for African Americans, 139 for Hispanic individuals, and 60 for Asians and Pacific Islanders. Compared with whites, African Americans were more likely (incidence risk ratio 1.27) and Hispanics and Asians and Pacific Islanders were less likely (incidence risk ratios 0.60 and 0.26, respectively) to have idiopathic DVT. Similarly, compared with whites, the relative risks for secondary thromboembolism were higher in African Americans (1.03) and lower in Hispanics (0.95) and Asians and Pacific Islanders (0.65).

Conclusions.—Hispanic individuals, Asians, and Pacific Islanders have a lower incidence of idiopathic DVT and a lower risk of secondary thromboembolism compared with white individuals. On the other hand, African Americans have a higher incidence of DVT and a higher relative risk for recurrence. These findings have relevance in the planning of prophylaxis in patients of different ethnic backgrounds.

► I have always been curious about the relationship between ethnicity and venous thrombosis. It seems crystal clear that individuals in Northern Euro-

quet release and embolic phenomenon in patients undergoing total knee arthroplasty.

Methods.—Fifty-five patients (22 men and 33 women, mean age 65.5 years) underwent 59 total knee arthroplasties with implants secured by cement. The operated limb was exsanguinated and kept free of blood by a tourniquet inflated to 50 mm Hg. After the implant was secured, 1 unit of autologous blood was given before the tourniquet was deflated. The right atrium and right ventricle were imaged via transesophageal echocardiography during the procedure and for 15 minutes after tourniquet release. Hemodynamic parameters were monitored in all patients, and 10 patients also had a femoral vein catheter placed in the operated limb to assess the embolic events that occurred immediately upon tourniquet release.

Findings.—After deflation of the tourniquet, each patient had showers of echogenic material in the right atrium, right ventricle, and pulmonary artery outflow tract. The intensity of the showers peaked 30 seconds after tourniquet release, and in some patients the showers continued for 15 minutes. In 35 patients in whom the size of the particles was measured, most (26, or 74%) had distinct particles that were 0.5 cm or greater in diameter along with smaller particles. Hemodynamics changed significantly immediately after tourniquet release compared with mean values before surgery. Mean arterial pressure dropped from 85 to 79 mm Hg, mixed venous oxygen saturation dropped from 83% to 72%, and mean pulmonary arterial systolic pressure increased from 20 to 24 mm Hg. Mean pulmonary arterial pressure was still significantly higher 3 minutes after tourniquet release (27 mm Hg). In the patients who had echogenic particles that were 0.5 cm or greater in diameter, mean pulmonary vascular resistance increased significantly by 5 minutes after tourniquet release (from 205 to 328 dyne·sec·cm^{-5}·m^2). Three patients had postoperative pulmonary embolism; all 3 had echogenic particles that were greater than 0.5 cm in diameter. In the 10 patients who supplied femoral catheter aspirates, half had fresh venous thrombi. The aspirates did not contain fat, marrow, or polymethylmethacrylate or its breakdown products.

Conclusions.—After total knee replacement, the release of the tourniquet causes showers of echogenic material and significant changes in cardiopulmonary parameters. The lack of a relationship between the length of tourniquet use and the intensity of the embolic showers suggests that tourniquet release has an "all-or-nothing" effect. However, there was an association between a larger size of the echogenic material and an increase in pulmonary vascular resistance.

► These investigators appear to have accurately diagnosed emboli showering the pulmonary circulation immediately upon releasing a tourniquet from the leg where a total knee replacement using cement had been performed. They suggest that a patient who has hemodynamic collapse immediately after tourniquet deflation following knee replacement should have the diagnosis of pulmonary embolism suspected. On balance, this is both fascinating and frightening new information. I had no idea that showers of clots were visibly occurring immediately after knee tourniquet release.

Management Strategies and Determinants of Outcome in Acute Major Pulmonary Embolism: Results of a Multicenter Registry

Kasper W, Konstantinides S, Geibel A, et al (St Josefs-Hosp, Wiesbaden, Germany; Universitätsklinik, Freiburg, Germany; Krankenhaus, Bruchsal, Germany; et al)

J Am Coll Cardiol 30:1165–1171, 1997 15–20

Introduction.—There is still a poor understanding of the prognosis of acute pulmonary embolism. Clinical presentation and the degree of hemodynamic instability of the patients largely influence diagnostic and therapeutic strategies for acute pulmonary thromboembolism. It has been difficult to assess the impact on patient management and outcome.

Methods.—There were 1,001 patients with major pulmonary embolism who were studied to determine current management strategies. Whether the extent of diagnostic workup, such as the frequency of pulmonary angiographic studies or nuclear imaging decreases as the severity of hemodynamic instability increases at presentation was determined. Whether patients who are most hemodynamically unstable are those who most frequently receive aggressive treatment was also studied. The degree of clinical hemodynamic instability attributable to acute right heart failure as the most important determinant of inhospital mortality was reviewed. The patients were categorized into 4 groups of increasing clinical and hemodynamic instability, indicating increasing severity of acute right heart failure.

Results.—The most frequently performed diagnostic procedure was echocardiography (74%). In 79% of clinically stable patients, lung scan or pulmonary angiography was performed, but in those with circulatory collapse at presentation, lung scan or pulmonary angiography was performed much less frequently (32%). About 48% of patients were given thrombolytic agents, despite 40% of these patients having contraindications. In clinically unstable patients, the frequency of initial thrombolysis was significantly higher than in normotensive patients (57% vs. 22%). In the group of stable patients, overall inhospital mortality rate was 8.1%. In those with cardiogenic shock, it was 25%, and in patients necessitating cardiopulmonary resuscitation, it was 65% (Table 6). In 9.2% of patients, major bleeding was reported, but cerebral bleeding (0.5%) was uncommon. In 17% of patients, recurrent pulmonary embolism occurred.

Conclusion.—The degree of hemodynamic instability at presentation influences current management strategies of acute major pulmonary embolism. Physicians often rely on the findings of bedside echocardiography in the presence of severe hemodynamic compromise. Without seeking further diagnostic certainty in nuclear imaging or angiographic studies, physicians then proceed to thrombolytic treatment.

TABLE 6.—Inhospital Clinical Course

Event	Group 1 (n = 407)	Group 2 (n = 316)	Group 3 (n = 102)	Group 4 (n = 176)
Overall mortality	33 (8.1%)	48 (15%)	25 (25%)	114 (65%)
Death due to PE	29 (7.1%)	43 (14%)	23 (23%)	106 (60%)
Death due to underlying disease	3 (0.7%)	3 (1.0%)	1 (1.0%)	2 (1.1%)
Death due to complications of diagnostic procedures or treatment	1 (0.3%)	2 (0.6%)	1 (1.0%)	6 (3.4%)
Nonfatal events				
Recurrent PE	57 (14%)	61 (19%)	22 (22%)	32 (18%)
Arterial thromboembolism	5 (1.2%)	4 (1.3%)	0	5 (2.8%)
Cerebral bleeding	1 (0.3%)	3 (1.0%)	0	1 (0.6%)
Other major bleeding*	30 (7.4%)	24 (7.6%)	12 (12%)	21 (12%)

*Bleeding requiring red blood cell transfusion or discontinuation of therapeutic anticoagulation or thrombolytic treatment. Data presented are number (%) of patients.

Abbreviation: PE, pulmonary embolism.

(Reprinted with permission from the American College of Cardiology from Kasper W, Konstantinides S, Geibel A, et al: Management strategies and determinants of outcome in acute major pulmonary embolism: Results of a multicenter registry. *Am Coll Cardiol* 30:1165–1171, 1997.)

▶ These authors appropriately note that current community treatment practice of acute pulmonary embolism is not known with certainty. They conducted a remarkable study of treatment methods for pulmonary embolism at 204 participating centers. Their conclusions were interesting and indicated that increasing clinical instability at presentation resulted in a dramatic decrease in the frequency with which invasive studies were obtained to confirm the diagnosis. In cases of clinical instability, thrombolytic therapy was frequently used even in the presence of contraindications to such therapy. Although possibly not terribly surprising, these results should prove especially helpful in planning prospective, randomized trials that will clarify the impact of widely used treatment modalities.

Low-Molecular-Weight Heparin in the Treatment of Patients With Venous Thromboembolism

The Columbus Investigators (Univ of Amsterdam)

N Engl J Med 337:657–662, 1997 15–21

Introduction.—Compared with unfractionated heparin, low–molecular weight heparins have a longer half-life and a more suitable anticoagulation response that make them more appropriate for subcutaneous administration without laboratory monitoring in patients with venous thromboembolism. The effectiveness of low–molecular weight heparin in patients with pulmonary embolism or previous episodes of thromboembolism are not known. The clinical outcomes of recurrent venous thromboembolism, hemorrhage, and death during 12-week follow-up was evaluated in a large, open, international, randomized clinical trial designed to determine whether fixed-dose, subcutaneous low–molecular weight heparin and adjusted-dose, continuous intravenous unfractionated heparin have equivalent efficacy in unselected patients with symptomatic venous thromboembolism.

Methods.—One thousand twenty-one patients with symptomatic venous thromboembolism were randomly assigned to either fixed-dose, subcutaneous low–molecular weight heparin (reviparin sodium) or adjusted-dose, intravenous unfractionated heparin. Concomitant oral anticoagulation therapy with Coumadin was given over a period of 12 weeks. Nearly one third of patients had associated pulmonary embolism.

Results.—Among 510 patients treated with low–molecular weight heparin, 27 patients had 29 episodes of recurrent thromboembolism, compared with 30 episodes in 25 patients of the 511 patients treated with unfractionated heparin (5.3% vs. 4.9%). Of 93 instances of clinically important bleeding, 46 were in patients treated with low–molecular weight heparin and 47 were in patients treated with unfractionated heparin; 16 and 12, respectively, were major bleeding episodes. During the 12-week follow-up period, 75 patients died: 36 (7.1%) treated with low–molecular weight heparin and 39 (7.6%) treated with unfractionated heparin. The relative effect of the 2 treatment approaches was similar in primary outcome events: symptomatic deep-vein thrombosis or pulmonary embolism and major bleeding.

Conclusions.—Unmonitored, subcutaneous low–molecular weight heparin may be considered a safe and effective treatment for patients with venous thromboembolism. It is an appropriate alternative to unfractionated heparin in these patients.

► This study adds a small slice of salami to the existing pile. We have known for some time that low–molecular weight heparin is effective both for deep venous thrombosis prophylaxis, as well as the initial treatment of patients with proximal deep vein thrombosis. As these authors note, however, we have previously not known with certainty that low–molecular weight heparin was effective in patients with pulmonary embolism or prior episodes of venous thrombosis. Not surprisingly, they concluded from this well-conducted study that it is at least as effective as unfractionated heparin in this setting. I continue to believe that low–molecular weight heparin represents a new therapeutic principle that will fundamentally alter the way we treat venous thromboembolism. (See also Abstract 15–22.)

A Comparison of Low-Molecular-Weight Heparin With Unfractionated Heparin for Acute Pulmonary Embolism

Simonneau G, for the THÉSÉE Study Group (Hôpital Antoine Béclère, Clamart, France; Hôpital Laennec, Paris; Hôpital Trousseau, Tours, France; et al)

N Engl J Med 337:663–669, 1997 15–22

Introduction.—Low–molecular weight heparin seems to be at least as effective and safe as standard, unfractionated heparin in the treatment of

TABLE 3.—Anticoagulant Therapy Provided to the Study Patients According to Treatment Group

Variable	Mean Value*
Unfractionated heparin	
Days of treatment	7.0±2.4
Dose on day 1 (IU)	32,439
Daily dose, days 1 to 8 (IU)	27,495
Days to start of oral anticoagulation	2.0±1.0
Low-molecular-weight heparin	
Days of treatment	7.3±2.3
Days to start of oral anticoagulation	2.0±1.0

*Plus-minus values are means ± SD.

(Courtesy of Simonneau G, for the THÉSÉE Study Group: A comparison of low-molecular-weight heparin with unfractionated heparin for acute pulmonary embolism. *N Engl J Med* 337:663–669.

deep-vein thrombosis. Data are scarce regarding the use of low–molecular weight heparin in the treatment of acute, symptomatic, pulmonary embolism. Six hundred twelve patients with symptomatic pulmonary embolism who did not require thrombolytic therapy or pulmonary embolectomy were randomly assigned to treatment with subcutaneous low–molecular weight heparin given in a fixed dose once daily, or an adjusted-dose, intravenous unfractionated heparin.

Methods.—In both sets of patients, oral anticoagulation therapy was initiated between the first and third days of the start of heparin therapy and was continued for at least 3 months on an open-label basis (Table 3). Treatments were compared on day 8 and day 90 for major end points: recurrent thromboembolism, major bleeding, and death.

Results.—At least 1 end point was reached within the first 8 days of treatment in 9 of 308 (2.9%) patients treated with unfractionated heparin and in 9 of 304 patients treated with low–molecular weight heparin (3.0%). By day 90, these numbers were 22 (7.1%) and 18 (5.9%), respectively. Both treatment groups had similar risks of major bleeding throughout follow-up.

Conclusions.—Subcutaneous therapy with low–molecular weight heparin seemed to be as effective and safe as intravenous unfractionated heparin in the treatment of patients with acute pulmonary embolism.

► Once again we have confirmation that low–molecular weight heparin is at least as effective as unfractionated heparin for the treatment of acute pulmonary embolism. I consider it established that low–molecular weight heparin is as effective as unfractionated heparin for thromboembolism prophylaxis, initial treatment of deep vein thrombosis, and initial treatment of pulmonary embolism. (See also Abstract 15–21.)

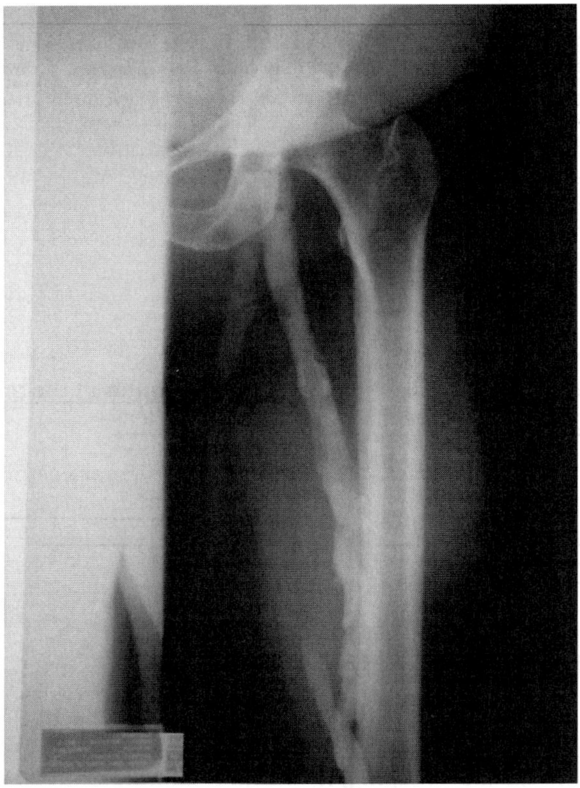

FIGURE 2.—Axial transformation of deep femoral vein through large profunda-popliteal connection. Major portion of superficial femoral vein, except distal portion, is occluded. Removal of saphenous vein is well tolerated because of presence of profunda-popliteal collateral connection. (Courtesy of Raju S, Easterwood L, Fountain T, et al: Saphenectomy in the presence of chronic venous obstruction. *Surgery* 123:637–644, 1998.)

icant improvement in obstructive grading, probably as a result of reflux flow elimination (Fig 2).

Conclusions.—The admonition against removing secondary varices should be reconsidered. Saphenectomy may be appropriate for patients with postthrombotic syndrome with mixed obstruction and reflux. Such patients tolerate the procedure well with no sequelae. Reflux parameters improved without significant worsening of objective measures of obstruction.

► For years, we have heard that secondary varicose veins should not be stripped in the presence of deep vein obstruction because, even if these veins are varicose, they function as essential collaterals and their interruption may result in marked patient decline. These investigators appear to have disproved this belief. Sixty-four saphenous vein removals were carried out in patients who had phlebographically proven significant deep vein obstruction.

Not only was saphenectomy well tolerated in the obstruction group, but most patients experienced a significant improvement in reflux and calf venous pump function. The authors conclude correctly that the traditional admonition against removal of secondary varicose veins in the presence of venous obstruction must be re-examined. Not only does the procedure cause no harm, it appears beneficial in most patients, if they are selected properly.

Subfascial Endoscopic Perforator Vein Surgery

Endoscopic Versus Open Subfascial Division of Incompetent Perforating Veins in the Treatment of Venous Leg Ulceration: A Randomized Trial

Pierik EGJM, van Urk H, Hop WCJ, et al (Hosp de Weezenlanden, The Netherlands; Univ Hosp Rotterdam-Dijkzigt, The Netherlands; Erasmus Univ Rotterdam, The Netherlands; et al)
J Vasc Surg 26:1049–1054, 1997 16–7

Introduction.—Venous ulceration is a common cause of serious disability. Most venous ulcers respond to conservative treatment, but recurrent ulceration is typical. Subfascial division of incompetent perforating veins can provide good long-term results, but the surgery involves long incisions through compromised cutaneous and subcutaneous layers. Postoperative wound complications are common. Endoscopic approaches have been developed that allow subfascial endoscopic interruption of incompetent perforating veins. No comparative trials have been performed between open and endoscopic subfascial explorations. This comparison was accomplished in a prospective, randomized trial evaluating ulcer healing and postoperative wound complications in a cohort of patients with chronic lower leg venous ulceration.

Methods.—Of 39 patients with venous ulceration on the medial side of the lower leg, 20 and 19, respectively, were randomized for endoscopic exploration by use of a mediastinoscope or for open exploration by the modified Linton approach.

Results.—The incidence of wound infections was 53% after open exploration and 0% after the endoscopic approach (Table 1). Mean length of

TABLE 1.—Postoperative Wound Complications After Open and Endoscopic Division of Perforating Veins

	Open approach *(n = 19)*	*Endoscopic approach* *(n = 20)*	*p*
Wound infection	10 (53%)	0 (0%)	<0.001
Superficial	3 (16%)	0 (0%)	0.11
Deep	7 (37%)	0 (0%)	0.003
Nerve injury	2 (11%)	0 (0%)	0.23

(Courtesy of Pierik EGJM, van Urk H, Hop WCJ, et al: Endoscopic vs. open subfascial division of incompetent perforating veins in the treatment of venous leg ulceration: A randomized trial. *J Vasc Surg* 26:1049–1054, 1997.)

hospital stay was significantly longer with open than with endoscopic procedures (7 and 4 days, respectively). At postoperative month 4, ulcers were healed in 17 patients each in the open and endoscopic groups. At a mean follow-up of 21 months, no patients in either group had recurrent ulcerations.

Conclusion.—Endoscopic and open subfascial divisions of incompetent perforating veins are similarly effective in the treatment of venous ulceration of the lower leg. Significantly fewer wound complications were observed in the endoscopic than in the open procedure group. Endoscopic division is the recommended method.

► On balance, this is one of the silliest studies I have seen in recent years. Let's think about this for a minute. If you make a massive incision directly through an infected ulcer, are you or are you not liable to have postoperative wound infection? Remarkably, it turns out that you are. For convincingly demonstrating this remarkable conclusion through the use of a prospective, randomized study, I am delighted to recognize these authors with a coveted Camel Dung Award. Is there a single non–brain-dead person in the world who would have suspected that SEPS would not produce a lower incidence of postoperative infection compared to a Linton carried out through an infected field?

Efficacy of Subfascial Endoscopy in Eradicating Perforating Veins of the Lower Leg and Its Relation With Venous Ulcer Healing

Pierik EGJM, van Urk H, Wittens CHA (Univ Hosp Rotterdam-Dijkzigt, The Netherlands)

J Vasc Surg 26:255–259, 1997 16–8

Background.—Early reports of subfascial endoscopy for venous ulceration indicated good clinical outcome in terms of newly formed varicosities, ulcer healing, and wound complications. In some cases, however, ulcers failed to heal or ulceration recurred after endoscopic treatment of incompetent perforating veins. A prospective study assessed the efficacy of subfascial endoscopy in eradicating perforating veins and examined the relationship between persistent incompetent perforating veins and problems with ulcer healing.

Methods.—Study participants were all consecutive patients who underwent subfascial endoscopy for venous ulceration of the lower leg over a 14-month period. All had class 6 chronic venous insufficiency; none had an arterial component to their ulceration. The patients underwent duplex US scans of the lower leg before and 6 weeks after operation. Findings during subfascial endoscopy, performed with a mediastinoscope and clipping instrument, were compared with the number and localization of the perforating veins on the mediodorsal side.

Results.—Patients were 11 men and 9 women with a mean age of 64. Preoperative duplex scanning identified 46 incompetent perforating veins (mean 2.3 per patient) on the mediodorsal side of the lower leg. Six competent perforating veins were found in 5 patients. A total of 54 perforating veins were identified and clipped during subfascial endoscopy. The site of 43 incompetent and all 6 competent perforating veins were confirmed during operation; 5 additional perforating veins found in 4 patients had not been visualized at preoperative duplex US. Postoperative duplex US scans identified 6 incompetent perforating veins in 4 patients, and the ulcers in 3 of these patients did not heal. All ulcers healed in the remaining 17 patients.

Conclusion.—Endoscopic subfascial division of perforating veins was confirmed to be an effective and safe procedure in the treatment of patients with venous ulceration of the lower leg. All existing perforating veins were identified and divided in 17 of 20 patients in this series. The failure of ulcers to heal after operation is related to the persistence of incompetent perforating veins.

► I have secretly suspected for years that duplex is not going to be able to accurately detect all perforating veins. This interesting study confirms my suspicion. I remain unconvinced that eradication of perforating veins results in any patient benefit. I wish we could have proof of the benefit of perforator interruption before we engage in widespread programs to annihilate them. Somehow, it seems that we have the cart and the horse in an inappropriate relationship.

Congenital

Klippel-Trénaunay Syndrome: Spectrum and Management

Jacob AG, Driscoll DJ, Shaughnessy WJ, et al (Mayo Clinic Rochester, Minn)

Mayo Clin Proc 73:28–36, 1998 16–9

Background.—Klippel-Trénaunay syndrome (KTS) has 3 key features: capillary malformations, soft tissue or bony hypertrophy and varicose veins or venous malformations. Other frequent findings are deep venous anomalies and lymphatic malformations. These authors describe the various manifestations of KTS and its treatment in a large group of patients.

Methods.—Over 39 years, 252 patients (136 females and 116 males, median age 11.9 years) with KTS were evaluated; 230 patients (91%) had signs of KTS at birth. When necessary, limb length was assessed by serial roentgenograms of the long bones. Other studies (arterial and venous Doppler, venograms, gastrointestinal tests, etc.) were undertaken as needed to explore the patient's symptoms. Patients were studied for a mean of 3.58 years.

Findings.—Most patients (159, or 63%) had all 3 key features of KTS, and 93 (37%) had 2 of them. The most common findings were port-wine stains (246, or 98%), varicosities or venous malformations (182, or 72%), atypical veins such as lateral veins and persistent sciatic vein (182, or 72%), and limb hypertrophy (170, or 67%) (Fig 1). Concomitant congenital defects (most commonly hip dysplasia or syndactyly) were found in 74

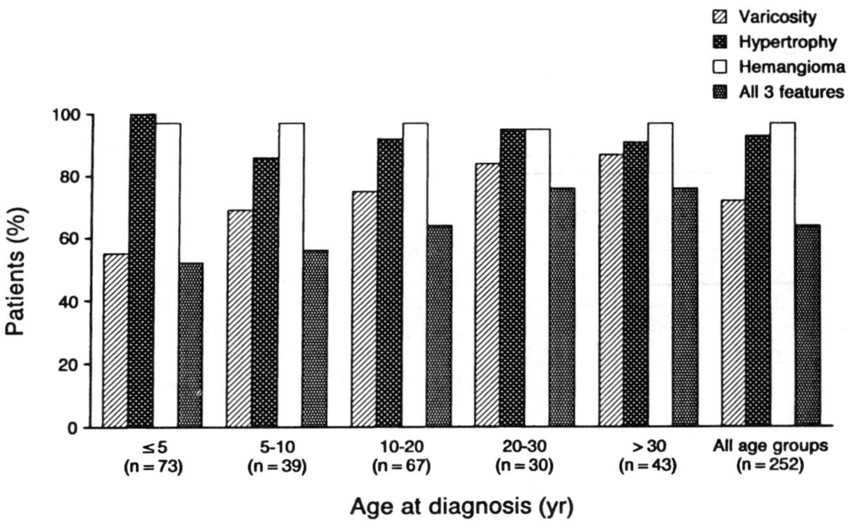

FIGURE 1.—Relative number of patients with principal features of Klippel-Trénaunay syndrome, stratified by age. (Courtesy of Jacob AG, Driscoll DJ, Shaughnessy WJ, et al: Klippel-Trénaunay syndrome: Spectrum and management. *Mayo Clin Proc* 73:28–36, 1998.)

patients (29%). Deep vein thrombosis was present in 11 patients (4%), and pulmonary embolism in 9 (4%). In most patients (177, or 70%), only the lower extremity was involved; in 28 patients (11%), only the upper extremity was involved. Discrepancies in limb length varied greatly and did not progress in a predictable manner. Fifty-four patients (21%) received no therapy, 166 (66%) received some type of medical treatment (mainly elastic support), and 145 patients (58%) underwent surgery. Operations included ligation and stripping of varicose veins, excision angioma, epiphysiodesis, and debulking. The most improvement was seen with epiphysiodesis, with the other 3 approaches providing improvement in less than 60% of patients.

Conclusions.—Klippel-Trénaunay syndrome is diagnosed by its 3 key features, and these are typically present at birth. Nonsurgical treatment is typically warranted. In a child with a limb length discrepancy, epiphysiodesis can be successful if the limb length discrepancy is expected to exceed 2.0 cm at skeletal maturity. Surgery to remove symptomatic varicosities or localized venous malformations can be useful, but only if the patient has a functioning deep vein system.

▶ The Mayo Clinic has undoubtedly had the largest experience with KTS in America, and probably in the world. We all continue to see afflicted patients occasionally, and it is well for us to be familiar with the tenets of this condition. I am especially impressed with the frequency of the persistence of the embryologic sciatic vein in many of these patients. Certainly, it appears that the surgery does not offer a good therapeutic alternative to

vein. With the 2 available foot devices, foot compressive devices 1 and 2, acceleration was greatest, compared with the other 3 devices at both levels. With the calf-only intermittent pneumatic compression device, the return time was significantly longer. Compared with the other 4 devices, return time was 4–10 times slower at the popliteal vein and 3–5 times slower at the common femoral vein.

Conclusion.—Significant alterations were produced in venous hemodynamics with the 2 commercially available foot devices, foot compression device 1 and foot compression device 2, and the calf-only intermittent pneumatic compression device. Changes produced by the foot and calf devices at the popliteal vein were seen proximally at the common femoral vein, but the changes were usually less. Rapid acceleration of venous flow to an elevated maximum venous velocity was produced by the mechanical devices. An elevated peak with a sustained period of flow above baseline return time was produced by the calf-only intermittent pneumatic compression device. Before widespread adaptation of these devices as an equivalent to existing calf-only intermittent pneumatic compression devices, further clinical comparison should be completed.

► It is obvious that the foot venous circulation is complex with normal blood flow from the deep veins to the superficial veins. Weight-bearing forces blood into the deep veins of the calf, as well as the saphenous veins without any muscular action. Numerous studies in recent years have indicated that compressive devices for the lower extremity represent effective prophylaxis for deep vein thrombosis (DVT), and new evidence suggests that application of a compressive device only to the foot may be equally effective in DVT prophylaxis. This study documents considerable alterations in venous dynamics with foot compressive devices. Available information suggests to me that in the future foot compression alone may come to be a preferred method for DVT prophylaxis. (See also Abstract 15–13.)

Collagen Subtype Pattern in Normal and Varicose Saphenous Veins in Humans

Waksman Y, Mashiah A, Hod I, et al (Hebrew Univ of Jerusalem, Rehovot; Kaplan Hosp, Rehovot, Jerusalem; Univ Hosp of South Manchester, England)

Isr J Med Sci 33:81–86, 1997 16–15

Background.—The development of varicose saphenous veins has been attributed to a number of causes, including incompetence of the venous valves, inherited abnormalities, and changes in venous wall architecture and in the composition of connective tissue extra-cellular matrix. A study of normal and varicose veins (VVs) of the lower limb was conducted to quantitatively determine the collagen subtype pattern and compare affected and unaffected segments of the diseased saphenous veins.

Methods.—Specimens of normal saphenous veins were obtained from 21 women undergoing coronary artery bypass grafting. Affected segments of greater saphenous veins were obtained from 37 women treated by ligation and stripping surgery for symptomatic primary VVs of the lower limb. Unaffected segments from these patients were collected from competent segments of the greater saphenous veins that were varicosed elsewhere. Types I, III, and V collagens (CI, CIII, CV) were extracted from the veins after elastase pretreatment and partial pepsin digestion for quantitative measurements.

Results.—All 3 collagen types were purified from both normal veins and VVs, and the relative amounts of CI were higher than CIII and CV, a finding that corresponds to previous data on human blood vessels. Compared to normal saphenous veins, the water content of VVs (both affected and unaffected segments) was significantly increased, a change that may reflect alterations in connective tissue content. Both affected and unaffected segments of VVs also exhibited significant increases in total collagen content compared to normal saphenous veins. Because the CIII and CV content of VVs was slightly reduced compared to normal veins, the CI/(CIII+CV) ratio in VVs increased significantly relative to normal veins.

Conclusion.—The findings of this study support the "weak wall" theory of VVs etiology, a weakness that may result from elevation of the CI/(CIII+CV) ratio. Both affected and unaffected segments of VVs contained abnormally elevated amounts of CI compared to normal saphenous veins.

▶ A careful study of the collagen content in varicose veins vs. nonvaricose veins revealed distinct abnormalities in the varicosities, consisting primarily of significant elevations of water and collagen type I. It is attractive to speculate that this may be a primary abnormality, perhaps related to genetic alterations, and may explain the spontaneous occurrence of varicose veins in certain patients. Of course, one has to guard against the possibility that long duration varicose veins result in phenotypic changes and that the collagen alterations detected may simply have resulted from secondary changes in longstanding dilated varicose veins.

Effective Treatment of Lymphedema of the Extremities

Ko DSC, Lerner R, Klose G, et al (Harvard Med School, Boston; Lerner Lymphedema Services, Boston)

Arch Surg 133:452–458, 1998 16–16

Introduction.—Most patients with chronic extremity lymphedema are advised to learn to live with the chronic swelling because of the lack of effective therapy. The Foeldi technique, or complete (or complex) decongestive physiotherapy (CDP) consists of skin care, eradicating infections, compression bandaging, and remedial exercises. The immediate and long-term volumetric reductions of upper and lower lymphedematous extremities were prospectively evaluated after a single course of CDP.

Methods.—Two hundred ninety-nine consecutive patients with lymphedema of the upper (2% primary, 98% secondary) or lower (61.3% primary, 38.7% secondary) extremities were treated with CDP for an average of 15.7 days. Patients underwent 2 phases of CDP. Phase 1 consisted of manual lymphatic massage, multilayered inelastic compression bandaging, remedial exercises, and meticulous skin care. Self-care was the focus of phase 2; it included the use of daytime elastic sleeve or stocking compression, nocturnal wrapping, and continued exercises. Patients were evaluated for lymphedema reduction at completion of phase 1 and at 6- and 12-month intervals during phase 2.

Results.—The average lymphedema reductions were 59.1% and 67.7%, respectively, after upper- and lower-extremity treatment. At an average follow-up of 9 months, the improvement was maintained within 95% of the initial volume reduction in 84% and 82% of patients for upper and lower extremities, respectively. The 33% of patients who were noncompliant lost part of their initial reduction. The rate of infections decreased from 1.10 to 0.65 infections per patient-year after a complete series of CDP treatments.

Conclusion.—Complete decongestive physiotherapy was highly effective in treating primary and secondary lymphedema. Initial volume reductions were maintained in most patients. Patients reported a significant recovery from their previous cosmetic and functional impairments and from the physical stigma they believed was frequently trivialized by the medical and payor communities.

▶ Massage and compression reduce edema! The harder and more diligently you do it, the greater the effect and the easier to maintain the effect. This is all that the Foeldi technique is. It is not a new approach, and there is no evidence to support Foeldi's claims that this method stimulates lymphatic contraction . I disagree that pneumatic pumps are not useful and should not be part of primary treatment. *Message*: What is needed is a proper randomized trial of complete decongestive physiotherapy vs. complete decongestive therapy *without manual lymph drainage* to prove the theory.

N. Browse, M.D.

Morphometric Assessment of the Dermal Microcirculation in Patients With Chronic Venous Insufficiency

Pappas PJ, DeFouw DO, Venezio LM, et al (UMDNJ-New Jersey Med School, Newark; Veterans Affairs Med Ctr, East Orange, NJ)
J Vasc Surg 26:784–795, 1997 16–17

Introduction.—Chronic venous insufficiency (CVI) is a well-known clinical entity, yet few trials have evaluated the ultrastructural changes of the microcirculation in this condition. Earlier trials limited their analyses to qualitative descriptions. Differences in endothelial cell structure and local

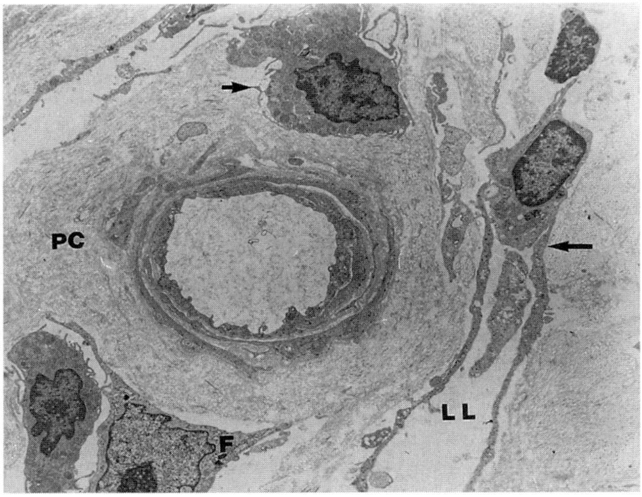

FIGURE 2.—Presence of a well-developed perivascular cuff (*PC*) in a patient with class 6 chronic venous insufficiency. Lymphatic vessel is at edge of perivascular cuff. *Long arrow* points at macrophage that appears to be entering lymphatic lumen (*LL*). Cell near this macrophage is a fibroblast. *Short arrow* indicates pericuff macrophage. *F* denotes a pericuff fibroblast. Original magnification, 4,300×. (Courtesy of Pappas PJ, DeFouw DO, Venezio LM, et al: Morphometric assessment of the dermal microcirculation in patients with chronic venous insufficiency. *J Vasc Surg* 26:784–795, 1997.)

cell type were quantified, with emphasis on leukocytes and their relationship to arterioles, capillaries, and postcapillary venules (PCVs).

Methods.—Thirty-five patients underwent two 4.0-mm punch biopsies from areas of dermal stasis skin changes in the gaiter region of the leg, and from noninvolved areas of skin of the ipsilateral thigh. Patients were grouped according to CEAP classification: 11 patients, class 4; 9 patients, class 5; 10 patients, class 6; and 5 patients without CVI who had normal skin biopsy specimens. At magnifications of 6,700× and 23,800×, electron microscopy was performed to determine endothelial cell thickness; number of fibroblasts, leukocytes, and mast cells and their proximity to arterioles, capillaries, and PCVs; endothelial cell vesicle density; interendothelial junctional widths; and basal lamina thickness. Three patients were evaluated for transforming growth factor-β1 (TGF-β1).

Results.—Quantitative measurements revealed a greater mast cell content for class 4 and class 5 patients around arterioles and PCVs and increased macrophage numbers for class 6 patients around PCVs (Fig 2). Fibroblasts were the most frequently observed cells. Basal lumina thickness was greater only at the capillary level. Three patients were positive for TGF-β1 messenger RNA.

Conclusions.—Mast cells are probably important in the pathogenesis of chronic venous insufficiency. Transforming growth factor-β1 may mediate the effects of mast cells and/or macrophages. There is no association between capillary cuff formation and widened interendothelial gap junctions. Enhanced vesicular transport rate or conformational changes in the interendothelial glycocalyx may cause capillary cuff formation.

► It is difficult to know what to make of these preliminary data. I suppose one may conclude that mast cells are prominent in the dermal microcirculation in patients with chronic venous insufficiency, but I am unable to take away much additional information.

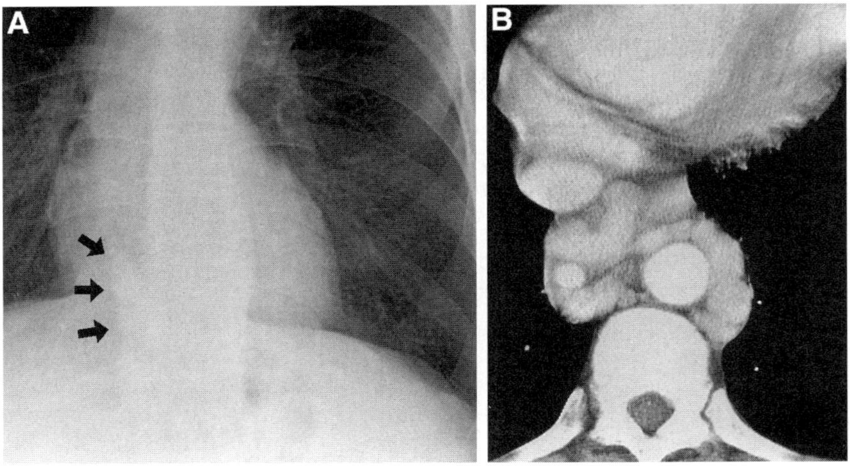

FIGURE 1.—Paraesophageal varices in a 68-year-old man. **A**, chest radiograph shows lateral bulging of right paraspinal interface (*arrows*). Descending thoracic aorta interface is not clearly shown. Also note marked splenomegaly with medial displacement of gastric air shadow. **B**, enhanced CT scan obtained at level of inferior vena cava reveals varices surrounding descending thoracic aorta. Right-sided varices are larger than left-sided varices. (Courtesy of Lee SJ, Lee KS, Kim SA, et al: Computed radiography of the chest in patients with paraesophageal varices: Diagnostic accuracy and characteristic findings. *AJR* 170:1527–1531, 1998.)

hepatic helical CT scans. Findings were compared with those of 20 controls by 2 chest radiologists. Observers decided on computed radiographic findings by consensus. They were blinded to findings of hepatic helical CT scans, number of patients with portal hypertension, and number of control subjects.

Results.—Paraesophageal varices were observed in 38 of 100 patients with portal hypertension (38%). Overall sensitivity, specificity, and accuracy were 53% (20/38), 90% (74/82), and 78% (94/120), respectively, for chest computed radiography in the detection of paraesophageal varices. In patients with paraesophageal varices, chest computed radiographs revealed 76% (29/38) with splenomegaly, 47% (18/38) with lateral displacement or obliteration of the inferior portion of the azygoesophageal interface, 24% (9/38) with obliteration or nodularity of the inferior portion of the descending thoracic aorta interface, 16% (6/38) with lateral displacement of the right inferior paraspinal interface, 11% (4/38) with lateral displacement of the left inferior paraspinal interface (Fig 1), and 3% (1/38) with varices in the left inferior pulmonary ligament. Paraesophageal varices of lesser diameter than the diameter of the descending thoracic aorta (typically smaller than 2.5 cm) could not be seen on chest computed radiography.

Conclusion.—Chest computed radiography was moderately sensitive for paraesophageal varices. When well developed, varices were characteristic and offered a limited differential diagnosis. Whether observed clinically or radiographically, splenomegaly eliminated almost all other diagnostic considerations.

► In patients with significant paraesophageal varices, a well-done chest x-ray study can detect the varices with a moderate sensitivity, a very high specificity, and reasonable accuracy. Interestingly, detection of paraesophageal varices by chest x-ray film appears to be limited to those masses of varices that are as large as or larger than the descending thoracic aorta. Interesting information, but of uncertain clinical significance.

Subject Index

A

Abdominal
  aneurysmal aortitis in Behçet's disease, endovascular treatment of, 130
  aortic aneurysm (*see* Aneurysm, aortic, abdominal)
Acidic
  fibroblast growth factor, angiogenic potential of (in rat), 1
Addicts
  drug, femoral pseudoaneurysm in, 413
Adhesion
  molecule-1, vascular cell, increase in chronic venous disease, 108
Adolescents
  palmar hyperhidrosis in, primary, thoracoscopic upper thoracic sympathectomy for, 210
α-Adrenergic
  receptors, role in ischemic preconditioning, 8
African-Americans
  renal artery repair in, 299
Age
  aortic diameter and, infrarenal, 267
  hemodialysis access survival and, 346
  as risk factor for endarterectomy for asymptomatic carotid stenosis, 375
Air
  plethysmography
    in diagnosis of chronic venous insufficiency, 181
    in venous disease, chronic, variability and reliability of, 452
Albumin
  -impregnated prosthetic graft for infrarenal aortic replacement, 402
Alcoholic
  solution of zein, percutaneous sclerotherapy for lymphangiomas with, in children, 208
Allograft, 394
  aortic, cryopreserved
    in situ repair of aortobronchial, aortoesophageal, and aortoenteric fistulae with, 397
    in situ replacement for vascular graft infection (in dog), 396
  arterial, in situ, for aortic prosthetic infection, 395
  saphenous vein, bypass surgery, immunosuppression for, 394
Alpha-adrenergic
  receptors, role in ischemic preconditioning, 8
Alpha-tocopherol
  supplements, effect on incidence of major coronary events in men with previous myocardial infarction, 17
Amputation
  rates, effects of vascular surgery on, 332
Amyloid
  A protein, serum, as marker of exercise-induced inflammatory response, effect of exercise training for intermittent claudication on, 26
Anastomosis
  aortoiliac, noninfected aneurysm of, endovascular grafts for, 123
  distal, vein interposition cuff at, infrainguinal polytetrafluoroethylene graft with, 324
Ancrod
  for digital ischemia and gangrene due to red cell aggregation induced by acquired dysfibrinogenemia, 354
Anesthesia
  leg bypass, 327
  local
    for arterial reconstruction, infrainguinal, 327
    for revascularization, lower limb, in high-risk patients, 328
AneuRx graft
  bifurcated, for abdominal aortic aneurysms, 127
Aneurysm
  aortic, 267
    abdominal (*see below*)
    descending, repairs, neurologic deficit after, effect of cerebrospinal fluid drainage and distal aortic perfusion on, 258
    epidemiology, 267
    graft repair of, endovascular, endoleak after (in dog), 121
    infected, surgical treatment of, 272
    inflammatory, 285
    "inoperable," complementary surgical/interventional techniques for nonresective management of, 282
    management, 271
    perivisceral, rupture of, 246
    ruptured, decision not to operate, 276
    thoracic, 245
    thoracic, extensive, staged repair of, effect on neurologic outcome, 253
    thoracic, resection of, appropriate size criterion for, 245

thoracoabdominal, 247
thoracoabdominal, repair, clamp-and-sew technique, 255
thoracoabdominal, repair, importance of intercostal artery reattachment during, 249
thoracoabdominal, repair, mesenteric shunting decreases visceral ischemia during, 261
thoracoabdominal, repair, neurologic deficit after, delayed, 260
thoracoabdominal, repair, neurologic deficit after, effect of cerebrospinal fluid drainage and distal aortic perfusion on, 258
thoracoabdominal, repair, perfusion during, retrograde aortic and selective organ, 257
aortic, abdominal
angiography of, CT, 124
in coronary bypass patients, 269
diameter of, 287
endoprosthesis for, modular bifurcation, 127
infrarenal, endovascular treatment by Stentor system, 120
infrarenal, repair, natural history of residual infrarenal aorta after, 278
prevalence in diabetic men, 269
repair, conversion from endoluminal to open, 125
repair, endovascular *vs.* open, postoperative fever, bowel ischemia, and cytokine response to, 133
repair, laparoscopically assisted, 279
rupture associated with
high-attenuating crescent sign, 188
rupture repair, long-term survival and late complications after, 274
small, expansion of, serum elastin peptides as predictor of, 106
small, very, long-term outcome, 271
stent-graft for, colonic ischemia after, fatal, 132
stent-graft for, covered, juxtarenal placement of, 119
wall stress, effect of intraluminal thrombus on, 114
aortoiliac, noninfected anastomotic, endovascular graft for, 123
false, noninfected, detected long after aortic prosthetic reconstruction, morbidity and mortality of reconstructive surgery for, 284
venous, presentation and management of, 464

Aneurysmal
aortitis, abdominal, in Behçet's disease, endovascular treatment of, 130
Angiogenesis, 1
therapeutic (in rat), 1
Angiogenic
potential of acidic fibroblast growth factor and heparin (in rat), 1
Angiography
(*See also* Arteriography)
carotid, cost savings associated with nonroutine use of, 361
completion, is it really necessary? 358
CT
of abdominal aortic aneurysms, 124
vs. intra-arterial digital subtraction angiography of aortoiliac occlusive disease, 190
digital subtraction, intra-arterial, *vs.* CT angiography of aortoiliac occlusive disease, 190
Doppler, three-dimensional power, in vitro evaluation of multiple arterial stenoses using, 172
magnetic resonance
of hand and wrist with severe ischemic disease, 352
of renal artery stenosis, hemodynamically significant atherosclerotic, 191
two-dimensional digital subtraction, of distal lower extremity arteries, 168
outcome, long-term, after percutaneous transluminal coronary angioplasty and intracoronary radiation therapy, 6
outcome of antiplatelet *vs.* anticoagulant therapy after coronary stent placement for myocardial infarction, 43
pulmonary, in acute major pulmonary embolism, 446
serial, natural history of stenosis from intracranial atherosclerosis by, 382
Angioplasty, 134
balloon *(see* percutaneous transluminal *below)*
coronary
ischemia during, phentolamine prevents adaptation to, 8
percutaneous transluminal, myocardial infarction and cardiac mortality rate after, 10
percutaneous transluminal, radiation therapy after, intracoronary, long-term angiographic and clinical outcome after, 6

Coagulation, 40
  profiles, abnormal, and saphenous vein thrombophlebitis, 434
Coil
  embolization for endoleak after endovascular graft repair of aortic aneurysms (in dog), 121
Colitis
  Clostridium difficile, after aortic surgery, 290
Collagen
  subtype pattern in normal and varicose saphenous veins, 471
Collars
  vein, for ePTFE grafts, myointimal hyperplasia in, 320
Colon
  ischemia
    after endovascular treatment of infrarenal abdominal aneurysms by Stentor system, 121
    fatal, after stent graft for aortic aneurysm, 132
Compression
  devices
    foot venous, hemodynamic evaluation of, 470
    sequential, *vs.* foot pumps for prophylaxis of deep venous thrombosis in high-risk trauma patients, 437
  pneumatic, intermittent, fibrinolytic effects of, 112
  popliteal artery, and force of active plantar flexion, 207
  therapy for femoral artery pseudoaneurysm, delayed rupture after, 175
Computed radiography
  chest, in paraesophageal varices, 483
Computed tomography
  angiography
    of abdominal aortic aneurysms, 124
    vs. intra-arterial digital subtraction angiography of aortoiliac occlusive disease, 190
  crescent sign on, high-attenuating, abdominal aortic aneurysm rupture associated with, 188
  helical
    after aortic injury, blunt, 411
    of pulmonary embolism, acute, 184
  of hematoma of aorta, intramural, 241
Contamination
  threshold for infection of laparotomies, electric cautery lowers (in rat), 232
Contrast
  agent, ultrasound, perflenapent emulsion as, 201
Coronary
  angioplasty (*see* Angioplasty, coronary)
  arterioles, integrin signaling transduces shear stress–dependent vasodilation of, 104
  artery disease
    endovascular presence of viable *Chlamydia pneumoniae* in, 35
    mortality, and plasma homocysteine levels, 61
    perioperative considerations, 213
    unstable, low-molecular-weight *vs.* unfractionated heparin for, 53
  atherosclerosis (*see* Atherosclerosis, coronary)
  bypass (*see* Bypass, coronary)
  events, major, incidence in men with previous myocardial infarction, effects of α-tocopherol and β-carotene supplements on, 17
  heart disease
    (See also Coronary, artery disease *above)*
    risk in women, relation to folate and vitamin B_6 intake, 54
  intracoronary radiation therapy after percutaneous transluminal angioplasty, long-term angiographic and clinical outcome after, 6
  stent placement for myocardial infarction, outcome with antiplatelet *vs.* anticoagulant therapy after, 43
Cost
  -effectiveness of screening for major deep vein thrombosis in seriously injured patients, 441
  efficacy of duplex surveillance and prophylactic angioplasty of arteriovenous ePTFE grafts, 351
  impact of clinical pathway for elective infrarenal aortic reconstructions on, 295
  savings associated with nonroutine use of carotid angiography, 361
  of stenting and balloon angioplasty *vs.* endarterectomy for carotid artery stenosis, 139
Counterpulsation
  intra-aortic balloon pump, prolonged, implications for vascular surgeon with, 331

CP101,606
  effect on volume of ischemic brain damage and cytotoxic brain edema after middle cerebral artery occlusion (in cat), 69
C-reactive protein
  as marker of exercise-induced inflammatory response, effect of exercise training for intermittent claudication on, 26
Crescent sign
  high-attenuating, abdominal aortic aneurysm rupture associated with, 188
Cryopreserved
  aortic allograft
    repair, in situ, of aortobronchial, aortoesophageal, and aortoenteric fistulae, 397
    replacement, in situ, for vascular graft infection (in dog), 396
CT (*see* Computed tomography)
Cuff
  vein interposition, at distal anastomosis, infrainguinal polytetrafluoroethylene graft with, 324
Cyclooxygenase
  -dependent mechanism, fatty acids augment endothelium-dependent dilation in hand veins by, 101
Cytokine
  response to endovascular *vs.* open abdominal aortic aneurysm repair, 133
Cytomegalovirus
  in atherosclerosis of carotid artery, 32
Cytotoxic
  brain edema after middle cerebral artery occlusion, effect of CP101,606 on (in cat), 69

D

D-dimer
  prediction of deep venous thrombosis by, 426, 428
Decision
  making, impact of noninvasive venous testing in diagnosis of pulmonary embolism on, 439
Decongestive
  physiotherapy, complete, for lymphedema of extremities, 472
Demographics
  valvular strands and cerebral ischemia and, 163
Dermal
  fibroblast growth in chronic venous ulcers, reduced, stimulation with growth factors, 107
  microcirculation, morphometric assessment in chronic venous insufficiency, 473
Diabetes mellitus, 55
  aneurysm and, abdominal aortic, in men, 269
  insulin-dependent, endothelial function in, effect of angiotensin-converting enzyme inhibition on, 57
  non–insulin-dependent, metabolic control and prevalent cardiovascular disease in, 55
Dialysis
  (*See also* Hemodialysis)
  access methods, longitudinal comparison of, 337
  dependence after renal artery repair failures, 303
  patients
    hyperhomocysteinemia as adverse cardiovascular risk factor in, 65
    leg ischemia in, critical, outcome of infrainguinal bypass for, 335
Diastolic
  velocities, importance in detection of celiac mesenteric artery disease by duplex ultrasound, 196
Digital
  ischemia and gangrene due to red cell aggregation induced by acquired dysfibrinogenemia, 353
Dilator
  responses of atherosclerotic epicardial coronary arteries, effects of conjugated estrogens and tamoxifen on (in monkey), 60
Discharge
  hospital, ultrasound screening for deep venous thrombosis after arthroplasty for, 442
Dodecafluoropentane
  emulsion and ultrasound, dissolution of thrombotic arterial occlusion by, 117
Doppler
  angiography, three-dimensional power, in vitro evaluation of multiple arterial stenoses using, 172
  ultrasound (*see* Ultrasound, Doppler)
Drug
  addicts, femoral pseudoaneurysm in, 413
  therapy, 216

Duplex imaging (*see* Ultrasound, duplex)
Dysfibrinogenemia
  red cell aggregation induced by, digital ischemia and gangrene due to, 353

E

ECG
  -gated 3D intravascular ultrasound of coronary atherosclerotic plaques, 198
  12-lead, preoperative, importance in predicting perioperative ischemia and cardiac complications in major vascular surgery, 213
Echocardiography
  in pulmonary embolism, acute major, 446
  transesophageal
    for emboli immediately after tourniquet release during total knee arthroplasty with cement, 444
    in patients with peripheral macroemboli from thoracic aortic pathology, 235
EchoGen
  ultrasound and, dissolution of thrombotic arterial occlusion by, 117
Echolucency
  of carotid artery plaques, lipid-rich, on ultrasound B-mode images, 383
  of computerized ultrasound images of carotid atherosclerotic plaques, association with increased levels of triglyceride-rich lipoproteins and increased plaque lipid content, 160
Economizing
  vein-graft surveillance programs, 389
Edema
  brain, cytotoxic, after middle cerebral artery occlusion, effect of CP101,606 on (in cat), 69
Elastin
  peptides, serum, as predictor of expansion of small abdominal aortic aneurysms, 106
Elderly
  aneurysm in, abdominal aortic
    prevalence in diabetic men, 269
    small, expansion of, serum elastin peptides as predictor of, 106
    stent graft for, fatal colonic ischemia after, 132
  aortic surgery in, *Clostridium difficile* colitis after, 290
  atrial fibrillation patients, warfarin use in, 217
  carotid endarterectomy in
    for asymptomatic stenosis, 375
    in octogenarians, 372
  vascular patients, coronary bypass in, 214
Electric
  cautery lowers contamination threshold for infection of laparotomies (in rat), 232
Electrocardiography
  -gated 3D intravascular ultrasound of coronary atherosclerotic plaques, 198
  12-lead, preoperative, importance in predicting perioperative ischemia and cardiac complications in major vascular surgery, 213
Elephant trunk procedure
  reversed, for mega aorta, 265
  staged, for extensive thoracic aortic aneurysms, 253
Emboli
  immediately after tourniquet release during total knee arthroplasty with cement, transesophageal echocardiography for, 444
  macroemboli, peripheral, from thoracic aortic pathology, diagnosis and management of patients with, 235
Embolic
  disease, distal vertebral artery reconstruction for, 378
Embolism
  pulmonary, 421
    acute, CT of, helical, 184
    acute, heparin for, low-molecular-weight *vs.* unfractionated, 448
    acute major, management strategies and determinants of outcome in, 446
    diagnosis, noninvasive, 439
    diagnosis, noninvasive, impact on decisionmaking, 439
    early after isolated calf vein thrombosis, 432
    risk of cancer diagnosis after, 425
  thromboembolism (*see* Thromboembolism)
Embolization
  atheroma of aortic arch as underestimated source of, mobile, 236
  during carotid endarterectomy with Javid *vs.* Pruitt-Inahara shunt, 153
  coil, for endoleak after endovascular graft repair of aortic aneurysms (in dog), 121

Enalapril
  effect on endothelial function in insulin-dependent diabetes mellitus, 58
Enalaprilat
  effect on endothelial function in insulin-dependent diabetes mellitus, 58
Encephalopathy
  after portosystemic shunt, transjugular intrahepatic, for prevention of recurrent variceal hemorrhage, 481
Endarterectomy
  of aorta, ascending, 237
  carotid
    angiography after, completion, is it really necessary? 358
    for asymptomatic stenosis, preoperative risk factors for, 375
    does not affect long-term blood pressure, 366
    epidemiology among Medicare beneficiaries, 376
    eversion *vs.* standard, 360
    hemodynamic cerebral ischemia and microembolic signals detected during, 140
    indications, outcomes, and provider volumes for, 365
    with Javid *vs.* Pruitt-Inahara shunt, middle cerebral artery blood velocity, embolization, and neurologic outcome during, 153
    mortality, in Medicare population, 364
    in octogenarians, 372
    outcome assessment, early, for 2228 consecutive procedures, 357
    outcomes, population-based *vs.* NASCET, 363
    for progressive stenosis, after angioplasty and stent placement, 141
    prophylactic, 369
    prophylactic, in patients with high-grade carotid stenosis undergoing coronary bypass, 371
    stenosis after, duplex imaging predicts, 155
    for symptomatic stenosis, recently, 380
    vs. balloon angioplasty and stenting for carotid artery stenosis, cost of, 139
Endograft (*see* Graft, endovascular)
Endoleak
  after endovascular graft repair of aortic aneurysms (in dog), 121
Endoluminal
  repair
    (*See also* Graft, endovascular)
    of abdominal aortic aneurysms, conversion to open repair, 125
Endoprosthesis (*see* Graft, endovascular)
Endoscopic
  perforating vein surgery, subfascial (*see* Perforating vein, surgery, endoscopic subfascial)
  sclerotherapy *vs.* transjugular intrahepatic portosystemic shunt for variceal hemorrhage
    acute, 479
    for prevention of recurrent hemorrhage, 480
Endothelium
  activation in patients with chronic venous disease, 108
  cell(s)
    adaptation to chronic thrombosis (in dog), 46
    cultured, hyperglycemia-induced migration defect in, nitric oxide mediation of, 85
    vascular, apolipoprotein(a) induces monocyte chemotactic activity in, 103
  -dependent dilation in hand veins, effect of fatty acids on, 101
  -dependent relaxation
    effect of red wine on (in rabbit), 86
    in vein grafts, effect of topical vascular endothelial growth factor on (in rabbit), 2
  dysfunction, arterial, hyperhomocysteinemia as risk factor for, 68
  function, in insulin-dependent diabetes mellitus, effect of angiotensin-converting enzyme inhibition on, 57
  growth factor, vascular (*see* Vascular, endothelial growth factor)
Endovascular
  graft (*see* Graft, endovascular)
  presence of viable *Chlamydia pneumoniae* in coronary artery disease, 35
  stents in combined approach to treatment of proximal arterial occlusions of upper limb, 138
  technique in hemodialysis access, 339
  treatment
    of aneurysms, infrarenal abdominal, by Stentor system, 120
    of aortitis, abdominal aneurysmal, in Behçet's disease, 130
  vs. surgical management of thrombosed dialysis access grafts, 350

Enoxaparin
- *vs.* unfractionated heparin for unstable coronary artery disease, 53

Enteritis
- *Salmonella,* causing infected aortic aneurysm, 272

Enzyme
- angiotensin-converting enzyme inhibition, effect on endothelial function in insulin-dependent diabetes mellitus, 57

Epidermal
- growth factor, dermal fibroblast growth in chronic venous ulcers stimulated by, 107

Epiphysiodesis
- in Klippel-Trénaunay syndrome, 462

Estrogen, 58
- conjugated, effect on dilator responses of atherosclerotic epicardial coronary arteries (in monkey), 60
- replacement therapy, postmenopausal
  - alone or combined with pravastatin for hypercholesterolemia, 58
  - duration in relation to risk of myocardial infarction, 216

Ethanol
- injection, direct, for venous malformations, 463

Ethibloc
- percutaneous sclerotherapy with, for lymphangiomas, in children, 208

Ethnicity
- incidence of idiopathic deep venous thrombosis and secondary thromboembolism and, 435

Exercise
- therapy for intermittent claudication, 228
- training for intermittent claudication, 26

Extracellular
- matrix
  - –basic fibroblast growth factor inactivation by photodynamic therapy, 102
  - production by infragenicular smooth muscle cells, effect of interleukin-1β on, 95
  - proteins and platelet-derived growth factor provide synergistic stimulus for vascular smooth muscle cell migration, 92
  - in vein grafts, effect of hypercholesterolemia on gene expression of novel components of (in rabbit), 23

Extremity
- hypertrophy in Klippel-Trénaunay syndrome, 461
- ischemia
  - acute, intramuscular injection of vascular endothelial growth factor gene for (in rabbit), 3
  - critical, diagnosis, skin perfusion pressure measurement in, 329
- lower
  - (*See also* Leg)
  - aneurysm in, venous, presentation and management of, 464
  - artery(ies), distal, evaluation with two-dimensional MR digital subtraction angiography, 168
  - artery(ies), evaluation, segmental arterial blood pressures in, 170
  - artery(ies) walls, detection of *Chlamydia pneumoniae* in atherosclerotic plaques in, 31
  - atherosclerosis, carotid duplex in, in young adults, 374
  - atherosclerotic disease progression, ability of ankle-brachial index to detect, 174
  - injury, venous, long-term results of, 419
  - ischemia, critical, subintimal angioplasty of infrapopliteal occlusion in, 135
  - ischemia, limitations of intra-arterial thrombolysis for, 149
  - ischemia/reperfusion of, causing lung injury, role of nitric oxide and tumor necrosis factor in (in rat), 80
  - malperfusion after acute aortic dissection, abdominal aortic tailoring for, 283
  - revascularization, arteriography in, MR, 202
  - revascularization, in high-risk patients, local anesthesia for, 328
  - salvage, prosthetic bypass with distal vein patch for, 322
  - thrombi, deep vein, origin in acute venous thrombosis 421
  - thrombosis, deep venous, *vs.* upper extremity thrombosis, 438
  - vascular reconstruction, based on color duplex imaging alone, 164
  - venous malformations in, direct injection of ethanol for, 463
- lymphedema, effective treatment of, 472
- salvage and dialysis access maintenance in ischemic steal syndrome, distal revascularization-interval ligation for, 344

Laser
  photocoagulation, interstitial Nd:YAG, for vascular malformations and hemangiomas, in children, 209
Lefradafiban
  platelet aggregation inhibited by, 40
Leg
  (*See also* Extremity, lower)
  bypass anesthesia, 327
  ischemia, 307
    critical, with chronic renal failure, outcome of infrainguinal bypass for, 335
  microcirculation in, leukocyte activity in, in chronic venous disease, 110
  microvascular permeability after aortic surgery in, 82
  ulcer, venous, subfascial endoscopic perforator vein surgery for
    efficacy and relation to venous ulcer healing, 460
    vs. open surgery, 459
  vein graft, 307
    saphenous bypass, effect of ticlopidine on long-term patency of, 315
    surveillance, 309
Leukocyte
  activity in microcirculation of leg in chronic venous disease, 110
  adhesion inhibition reduces neointimal hyperplasia after arterial injury (in rabbit), 45
Ligation
  distal revascularization-interval ligation for limb salvage and maintenance of dialysis access in ischemic steal syndrome, 344
  femoral artery, for pseudoaneurysm in drug addicts, 413
  vein, for lower extremity venous injuries, long-term results of, 419
Limb (*see* Extremity)
Lipid
  content of carotid atherosclerotic plaques associated with echolucency of computerized ultrasound images, 160
  -rich carotid artery plaques appear echolucent on ultrasound B-mode images and may be associated with intraplaque hemorrhage, 383
Lipids, 5
Lipoproteins
  triglyceride rich-, association with echolucency of computerized ultrasound images of carotid atherosclerotic plaques, 160
Livedo
  reticularis after carbon dioxide arteriography, 203
Liver
  function during thoracoabdominal and descending thoracic aortic repair, impact of distal aortic and visceral perfusion on, 251
  transplantation, shunt surgery during era of, 482
Lumbar
  sympathectomy for focal ischemic necrosis, foot $TcPO_2$ response to, 334
Lung
  (*See also* Pulmonary)
  injury
    acute, after aortic surgery, 82
    ischemia/reperfusion of lower extremities causing, role of nitric oxide and tumor necrosis factor in (in rat), 80
  scan in acute major pulmonary embolism, 446
Lymphangioma
  percutaneous sclerotherapy with alcoholic solution of zein for, in children, 208
Lymphatic
  disease, chronic, 451
Lymphedema
  extremity, effective treatment of, 472

M

Macroemboli
  peripheral, from thoracic aortic pathology, diagnosis and management of patients with, 235
Magnetic resonance angiography (*see* Angiography, magnetic resonance)
Magnetic resonance arteriography
  in revascularization, distal lower extremity, 202
Magnetic resonance imaging
  of aortic dissection, acute type A, in 20-year follow-up, 263
  of hematoma of thoracic aorta, 243
  measurements, in vivo, of blood oxygen saturation in superior mesenteric vein for diagnosis of chronic mesenteric ischemia, 195
Magnetic resonance spectroscopy
  phosphorus-31, dynamic, in arterial occlusive disease, 87

Magnetic resonance venography
  gadolinium-enhanced, "bull's-eye" sign determines thrombus presence and age on, 185
Malformations
  vascular, interstitial Nd:YAG photocoagulation for, in children, 209
  venous
    ethanol injection for, direct, 463
    in Klippel-Trénaunay syndrome, 461
Malignancy
  neck, operation for, carotid resection and replacement with autogenous arterial graft during, 368
Malperfusion
  renal, visceral, and lower extremity, after acute aortic dissection, abdominal aortic tailoring for, 283
Mast cells
  in dermal microcirculation in chronic venous insufficiency, 474
  distribution, activation, and phenotype in carotid atherosclerosis, 116
Medicare
  population, carotid endarterectomy among
    epidemiology of, 376
    mortality of, 364
Medtronic AneuRx graft
  bifurcated, for abdominal aortic aneurysms, 127
Mega aorta
  reversed elephant trunk procedure for, 265
Membrane
  polytetrafluoroethylene pericardial, for retroperitoneal closure after abdominal aortic surgery, 289
Mesenteric
  artery disease, detection by duplex ultrasound, importance of diastolic velocities in, 196
  ischemia, chronic
    MRI measurements of blood oxygen saturation in superior mesenteric vein for diagnosis, in vivo, 195
    surgical therapy results for, 304
  resistance arteries, nitric oxide production in, flow-dependent, direct in vivo measurement of (in dog), 83
  shunting decreases visceral ischemia during thoracoabdominal aneurysm repair, 261
Metabolic
  control in non–insulin-dependent diabetes, and prevalent cardiovascular disease, 55
  results of side-to-side portacaval shunt for intractable cirrhotic ascites, 477
Methicillin
  -resistant *Staphylococcus aureus* infection of femoral pseudoaneurysm in drug addicts, 414
Methylenetetrahydrofolate
  reductase gene variant related to plasma total homocysteine and plasma folate, and myocardial infarction in young women, 63
Microcirculation
  dermal, morphometric assessment in chronic venous insufficiency, 473
  leg, leukocyte activity in, in chronic venous disease, 110
Microemboli
  detection, transcranial Doppler
    in identification of patients at high risk of perioperative stroke, 151
    oxygen inhalation differentiates gaseous from nongaseous, 162
Microembolic
  signals detected during carotid endarterectomy and carotid angioplasty, 140
Microvascular
  permeability in lung and leg after aortic surgery, 82
Mitogen
  -activated protein kinase
    activation of, smooth muscle cell migration and proliferation mediated by, 93
    signaling in arterial smooth muscle cells, thrombin-induced, heparin inhibits (in baboon), 50
Modular
  bifurcation endoprosthesis for abdominal aortic aneurysms, 127
Monocyte
  chemotactic activity in vascular endothelial cells induced by apolipoprotein(a), 103
Morbidity
  cardiac, effect of perioperative maintenance of normothermia on, 221
  of reconstructive surgery for noninfected false aneurysms detected long after aortic prosthetic reconstruction, 284

of vascular surgery, elective, effect of routine pulmonary artery catheterization on, 224
Morphology
carotid plaque, correlation with presenting symptomatology, 377
Morphometric
assessment of dermal microcirculation in chronic venous insufficiency, 473
Mortality
of allograft treatment, in situ arterial, for aortic prosthetic infection, 395
among retired men, nonsmoking, effects of walking on, 227
after arteriography, carbon dioxide, 203
cardiac, rate after bypass surgery or angioplasty, 10
coronary artery disease, and plasma homocysteine levels, 61
effects of vascular surgery on, 332
of endarterectomy, carotid, in Medicare population, 364
after myocardial infarction, and β-blocker dosages, 233
of reconstructive surgery for noninfected false aneurysms detected long after aortic prosthetic reconstruction, 284
surgical, of endovascular treatment of infrarenal abdominal aneurysms by Stentor system, 121
of vascular surgery, elective, effect of routine pulmonary artery catheterization on, 224
MRI (*see* Magnetic resonance imaging)
Multivitamins
in prevention of restenosis after coronary angioplasty, 7
Muscle
smooth muscle cells (*see* Smooth muscle, cells)
Mycotic
aneurysm in perivisceral aorta, rupture of, 246
Myocardial
infarction
coronary stent placement for, outcome with antiplatelet *vs.* anticoagulant therapy after, 43
heart failure after, effect of ramipril on, follow-up study, 18
mortality after, and β-blocker dosages, 233
previous, incidence of major coronary events in men with, effects of α-tocopherol and β-carotene supplements on, 17
rate after bypass surgery or angioplasty, 10
risk, and body iron stores, in men, 21
risk, and common carotid intima-media thickness, 11
risk, and estrogen replacement therapy duration, 216
survivors, elevated *Chlamydia pneumoniae* antibodies, cardiovascular events, and azithromycin in, 38
in women, young, relation to plasma total homocysteine, folate, and methylenetetrahydrofolate reductase gene variant, 63
viability, residual, in patients with ischemic cardiomyopathy, improved outcome after coronary bypass surgery, 5
Myointimal
hyperplasia in vein collars for ePTFE grafts, 320

N

Naloxone
in prevention of paralysis in thoracoabdominal aortic replacement, 262
Nd:YAG
photocoagulation, interstitial, for vascular malformations and hemangiomas, in children, 209
Near-infrared spectroscopy (*see* Spectroscopy, near-infrared)
Neck
malignancy, operation for, carotid resection and replacement with autogenous arterial graft during, 368
Necrosis
ischemic, focal, foot $TcPO_2$ response to lumbar sympathectomy for, 334
Neural
-vascular trauma, combined, 416
lower extremity, management of, 416
Neurologic
deficit
after aortic aneurysm repairs, effect of cerebrospinal fluid drainage and distal aortic perfusion on, 258
delayed, after thoracoabdominal aneurysm repair, 260
outcome
of carotid endarterectomy with Javid *vs.* Pruitt-Inahara shunt, 153
of staged repair of extensive thoracic aortic aneurysm, 253

Nitinol
  stent-grafts, polyester-covered, juxtarenal placement for abdominal aortic aneurysms, 119
Nitric oxide, 75
  dilatation of saphenous vein grafts by, 76
  mediates hyperglycemia-induced defective migration in cultured endothelial cells, 85
  production, flow-dependent, in mesenteric resistance arteries, direct in vivo measurement of (in dog), 83
  role in lung injury due to ischemia/reperfusion of lower extremities (in rat), 80
  supplementation and suppression, effects on development of intimal hyperplasia in vein grafts (in rabbit), 77
  synthase
    activity, suppression of, effect on flow-induced arterial enlargement (in rat), 79
    inducible, expression in vein grafts, 75
Nitroprusside
  with beta-blockers reduces aortic rupture after blunt injury, 411
N-Methyl-D-aspartate
  receptor antagonist CP101,606, effect on volume of ischemic brain damage and cytotoxic brain edema after middle cerebral artery occlusion (in cat), 69
Nonatherosclerotic
  conditions, 213
Normothermia
  maintenance, perioperative, reduces incidence of morbid cardiac events, 221

O

Occlusion
  arterial
    proximal, upper limb, combined treatment approach with endovascular stents, 138
    thrombotic, dissolution by ultrasound and dodecafluoropentane emulsion, 117
  cerebral artery, middle
    effect of CP101,606 on volume of ischemic brain damage and cytotoxic brain edema after (in cat), 69
    effect of ZD9379 on number of spreading depressions and infarct size after (in rat), 70
  infrapopliteal, in critically ischemic limbs, subintimal angioplasty of, 135
  vein graft, thrombectomy *vs.* thrombolysis in, intimal hyperplasia after (in dog), 313
Occlusive disease
  aortoiliac, angiography of, CT *vs.* intra-arterial digital subtraction, 190
  arterial
    innominate, central reconstruction techniques for, 240
    magnetic resonance spectroscopy in, dynamic phosphorus-31, 87
  venous, iliac vein reconstructions in, 468
Octogenarians
  carotid endarterectomy in, 372
Organ
  perfusion, selective, during thoracoabdominal aortic aneurysm repair, 257
Ovarian
  cancer and venous thromboembolism, 424
Oxygen
  inhalation differentiates gaseous from nongaseous microemboli detected by transcranial Doppler ultrasound, 162
  saturation, blood, in superior mesenteric vein, in vivo MR imaging measurements for diagnosis of chronic mesenteric ischemia, 195
  tension, transcutaneous tissue, foot, response to lumbar sympathectomy for focal ischemic necrosis, 334

P

Pacific Islanders
  incidence of idiopathic deep venous thrombosis and secondary thromboembolism in, 435
Pain
  after endoscopic therapy for prevention of recurrent variceal hemorrhage, 481
Palmar
  hyperhidrosis, primary, thoracoscopic upper thoracic sympathectomy for, 210

Palmaz-Schatz stent placement
  for myocardial infarction, outcome of antiplatelet *vs.* anticoagulant therapy after, 43
Pancreas
  cancer and venous thromboembolism, 422
Paraesophageal
  varices, chest computed radiography in, 483
Paralysis
  in thoracoabdominal aortic replacement, cardiac function as risk factor for, 262
Patch
  distal vein, with prosthetic bypass for limb salvage, 322
Pathway
  clinical, for elective infrarenal aortic reconstructions, impact of, 295
Peptides
  serum elastin, as predictor of expansion of small abdominal aortic aneurysms, 106
Percutaneous
  angioplasty, transluminal (*see* Angioplasty, percutaneous transluminal)
  sclerotherapy with alcoholic solution of zein for lymphangiomas, in children, 208
  thrombin injection for iatrogenic femoral pseudoaneurysm, 415
Perflenapent
  emulsion as ultrasound contrast agent, 201
Perforating vein
  surgery, subfascial endoscopic, 459
    efficacy and relation to venous ulcer healing, 460
    vs. open subfascial surgery, for venous leg ulceration, 459
Perfusion
  aortic (*see* Aorta, perfusion)
  organ, selective, during thoracoabdominal aortic aneurysm repair, 257
  skin, pressure measurement, in diagnosis of critical limb ischemia, 329
  visceral, distal, impact on liver function during thoracoabdominal and descending thoracic aortic repair, 251
Pericardial
  membrane, polytetrafluoroethylene, for retroperitoneal closure after abdominal aortic surgery, 289
Perioperative
  conditions, 213
  ischemia in major vascular surgery, importance of preoperative 12-lead ECG in predicting, 213
  maintenance of normothermia reduces incidence of morbid cardiac events, 221
  stroke
    does prophylactic carotid endarterectomy in patients with high-grade stenosis undergoing coronary bypass decrease? 371
    microembolus detection by transcranial Doppler in identification of patients at high risk of, 151
  transfusion incidence and volume, effects of albumin-impregnated prosthetic graft for infrarenal aortic replacement on, 402
Peripheral
  arteries, biochemical composition of, as examined with near-infrared Raman spectroscopy, 89
  vascular disease
    activated protein C resistance and factor V Leiden and, 52
    risk of, and plasma C-reactive protein, 97
  vein bypasses, failure of, and antibodies to cardiolipin, 310
Peritoneal
  dialysis patients, hyperhomocysteinemia as adverse cardiovascular risk factor in, 65
Perivisceral
  aorta, rupture of, 246
Phenotype
  mast cell, in carotid atherosclerosis, 116
Phentolamine
  prevents adaptation to ischemia during coronary angioplasty, 8
Phosphorus-31
  magnetic resonance spectroscopy, dynamic, in arterial occlusive disease, 87
Photocoagulation
  laser, interstitial Nd:YAG, for vascular malformations and hemangiomas, in children, 209
Photodynamic therapy
  inactivates extracellular matrix–basic fibroblast growth factor, 102
Physiotherapy
  complete decongestive, for lymphedema of extremities, 472

high-risk, prophylaxis of deep venous thrombosis in, sequential compression devices *vs.* foot pumps for, 437
serious, screening for major deep vein thrombosis in, 441
vascular, 407
combined with neural trauma, 416
combined with neural trauma, lower extremity, management of, 416
thoracic outlet, aggressive management of, 418
venous, 419
lower extremity, long-term results of, 419
Treadmill
testing for evaluation of claudication, 176
Triglyceride
-rich lipoprotein levels, increased, association with echolucency of computerized ultrasound images of carotid atherosclerotic plaques, 160
Tumor
necrosis factor role in lung injury due to ischemia/reperfusion of lower extremities (in rat), 80

U

Ulcer
venous
chronic, dermal fibroblast growth in, reduced, stimulation with growth factors, 107
leg, subfascial endoscopic perforator vein surgery for, efficacy and relation to venous ulcer healing, 460
leg, subfascial endoscopic *vs.* open perforator vein surgery for, 459
Ultrasound
B-mode
atherosclerotic changes in carotid artery bulb measured by, association with extent of coronary atherosclerosis, 12
echolucency of lipid-rich carotid artery plaques on, 383
contrast agent, perflenapent emulsion as, 201
dodecafluoropentane emulsion and, dissolution of thrombotic arterial occlusion by, 117
Doppler
power, of carotid artery stenosis, 157
renal hilar, in management of renovascular disease, 193
transcranial, for hemodynamic cerebral ischemia and microembolic signals during carotid endarterectomy and carotid angioplasty, 140
transcranial, microemboli detected by, oxygen inhalation differentiates gaseous from nongaseous, 162
transcranial, microembolus detection on, in identification of patients at high risk of perioperative stroke, 151
duplex
carotid, in young adults with lower extremity atherosclerosis, 374
carotid stenosis after carotid endarterectomy predicted with, 155
celiac mesenteric artery disease detected by, importance of diastolic velocities in, 196
color, for surveillance of infrainguinal polytetrafluoroethylene grafts, 205
color, in temporal arteritis diagnosis, 158
color, lower limb vascular reconstruction based on, 164
color, *vs.* arteriography, for imaging infrapopliteal arterial lesions, 165
in hemodynamic evaluation of late sequelae of deep venous thrombosis, 456
predictive ability for internal carotid artery stenosis of 70%–99%, 154
for renal parenchymal injury, contralateral, with unilateral atherosclerotic renal artery stenosis, 300
of run-off before femorocrural reconstruction, 167
selective use to replace preoperative arteriography for failing grafts, 390
surveillance of arteriovenous ePTFE grafts, cost efficacy of, 351
surveillance protocol, natural history of failing grafts in, 392
venous, for unilateral symptoms, 186
echolucency of computerized images of carotid atherosclerotic plaques are associated with increased levels of triglyceride-rich lipoproteins and increased plaque lipid content, 160
-guided percutaneous thrombin injection for iatrogenic femoral pseudoaneurysm, 416
intravascular, ECG-gated 3D, of coronary atherosclerotic plaques, 198
screening

for abdominal aortic aneurysms in diabetic men, 269
before hospital discharge for deep venous thrombosis after arthroplasty, 442
Urokinase
intra-arterial, limitations of, 149
intraoperative, after popliteal artery trauma improves limb salvage, 408
in occluded vein grafts, intimal hyperplasia after (in dog), 314

V

Valve
aortic, replacement, endarterectomy of ascending aorta in patients with porcelain aorta requiring, 237
incompetence early after isolated calf vein thrombosis, 432
vein, insufficiency, mild to moderate, after isolated calf vein thrombosis, 455
Valvular
strands and cerebral ischemia, 163
Varices
hemorrhage
acute, sclerotherapy in, endoscopic, *vs.* transjugular intrahepatic portosystemic shunt for, 479
recurrent, endoscopic sclerotherapy *vs.* transjugular intrahepatic portosystemic shunt for prevention of, 480
paraesophageal, chest computed radiography in, 483
Varicose veins
in Klippel-Trénaunay syndrome, 461
primary, venous insufficiency in, near-infrared spectroscopy of, 182
saphenous, collagen subtype in, 471
Vascular
access
for hemodialysis (*see* Hemodialysis, access)
upper extremity, 337
biology, 92
cardiovascular (*see* Cardiovascular)
cell adhesion molecule-1 increase in chronic venous disease, 108
disease, peripheral
activated protein C resistance and factor V Leiden and, 52
risk of, and plasma C-reactive protein, 97
endothelial cells, apolipoprotein(a) induces monocyte chemotactic activity in, 103
endothelial growth factor
expression in peripheral vein bypass grafts (in dog), 98
gene, intramuscular injection of, for acute limb ischemia (in rabbit), 3
topical, effect on vein graft intimal hyperplasia and endothelium-dependent relaxation (in rabbit), 2
endovascular (*see* Endovascular)
imaging, 151
intravascular ultrasound, ECG-gated 3D, of coronary atherosclerotic plaques, 198
laboratory, 151
malformations, interstitial Nd:YAG photocoagulation for, in children, 209
microvascular permeability in lung and leg after aortic surgery, 82
patients, coronary bypass in, 214
reconstruction
central, for innominate artery occlusive disease, 240
lower extremity, based on color duplex imaging alone, 164
renovascular disease management, renal hilar Doppler analysis in, 193
smooth muscle cells (*see* Smooth muscle, cells, vascular)
surgeon, implications of prolonged intra-aortic balloon pump counterpulsation for, 331
surgery, 218
antimicrobial prophylaxis in, duration of, 229
effects on amputation rates and mortality, 332
elective, effect of routine pulmonary artery catheterization on morbidity and mortality of, 224
major, perioperative ischemia and cardiac complications in, importance of preoperative 12-lead ECG in predicting, 213
patients, transfusions in, perioperative red cell, limiting, 220
reoperations, redo surgery and other interventions constitute more than one-third of, 218
trauma (*see* Trauma, vascular)
Vasodilation
of coronary arterioles, shear stress–dependent, integrin signaling transduces, 104
VCAM-1
increase in chronic venous disease, 108

Vein(s)
  aneurysms, presentation and management of, 464
  arteriovenous (*see* Arteriovenous)
  bypasses, peripheral, failure, and antibodies to cardiolipin, 310
  collars for ePTFE grafts, myointimal hyperplasia in, 320
  compression devices, foot, hemodynamic evaluation of, 470
  disease
    chronic, 451
    chronic, air plethysmography in, variability and reliability of, 452
    chronic, endothelial activation in, 108
    chronic, leukocyte activity in microcirculation of leg in, 110
    congenital, 461
    occlusive, iliac vein reconstructions in, 468
  femoral, catheterization, incidence of deep venous thrombosis after, 433
  graft (*see* Graft, vein)
  hand, fatty acids augment endothelium-dependent dilation in, 101
  imaging, 178
  insufficiency
    chronic, air plethysmography in diagnosis, 181
    chronic, dermal microcirculation in, morphometric assessment of, 473
    in varicose veins, primary, near-infrared spectroscopy of, 182
  interposition cuff at distal anastomosis, infrainguinal polytetrafluoroethylene graft with, 324
  lateral, in Klippel-Trénaunay syndrome, 461
  malformations
    ethanol injection for, direct, 463
    in Klippel-Trénaunay syndrome, 461
  mesenteric, superior, in vivo MR imaging measurements of blood oxygen saturation in, for diagnosis of chronic mesenteric ischemia, 195
  obstruction
    central upper extremity, interventional radiology in management of, 143
    chronic, saphenectomy in presence of, 457
  patch, distal, with prosthetic bypass for limb salvage, 322
  perforating (*see* Perforating vein)
  reconstruction, 466
    femoral-popliteal vein in, superficial, 466
    iliac, in venous occlusive disease, 468
  reflux, 451
    origin of, 453
    after thrombosis, deep venous, duplex ultrasound in evaluation of, 456
  saphenous (*see* Saphenous vein)
  sciatic, persistent, in Klippel-Trénaunay syndrome, 461
  testing, noninvasive, in diagnosis of pulmonary embolism, impact on decisionmaking, 439
  thrombectomy for iliofemoral vein thrombosis, 429
  thrombi, deep lower extremity, origin in acute venous thrombosis, 421
  thromboembolism (*see* Thromboembolism, venous)
  thrombosis (*see* Thrombosis, venous)
  transposition in forearm for autogenous hemodialysis access, 341
  trauma, 419
    lower extremity, long-term results of, 419
  ulcer (*see* Ulcer, venous)
  ultrasound, duplex, for unilateral symptoms, 186
  valvular insufficiency, mild to moderate, after isolated calf vein thrombosis, 455
  varicose
    in Klippel-Trénaunay syndrome, 461
    primary, venous insufficiency in, near-infrared spectroscopy of, 182
Venography
  magnetic resonance, gadolinium-enhanced, "bull's eye" sign determines thrombus presence and age on, 185
Vertebral
  artery, distal, reconstruction for embolic and hemodynamic disease, 378
Video
  -assisted saphenous vein harvest, 311
Virus
  cytomegalovirus in atherosclerosis of carotid artery, 32
  herpes simplex, in atherosclerosis of carotid artery, 32
Visceral
  ischemia, 304
    during thoracoabdominal aneurysm repair, mesenteric shunting decreases, 261
  malperfusion after acute aortic dissection, abdominal aortic tailoring for, 283

perfusion, distal, impact on liver function during thoracoabdominal and descending thoracic aortic repair, 251
renal artery disease, 297
Vitamin
B_6 intake and risk of coronary heart disease in women, 64
K reduction with long-term oral anticoagulation reduces bone mass in patients with previous hemispheric infarction and nonrheumatic atrial fibrillation, 49
multivitamins in prevention of restenosis after coronary angioplasty, 7
von Willebrand factor
increase in chronic venous disease, 108

W

Walking, 227
effects on mortality among nonsmoking retired men, 227
Warfarin
for atheroma of aortic arch, mobile, 236
long-term, reduces bone mass in patients with previous hemispheric infarction and nonrheumatic atrial fibrillation, 49
use in atrial fibrillation patients, 217
Wine
red, effect on endothelium-dependent relaxation (in rabbit), 86
Women
endarterectomy for asymptomatic carotid stenosis in, 375
heart disease risk in, coronary, relation to folate and vitamin B_6 intake, 64
postmenopausal
estrogen replacement therapy in, duration in relation to risk of myocardial infarction, 216
hypercholesterolemia in, estrogen replacement and pravastatin for, 58
young, myocardial infarction in, relation to plasma total homocysteine, folate, and methylenetetrahydrofolate reductase gene variant, 63
Workload
required to maintain infrainguinal bypass graft patency, 388
Wound
infection, groin, after bifurcated AneuRx graft for abdominal aortic aneurysm, 127
Wrist
ischemia, severe, magnetic resonance angiography of, 352

Y

YAG
Nd:YAG photocoagulation, interstitial, for vascular malformations and hemangiomas, in children, 209

Z

ZD9379
effect on number of spreading depressions and infarct size after middle cerebral artery occlusion (in rat), 70
Zein
alcoholic solution of, percutaneous sclerotherapy for lymphangiomas with, in children, 208

Author Index

A

Abad C, 289
Abe K, 71, 79
Abela A, 208
Acher CW, 262
Adams MR, 60
Adera HM, 329
Adili F, 102
Ahn SS, 147
Aiello LP, 98
Akins PT, 382
Alimi YS, 468
Allard L, 172
Almeida JI, 399
Aly HM, 95
Ambrosio G, 45
Anderson DR, 442
Anderson JL, 36
Andrades JA, 85
Arita T, 188
Arko F, 236
Artemis N, 157
Asahara T, 2
Ascher E, 434, 438
Atkinson JLD, 409
Attinger C, 322
Azizzadeh A, 260

B

Baca-Regen LM, 96
Back MR, 202
Bacourt F, 401
Badosa F, 349
Bahnini A, 395
Bainbridge JS, 30
Baisden C, 236
Baldwin D, 334
Ballinger BA, 361
Ballinger J, 202
Balm R, 124
Barber L, 77
Barkmeier LD, 327
Baron JA, 423
Barrett S, 290
Barron DJ, 263
Barron HV, 233
Bartels C, 35
Bartleson JD, 409
Bayly R, 433
Beard JD, 138
Beaufigeau M, 402
Becquemin J-P, 315
Belkin M, 318
Bell PRF, 135
Beller GA, 5
Bender JS, 224
Bengtson TD, 466
Beregi JP, 130
Bergamini TM, 437
Bergelin RO, 302, 431
Bergersen L, 269
Bergqvist D, 332
Berguer R, 238, 368, 378
Bergvist D, 218
Berman AT, 444
Berman JA, 343
Berman SS, 344
Bermudez KM, 419
Biancari F, 335
Birchall D, 175
Birkmeyer JD, 364
Bitar G, 349
Bitsch M, 285
Blanchard DG, 235
Bonora E, 56
Booth FV, 440
Bosson J-L, 184
Bots ML, 11
Boyd PI, 374
Boyd SJ, 178
Bradbury AW, 290
Brandsma JW, 228
Brass LM, 217
Brennan JF III, 89
Breslow MJ, 221
Brickl R, 40
Broderick JP, 73
Brouwer KJ, 292
Brown IW, 263
Brunkwall J, 133
Buckenham T, 140
Buckley C, 236
Budenbender KT, 1
Buffaz P-D, 184
Bullock R, 69
Bulstrode NW, 290
Burchfiel CM, 227
Bush RL, 220
Buth J, 309, 389
Butler SP, 178

C

Cachovan M, 176
Calligaro KD, 146, 390, 392
Cambria RP, 247, 255, 261
Campbell LA, 31
Campbell MP, 258
Campbell WB, 276
Cao P, 360
Caps MT, 300, 431
Carlin RE, 80
Carlton LM, 295
Carmody TP, 231
Carpenter JP, 394
Carr C, 249
Carrington D, 38
Castronuovo JJ Jr, 329
Cebul RD, 365
Cello JP, 479
Chaitman BR, 10
Chakfé N, 402
Chalmers N, 175
Chang BB, 323
Chen D, 3
Ch'en IY, 195
Chen JC, 154
Chen M-F, 415
Chen MHM, 279
Chen Z-M, 42
Cheng SWK, 413
Chilian WM, 104
Chiu B, 32
Cho J-S, 274
Chook P, 68
Chouhan V, 112
Christiansen KJ, 229
Christopherson R, 213
Chulakadabba A, 26
Cikrit DF, 418
Cishek MB, 86
Clagett GP, 297
Clarke K, 143
Cleveland TJ, 138
Clifton A, 140
Clowes AW, 50
Clymer MA, 209
Cmolik BL, 214
Coady MA, 245
Cohen M, 53
Cohen Z, 210
Colier WNJM, 28
Comerota AJ, 112
Condado JA, 6
Coselli JS, 265
Coulson AS, 31
Counsell C, 74
Cox K, 430
Craven TE, 299
Crawley F, 140
Crea F, 8
Creutzig A, 176
Criado E, 181, 240, 350
Croce MA, 407
Cross DT III, 382

Cruz HA, 237
Cuming R, 155
Curl GR, 440
Cushman M, 97
Cuypers P, 389

D

Dalman RL, 195
Dalsing MC, 83
D'Angelo AJ, 279
Darling RC III, 323
Dattilo JB, 23, 75, 316
Dattilo MPM, 23, 75
Daum G, 50
Davda RK, 101
Davidson MH, 58
Davies JN, 223
Davies MG, 77
Davis KA, 411
Davis MJ, 104
Davis TME, 269
Davison JK, 247, 255, 261
DeFouw DO, 473
Deitch JS, 299, 303
DeLaurentis DA, 392
Delis K, 453
de Mol BAJM, 257
DePippo P, 434
DeRose JJ, 282
de Vrey EA, 198
Di X, 69
Di Bartolomeo R, 412
DiMauro P, 468
Di Tullio MR, 163
Dobrin PB, 313
Does RTC, 292
Donayre CE, 127
Dougherty MJ, 146, 390, 392
Driscoll DJ, 461
Droste DW, 162
Düber C, 190
Dubois J, 208
Duda SH, 119
Duenas M, 1
Dunsky KG, 103
Durand L-G, 172

E

Eagleton MJ, 387
Easterwood L, 457
Edmondson RA, 132
Egger G, 19
Einav S, 213
Eisenbud DE, 46
Eklöf B, 429
Eklof B, 339
Eliasziw M, 366
Ellis M, 76, 155
Emanuelsson H, 12
Engel PM, 35
Ernst CB, 278
Eslami MH, 318

F

Fabian TC, 411
Fabre D, 468
Falcone R, 441
Farber MA, 181
Fell G, 151
Fernandez-Llamazares J, 422
Ferretti GR, 184
Fields JM, 175
Fillinger MF, 337
Fishbein MC, 117
Fisher CM, 149
Fisher WS III, 139, 141
Fishwick G, 165
Fisk P, 470
Flamm SD, 243
Fleisher LA, 221
Flemmer MC, 426
Flores RM, 291
Foley PWX, 52
Forsyth EA, 95
Fortune DS, 209
Fosdick DA, 466
Fountain T, 457
Fowkes FGR, 134
Frank SM, 221
Frazier OH, 264
Freedman AM, 480
Froehlich JB, 185
Fulton GJ, 77

G

Gade PV, 85
Gale SS, 170
Gallagher C, 464
Galli R, 412
Galloway MT, 86
Gambhir SS, 114
Gao Y, 80
Garb JL, 343
Garel L, 208
Garrard CL, 331, 361, 416
Gaspardone A, 8
Gavant ML, 411
Geibel A, 446
Gelabert HA, 246
Gentile AT, 344
George JK, 167
Georgiannos SN, 108
Giannoukas AD, 453
Giglia JS, 261
Gillespie DL, 464
Glickman MH, 344
Gloviczki P, 274
Goëau-Brissonnière O, 396
Goldstein DJ, 291
Goldstein LB, 375
Golino P, 45
Golledge J, 76, 155
Goodman M, 229
Grange JJ, 96
Green D, 57
Green RM, 387
Greenfield LJ, 185
Gregory RT, 307
Gridley G, 423
Groeneveld ABJ, 82
Grønholdt M-LM, 383
Grønholdt MM, 160
Gross M, 442
Guo Z, 172
Gupta S, 38
Gurdiel O, 6
Guzman RJ, 79

H

Haenen JH, 451, 456
Hagino RT, 297, 374, 466
Hakim AA, 227
Hall AS, 18
Hall JC, 229
Hallett JW Jr, 363
Hamdan AD, 98
Hammond EH, 36
Hammond GL, 245
Hands L, 25
Hanna AK, 100
Hansberg T, 162
Hansen KJ, 299, 303
Hanson J, 438
Hanson JN, 434
Harada RN, 112
Harding SP, 444
Harris LM, 440
Hartshorne T, 135, 164
Harward TRS, 295
Haulon S, 130
Hayashi T, 71
Hayward I, 232
Heckbert SR, 216
Hedin U, 50
Heickendorff L, 106

Henneberg EW, 106
Hertz SM, 46
Hertzer NR, 357, 372
Hewin DF, 276
Hiatt WR, 30
Hicks RCJ, 76
Hill SL, 421
Hines GL, 371
Hingorani A, 438
Hirschl M, 67
Hiyama DT, 147
Ho F-M, 415
Hoballah JJ, 193, 205
Hobson RW II, 341
Hoch JR, 262
Hod I, 471
Hodges TC, 337
Hoes AW, 11
Hoffman U, 207
Hoffmann JF, 437
Holcroft JW, 220
Holtzman GI, 421
Honda Y, 49
Honoré EK, 60
Hood DB, 327
Hop WCJ, 309, 459
Hopman MTE, 28
Hosoi Y, 182
Houghton AD, 393
Howard G, 15
Hsia DC, 376
Hu FB, 64
Huber TS, 202, 295
Hudoba M, 47
Hulse M, 26
Hulthe J, 12
Hye RJ, 235
Hyre CE, 83, 418

I

Idu MM, 309, 389
Iliopoulos DC, 253
Illig KA, 387
Ilstrup DM, 363
Imig H, 403
Irvine CD, 52
Ivancev K, 133

J

Jacob AG, 461
Jacobs MJHM, 257
Jain KM, 293
Janssen MCH, 451, 456
Jaques PF, 350
Jeziorska M, 116
Jin G, 482
Johnson WC, 334
Jones CE, 224
Jordan WD Jr, 139, 141, 311
Just S, 196

K

Kaatee R, 124
Kalman PG, 143
Karim M, 86
Karlström L, 332
Karp SJ, 102
Kashyap VS, 247
Kasper W, 446
Kaufman JL, 343
Keagy BA, 240
Kearney M, 3
Kemény V, 162
Kent KC, 92
Kerracher EMG, 134
Khaira HS, 428
Kiechl S, 19, 56
Kiernan S, 269
Kikeri D, 347, 351
Killewich LA, 430
Kim SA, 483
Kistner RL, 339
Kline DG, 416
Kline RA, 238, 378
Kline RG, 279
Klose G, 472
Knight S, 470
Knosalla C, 396
Knudson MM, 419
Ko DSC, 472
Koepsell TD, 216
Konstantinides S, 446
Kooijman HM, 28
Koudstaal PJ, 11
Kozman H, 426
Kraft HE, 158
Kransdorf MJ, 352
Krumholz HM, 217
Krushat WM, 376
Kuivenhoven JA, 22
Kumar M, 226
Kunoh H, 49
Kuo C-c, 31
Kwaan HC, 353
Kyrle PA, 67

L

Labropoulos N, 453
Lalka SG, 418
Lamparello PJ, 369
LaMuraglia GM, 102
Landesberg G, 213
Langnas AN, 482
Länne T, 287
Lau LS, 235
Laursen H, 383
Leatham EW, 38
Lederle FA, 267
Lee AJ, [illegible]4
Lee HM, 168
Lee KS, 483
Lee SJ, 483
Leflon V, 396
Legemate DA, 257
Lerner R, 472
Leslie B, 47
Levi CR, 151
Levi I, 210
Levin M, 353
Li KCP, 195
Liau C-S, 415
Liem TK, 399
Ligush J Jr, 240
Lindgren L, 335
Lindholt JS, 106
Lindsay TF, 143
Lipski DA, 278, 439
Livesey SA, 263
Loftus IM, 388
Lolin YL, 68
Loos J, 403
Lowe GDO, 14
Lu G, 101
Lucas FL, 364
Luketic VA, 480
Lumsden AB, 347, 351
Lundstrom RJ, 233
Luo H, 117
Luo Z, [illegible]

M

Maas J, 284
Maass M, 35
MacDonald MJ, 347, 351
Mackay CA, 328
Macko RF, 430
Maki KC, 58
Malinow MR, 63
Manisali M, 243
Mann J, 428
Mannick JA, 318
Manord JD, 331, 361, 416
Marin ML, 123
Marston WA, 181, 350
Martelli E, 274
Martin D, 421

Martin EC, 282
Marty B, 121
Mascha EJ, 357, 372
Mashiah A, 471
Masuda EM, 339
Matchar DB, 375
Matsunaga N, 188
Matsuoka Y, 241
Matsuura JH, 316
Mattes E, 269
May J, 125
McCarthy BD, 439
McCarthy WJ, 377, 463
McCollum C, 116
McFarlane G, 269
McKinsey JF, 304
McLafferty RB, 174, 455
Mehra MR, 331
Meigs JB, 55
Meiler MR, 70
Meissner MH, 431
Mellemkjær L, 425
Melton SM, 407
Menard J-F, 385
Merritt WH, 352
Mesh CL, 214
Mialhe C, 120
Mian NZ, 433
Mildenberger P, 87
Miller A, 89
Miller CC III, 249, 251, 253, 258, 260
Miller EV, 193
Miller N, 186
Mintz GS, 198
Misare BD, 98
Moawad J, 304
Moneta GL, 174, 272, 455
Monreal M, 422
Morasch MD, 238, 313, 368, 378
Moscoe LM, 376
Mostafa G, 226
Moustapha A, 65
Mowbray PI, 14
Mower WR, 114
Muhlestein JB, 36
Mulder EJ, 284
Muller JM, 104
Müller TH, 40
Munn JS, 293
Mureebe L, 93, 94
Murray JG, 243

N

Nahlawi M, 65
Naso A, 65
Nazzal MM, 205
Nazzal MMS, 193
Nelken NA, 419
Nelson PR, 92, 93, 94
Nene SM, 246
Neschis DG, 100
Neufang A, 190
Neumann FJ, 43
Neville RF, 95, 322
Nicolini P, 402
Nielsen TG, 310
Nimbkar NV, 232
Nimni ME, 85
Nishioka T, 117
Nollendorfs AJ, 96
Nordestgaard BG, 160, 310
Nordrehaug JE, 61
Nørgaard HH, 285
Norgren L, 429
Nydahl S, 135, 164
Nygård O, 61
Nyyssönen K, 21

O

Oberwalder P, 265
Obrand D, 186
O'Brien SP, 293
O'Brien-Irr MS, 358
O'Driscoll G, 57
O'Hara PJ, 357, 372
Ohki T, 121
Olcott EW, 479
Omarali I, 163
Orloff MJ, 477
Orloff MS, 477
Orloff SL, 477
Oskin TC, 303
Ouchi K, 34
Owen R, 165

P

Pacini D, 412
Pagley PR, 5
Panayiotopoulos YP, 132
Pappas PJ, 341, 473
Pardy B, 393
Park AE, 377
Park H-Y, 107
Parmet JL, 444
Passman MA, 455
Patton JH Jr, 407
Pearce WH, 377
Peltonen S, 335
Pemberton M, 164
Perandreu J, 422
Perko MJ, 196
Petrovitch H, 227
Pevec WC, 220
Pfammatter T, 397
Phillips D, 25
Phillips TJ, 107
Pierik EGJM, 459, 460
Pietropaoli JA Jr, 363
Pilgram TK, 382
Pine R, 365
Pinsk I, 210
Plate G, 429
Plissonnier D, 395
Poletti LF, 316
Polissar NL, 302
Poon M, 103
Porter JB, 110
Prince MR, 185, 191
Punnonen K, 21

Q

Quiñones WJ, 114
Quiñones-Baldrich WJ, 246

R

Ragni M, 45
Rahman T, 178
Rahnama M, 426
Raijmakers PGHM, 82
Rainoni L, 207
Raju S, 457
Ranaboldo CJ, 223
Rankin J, 57
Rapola JM, 17
Rauwerda JA, 82
Raygrotzki S, 119
Razik W, 328
Refsum H, 61
Reid A, 388
Reinisch L, 209
Ricci MA, 470
Rickard MJFX, 149
Ricotta JJ, 358
Ridker PM, 97
Rieker O, 190
Riepe G, 403
Ries S, 157
Rikkers LF, 482
Riles TS, 369
Rimm EB, 64
Ring EJ, 479
Ripatti S, 17
Rizzo JA, 245

Robbin ML, 201
Robeer GG, 228
Roberts AK, 151
Roberts JK, 163
Robinson KD, 307
Robinson KS, 442
Rochester JR, 153
Rockman CB, 369
Røder O, 285
Rogatti W, 176
Romaneehsen B, 87
Romano PS, 435
Rose DA, 46
Rosengart TK, 1
Roye GD, 139
Rua I, 146
Rudkin GH, 147
Rundback JH, 203
Ruotolo C, 395
Ryan SM, 205

S

Safford SD, 100
Safi HJ, 249, 251, 253, 258, 260
Saharay M, 108, 110
Sakamoto I, 241
Sakurai M, 71
Sakurai S, 353
Salenius JP, 89
Salles-Cunha SX, 170
Salvian AJ, 154
Samsa GP, 375
Sanchez LA, 121
Sandgren T, 287
Sandison AJP, 132
Sandmann W, 398
Sanyal AJ, 480
Satiani B, 441
Sato DT, 307
Sato Y, 49
Scherer SA, 30
Schievink WI, 409
Schlotthauer J, 226
Schlumpf R, 397
Schmidt WA, 158
Schoenberg SO, 191
Schömig A, 43
Schreck DM, 433
Schroeder PT, 311
Schroeder TV, 196
Schubach SL, 371
Schunk K, 87
Schwartz SM, 63
Scinto JM, 217
Scissons RP, 170
Scott WC, 371
Sensier Y, 165
Sessa CN, 368
Shah PM, 203
Shapira OM, 237
Shaughnessy WJ, 461
Shaw E, 271
Shemin RJ, 237
Shepard AD, 439
Shields DA, 108, 110
Shigematsu H, 182
Shirai M, 34
Shireman PK, 463
Shook L, 441
Sidawy AN, 322
Silva MB Jr, 341
Silver D, 399
Simms MH, 328
Simon JA, 231
Simonneau G, 448
Singer DE, 55
Siscovick DS, 63
Sivaguru A, 153
Smiell JM, 329
Smith-Meek MA, 224
Snow RJ, 365
Soballe PW, 232
Solkowitz SN, 231
Sonesson B, 287
Soong CV, 149
Sørensen HT, 425
Sostman HD, 168
Soury P, 385
Spain DA, 437
Spratt JA, 75
Stacey MC, 452
Stampfer MJ, 97
Standen GR, 52
Stanley AC, 107
Steffensen FH, 425
Steinke W, 157
Stepniakowski KT, 101
Stokking R, 124
Stonebridge PA, 324
Strawderman RL, 346
Stümpflen A, 67
Sueyoshi E, 241
Sullivan LM, 55
Sumner DS, 327
Sweeney MS, 264
Syk I, 133
Syrek JR, 390

T

Takano K, 70, 188
Tardif J-C, 7
Tassiopoulos AK, 80
Tatlisumak T, 70
Taylor DC, 154
Taylor LM Jr, 174, 272
Testolin LM, 58
Thompson JF, 223
Thompson MM, 388
Tielbeek AV, 144
Ting ACW, 413
Tisi PV, 26
Todd C, 393
Todd GJ, 282, 291
Tomai F, 8
Tomaszewski JE, 394
Torsello G, 398
Tousignant L, 186
Tsurumi Y, 2, 3
Tucker W, 32
Tullis MJ, 300
Tuomainen T-P, 21
Turenne MN, 346
Turner-Stepahin S, 352
Tyrrell MR, 320

U

Unthank JL, 83

V

Vale FL, 141
Valentine RJ, 297, 374
van Asten WNJC, 451
van Bockel JH, 284
van den Heuvel SP, 228
Vandongen YK, 452
Van Heekeren DW, 214
van Langen H, 456
van Urk H, 459, 460
Vasseur M-A, 130
Veith FJ, 123
Venezic LM, 473
Verstraete M, 211
Vetter J, 207
Viira E, 32
Villavicencio JL, 464
Virtamo J, 17
Viskin S, 233
Voellinger DC, 311
Vogt PR, 397
von Birgelen C, 198
von Jessen F, 310
Vorpahl K, 158
Vos LD, 144
Vroegindeweij D, 144

W

Waksman R, 6
Waksman Y, 471
Walot I, 127
Walter H, 43
Walton J, 271
Wang Y, 168
Ward JS, 191
Wardlaw JM, 74
Warlow C, 380
Warlow CP, 74
Watelet J, 385
Watkins MT, 334
Watson CJE, 25, 271
Watson DD, 5
Watson J, 69
Webb TH, 283
Weiderpass E, 423
Weisenberger H, 40
Weiss NS, 216
Weitz JI, 47
Wennberg DE, 364
Whitbread T, 138
White GH, 125
White RA, 127
White RH, 435
Whyman MR, 134
Wiebe BM, 160, 383
Wikstrand J, 12
Wilkins DC, 167
Wilkinson JM, 153
Willeit J, 19, 56
Willett WC, 64
Williams GM, 283
Williams JK, 60
Wilson YG, 167
Wiskirchen J, 119
Wittens CHA, 460
Wolfe JHN, 320
Wong J, 203
Woo KS, 68
Woods JD, 346
Woolley DE, 116
Woratyla SP, 323
Wyble CW, 304
Wynn MM, 262

Y

Yager DR, 23
Yamamura S, 92, 93, 94
Yamashita K, 34
Yang D, 269, 452
Yang S, 349
Yao JST, 463
Yasuhara H, 182
Yawn DH, 251
Yeager RA, 272
Young DJ, 264
Yu W, 125
Yuan JG, 123

Z

Zannetti S, 255
Zarins CK, 79
Zenni GC, 313
Zhang X, 103
Zhou H, 435
Zierler RE, 300, 302
Zwolak RM, 337